MANAGEMENT OF MOTOR SPEECH DISORDERS IN CHILDREN AND ADULTS

Management of Motor Speech Disorders in Children and Adults

SECOND EDITION

Kathryn M. Yorkston,
David R. Beukelman,
Edythe A. Strand,
and
Kathleen R. Bell

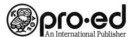
pro·ed
An International Publisher

8700 Shoal Creek Boulevard
Austin, Texas 78757-6897
800/897-3202 Fax 800/397-7633
Order online at http://www.proedinc.com

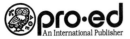

© 1999, 1988 by PRO-ED, Inc.
8700 Shoal Creek Boulevard
Austin, Texas 78757-6897
800/897-3202 Fax 800/397-7633
Order online at http://www.proedinc.com

This book is designed in Goudy.

Printed in the United States of America

7 8 9 10   08 07 06 05

Dedicated to the speech–language pathologists
of the University of Washington Medical Center
and Harborview Medical Center,
the Madonna Rehabilitation Hospital,
and the Munroe–Meyer Institute for Genetics and
Rehabilitation, whose commitment to clinical service
has created wonderful settings in which to
learn about motor speech disorders.

Dedicated to our families who have understood
and supported our personal commitments
to persons with severe communication disorders.

CONTENTS

PREFACE

Management of Motor Speech Disorders in Children and Adults was written for graduate students and practicing speech–language pathologists interested in neurologic communication disorders. This revision of a book first published in 1988 contains several noteworthy modifications. First, content was expanded to include not only dysarthria but also apraxia of speech. Thus, the text represents a general source of clinical information about motor speech disorders. Second, issues related to developmental dysarthria and apraxia of speech have been highlighted. Thus, unique issues related to children with motor speech disorders are addressed.

Finally, we have attempted to reflect a trend in medical education that emphasizes clinical decision making. It has been suggested that medical management has gone through several eras or phases. The first phase can be described as the *era of diagnosis* in which a disorder is described and differentiated from other disorders. The next phase can be described as the *era of treatment* in which a repertoire of interventions are developed and tested. The most sophisticated phase of medical management can be described as the *era of clinical decisions* in which a logic is provided to the clinician for the selection and timing of the various interventions. The field of motor speech disorders can also be characterized by a series of phases. The first era, culminating in the mid-1970s by the classical Mayo Clinic studies, was the era of diagnosis. This was followed by an era of treatment in which various intervention strategies were described. The field is now entering the era of clinical decisions. Readers will note that many of the descriptions of populations are organized into levels or stages in which speakers are characterized across a continuum of severity. Further, approaches to intervention are also organized by stages of the disorders so that clinical decisions vary depending on the level of functional limitation.

In this text, we summarize the basic neurologic and medical information associated with the various diseases, disorders, and syndromes that cause motor speech disorders. In addition, we review and organize the available literature and relate it to the clinical management of speakers with motor speech disorders. Finally, the clinical management chapters contain discussion of clinical practice that we have developed or adopted while treating speakers with motor speech disorders in a hospital-based speech–language pathology service.

The first chapter, "Perspectives on Motor Speech Disorders—A Clinical Point of View," reviews the perspectives from which motor speech disorders can be viewed, including the viewpoints of the neurologist, the speech physiologists, the rehabilitationists, and the individuals experiencing the disorder. Motor speech disorders are defined within the framework of a model of chronic disease as an impairment, functional limitation, disability, and social limitation.

Individuals with motor speech disorders frequently have serious underlying neurologic diseases and syndromes. Therefore, speech–language pathology services are often delivered in conjunction with other medically related services. Chapters 2, 3, and 4 are provided as a resource guide to speech–language pathologists serving individuals with neurologic disorders. They contain information about the pathology of disease; typical impairments of the subsystems of speech, including respiratory, laryngeal, velopharyngeal, and oral function; and levels or stages of speech function associated with the disease. Motor speech disorders are grouped according to their age of onset and the natural course of the disorder because these two features are important to clinical management. Chapter 2, "Developmental Motor Speech Disorders," contains a discussion of cerebral palsy and developmental apraxia of speech. Chapter 3, "Adult-Onset, Nonprogressive Dysarthria and Apraxia of Speech," contains a discussion of stroke and traumatic brain injury. Chapter 4, "Dysarthria in Degenerative Disease," contains a discussion of those dysarthrias with a progressive course, including Parkinsonism, parkinsonism-plus syndromes, hereditary diseases, dystonia, Huntington's disease, amyotrophic lateral sclerosis, and multiple sclerosis.

Chapters 5 and 6 contain an overview of the assessment process. In Chapter 5, "Clinical Examination of Motor Speech Disorders," the components of the clinical examination are described, including the history, the physical examination, and the motor speech examination. In Chapter 6, "Interpreting the Clinical Examination," the topics of differential diagnosis and treatment planning in dysarthria are discussed.

The remaining chapters in this text provide detailed discussion of specific areas of intervention. Chapter 7, "Respiration," outlines approaches for assessment and training of the respiratory aspects of speech, including establishing respiratory support, stabilizing the respiratory pattern, and increasing respiratory flexibility. Chapter 8, "Laryngeal Function," reviews such management topics as establishing voluntary phonation, increasing loudness, reducing hyperadduction of the vocal folds, and improving laryngeal coordination. Chapter 9, "Velopharyngeal Function," reviews the assessment and intervention of velopharyngeal dysfunction in dysarthria, including behavioral, prosthetic, and surgical methods. Chapter 10, "Speaking Rate Control," reviews topics including candidacy for rate control and selection of appropriate techniques. Included is a discussion both of the rigid rate control techniques used with the speakers with severe impairment and those techniques that attempt to preserve prosody. Chapter 11, "Articulation and Prosody: Segmental and Suprasegmental Aspects of Dysarthric Speech," presents management techniques designed to improve the production of speech and sounds and management techniques that focus on the prosodic aspects of speech, including stress patterning, intonation, and rate–rhythm. Chapter 12, "Optimizing Communicative Effectiveness: Bringing It Together," was co-authored with Katherine C. Hustad. In this chapter, the staging of intervention is described in order to reduce disability and social limitations experienced by speakers with dysarthria. Finally, Chapter 13, "Treatment of Developmental and Acquired Apraxia of Speech," summarizes treatment approaches for children and adults with apraxia. Principles of motor learning are reviewed as they relate to a variety of clinical decisions associated with treatment planning.

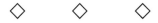

A project such as *Management of Motor Speech Disorders in Children and Adults* reflects the contributions of many individuals. The work of numerous colleagues is referenced throughout the text. We are indebted to those clinicians and researchers who have been disciplined enough to record their observations, insights, and conclusions. Unfortunately, space and confidentiality do not permit a listing of clients who have served as our "teachers." We also acknowledge the pervasive influence of the speech pathology staff of the University of Washington Medical Center, Seattle; the Harborview Medical Center, Seattle; the Barkley Memorial Center, Lincoln; the Madonna Rehabilitation Hospital, Lincoln; and the Munroe–Meyer Institute for Genetics and Rehabilitation and University of Nebraska Medical Center, Omaha. Although their contributions are rarely referenced directly in this text, they have encouraged us, challenged us, listened to seemingly endless audio recordings of speakers with dysarthria, critiqued early versions of tests and software, and provided wonderful settings in which to learn about dysarthria. Finally, we wish to thank Nancy Brown for her unfailing efforts to keep us organized.

KMY
DRB

PERSPECTIVES ON MOTOR SPEECH DISORDERS— A CLINICAL POINT OF VIEW

Clinical Issues: Family conferences in which the patients and their families have the opportunity to meet with the entire team are frequent occurrences on our rehabilitation unit. After one such conference, which began on a particularly discordant note, a student asked, "How do you prepare yourself for such a confrontation?" Our advice was to try to understand the interaction from the viewpoints of the various participants. In this particular case, Sam was diagnosed over 12 years ago as having Parkinson's disease. He was being discharged from a 2-week hospitalization for adjustment of his medication. The physician considered the hospitalization a success in that Sam's rigidity, and the excessive movements that were a side effect of his former medication schedule, were reduced. The occupational therapist also considered it successful because Sam could more safely perform some activities of daily living. His speech was considered functional if the family modified their communication style. This required that his partners be face to face with Sam when he was attempting to speak, that they clearly signaled when they were not understanding, and that they took an active role in resolving communication breakdowns. However, Sam's wife and son were less positive. They concluded that Sam had not changed in any important ways and that the hospitalization was a waste of time and money. Sam still required a wheelchair for mobility, he needed some supervision when carrying out many activities of daily living, and his speech was still extremely difficult to understand. The family's disappointment with the intervention was clear. Sam could not return to work or even to an independent lifestyle.

- How could people observe the same events and interpret them so differently?

- Was the family less observant than the rehabilitation staff?

- Was the rehabilitation staff exaggerating the changes that had occurred?

Perspectives are standpoints from which a problem may be viewed. They provide a means for understanding or judging observations and for showing those observations in relationship with one another. This chapter presents a number of perspectives from which the speech–language clinician can view and understand motor speech disorders. Each perspective is valid for its own purposes. Before proceeding, an overview of some characteristics of motor speech disorders is discussed.

CHARACTERISTICS OF MOTOR SPEECH DISORDERS

Speech production occurs because of a complicated series of interactive cognitive, linguistic, and motor processes. A brief review of a basic model of how speech is produced helps one understand the processing deficits that result in motor speech disorders. Figure 1.1 illustrates a simple example of such a model that will be referred to throughout this book. The act of speaking begins with the intent to communicate a particular idea or message. This ideation leads to the linguistic level where a variety of language processes occur. Speakers must retrieve words from some storage mechanism, perform the appropriate phonologic encoding, and assemble the words into syntactic frames. Interactive with this linguistic processing, the speaker assembles and retrieves motor plans before executing them. Execution involves contraction of muscle fibers, causing the movements of structures responsible for modulating the airstream and the acoustic speech signal. Although this discussion will focus primarily on the two motor levels of this basic model, it is important to realize that speech motor control processes are influenced by and interactive with the cognitive and linguistic levels of processing that occur when people talk.

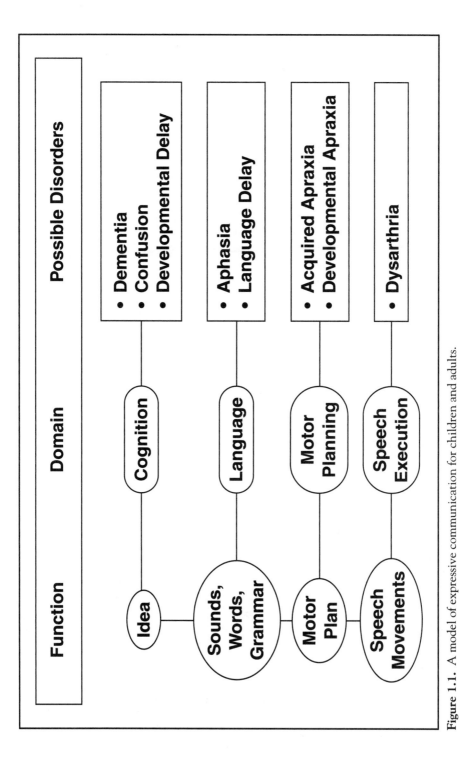

Figure 1.1. A model of expressive communication for children and adults.

Motor planning or *motor programming* are the terms most frequently used to designate the "translation" between language forms and the movement that occurs to create the sounds that are understood by the listener. Although specific aspects of motor planning are still open to debate, it is clear that some mechanism is at work to specify movement parameters. That is, certain areas of the brain must specify how far, how fast, in what direction, and with how much muscle contraction each muscle must move. Also, each muscle must move in a temporal relationship with all of the other muscles. The term *apraxia of speech* is used to designate a problem at this level of processing—the ability to program the movements that must occur for a particular acoustic result.

Motor execution refers to the complex processes by which the motor plan results in actual muscle contractions. It is overly simplistic to view the execution phase of motor control as a system of "neuro-electrical lines" in which the motor control signals pass from the primary motor cortex to the lower motor neuron pool, activating peripheral nerves such that peripheral fibers wrap around one or more muscle fibers and release acetylcholine, causing the muscle fibers to contract. Motor execution also involves a sophisticated system for refining the neuromotor signal with a variety of feedback and coordinative networks. These include proprioceptive and tactile sensory systems, extrapyramidal descending tracts, and the basal ganglia and cerebellar circuits. A pathology in the central or peripheral nervous system involved in motor execution can cause a communication disorder that is called *dysarthria*.

Question: Isn't the model presented in Figure 1.1 very simplistic, given that it attempts to represent cognitive, linguistic, and motor functions?

Yes. We develop models to help us understand concepts that in reality are very complex and interrelated. We are aware that speech—that is, the expression of ideas—is a complicated process or a series of complicated processes, depending on how one chooses to think about it. In an effort to understand a complicated process like speech production, we attempt to categorize it into "manageable chunks." While our categorization efforts, such as language, motor programming, and motor execution, aid our understanding in some ways, they often cause controversy as well. For example, later in this book we will discuss the long-standing argument as to whether or not apraxia of speech is a linguistic disorder or a motor disorder.

Keep in mind that a simplified model such as this is useful for patient and family education, such as helping children understand why their dad

(continues)

can understand them, but cannot talk. The model is also useful in pediatric populations. For example, the pediatrician or speech–language pathologist may have given the label "developmental apraxia" to a child with severe articulatory problems. Parents would ask, "What is that? Does that mean he has a problem with his brain?" The model can be helpful in explaining that there are different levels of processing, and that the child might be experiencing deficits at certain of those levels (i.e., phonologic or motor planning).

The Dysarthrias

Dysarthria is a neurologic motor speech impairment that is characterized by slow, weak, imprecise, and/or uncoordinated movements of the speech musculature. Literally, the term comes from the Greek *dys + arthroun*, which means "inability to utter distinctly." The dysarthrias form a group of disorders marked by impaired execution of the movements of speech production. Rather than being described by a single set of characteristics, different types of dysarthria vary along a number of dimensions:

- *Age of Onset*—The dysarthrias can be either congenital or acquired at any age.

- *Cause*—The origin of the underlying neuromotor problem can be vascular, traumatic, infectious, neoplastic, metabolic, and so on. Any trauma, lesion, or disease that causes central or peripheral nervous system damage may result in dysarthria.

- *Natural Course*—The course of the dysarthria may follow a number of patterns, including developmental (as in cerebral palsy in children), recovering (as in early post-onset traumatic head injury and stroke), stable (as in cerebral palsy in adults), degenerative (as in amyotrophic lateral sclerosis), or exacerbating–remitting (as in some cases of multiple sclerosis).

- *Site of Lesion*—The neuroanatomic site of lesion may be either the central or the peripheral nervous system or both, including the cerebrum, cerebellum, basal ganglia, brain stem, and cranial nerves.

- *Neurological Diagnosis of Disease*—A number of diagnoses may be associated with dysarthria, including cerebral palsy; Parkinson's disease; multiple sclerosis; amyotrophic lateral sclerosis; and unilateral, bilateral, or brain-stem stroke. See Table 1.1 for a more complete listing.

- *Pathophysiology*—One or a combination of pathophysiological processes may be involved, including spasticity, flaccidity, ataxia, tremor, rigidity, dysmetria, and involuntary movements such as tremor.

Table 1.1
Characteristics of the Dysarthrias and Apraxia of Speech

Type	Etiology	Location	Neuromuscular Condition
Dysarthrias			
Flaccid dysarthria	Poliomyelitis Stroke Congenital conditions Myasthenia gravis Bulbar palsy Facial palsy Trauma	Lower motor neuron	Flaccid paralysis Weakness Hypotonia Muscle atrophy Fasciculations
Spastic dysarthria	Stroke Tumor Encephalitis Trauma Spastic cerebral palsy	Upper motor neuron	Spastic paralysis Weakness Limited range of motion Slowness of movement
Ataxic dysarthria	Stroke Tumor Trauma Ataxic cerebral palsy Friedreich's ataxia Infection Toxic effects (e.g., alcohol)	Cerebellar system	Inaccurate movement Slow movement Hypotonia
Hypokinetic dysarthria	Parkinson's disease Drug induced	Extrapyramidal system	Slow movements Limited range of movement Immobility Paucity of movement Rigidity Loss of automatic aspects of movements

(continues)

Table 1.1 (*continued*)

Type	Etiology	Location	Neuromuscular Condition
Dysarthrias (*continued*)			
Hyperkinetic dysarthria			
Predominantly quick	Chorea Infection Gilles de la Tourette's syndrome Ballism	Extrapyramidal system	Quick involuntary movements Variable muscle tone
Predominantly slow	Athetosis Infection Stroke Tumor Dystonia Drug induced Dyskinesia	Extrapyramidal system	Twisting and writhing movements Slow movements Involuntary movements Hypertonia
Mixed dysarthria			
Spastic–flaccid	ALS Trauma Stroke	Upper and lower motor neuron	Weakness Slow movement Limited range of movement
Spastic–ataxic– hypokinetic	Wilson's disease	Upper motor neuron, cerebellar, and extrapyramidal	Intention tremor Rigidity Spasticity Slow movement
Variable (Spastic–ataxic– flaccid)	Multiple sclerosis	Variable	Variable
Apraxia of Speech	Stroke Tumors Trauma	Dominant hemisphere lesion	Reduced ability in programming the sequence of speech movements

Note. Based on work of Darley, Aronson, and Brown (1975), cited in "Neuropathologies of Speech and Language: Introduction to Patient Management," by R. T. Wertz, 1985, in *Clinical Management of Neurogenic Communicative Disorders* (2nd ed., pp. 1–96), Boston: Little, Brown.

- *Speech Components Involved*—All or several of the speech components may be involved to varying degrees. These include the respiratory, phonatory, velopharyngeal, and oral articulatory (lip, tongue, and jaw) components.

- *Perceptual Characteristics*—The various dysarthrias have unique perceptual features.

- *Severity*—Dysarthria may range in severity from a disorder so mild that it is just noticeable during connected speech to a disorder so severe that no functional speech is present.

Differences among the dysarthrias have an impact on nearly every aspect of clinical management; for example, different medical courses influence sequence for treatment. In recovering or developmental dysarthria, an extended period of intervention may be appropriate. Degenerative disorders, on the other hand, usually warrant a different approach involving short, intensive periods of intervention at critical points during the course of the disorder. Different underlying pathophysiological problems may dictate quite different intervention techniques. For example, the reduction of habitual speaking rate, which brings about an important increase in intelligibility for certain ataxic or hypokinetic dysarthric speakers, may not be appropriate for individuals with flaccid dysarthria. Strengthening exercises may be contraindicated for individuals with amyotrophic lateral sclerosis but appropriate for individuals with brain-stem stroke. Biofeedback programs designed to reduce overall muscle tone may be appropriate for those dysarthric individuals with increased spasticity but contraindicated for those with weakness. Knowing the pattern of speech component breakdown is critical in knowing where to intervene. For example, when developing a management program for velopharyngeal incompetency, the appropriateness of palatal lift may be dependent on the level of function of other speech components, including respiration and oral articulation. Thus, appreciation of the diversity of the dysarthrias is critical for management. Rather than developing a generic dysarthria treatment, the field is very rightfully developing specific interventions for specific patterns of impairment.

Apraxia of Speech

Apraxia of speech is a motor speech disorder caused by a disturbance in motor planning or programming of sequential movement for volitional speech production. Although the musculature itself is not impaired, individuals with apraxia of speech will have difficulty completing sequences of movements for sound production. Apraxia of speech often occurs concomitantly with aphasia or language delay and less frequently with dysarthria. The perceptual characteristics of apraxia of speech include disturbances in articulation, rate, and prosody, or in the rhythm of the spoken utterance (Wertz, LaPointe, & Rosenbek, 1984). Articulatory errors consist primarily of vowel and consonant distortions, although substitutions, additions, and omissions of sounds may be present. Articulatory errors are inconsistent. Some speakers with apraxia will have great difficulty initiating utterances, due to their inability to achieve initial articulatory configurations. Transitions of movement out of one sound and into the next will also be difficult, and these distorted transitions add to the perception of dysprosody. In addition to slower rate, prosody is affected by the tendency to equalize stress across syllables and words.

Articulatory errors are often perceived as approximations of target sounds as the speaker produces effortful groping for accurate movement of articulators into a particular position. Errors often increase as the length or phonetic complexity of the utterance increases. Speakers with apraxia exhibit more accuracy in well-practiced habituated utterances, such as counting, than during spontaneous speech. Speakers with apraxia are often aware of their errors and frequently attempt to correct error productions. Oral apraxia (difficulty planning volitional movement of oral structures for nonspeech movement tasks) may or may not be present with verbal apraxia.

Developmental apraxia of speech is the term used for the developmental counterpart of acquired apraxia of speech (Crary, 1984, 1993). Most definitions of developmental verbal apraxia focus on the inability or difficulty with the ability to carry out purposeful voluntary movements for speech, in the absence of a paralysis of the speech musculature (Chappell, 1973; Crary, 1993; Edwards, 1973; Hayden, 1994; Morley, 1972; Rosenbek & Wertz, 1972; Yoss & Darley, 1974). Most definitions also point out the articulatory aspects and the inability to sequence speech movements.

A problem with speech motor planning and programming during the early stages of language and speech acquisition will necessarily affect the development of the child's expressive phonologic system. Consequently, it is sometimes difficult to determine how much of a severe delay or deviancy in articulatory skill is due to motor planning problems or phonologic processing. Procedures for determining whether motor planning problems are contributing to delays or deviancies in speech development will be discussed in Chapter 13. For now, it is important to recognize that this term is useful to delineate a subgroup of children who present with severe articulatory performance deficits and who seem to have a variety of associated characteristics in common. Developmental verbal apraxia may be exhibited along with other deficits and strengths for a particular child. Our goal as clinicians is to be as informed as possible regarding the nature of the motor planning deficit so that we may make reasonable decisions as to the relative contribution of the disorder to the child's overall communicative performance.

> *Question: Are dysarthria and apraxia of speech medical diagnoses?*
>
> No, these terms are used to designate the type of communication disorder. The medical diagnoses related to the neuropathology that is causing the motor speech disorders include amyotrophic lateral sclerosis, stroke, and traumatic brain injury.

PERSPECTIVES ON DYSARTHRIA AND APRAXIA OF SPEECH

Like every complex phenomenon, motor speech disorders may be viewed from a variety of perspectives. Although the point of view of the rehabilitationist is the focus of this text, other perspectives must also be acknowledged.

The Neurologist's Point of View

Historically, the dysarthrias and apraxia of speech have been viewed by neurologists as signs or symptoms of disease. The term *disease* has been defined by Wood (1980) as a disruption of normal body processes that results in changes in the structure or functioning of the body. For the speaker with dysarthria, the disease may be multiple sclerosis, Parkinson's disease, amyotrophic lateral sclerosis, cerebral palsy, or stroke. For apraxia of speech, the disease is typically a left hemisphere stroke. At times, these neurologic changes result in signs and symptoms. The *signs* of a disease are those characteristics observed by others, including professionals examining the patient. The *symptoms* of a disease are those characteristics perceived by the individuals with the disabilities.

For nearly 120 years, the characteristics of speech have been used to describe neurologic disease. For example, in 1877 Charcot described a triad of symptoms that were characteristic of disseminated sclerosis, now known as multiple sclerosis. These symptoms included tremor, nystagmus, and scanning speech. In 1929, Hiller studied the dysarthria of Friedreich's ataxia and concluded that the primary speech problem of patients with cerebellar lesion is one of respiratory control. In 1937, Zentay classified the dysarthric speech resulting from cerebellar lesions as ataxic speech, adiadochokinesis, explosive speech, and scanning speech.

Early descriptions of dysarthria were associated with impairments of the nervous system that were diagnosed by medical professionals. Therefore, the illness or disease model, which is frequently employed in the medical field, has been applied to the dysarthrias. According to the illness model, the severity of the dysarthria is associated with the severity of the illness or disease process, and the dysarthria is managed by treating the disease. Thus, dysarthria has been used as an index of disease severity through the years, with little attention focused on remediation of the speech disorder itself.

The practice of describing neurologic disease in terms of speech characteristics continued in a rather unsystematic fashion until the late 1960s. It was then that Darley, Aronson, and Brown (1969a, 1969b, 1975) studied the perceptual speech characteristics associated with a wide variety of neurologic conditions. This work is referenced throughout this text, and the characteristics associated with various neurologic conditions are summarized in Chapters 2, 3, and 4.

At times, speech–language pathologists need to take the point of view that dysarthria or apraxia of speech is a sign or symptom of a neurologic disease or condition. This leads them to seek answers to specific types of questions:

- Is dysarthria or apraxia of speech present, or are the signs and symptoms characteristic of some other communication problem? This line of questioning eventually leads to a differential diagnosis of motor speech disorders from other neurologic communication problems, including aphasia and dementia.

- If motor speech disorders are present, are the features consistent with those typically observed in speakers with the proposed diagnosis? This line of questioning leads to a differential diagnosis among the dysarthrias and may contribute eventually to a differential diagnosis of the neurologic disorder.

- How severe are the signs and symptoms and are they changing? Answers to these questions will eventually lead to an index of the severity of the neurologic disease and a means of monitoring the course of the disease or response to medication.

The Basic Scientist's Point of View

Motor speech disorders can be viewed from the perspective of those who study speech processes. For example, the neurolinguist may be interested in apraxia of speech because it provides insight into the organization of language processes, and the speech physiologist may be interested in dysarthria because it provides insights into how speech movements are learned and executed. The viewpoints adopted by basic scientists such as neurolinguists and speech physiologists are equally valid but quite different from the one taken by neurologists. Speech is a wonderfully complex phenomenon: Consider the rapid, precise, well-coordinated sequences of movements required to produce understandable speech. Speakers use approximately 100 different muscles and produce recognizable sounds at a rate as high as 14 per second. Each of these sounds requires specific respiratory, laryngeal, and oral articulatory postures. Sound productions are not based on fixed patterns; rather, speakers appear to have the ability to produce a sound acceptable to the listener in a number of different ways. Perhaps most remarkably, the speech motor activity is almost completely automatic. Although speakers may be consciously aware of formulating a message, they devote almost no conscious effort to planning motor speech activities. Given the complexity of motor speech, one would expect that impairment in motor control would have negative consequences in the form of reduced intelligibility, naturalness, and articulatory adequacy.

During the 1960s a new, physiologic perspective on dysarthria appeared. Perhaps this position was articulated initially by Hardy (1967) when he wrote the article "Suggestions for Physiologic Research in Dysarthria" to demonstrate the value of studying dysarthric speakers using the principles of experimental phonetics. In developing a research orientation, Hardy highlighted principles that continue to guide dysarthria research. Included among these are the following:

1. The physiology of one mechanism (respiratory, phonatory, or articulatory) interacts with all others to produce the speech signal.

2. Study of physiologic aberrations of only one of these mechanisms without regard to the role of the others, or their compensatory capabilities for speech production, will allow only limited conclusions about speech problems of interest.

3. Many of the speech disorders that result from neuromuscular deficits may be studied advantageously by viewing the entire speech production system as an aerodynamic–mechanical system.

Focus on the physiologic aspects of speech production has contributed to the understanding of many types of motor speech disorders. For example, individuals with Parkinson's disease have reported frequent problems with weak or hoarse voice, imprecise articulation, and difficulty getting speech started (Hartelius & Svensson, 1994). These problems have been studied from a physiologic perspective. Respiratory contributions to parkinsonian dysarthria have been evaluated (Murdoch, Chenery, Bowler, & Ingram, 1989; Solomon & Hixon, 1993). Cinegraphic observation of laryngeal function (Hanson, Gerratt, & Ward, 1984) suggests a direct relationship between features of breathiness and reduced loudness and increasing amounts of glottal gap and bowing of the vocal folds. Acoustic features of parkinsonian dysarthria are consistent with perceptual features in that there is evidence in individuals with Parkinson's disease, compared with individuals who are aging normally, of reduced duration of vocalic segments, reduced formant transitions, and increased voice onset time (Forrest, Weismer, & Turner, 1989). Other researchers have concluded that persons with Parkinson's disease have reduced articulatory displacements compared with normal speakers and incoordination of agonist and antagonist muscle groups (Hirose, Kiritani, & Sawashima, 1982; Hunker, Abbs, & Barlow, 1982; Moore & Scudder, 1989).

At times, especially when developing specific intervention plans, the speech–language pathologist must take the speech physiologist's viewpoint. The physiologic examination of speakers with dysarthria has been described by Netsell, Lotz, and Barlow (1989). A variety of instrumental approaches are used to describe the aerodynamic, kinematic, and acoustic properties of speech. This type of evaluation leads to questions quite different from those posed from the neurologic perspective.

- How can aspects of speech mechanism performance be objectively measured during speech production activities? Answers to this question have led to the development of techniques for measuring physiologic aspects of speech and for comparing the performance of the various aspects of speech production. In addition, this approach has allowed for comparison of the performance of dysarthric speakers with that of normal individuals.

- Are there means of compensating for the abnormal performance of the speech mechanism? Answers to this question have led to the development of a series of behavioral or prosthetic approaches to intervention.

- What malfunctions of the speech mechanism contribute substantially to reduced intelligibility? Answers to this question may form part of the strategy for sequencing of intervention tasks.

The Rehabilitationist's Point of View

Undoubtedly a speech–language pathologist managing a caseload of individuals with motor speech disorders must be familiar with a number of perspectives to understand the disorder. Clinicians must be thoroughly familiar with the viewpoint of the neurologist in order to plan intervention that is compatible with the underlying neuropathology, and is appropriate considering the natural course of the disorder. In addition, this viewpoint is required for the clinician to participate in the differential diagnosis process. Likewise, the clinician must have an understanding of the speech physiologist's viewpoint to be able to select and sequence intervention tasks appropriately. The viewpoint taken by the speech–language clinician planning rehabilitation programs is somewhat different from the one taken by either the neurologist, who wishes to identify the disease or disorder and to treat that condition, or the basic scientist, who wishes to understand both the normal and abnormal speech processes. The following are among the types of questions asked by the clinician in the rehabilitation setting:

- How is the motor speech disorder affecting the individual's lifestyle?

- How can that effect be lessened?

- What are reasonable goals for intervention?

- What are important measures of successful intervention?

- How can these goals be achieved? Does this individual need an augmentative communication system, or a palatal lift, or an amplifier, and so on?

The Speakers' Point of View

The viewpoint of speakers with motor speech disorders is variable depending on many different issues. Early in the course of a progressive condition such as Parkinson's disease, for example, individuals with the disorder are very focused on the perspective of the neurologist as attempts are made to diagnose the symptoms that they are experiencing. Once the diagnosis is made and confirmed, the speakers and their families become very interested in what is known (the science) of the disease or condition. The search for information often involves many family members and at times members from the larger community. As function begins to deteriorate, individuals with disabilities become increasingly focused on the rehabilitationist's perspective as they strive to learn compensatory skills and to maximize function. Eventually, the point of view of the speaker with a disability shifts to a perspective that focuses on "living with the condition." In this phase, the speaker may be resistant to additional medical diagnostic or rehabilitation-related activities.

This description of the perspective of a person with a motor speech disorder is brief and linear; however, life does not work that way. Individuals with disabilities may shift through this sequence of perspectives several times. In addition, family members or others who are influential in the lives of these individuals may not work their way through this process in similar schedules.

Question asked at a presentation: I have listened today for the way you refer to yourself and the persons with whom you work. In our rehabilitation center, we are trying to use a "people-first" terminology. What are you doing in your work settings?

Most of the time, we use people-first terminology and say "persons with dysarthria" or "individuals with dysarthria." That works pretty well when we are referring to individuals with a specific condition, such as "individuals with multiple sclerosis." However, when talking generally about persons who are under current medical care, we refer to them as "patients" or "clients." You will notice that in the context of this text in which we are concerned about their ability to communicate, we often refer to them simply as "speakers." By the way, we refer to persons in my profession as "speech–language pathologists," reserving the generic term, *clinicians*, to refer to persons from a variety of professions who provide assessments and intervention services.

MOTOR SPEECH DISORDERS AS CHRONIC CONDITIONS

Almost without exception, motor speech disorders are associated with diseases and conditions that are chronic or long term. Therefore, a model of the consequences of chronic disorder is helpful in developing a clinical perspective for management of individuals with dysarthria (Nagi, 1977, 1991; Wood, 1980). This model contains five parameters: (1) *pathophysiology* (changes in basic cell or functional physiology); (2) *impairment* (loss or change in physiologic function); (3) *functional limitation* (restriction or lack of ability to perform an action or function because of the impairment); (4) *disability* (limitations in performance of specific functions within a natural context); and (5) *societal limitation* (changes in performance that limit fulfillment of social roles or deny access to services). See Table 1.2 for definitions of dysarthria and apraxia of speech within the framework of the model of chronic disease. Each of these parameters is also discussed further in the following paragraphs.

Pathophysiology (Cellular or Tissue Level)

According to the model of chronic disease, the first level at which dysarthria and apraxia of speech can be defined relates to the underlying pathophysiology.

Table 1.2
Dysarthria and Apraxia of Speech as Chronic Disorder

Parameter	Definition	Motor Speech Disorders	Measures
Pathophysiology	Interruption or interference of normal physiologic and developmental processes or structures	Alterations in the nervous system	Abnormalities at the cell or tissue level
Impairment	Loss or abnormality of psychological, physiologic, or anatomical structure or function	A neurologic speech impairment that is characterized by slow, weak, imprecise, and/or uncoordinated movements of the speech musculature or inability to plan sequence of speech movements	Respiratory control Phonatory function Velopharyngeal function Oral articulation
Functional limitation	Restriction or lack (resulting from an impairment) of ability to perform an activity in the manner or within the range considered normal	The disability resulting from the motor speech impairment includes reduced speech intelligibility and rate and abnormal prosodic patterns	Speech intelligibility Speaking rate Articulatory adequacy Naturalness
Disability	Inability or limitation in performing socially defined activities and roles within a social and physical environment as a result of internal or external factors and their interplay	Speech performance in a physical and social context	Comprehensibility
Societal limitation	Restriction, attributable to social policy or barriers (structural or attitudinal), that limits fulfillment of roles or denies access to services or opportunities	Performance of roles by speakers with motor speech disorders in social context	Anecdotal reports

Note. Adapted from Disability in America: Toward a National Agenda for Prevention, by A. M. Pope and A. R. Tarlov (Eds.), 1991, Washington, DC: National Academy Press.

The level of deficit is at the neurologic cell or tissue level. For example, in amyotrophic lateral sclerosis (ALS), there is degeneration of upper and lower motor neurons. These deficits may be identified during the clinical neurologic examination and observed with techniques such as electromyography. Medical interventions may or may not be available for targeting this level of deficits. In the case of neuronal degeneration in ALS, there is currently no medical treatment. On the other hand, pharmacological interventions are successful in Parkinson's disease to compensate for abnormalities in the level of the neurotransmitter dopamine.

Impairment (Subsystem Level)

Dysarthria and apraxia of speech are neurologic speech disorders characterized by abnormalities in movement rate, precision, coordination, and sequencing of movements that can result in impairment of any combination of the subsystems of the speech mechanism, including respiration, phonation, velopharyngeal function, and articulation. When attempting to describe the impairment of individuals with motor speech disorders, measures of physiologic control and support are needed. These measures may include those that supply information about speech mechanism subsystems as they function during speech and non-speech tasks. Many of the measures of impairment involve use of instrumentation to make physiologic measures. However, certain aspects of the impairment, such as voice quality, may also be measured perceptually using rating scales. Approaches to the measurement of specific aspects of impairment will be described in Chapter 5. To date, a large part of the research literature in motor speech disorders has focused on impairment. Although it is beyond the scope of this chapter to review this extensive literature, references to research focusing on the underlying motor dysfunction of the various motor speech disorders is included in many of the chapters that follow.

Functional Limitation (Organism or Person Level)

Dysarthria and apraxia of speech can also be defined as a functional limitation resulting from motor impairment. The functional limitations refer to overall measures of personal performance and are characterized by reduced speech intelligibility and rate and by abnormal prosodic patterns. When attempting to describe the functional limitation, a number of overall measures of speech performance are available. These will be discussed in more detail in Chapter 6. Briefly, these include measures of speech intelligibility and rate, perceptual judgments of overall articulatory adequacy, and prosody. The majority of these measures are perceptually derived; however, certain aspects of prosody lend themselves to acoustic analysis.

Reduction or stabilization of a speaker's functional limitation is the primary goal of speech intervention for persons with motor speech disorders. Therefore, measures of functional limitation are frequently considered the outcome measures of dysarthria or apraxia treatment, and also serve as an overall index of the severity of the disorder. The relationship between impairment and functional limitation is not always simple or straightforward. For example, a preliminary report is available that examines the relationship between impairment and functional limitations in speakers with ALS (Yorkston, Strand, & Hume, 1998). Our clinical experience suggests that relatively severe impairment of single subsystems of speech may not result in severe functional limitation. For example, severely restricted lip movement in the presence of adequate functioning of other speech components will not result in a severe disability. However, even moderate impairment in multiple speech components may result in severe disability. Clinical experience also suggests that severe impairment of certain speech components may be particularly devastating in terms of impact on functional limitation. For example, severe respiratory timing and coordination problems may result in severe disability.

Disability (Contextual Level)

Dysarthria and apraxia of speech may be defined as a disability. The disability resulting from a motor speech disorder involves the reduced ability to function in physical and social contexts that require understandable, efficient, and natural sounding speech. Disability, then, involves not only speakers with motor speech disorders but also their communication partners. The term *comprehensibility* has been used to indicate the adequacy of speech performance in a social context (Yorkston, Strand, & Kennedy, 1996) and will be discussed in detail in Chapters 6 and 12. Because few standardized measures are available in this area, clinicians must rely on activities such as checklists and interviews regarding communication in natural settings.

Societal Limitation (Societal Level)

The final level described in the model of chronic disease, societal limitation, relates to policies, practices (group attitudes that are not official policies), and individual attitudes. An individual with a motor speech disorder may be prevented from participating in a desired role because of the biases and attitudes of individuals in the society. An intelligible speaker who does not sound natural might not be hired in an occupation involving public contact, even though that individual possesses all of the skills required for the job. A teenager with a motor speech disorder may be excluded from a social group because of the attitudes of the group. An individual can be prevented from participating in desired roles because of the severity of the disability. An unintelligible speaker cannot function adequately in the role of a telephone operator. No standard technique is currently available to the clinician for measurement of social limitation.

Although documentation of the societal limitation associated with motor speech disorder is rare, a few examples of such efforts can be found in the literature. For example, Hooks (1984) explored the impact of societal biases toward dysarthric speakers. He demonstrated that vocational counselors discriminated against speakers with dysarthria by suggesting that these individuals not only would be unsuccessful at jobs with high speaking requirements, but also would be unsuccessful at jobs with minimal speaking requirements. This social limitation was imposed by the vocational counselors even though the personnel files of the dysarthric individuals contained information showing them to be qualified to successfully perform the work described for the jobs with minimal speech requirements. Gies-Zaborowski and Silverman (1986) used a semantic differential scale to document the impact of mild dysarthria on peer perceptions of an 11-year-old girl with mild cerebral palsy. Their results indicated that "her speech caused her to be perceived as frightened, nervous, tense, and unlovable" (p. 143). For a more detailed discussion of this topic, see Chapter 11.

Question: Can you give me an example of how a disorder might be considered an impairment by one person and a societal limitation by another?

We received a phone call from the parents of a 13-year-old child who was not socially accepted in junior high. In their call, they indicated that they wanted a speech evaluation for their son because they wanted him to become involved in speech intervention again. The results of the assessment revealed that the young man's speech was 96% intelligible, yet his dysarthria, due to athetoid cerebral palsy, was obvious. He had received speech intervention services since he was a toddler and at the time of the assessment was not interested in more intervention. Academically, he was a strong student. Through the years, he had attended a local neighborhood elementary school with two sections of each grade. His peers knew him, understood his speech, and accepted him socially. A few months before his parents called us, he had entered a regional junior high school, and in that social environment his speech was disvalued by his fellow students who excluded him from their social groups and verbally abused him about the way he spoke.

(continues)

By requesting a speech evaluation to encourage their son to "work on his speech," the parents were focusing on his speech impairment or his functional limitation. However, in our opinion, the societal limitation that he was experiencing needed to be addressed by focusing on the attitudes, practices, and policies of his school and its students rather than focusing primarily on his speech.

THE CLINICAL PROCESS

For the speech–language pathologist, a clinical intervention may be thought of as a process of observing behavior, gathering pertinent information, and making decisions about the management of the communication problems of the individual with motor speech disorders. The decisions made by speech–language pathologists in the clinical setting can be characterized by three features. First, they are individualized. Almost without exception, the clinician is faced with decisions that relate to a single individual, who may or may not exhibit a classic pattern of impairment, functional limitation, and disability that is associated with a particular neurologic disorder. Typically in clinical management, complicating factors or special considerations make each individual unique. Second, there is almost always an urgency to make clinical decisions. Rather than waiting until research has provided better measurement techniques or a more complete understanding of the disorder, the clinician is forced to do the best job with the knowledge and tools available at the moment. Third, the clinician must make decisions based on the broadest possible perspective. The researcher may quite rightfully choose to focus on a limited aspect of this complex disorder and to study that aspect both systematically and in great detail, but the clinician usually does not have this option. Viewing motor speech disorders as chronic disorders serves a number of clinical purposes. We will close this chapter by identifying some pressing clinical issues and discussing how the perspective of the chronic disorder model may help to resolve these issues.

Identifying Perspectives

The model of chronic disorders provides a vocabulary for communicating with other professionals and with speakers with motor speech disorders and their families. It allows the clinician to identify the perspectives of others. In the introduction to this chapter, we described a family conference in which there was an apparent disagreement about the outcome of intervention. Reviewing that situation from the perspective of a model of chronic disorder suggests that each participant in the family conference may have been viewing dysarthria from a different perspective. The physician was viewing it as an impairment; thus, demonstrable changes in rigidity were a signal of successful intervention. The rehabilitation clinicians, including the occupational therapist and the speech–language pathologist, viewed the dysarthria as a functional limitation; thus, the patient's ability to perform more activities of daily living signaled successful intervention. On the other hand, the family viewed the dysarthria as a disability; thus, because the individual with Parkinson's disease was no longer able to return to his former occupation or to carry out his role as husband and father as he had before, the family felt that intervention had fallen short of its target. Although it may be true that recognizing the viewpoints of others may not change the reality of the outcome, the level of discontent may have been reduced if communication had been clearer. The lack of close relationship between impairment, functional limitations, and disability makes it mandatory for professionals to communicate clearly the point of view from which they are discussing the disorder.

Obviously, changes in impairment do not always result in immediate changes in the functional limitation. At times, improvement in the performance of several aspects of the impairment is required before a reduction in the functional limitation can be observed. Nevertheless, the ultimate goal of intervention is either stabilization or reduction in functional limitation, depending on the natural course of the individual's disorder.

Identification of the perspectives of others is also important when attempting to read, understand, and interpret the literature in motor speech disorders. Students given the task of reviewing research literature in this area are quickly impressed with the diversity of approaches to measurement. Any number of physiologic, acoustic, and perceptual measures have been used to understand the nature of the disorder. This diversity may at first give the impression that there is little agreement as to the single best way of understanding dysarthria, so writers simply choose the measures they prefer. We do not believe that this is the case. Rather, the diversity of approaches to measurement may simply reflect the differing perspectives from which the problem is being viewed. The vocabulary used in the model of chronic disorders may enable the reader to critically evaluate the adequacy of the measures employed in research, in other words, to determine whether the measures are well suited to their intended purpose. For example, aerodynamic measures of velopharyngeal resistance are frequently used as an indicator of velopharyngeal impairment. However, these measures alone, without corroborating measures of functional limitations such as speech intelligibility, may not be sufficient to document the effectiveness of an intervention program. Because the ultimate goal of intervention is more intelligible speech, and not better velopharyngeal performance, the measures of change in functional limitation and disability must accompany the measures that reflect a change in the impairment.

Identifying Treatment Candidates

The presence of motor speech disorders can be easily documented by listening to the speaker or by obtaining any number of measures of motor performance of the various speech components. However, merely knowing that the disorder is present does not help the clinician decide how important it is to treat the individual. The chronic disease model of motor speech disorder may provide some assistance in this area. Consider the case of two dysarthric speakers each having moderately severe impairment and disability. The urgency of treatment for these individuals does not depend entirely on the impairment or the functional limitation, but on the disability. Suppose that the first speaker is a retired individual living at home with his wife. His intelligible but slow speech may be sufficient to support his conversational needs. His level of functional limitation may be mild because he only has occasion to speak with those who are familiar with him, and rapid, efficient, and natural sounding speech is not mandatory. However, suppose the second speaker is a minister whose duties require extensive public speaking. Intelligible speech is of course required, but rapid, efficient, natural sounding speech is also mandatory. Thus, even a moderate level of functional limitation would cause a severe disability for this individual. The severity of the impairment, functional limitation, and disability are not as closely correlated as they may first appear. An individual with minimal communication needs may experience a substantial impairment before the functional limitation becomes a disability. For other individuals, even the mildest of impairment may be of real concern.

Setting Treatment Goals

There are many different approaches to goal setting in treatment. One of the most common is to set goals in relation to normal performance. This approach to goal setting is not appropriate in dysarthria or apraxia intervention for at least two reasons. First, because of the nature of underlying neuropathology, normal performance can almost never be achieved. Second, some of the specific treatment techniques described in this text actually move at least some aspects of performance in a direction that is away from normal. An example of such a technique is rate reduction, in which speakers learn to slow their already slower than normal speech to increase intelligibility.

One alternative to setting normalcy as a general goal for speakers with motor speech disorders is to set highly specific task-related goals for performance. For example, when planning intervention with severe dysarthria, a treatment goal might be to sustain 5 centimeters of water pressure for 5 seconds. Unfortunately, specific goals may not be functionally important. Although setting treatment goals such as these is necessary to document recovery or learning rates, achieving these goals is important clinically only if they are also associated with some reduction of functional limitation. Using the vocabulary of this model of chronic disorders, the goals of intervention are to decrease or stabilize the functional limitation, thus improving such overall aspects of speech as intelligibility, rate, and naturalness. Setting goals related to functional limitation may be an acceptable compromise between the general goals of normalcy, which may not be achievable, and the specific goals of changing a single component of speech production, which may not be functionally important.

Assessing Treatment Efficacy

The model of chronic disorder may also be applied when studying treatment efficacy. A review of the literature reveals many articles describing various aspects of dysarthria and apraxia of speech and relatively few articles outlining treatment approaches. Still fewer articles document efficacy of treatment (Yorkston, 1996). This is not surprising in a field where attention has only recently turned to intervention. Documentation of treatment effectiveness progresses through a number of phases as a field of therapy matures. In the first phase, possible approaches to intervention are described. These descriptions are usually based on theoretical models of the disorder which suggest that a series of approaches "should work" if the understanding of the disorder is adequate. Darley and colleagues (1975), Rosenbek and LaPointe (1985), Perkins (1983), Hardy (1983), and Vogel and Cannito (1991) have described approaches that have been used with individuals with dysarthria. Although these descriptions are an important first step, a review of the literature shows a steady increase in the number of case studies being reported. This phase of efficacy studies is more specific than the first phase because, by describing the cases in detail, readers are provided some general guidelines for candidacy that are for the most part absent in the first phase of treatment outcome studies. Because of the heterogeneous nature of the dysarthric and apraxic populations, single case design research (McNeil & Kennedy, 1984; McReynolds & Kearns, 1983) holds great potential for documenting the impact of treatment for motor speech disorders.

The third phase of efficacy studies involves those that examine groups of individuals. There have been almost no group studies investigating the efficacy of dysarthria or apraxia treatment. As is obvious to those familiar with the aphasia literature, well-constructed group efficacy studies are difficult to carry out. One of the most challenging aspects of this type of study is to separate factors that are related to the natural course of the disorder from those that relate specifically to the impact of treatment. For example, spontaneous recovery in an individual with aphasia following stroke frequently prevents a clear interpretation of data describing the treatment outcomes. The model of chronic disorder may provide some guidelines for clearly interpreting treatment outcome data. The potential for independent measurement of the impairment and the disability provides some intriguing opportunities for documenting the impact of treatment. For example, consider the speaker with a degenerative disorder. In this case, increasing impairment is an inevitable consequence of the disease. However, if the clinician can document a stable disability in the face of increasing impairment, treatment effectiveness may be suggested. Likewise, a decrease in functional limitation in the presence of a stable impairment would imply that intervention was effective. The important implications for efficacy studies provide another reason to encourage research investigating the relationship between impairment, functional limitation, and disability in speakers with motor speech disorders.

REFERENCES

Chappell, G. E. (1973). Childhood verbal apraxia and its treatment. *Journal of Speech and Hearing Disorders, 38,* 362–368.

Charcot, J. M. (1877). *Lectures on the diseases of the nervous system* (Vol. 1). London: The New Sydenham Society.

Crary, M. (1984). Phonological characteristics of developmental verbal apraxia. *Seminars in Speech and Language, 5,* 71–83.

Crary, M. A. (1993). *Developmental motor speech disorders.* San Diego: Singular.

Darley, F., Aronson, A., & Brown, J. (1969a). Clusters of deviant speech dimensions in the dysarthrias. *Journal of Speech and Hearing Research, 12,* 462–496.

Darley, F., Aronson, A., & Brown, J. (1969b). Differential diagnostics patterns of dysarthria. *Journal of Speech and Hearing Research, 12,* 224.

Darley, F. L., Aronson, A. E., & Brown, J. R. (1975). *Motor speech disorders.* Philadelphia: Saunders.

Edwards, M. (1973). Developmental verbal dyspraxia. *British Journal of Disorders of Communication, 8,* 64–70.

Forrest, K., Weismer, G., & Turner, G. S. (1989). Kinematic, acoustic, and perceptual analyses of connected speech produced by Parkinsonian and normal geriatric adults. *Journal of the Acoustic Society of America, 85*(6), 2608–2622.

Gies-Zaborowski, J., & Silverman, F. (1986). Documenting the impact of a mild dysarthria on peer perception. *Speech and Hearing Services in Schools, 17*(2), 143.

Hanson, D., Gerratt, B. R., & Ward, P. H. (1984). Cinegraphic observations of laryngeal function in Parkinson's disease. *Laryngoscope, 94,* 348–353.

Hardy, J. C. (1967). Suggestions for physiologic research in dysarthria. *Cortex, 3,* 128.

Hardy, J. C. (1983). *Cerebral palsy.* Englewood Cliffs, NJ: Prentice-Hall.

Hartelius, L., & Svensson, P. (1994). Speech and swallowing symptoms associated with Parkinson's disease and multiple sclerosis: A survey. *Phoniatrica et Logopaedica, 46,* 9–17.

Hayden, D. A. (1994). Differential diagnosis of motor speech dysfunction in children. *Clinics in Communication Disorders, 4,* 119–141.

Hiller, H. (1929). A study of speech disorders in Friedreich's ataxia. *Archives of Neurology and Psychiatry, 22,* 75–90.

Hirose, H., Kiritani, S., & Sawashima, M. (1982). Velocity of articulatory movements in normal and dysarthric subjects. *Folia Phoniatrica, 34,* 210–215.

Hooks, D. (1984). The effects of dysarthric speaking voice on counselor's evaluation. *Dissertation Abstracts International, Nov 45.*

Hunker, C. J., Abbs, J. H., & Barlow, S. M. (1982). The relationship between Parkinsonism rigidity and hypokinesia in the orofacial system: A quantitative analysis. *Neurology, 32,* 749–754.

McNeil, M. R., & Kennedy, J. G. (1984). Measuring the effects of treatment for dysarthia: Knowing when to change or terminate. *Seminars in Speech and Language, 4,* 337–358.

McReynolds, L. V., & Kearns, K. (1983). *Single subject experimental design in speech pathology.* Baltimore: University Park Press.

Moore, C. A., & Scudder, R. R. (1989). Coordination of jaw muscle activity in Parkinsonian movement: Description and response to traditional treatment. In K. M. Yorkston & D. R. Beukelman (Eds.), *Recent advances in clinical dysarthria* (pp. 147–164). Austin, TX: PRO-ED.

Morley, M. E. (1972). *The development and disorders of speech in childhood* (3rd ed.). London: Livingstone.

Murdoch, B. E., Chenery, H. J., Bowler, S., & Ingram, J. C. L. (1989). Respiratory function in Parkinson's subjects exhibiting a perceptible speech deficit: A kinematic and spirometric analysis. *Journal of Speech and Hearing Disorders, 54,* 610–626.

Nagi, S. Z. (1977). The disabled and rehabilitation services: A national overview. *American Rehabilitation, 2*(5), 26–33.

Nagi, S. Z. (1991). Disability concepts revisited: Implications for prevention. In A. M. Pope & A. R. Tarlov (Eds.), *Disability in America: Toward national agenda for prevention* (pp. 309–327). Washington, DC: National Academy Press.

Netsell, R., Lotz, W. K., & Barlow, S. M. (1989). A speech physiology examination for individuals with dysarthria. In K. M. Yorkston & D. R. Beukelman (Eds.), *Recent advances in clinical dysarthria* (pp. 3–33). Austin, TX: PRO-ED.

Perkins, W. H. (1983). *Dysarthria and apraxia: Current therapy of communication disorders.* New York: Thieme-Stratton.

Pope, A. M., & Tarlov, A. R. (Eds.). (1991). *Disability in America: Toward a national agenda for prevention.* Washington, DC: National Academy Press.

Rosenbek, J. C., & LaPointe, L. L. (1985). The dysarthrias: Description, diagnosis, and treatment. In D. Johns (Ed.), *Clinical management of neurogenic communication disorders* (pp. 97–152). Boston: Little, Brown.

Rosenbek, J. C., & Wertz, R. T. (1972). A review of 50 cases of developmental apraxia of speech. *Language, Speech and Hearing Services in Schools, 3,* 23–33.

Solomon, N. P., & Hixon, T. J. (1993). Speech breathing in Parkinson's disease. *Journal of Speech and Hearing Research, 36,* 294–310.

Vogel, D., & Cannito, M. (1991). *Treating disordered speech motor control.* Austin, TX: PRO-ED.

Wertz, R. T. (1985). Neuropathologies of speech and language: An introduction to patient management. In D. F. Johns (Ed.), *Clinical management of neurogenic communicative disorders* (2nd ed., pp. 1–96). Boston: Little, Brown.

Wertz, R. T., LaPointe, L., & Rosenbek, J. (1984). *Apraxia of speech in adults: The disorder and its management.* Orlando, FL: Grune & Stratton.

Wood, P. H. N. (1980). Appreciating the consequences of disease: The classification of impairments, disability and handicaps. *The WHO Chronicle, 43,* 376–380.

Yorkston, K. M. (1996). Treatment efficacy: Dysarthria. *Journal of Speech and Hearing Research, 39*(5), S46–S57.

Yorkston, K. M., Strand, E. A., & Hume, J. (1998). The relationship between motor function and speech function in amyotrophic lateral sclerosis. In M. Cannito, K. M. Yorkston, & D. R. Beukelman (Eds.), *Neuromotor speech disorders: Nature, assessment, and management* (pp. 85–98). Baltimore: Brookes.

Yorkston, K. M., Strand, E. A., & Kennedy, M. R. T. (1996). Comprehensibility of dysarthric speech: Implications for assessment and treatment planning. *American Journal of Speech–Language Pathology, 5*(1), 55–66.

Yoss, K. A., & Darley, F. (1974). Developmental apraxia of speech in children with defective articulation. *Journal of Speech and Hearing Research, 17,* 399–416.

Zentay, P. J. (1937). Motor disorders of the nervous system and their signficance for speech: Part I. Cerebral and cerebellar dysarthria. *Laryngoscope, 47,* 147–156.

CHAPTER

DEVELOPMENTAL
MOTOR SPEECH DISORDERS

Preface: Individuals with motor speech disorders frequently have serious neurologic disorders. Therefore, speech–language pathology services are often delivered in conjunction with other medically related services. To provide a resource guide for speech–language pathologists, each of the following three chapters contains a review of medical issues related to those neurologic conditions that are frequently associated with motor speech disorders, including a description of the disorder, underlying neuropathology, differential diagnosis, natural course, and medical management. A summary of research describing the speech characteristics related to selected neurologic conditions is included to assist the reader in integrating the speech consequences and characteristics of the neurologic disorders. In several cases, a staging of speech intervention will provide details of intervention as a function of the severity of the disorder. Reference to the speech symptoms will be made throughout the book during discussions of specific assessment and intervention procedures. Citations are provided so that interested readers can pursue the in-depth study of specific disorders.

This chapter reviews those motor speech disorders that are developmental, Chapter 3 contains a review of disorders with an adult onset and a nonprogressive course, and Chapter 4 contains a review of the degenerative motor speech disorders. We adopted this organizational approach because the age of onset and natural course has a strong impact on characteristics of the disorders and their management. For example, although we will focus exclusively on the speech aspects of cerebral palsy, the onset of the disorder before language has developed has important implications. Thus, the need to attend to the issue of language development becomes critical in this population when it is not in disorders that have their onset in adulthood.

The term *motor speech disorders* is used to describe a group of disorders characterized by difficulty with either planning or executing sequential movements during speech. When the disorder occurs during early childhood, the term *developmental motor speech disorder* is often used. The distinction between developmental and acquired disorders is an important one because of the complex interactions that occur among motor, cognitive, and linguistic processes in the developing child (Strand, 1992). When something delays or impedes the development of movement, it is clear that speech will be delayed. Moreover, delays in the development of movement will also have an impact on the ongoing development of language, including phonology. This makes assessment and treatment of developmental motor speech disorders complex and different from the management of acquired disorders. This chapter will focus on descriptions of the nature and characteristics of developmental motor speech disorders.

Question: I am having difficulty differentiating a developmental from an acquired disorder in childhood. When do you use each of these terms?

We usually use the term *acquired disorder* in the case where the child is developing speech and language normally, then something happens (e.g., brain injury, tumor, or stroke) to impede that development. The term *developmental* is usually used when speech and language development is delayed or deviant; that is, there is no period of time in which things were progressing as expected. The term *congenital* also comes into play here. This term is used when a particular condition, such as cerebral palsy or cleft palate, exists at birth. In this case, something has occurred that accounts for the speech problem. Because it exists from the time of birth, the term congenital is used. In this chapter, we are describing motor speech disorders that occur in childhood, whether congenital, acquired, or developmental.

Children may fail to speak normally for a variety of reasons. For example, in cerebral palsy, a particular problem in the central or peripheral nervous system occurs. Trauma to the brain, such as may occur in a motor vehicle accident, can cause failure of speech development. Sometimes abnormal speech development may be due to severe delays that impede the development of all cognitive, linguistic, and motor processing. At other times, it is difficult to determine any particular reason why the child does not develop functional verbal communication or why the child's speech is difficult to understand. In any case, the problem facing the speech–language pathologist who works with children who have severe articulatory output problems is to determine what is contributing to the child's problems with speech. That is, one has to determine if the primary problem is at the linguistic level of phonological processing, at the level of motor planning (often called a developmental apraxia of speech), and/or at the level of motor execution (a dysarthria).

In Chapter 1, definitions were given and distinctions were made between apraxia of speech and dysarthria. These distinctions must be viewed slightly differently when examined from the developmental perspective. The complicating factor is that they occur while the linguistic processes of phonology, semantics, and syntax are still emerging. *Developmental apraxia of speech* is the term most often used to refer to children who have severe articulatory output problems due primarily to difficulty with planning sequential movements of the articulators for speech purposes, even though the musculature is normal for nonspeech movement, such as smiling, chewing, and swallowing. *Acquired apraxia* also occurs in childhood, usually as a result of trauma. The earlier the acquired apraxia occurs, the more it will influence the development of phonology and language.

Question: Is there a difference between apraxia of speech and oral apraxia?

Yes, it is important to differentiate the terms *apraxia of speech* (sometimes called verbal apraxia) from *oral apraxia*. Children who have difficulty planning sequences of movement for direct imitation of nonspeech movement of oral structures are said to have an oral apraxia. That is, the tongue may move easily in all directions during play, chewing, and swallowing, but when shown or asked to elevate the tongue to the alveolar ridge, the child may grope or exhibit trial-and-error behavior and not be able to achieve the correct position. The term apraxia of speech is used only when movement planning is impaired for speech. Children who have oral apraxia may also have apraxia of speech. Not all children with apraxia of speech have oral apraxia. In our clinical experience, if a child with apraxia of speech has coexisting oral apraxia, treatment will be more difficult and progress may be slower at first.

The other category of motor speech disorder to be discussed in this chapter is *dysarthria*. In Chapter 1, dysarthria was described as a motor speech disorder resulting from disturbed neuromuscular control of the speech mechanism itself. The deficits are seen in both speech and nonspeech movement and may involve respiration, phonation, resonance, articulation, and prosody. Childhood dysarthria can result from a congenital etiology, such as cerebral palsy, or from developmental delay. Acquired dysarthrias also occur, due to tumor, traumatic brain injury, anoxia, or infectious disease. Like developmental apraxia of speech, factors complicating assessment and treatment include the emerging language and speech processing system.

In this chapter, we begin by reviewing the most common etiology of childhood dysarthria, cerebral palsy. The focus is on the nature of the disorder and the associated motor speech characteristics. We follow this with a brief description of several other etiologies of the dysarthrias seen in childhood. We then provide a description of the nature of developmental apraxia of speech, including a discussion of the specific speech characteristics and how those vary with changes in phonetic or linguistic context.

CEREBRAL PALSY

Pathology—Nature of the Disorder

DESCRIPTION AND DIAGNOSIS

Cerebral palsy can be defined as a nonprogressive motor disorder that stems from an insult to the central nervous system during the prenatal or perinatal period. It is important to realize, however, that even though cerebral palsy stems from a static lesion of the nervous system, the manifestations and complications of the disorder will change with the growth of the child into adolescence and adulthood. Although the incidence of cerebral palsy is between 1.5 and 3.0 per 1,000 individuals, prevalence figures for adults are difficult to obtain (Dabney, Lyston, & Miller, 1997). However, studies suggest that the majority of even the most severely affected individuals survive to adulthood (Evans, Evans, & Alberman, 1990). The population most at risk for cerebral palsy are infants with low birth weight and those with preterm delivery (Eicher & Batshaw, 1993). Other causal factors associated with the presence of cerebral palsy are hypoxia, periventricular hemorrhage (hemorrhage around the ventricles), mechanical birth trauma, intrauterine infection, and kernicterus (caused by Rh incompatibility with the mother); however, in almost 25% of the cases, there are no identified perinatal complications (Eicher & Batshaw, 1993).

Question: What is the difference between incidence and prevalence of a disorder?

We use the terms incidence and prevalence when discussing the demographics of various clinical populations. Prevalence refers to the number of cases of a disease or disorder that occur at a given time. Incidence, on the other hand, is the number of new cases that occur during a specific time frame. When reviewing the disorder cerebral palsy, Erenberg (1984) reported a prevalence of 400,000 school-aged children, which means that when the study was reported, there were about that number of cases in the United States. Erenberg also reported an incidence rate of 2 to 2.5 per 1,000, which means that about 2 new cases occur per 1,000 people per year.

The diagnosis of cerebral palsy rests primarily on clinical information and observation of a child's development over time. The hallmarks of cerebral palsy are the persistence of primitive reflexes in the child and delays in achieving developmental milestones. For instance, the Moro or startle reflex, which usually becomes difficult to elicit after 2 to 3 months of age in an unimpaired child, may last indefinitely in an individual with cerebral palsy. More mature postural mechanisms (e.g., the equilibrium response) may fail to develop. The infant may display poor feeding ability, unexplained irritability, or disordered sleep patterns, and as he or she grows, may have poor balance and an early hand preference (before 1 year). Diagnostic studies such as computerized tomography and electroencephalography are not always correlated with the clinical picture.

PATHOPHYSIOLOGY

The etiology and neuropathology of cerebral palsy have been the subjects of some confusion, probably because the term cerebral palsy is used in relation to a heterogeneous group of deficits (Towbin, 1960). In fact, because of the variety of etiologies that may result in cerebral palsy and the diffuse nature of neuropathological impairment, the term cerebral palsy has somewhat reduced clinical significance (Hardy, 1983). The pathophysiology in cerebral palsy may be diffuse (e.g., in precipitating conditions such as anoxia) or focal (e.g., in conditions such as intracranial injury or ischemic event). The precipitating pathophysiologic condition may occur at different time periods: prenatal, perinatal, or within the first few years after birth. There is increasing evidence that the initial process causes brain damage in utero and that problems related to delivery may be in part a result of the initial damage (Stempien & Gaebler-Spira,

1996). Prenatal factors may include genetic factors, agenesis (failure of part of the brain to develop), viruses, anoxia, or rarely genetic factors. Perinatal factors, or those that happen just before, during, or just after birth, often result in anoxia. These can include cord compression, mucous blockage of the airways, or aspiration pneumonia. The use of narcotics during the birth process may also depress the infant's respiratory function, resulting in hypoxia. Trauma that occurs shortly before, during, or after birth is another major cause of disorders during the perinatal stage. Postnatal factors include brain injury, high fevers, and diseases such as meningitis and encephalitis (Eicher & Batshaw, 1993).

The site of neural damage in cerebral palsy varies extensively. The specific movement characteristics exhibited by a child with cerebral palsy depend on which neural systems are involved. Those neural systems most important to movement and motor control are the pyramidal and extrapyramidal descending systems, the basal ganglia, and the cerebellum. In addition, reflex activity is important for the maintenance of posture, muscle tone, and eventually coordinated movement.

Question: I am confused by the term extrapyramidal. *I have heard it used for descending motor systems and for the basal ganglia. Which is correct?*

The extrapyramidal system refers to those fiber tracts that lie outside the pyramidal tracts. The term is often used to denote tracts whose cell bodies lie in the brain stem and project to lower motor neurons in the spinal cord. These pathways, including the reticulospinal, vestibulospinal, and tectospinal, have to do with postural control, whereas the pyramidal (corticospinal and corticobulbar) tracts are important for voluntary movement. The basal ganglia, a group of nuclei at the base of the cerebral hemispheres, are also referred to as an extrapyramidal system. This system facilitates the initiation and control of movement.

Although damage to the motor systems results in predictable motor deficits, keep in mind that there is no one characteristic finding regarding neuropathology in the population of individuals with cerebral palsy, nor is there a single or typical postmortem pathologic finding in children with cerebral palsy (Denhoff, 1976). Generalized cortical atrophy is common, as is focal atrophy. Some gyri seem swollen because adjacent cerebral gyri are undeveloped. Some myelin sheaths become prominent while others are destroyed. Most children with cerebral palsy have damage to a number of cortical and subcortical areas, resulting in significant impairment of voluntary movement, without complete loss of movement. Because the nervous system continues to develop after birth, the effects of damage before or during birth may alter the continued course of neural development. Therefore, the behavioral character-istics of the disorder may change over time until stabilizing as a definite clinical picture (Hardy, 1983). The most typical change is from dramatically reduced muscle tone to some form of spasticity or involuntary movement. It is impor-tant to remember that the movement disorders in cerebral palsy represent a dis-ruption in the dynamics of the interaction of motor systems, more than specific dysfunction of one or more unrelated neural systems.

To summarize the pathophysiology related to cerebral palsy, it is helpful to describe particular aspects of movement disorders in general, and the specific neuropathology that is most often associated with those behaviors. Specific terms are used to denote types of movement disorders, and many of these terms are used to describe specific types of cerebral palsy. In general, these terms refer to disorders of too much or too little muscle contraction that yield limited or weak movement, involuntary "extra" movement, uncoordinated movement, or a combination of all of these. See Table 2.1 for a summary of these terms. In

Table 2.1
Terms Relating to Types of Movement Disorder in Cerebral Palsy

Term	Description	Neural System Involved
Spasticity (Hypertonicity)	State of the muscles in which there is too much contraction. Individuals with spas-ticity exhibit hyperactive deep reflexes, and exaggerated contraction when stretched.	Upper motor neuron
Flaccidity (Hypotonicity)	State of the muscles in which there is too little contraction. Muscles have low muscle tone and do not respond to stimulation. There is a decrease or absence of reflexes.	Lower motor neuron
Ataxia	Impairment in ability for muscle groups to work in a coordinated fashion. It is a general term used to denote a number of deficits in executing voluntary movement, including the following:	Cerebellum
Dysmetria	Errors in range, rate, and force of movement	
Dysdiadochokinesia	Difficulty maintaining regular movement patterns during rapid alternating movement	
Asynergia	Errors in the relative timing of the compo-nents of complex movement	

(continues)

Table 2.1 (*continued*)

Term	Description	Neural System Involved
Dyskinesia	Involuntary extraneous motor activity of the following types:	Basal ganglia and their connections
Athetosis	Slow, writhing, irregular movements, especially in the hands, fingers, and wrists	
Dystonia	Similar to athetosis, but abnormal movements may involve the trunk muscles more than the extremities	
Chorea	Quick, jerky, involuntary movements of the extremities, head, or trunk	
Tremor	Rhythmic oscillation of an extremity, head, or trunk	
Rigidity	Increased resistance to passive movement through an entire range of movement	Basal ganglia

cerebral palsy, it is very difficult to establish specific correlations between movement disorders and specific pathologic findings. In general, damage to upper motor neurons (pyramidal tracts, extrapyramidal tracts) is responsible for spasticity, damage to the cerebellum results in ataxia, and damage to the basal ganglia results in dyskinesias.

Pyramidal System

The pyramidal system (corticobulbar and corticospinal systems) is excitatory in function and is responsible for fine, rapid, voluntary movement. The neuron cell bodies are located in the motor cortex, pass through the internal capsule, and send axons down to end in lower motor neuron pools in the brain stem (corticobulbar tract) or the spinal cord (corticospinal tract) (see Figure 2.1). In the corticobulbar tract, the axons travel only to the brain stem, where they synapse with lower motor neurons in the motor nuclei of the cranial nerves. Most of these motor neuron pools are bilaterally innervated (except for the lower part of Cranial Nerve VII, which innervates the lower half of the face). The extrapyramidal tracts descend from primarily brain stem nerve nuclei and also enter the ventral part of spinal gray matter. For children who exhibit spastic cerebral palsy, there is usually damage within the extrapyramidal system. This results in spasticity, or too much muscle tone. Damage to the corticospinal tract

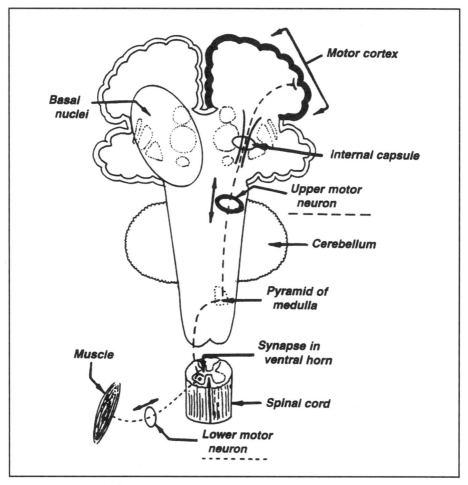

Figure 2.1. Pyramidal motor system represented as an upper motor neuron and lower motor neuron. From *The Speech Sciences* (p. 280), by R. D. Kent, 1997, San Diego: Singular. Copyright 1997 by Singular Publishing Group. Reprinted with permission.

Question: What does the term muscle tone really mean? I am also having difficulty differentiating spasticity and flaccidity from paralysis and weakness. How do these terms relate to each other?

Muscle tone is the term used to denote the current state of muscle contraction when the muscle is at rest, as well as when that muscle is contracting during movement. When there is no (or too little) muscle

(continues)

contraction, that is called flaccidity. If there is too much contraction of muscle fibers when the muscle is at rest, it is called spasticity. Flaccidity occurs when there is interruption of the innervation of the muscle by the lower motor neuron and is often associated with atrophy (muscle wasting). Spasticity occurs when upper motor neurons are damaged, primarily because tracts that are inhibitory are affected and cannot do their job. Both flaccidity and spasticity may be mild, moderate, or severe.

It is important to differentiate between the "state of the muscle" at rest, and the resulting difficulty with movement of a structure, such as an arm or leg. Both flaccidity and spasticity will result in weak and perhaps reduced range of movement. So, weakness is the result of aberrant muscle tone, whether there is too much or too little tone. Paralysis is when there is no voluntary movement. For example, a person with flaccidity or spasticity that is so severe that no movement of an extremity will occur has paralysis of that extremity. The word *paresis* is also used, usually to denote partial paralysis of the extremity. There are also different terms used to refer to which extremities are paralyzed. For example, when all four limbs are paralyzed, it is called *quadriplegia*. *Diplegia* involves the two legs, whereas *hemiplegia* refers to the arm and leg on one side of the body. The term *tetraplegia* is sometimes used when spasticity is distributed all over the body musculature.

alone may initially result in flaccidity, and spasticity later becomes evident. It is improbable, however, to have a lesion affecting only the corticospinal tract.

The Basal Ganglia

The basal ganglia are a group of subcortical nuclei that are important to motor control. These nuclei are the caudate nucleus, the putamen, the globus pallidus, and the substantia nigra. There is a delicate balance of excitatory and inhibitory neurotransmitters that work in the basal ganglia and play an essential role in motor control. There are major projections from frontal cortex to the basal ganglia, which in turn send projections back up to supplementary and primary motor cortex through the thalamus. These nuclei seem to play an important role in the planning and execution of learned movements, including initiating and regulating amount of movement. Lesions to the basal ganglia will typically result in involuntary movement, with both reductions and exaggerations in the amount of movement. In cerebral palsy, involvement of the basal ganglia will often result in the involuntary movement associated with athetosis and a characteristic speech pattern that is distinguishable from other types of dysarthria in cerebral palsy.

The Cerebellum

The cerebellum is integral to motor control, as it plays an important role in maintaining muscle tone and coordinated movement. In particular, the cerebellum helps maintain equilibrium, coordinates muscle action for both stereotyped and nonstereotyped movement, and makes an important contribution to the synergy of muscle action. That is, it helps make sure muscles contract at the right time and with the right force in synchrony with other muscles. This synchrony is critical in coordinating the finely controlled, rapid voluntary movements of speech. It has influence over both postural and voluntary movement. The cerebellum receives information from cortex, the spinal cord, and the vestibular system. From cortex, it receives information regarding the initiation of movement, so that it can make appropriate adjustments in muscle activity. Information comes from proprioceptors (muscle spindles and golgi tendon organs) via the spinal cord. This information helps the cerebellum in its role in maintaining appropriate muscle tone. The vestibular nerve gives the cerebellum information regarding linear and angular movement acceleration so that balance can be maintained. The cerebellum sends information back to cortex, particularly motor cortex, in order to facilitate coordinated muscle activity. Information from cerebellum also goes back to the spinal cord to influence spinal segmental motor activity. Lesions to the cerebellum usually result in ataxia and hypotonia. Thus, children with ataxic cerebral palsy will exhibit errors in rate, range, force, and direction of movement. They may overshoot or undershoot spatial targets, will walk with a wide-based ataxic gait, and may be hypotonic. Their speech will also reflect impairment in the coordination of movement. For example, children with cerebral palsy may have particular difficulty coordinating respiratory activity with other aspects of speech.

Reflex Activity

It is also important to consider reflex activity and how that is affected in cerebral palsy. There is integration of specific stimuli, especially in the brain stem and spinal cord, that is responsible for predictable, patterned responses called reflexes. These reflexes are important to maintaining muscle tone, posture, and coordinated movement. Some reflexes are abnormal at any time during development. Other reflexes are normal in early infancy, but cannot be elicited later, as maturation of the central and peripheral nervous system proceeds. It is the exaggeration or continued presence (beyond expected ages) of these reflexes that is typically seen in children with cerebral palsy. These primitive reflexes interfere with normal movement.

The following primitive postural reflexes are normally elicited only in infancy but are frequently seen in children with cerebral palsy.

1. *The tonic neck reflex* includes both asymmetrical and symmetrical types, and is normal until 6 or 7 months of age. If the duration of the response lasts more than 30 seconds, this is abnormal, even for infants, who usually exhibit the response only for a few seconds. In the symmetrical type, when the infant is placed in the prone position, flexion of the head elicits flexion of the arms and extension of the legs. Head exten-sion elicits extension of the arms and legs. The asymmetrical tonic neck reflex is most common and may be elicited with rotation of the head to one side. This results in extension of the arm and leg on the side to which the head is turned, with flexion on the other side (see Figure 2.2).

2. In the *positive supporting reaction,* the infant will make automatic step-ping movements when suspended vertically. This leads to the ability of

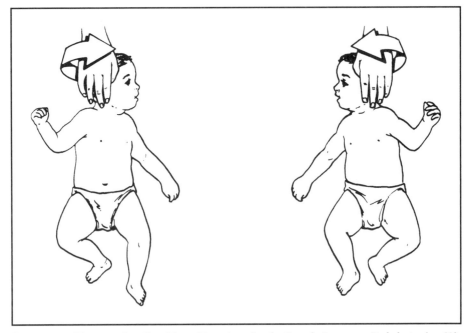

Figure 2.2. Tonic neck reflex. From *Neurology for the Speech–Language Pathologist* (p. 60), by R. J. Love and W. G. Webb, 1986, Stoneham, MA: Butterworth. Copyright 1986 by Butterworth. Reprinted with permission.

the child to stand. If there is an exaggeration of this reflex, combined with hypertonicity of trunk muscles, as is seen in spastic cerebral palsy, sequential movement will be very difficult.

3. The *Moro reflex* is also called the startle reflex. It is elicited when the infant's head is dropped back or with a loud noise. The infant will move the arms up and open them, followed by sudden movement of the arms together.

4. The *sucking and rooting response* is elicited by stroking the infant's cheek. The infant will turn toward the stimulus and begin sucking. In those children with cerebral palsy who have cortical lesions, this reflex may interfere with oral facial movement and phonation. This will, therefore, hamper the development of speech motor control and contribute to the presence of dysarthria.

The persistence of those reflexes that are normal only in early infancy, then, will influence the development of motor control and hamper voluntary motor activity.

Major Classification

There are four overall classes of cerebral palsy, with the spastic variety accounting for the majority of cases (75%). In this form of cerebral palsy, there is increased muscle tone with hyperactivity of the stretch reflexes and a Babinski reflex. Many children with spastic cerebral palsy retain some primitive reflexes, such as Moro, tonic neck, or grasp. The distal portions of the arms and legs are usually more affected than the trunk. This makes walking or fine-skilled hand movements very difficult or impossible. Within the spastic category are the subclasses of hemiparesis (21%), diplegia (21%), and quadriparesis (27%). Other classes include dyskinetic (athetoid), ataxic (dystonic), and mixed variety (Eicher & Batshaw, 1993).

The infant may initially demonstrate normal or even decreased muscle tone because of damage primarily to pyramidal tracts. Therefore, hemiplegia is often undiagnosed at birth and is usually brought to the physician's attention when the infant fails to match peer development at 3 to 9 months. Later, however, spasticity gradually emerges due to the damage to the extrapyramidal system. While hemiplegia refers to impairment on one side of the body, it usually involves the arm to a greater extent than the leg and may also occur with a sensory deficit. This sensory deficit is usually one of proprioception, but impaired awareness of the affected limb may also occur and may also contribute to the movement disorder. Children with spastic hemiplegia may or may not show symptoms of corticobulbar involvement. If there is some involvement, dysarthria and dysphagia may not be important problems because of bilateral innervation of most of the cranial nerves. Mental retardation is less common in this form than with quadriplegia or diplegia.

Quadriplegia (or quadriparesis) is characterized by spasticity and weakness in all four limbs. This form is due to bilateral damage to the pyramidal and extrapyramidal tracts, although one side may be more severely involved than the other. Sometimes the word tetraplegia is used when the spasticity is distributed over all the body's musculature. Due to the bilateral cortical damage, it is likely that both dysarthria and dysphagia will occur, and may be quite severe, because of spasticity in the cranial nerve system. Quadriplegia is more severe in the upper extremities.

Diplegia (also called Little's disease) is most closely associated with a low birth weight. It typically results in spasticity of all four limbs, but the legs are much more involved. Because of weakness or paralysis, children with spastic diplegia will have difficulties sitting, walking, and running, but will usually have little difficulty with skilled movement involving their hands. In very mild form, there may be only spasticity in the ankle and plantarflexion (toe walking) of the foot. Most children with spastic diplegia will not exhibit dysarthria, although some may if the lesions are large enough to affect the corticobulbar system.

Ataxic and dystonic cerebral palsy are due to lesions in the cerebellum, although less is known about anatomical correlates than with the other types of cerebral palsy. Children with ataxic cerebral palsy are often hypotonic at birth and may, therefore, be diagnosed late because slight hypotonia is so common at birth. Later in life, they typically exhibit a wide stance and ataxic gait. Perceptual deficits also may be present, including poor orientation of the body in space. These children often exhibit incoordination of movement, action tremor, and dysmetria.

Athetoid cerebral palsy results from damage to the basal ganglia, and is characterized by disorders of posture and involuntary movement. Like the ataxic syndromes, athetoid cerebral palsy may not be fully apparent for a year or two after birth, with initial hypotonia and gradual onset of involvement of involuntary athetoid and choreic movements. In this form of cerebral palsy, many primitive postural reflexes are retained, especially the tonic neck reflex. Emotional tension and other stimuli may aggravate the involuntary movement. Feeding and walking may be very difficult. Dysarthria and dysphagia are common in children who exhibit the athetoid syndrome in cerebral palsy. Children may display combinations of spasticity and dyskinesia, or dyskinesia and ataxia as well.

ASSOCIATED PROBLEMS

Some limitation in intellectual and cognitive functioning occurs in 30% to 70% of individuals with cerebral palsy. Behavioral problems, perhaps linked with intellectual deficits, are less frequently seen. These include hyperactivity, decreased attention span, or emotional lability. Depression may occur, especially in adolescents coping with body image issues. Various ocular abnormalities, such as refractive errors, visual field defects, and extraocular muscle imbalances, may interfere with learning and movement abilities. Deafness is now rarely associated with cerebral palsy and is mostly seen in the dyskinetic type of cerebral palsy. Seizure disorders may be present in 30% or more. Bowel and bladder control may be impaired. Orthopedic complications occur in response to chronic muscle imbalances and involuntary movement. Scoliosis, hip dislocations, and muscle/tendon contractures are examples that frequently require correction; uncorrected, these can lead to osteoarthritis, seating problems, pressure sores, and additional problems with secondary scoliosis. Dental needs in addition to those normally exhibited by the growing child may also result from chronic involuntary movements (Erenberg, 1984; Lord, 1984; Stempien & Gaebler-Spira, 1996).

SWALLOWING PROBLEMS

Swallowing problems, and therefore saliva management and nutritional problems, are common in children with dysarthria and cerebral palsy. Recent studies have expanded our understanding of these problems. In a study of 35 children with cerebral palsy (mean age of 8 years), 60% were reported by parents to have current feeding problems (Dahl, Thommeseen, Rasmussen, & Selberg, 1996). Children in the youngest age group with severe involvement were most at risk for nutritional problems. Sucking and swallowing problems are reported to be common in the first year of life (Reilly, Skuse, & Poblete, 1996). Reilly and colleagues reported that 90% of children with cerebral palsy had clinically significant oral-motor dysfunction and 80% had been fed nonorally on at least one occasion. Individuals with marginally effective swallowing and oral-motor skills may be particularly at risk when calorie demands increase during periods of growth, such as the teenage years (Gisel, 1994; Gisel, Applegate-Ferrante, Benson, & Bosma, 1995). In fact, nutritionally based growth failure and abnormal resting energy expenditure have been related to inadequate calorie intake in children and adolescents with cerebral palsy (Stalling, Zemel, Davies, Cronk, & Charney, 1996).

Characteristics of swallowing disorders in children with cerebral palsy have been studied radiologically (Kramer, 1988; Rogers, Arvedson, Buck, Smart, & Msall, 1994). Problems may occur during any phase of swallowing. For example, during the oral phase, deficient suckling or premature leakage into the pharynx may occur. Children with cerebral palsy require more time than noninvolved children for collection and organization of the bolus (Casas, Kenny, & McPherson, 1994; Casas, McPherson, & Kenny, 1995). The pharyngeal phase may be delayed or cricopharyngeal sphincter abnormalities may be present. During the esophageal phase, gastroesophageal reflux may occur.

In a study of 56 individuals with cerebral palsy, ranging in age from 5 to 21 years, a number of factors were found to contribute to dysphagia, including abnormal bite reflexes, slowness of oral intake, poor trunk control, inability to feed independently, anticonvulsant medication, coughing with meals, choking, and pneumonia (Waterman, Koltai, Downey, & Cacace, 1992). The importance of clinical examination was stressed by Rogers and colleagues (1994). They found abnormalities only while swallowing specific food textures in the majority of the 90 consecutive individuals they studied. Further, they suggested that aspiration of specific food textures was significantly more common than aspiration of all food textures and that aspiration was silent in 97% of the children.

The interaction between swallowing and respiratory function in children with cerebral palsy has also been examined. The ventilatory preparation phase and the recovery to baseline ventilatory patterns after swallowing was found to be longer for children with cerebral palsy (Casas et al., 1994). The coordination of swallowing and breathing may be difficult. While noninvolved children tend to swallow at or near the peak of inspiration, children with cerebral palsy have supplementary swallows and solid bolus swallows at any point in the ventilatory cycle.

Drooling is a problem frequently associated with poor oral motor control in cerebral palsy. It may be associated with a number of disturbances, including incomplete lip closure during swallowing, low suction pressure, and prolonged delay between the suction phase and propelling stages of swallowing (Lespargot, Langevin, Muller, & Guillemont, 1993) as well as both inefficient and infrequent swallowing (Sochaniwskyj, Koheil, Bablich, Milner, & Kenny, 1986). Intervention for drooling has been approached from the perspectives of behavioral, biofeedback training (Koheil, Sochaniwskyj, Bablich, Kenny, & Milner, 1987), and medication (Blasco & Stansbury, 1996).

Management of swallowing and eating impairment in children with cerebral palsy must take into account both issues related to growing (e.g., weight, height, skinfold thickness) and eating skills (e.g., eating efficiency, oral motor skills, safety) (Gisel & Alphonce, 1995). When problems are severe, intervention may take the form of alternative means of feeding, such as a gastrostomy (McGrath, Splaingard, Alba, Kaufman, & Glicklick, 1992; Meek, 1991). Both positioning (Larnert & Bkberg, 1995) and oral sensorimotor training (Gisel et al., 1995) have been used to improve swallowing and eating function. Excellent sources are available that describe the complex issue of intervention for swallowing disorders in children (e.g., Arvedson & Brodsky, 1993).

NATURAL COURSE

As mentioned previously, although the definition of cerebral palsy contains the term *nonprogressive*, the manifestations of this primarily motor disorder change as the body grows and ages. Periods of rapid growth, such as infancy and adolescence, may bring an exacerbation of symptoms and a regression of functional status until new skills are acquired and a new level of neuromuscular equilibrium is attained. Over time, new complications of spasticity and dystonia may become evident as the orthopedic disorders mentioned earlier occur in response to overuse and postural abnormalities. However, the basic level of intellectual functioning and neurologic dysfunction should remain relatively unchanged.

Virtually all hemiplegic children will walk in time; the functional use of the hemiplegic arm, however, depends largely on the degree of sensory deficit (especially proprioception) present, as well as the motor impairment. Current figures indicate that about 50% of hemiplegic children are employable as adults. Most diplegic children can walk during childhood; however, it is not uncommon to see them begin to use a wheelchair during adolescence because of the increased efficiency of mobility provided. Diplegic children tend to integrate well into the mainstream classroom situations and about one third will later be employed. The outlook for quadriplegia is less optimistic. In mild cases, ambulation and at least some level of independence in self-care are possible; in one quarter of the cases of quadriplegia, total care is needed to sustain life (Eicher & Batshaw, 1993; Lord, 1984).

Question: Aren't the less than optimistic employment figures for individuals with cerebral palsy reflective of a combination of personal and social factors?

Undoubtedly, one would expect that, as schools educate students with cerebral palsy in more inclusive environments with academic standards more similar to those for typical children, they will be increasingly well prepared for employment in the future. However, the acceptance of persons with cerebral palsy into the workforce is also a difficult transition. For example, currently we are attempting to mentor a young man with cerebral palsy who has graduated from college. His speech is understandable, with careful listening, to those who are familiar with him. Although his athetoid movements are very obvious, he has learned to drive and has actually ridden his bike across the state. However, employment has been difficult for him, as human resource offices tend to screen him out of consideration following the application phase before he even gets to the interview phase.

Therapy and Other Management Issues

The family outlook and support system is crucial to successfully habilitating the child or adult with cerebral palsy. Therefore, families should be included early in educational efforts, to alert them to expected developmental crises and achievements, and they should be urged to participate in peer support groups for encouragement and practical advice on the care of the child with disability. Physical therapy, in the form of early intervention programs, is a controversial but common ingredient in the management of cerebral palsy. The child and family are encouraged, via various techniques, to facilitate normal patterns of sensation and movement and to inhibit abnormal reflexes and postures. As these are often applied in groups, opportunities for fostering socialization are present. Early and aggressive orthopedic surgery is called for to prevent childhood hip dislocation with its resultant problems, and to correct fixed deformities, aid in restoring muscle balance, improve postural stability, and maximize function (Bleck, 1984; DeLuca, 1996). Training in functional activities, as well as environmental adaptation to achieve the optimal level of independence in self-care activities, is mandatory to allow development of the child's sense of mastery and achievement. In the area of adaptive equipment, motorized mobility devices have been prescribed for increasingly younger children, allowing access to the community and enhancing the child's ability to explore the environment.

Specific therapies to control spasticity and involuntary movement have been moderately successful. Various splints and casts are used to control tone, prevent contracture, and improve function. Neuromuscular biofeedback has had some limited success in head control and the treatment of certain gait abnormalities. A decade of experience with selective dorsal rhizotomy indicates that the best results in spasticity control and ambulation occur in young children with spastic diplegia and good intelligence. Although oral medications (diazepam, dantrolene, and baclofen) are used to treat spasticity, none have been ideal. All cause drowsiness in sufficient doses to affect muscle tone. The use of intrathecal baclofen pumps for spasticity is still being investigated in children. Injections of phenol or botulinum toxin A may be helpful on a relatively temporary basis (Dabney, Lyston, & Miller, 1997; DeLuca, 1996; Stempien & Gaebler-Spira, 1996). Most of the anticonvulsants (especially diphenytoin and phenobarbital; carbamazepine, valproic acid, and primidone to a lesser degree) can cause central nervous system effects such as drowsiness and ataxia; learning potential may be adversely affected. New anticonvulsants (gabapentin, lamotrigine, vigabatrin, and topiramate) are still being investigated in children and are used mostly for resistant forms of epilepsy (American Academy of Pediatrics Committee on Drugs, 1995; Bourgeois, 1996).

Speech Characteristics

Many early studies of dysarthria focused on speakers with cerebral palsy (Achilles, 1955; Blumberg, 1955; Byrne, 1959; Clement & Twitchell, 1959; Hardy, 1961, 1964, 1967; Hixon & Hardy, 1964; Irwin, 1955; Rutherford, 1944; Wolfe, 1950). These studies formed the foundation on which later studies of the physiologic and perceptual aspects of dysarthric speech are based. Although the reported incidence of speech disorders associated with cerebral palsy varies, a review shows that speech disorders are a common sequela of this neurologic disorder. Reports of the frequency of dysarthria in cerebral palsy range from a low of 31% (Wolfe, 1950) to as high as 88% (Achilles, 1955).

No pattern of speech is typical of all individuals with cerebral palsy. The pattern and severity of dysarthria are dependent upon the underlying pathophysiology. Spastic cerebral palsy, by far the most frequent type, results in abnormalities of voluntary movement including spasticity, weakness, limitation of range, and slowness of movement. The speech patterns associated with spastic cerebral palsy are characterized by low pitch, hypernasality, pitch breaks, breathy voice, and excess and equal stress (Workinger & Kent, 1991). Athetosis occurs in approximately 5% of individuals with cerebral palsy and results in a pattern of speech different from that of spastic cerebral palsy. Speech in athetoid cerebral palsy is characterized by irregular articulatory breakdowns, inappropriate silences, prolonged intervals and speech sounds, excessive loudness variation, and voice stoppage. There also appear to be differences between the two groups in the severity and natural course of the dysarthria. Workinger and Kent (1991) suggested that children with spastic cerebral palsy may develop speech relatively early but that, as they grow, respiratory support for speech becomes more impaired, perhaps because of abnormalities in posture and positioning. Consequently, the speech performance of persons with spastic cerebral palsy *may* deteriorate as they progress toward adulthood. Children with athetosis, on the other hand, may be late to speak, but their speech improves as they grow and gain control.

Question: What are the clinical implications of the differing natural courses of speakers with dysarthria due to spastic and athetoid cerebral palsy?

This information should inform these speakers, their parents, and their clinicians about future expectations for these children's communication skills. At times, children and their parents will resist the use of augmen-

(continues)

tative communication systems in the hope that, as the children grow into teenagers and adults, their natural speech will continue to improve. Especially for those children with spastic cerebral palsy, these hopes must be tempered with practical considerations. It is our observation that for children with athetoid cerebral palsy, speech improvements that do occur during the late elementary, teenage, and young adults years are very gradual. Occasionally, those individuals who are understandable by those who are familiar with them, may become somewhat more intelligible to strangers. Also, if children with spastic cerebral palsy, as well as their parents, teachers, and clinicians, realize that their speech may deteriorate as they grow, all involved will hopefully be less inclined to blame reductions in speech performance on other potential causes, such as progression of symptoms, laziness, depression, and so on.

IMPAIRMENT OF SPEECH COMPONENTS

Respiratory Function

In early studies that investigated speech characteristics in cerebral palsy, individuals with athetosis were reported to have poorer respiration control than do individuals with spasticity (Achilles, 1955; Blumberg, 1955). In a series of studies that examined the respiratory function of speakers with cerebral palsy, Hardy (1964) reported that the breathing rates of children with spastic cerebral palsy demonstrated significantly reduced respiratory reserve and, therefore, reduced vital capacities. He also reported that the respiratory patterns of children with cerebral palsy were less flexible than those of normal children. This reduction in flexibility may result from a number of different factors, including muscular weakness and excessive involuntary oppositions of antagonistic muscles in addition to posture. Hardy (1983) expanded these observations by writing that the group with spasticity demonstrated reduced ability to expire below their resting respiratory levels due to the involvement of their abdominal muscles.

A reduction in vital capacity is not necessarily associated with inadequate respiratory support for speech. Hardy (1961) indicated that the absolute volume of air capacity does not determine whether or not speakers with cerebral palsy have severe dysarthria. Rather, he observed that children with cerebral palsy utilized more air volume per syllable than other speakers with dysarthria. Together with a reduced vital capacity, the inefficient valving of the breath stream results in respiratory support for speech that is often inadequate. For example, 16 of 41 children were found to have problems with velopharyngeal closure. In addition to velopharyngeal dysfunction, laryngeal and oral articulation dysfunction may contribute to insufficient intraoral air pressure.

Laryngeal Function

A number of early studies reported laryngeal dysfunction in speakers with cerebral palsy including monotonous pitch level (Rutherford, 1944); low pitch with a weak intensity, and a "throaty" voice quality (Clement & Twitchell, 1959); and whispered, hoarse phonation (Berry & Eisenson, 1956). Others reported excessive laryngeal adduction (Ingram & Barn, 1961). Adductor spasm of laryngeal muscles in cerebral palsy may prevent the initiation of voicing or interrupt phonation during speech (McDonald & Chance, 1964). Although informal observations of phonatory performance of speakers with cerebral palsy have been reported, little instrumental research has been completed in this area.

Velopharyngeal Function

Although velopharyngeal dysfunction in many speakers with cerebral palsy has been reported clinically, careful study of this speech component in this population has been quite limited. Speakers with athetosis exhibit velopharyngeal function described as inconsistent and uncoordinated when studied using cinefluorography (Hardy, 1961). Studies of the vowel positions of children with cerebral palsy have been reported (Netsell, 1969). Results indicate a larger oral opening without palatal lifts and smaller oral openings when the palatal lift was in place. It was hypothesized that the speakers attempt to radiate more sound orally in the presence of velopharyngeal incompetence. Kent and Netsell (1978) studied articulatory abnormality in five subjects with athetoid cerebral palsy and concluded that all five demonstrated some difficulty in achieving velopharyngeal closure, as they exhibited instability of velar position.

Oral Articulation

Of all the speech components, oral articulation has received the most systematic study. The articulatory performance of speakers with spastic cerebral palsy, speakers with athetoid cerebral palsy, and speakers with tension athetosis has been studied (Irwin, 1955). No strong statistical differences between the three subgroups were found. However, a significant increase in the mastery of speech sounds was observed with increasing age. These early studies also reported that speech elements involving the movement of the tongue tip were the most frequently misarticulated in children with cerebral palsy and that these children misarticulated voiceless sounds more frequently than the voiced cognates (Byrne, 1959; Irwin, 1955). This may occur as a function of the increased spasticity in the larynx. The relationship among speech defectiveness, rates of repetition of consonant–vowel syllables, and rates of repetitive nonspeech movements has also been reported (Hixon & Hardy, 1964). Results indicated that restrictions of mobility in the posterior portion of the tongue may exert important influences on the production of the speech of individuals with spastic or athetoid cerebral palsy.

The articulatory performance of adults with cerebral palsy has also been studied using cinefluorography (Kent & Netsell, 1978). Findings include large ranges of jaw movements, inappropriate tongue positioning, and abnormalities in the timing and range of velopharyngeal movements. In addition, articulatory transition times were prolonged. Adults with spastic cerebral palsy were found to differ from speakers with athetoid cerebral palsy in articulatory error pattern (Platt, Andrews, & Howie, 1980; Platt, Andrews, Young, & Quinn, 1980). In addition, Platt and colleagues reported that both groups of speakers with cerebral palsy demonstrated imprecision of fricative and affricate manner of articulation, and inability to achieve the extreme positions in the articulatory space. Their subjects demonstrated a predominance of within-manner errors. Errors that cross manner of articulation boundaries were uncommon. More errors occurred in word-final as compared to word-initial positions.

OVERALL ADEQUACY

The overall performance of subgroups of speakers with cerebral palsy has also been investigated. Platt and colleagues (Platt, Andrews, & Howie, 1980; Platt, Andrews, Young, & Quinn, 1980) reported that the speech of individuals with spastic cerebral palsy was more intelligible and less articulatorily impaired than that of speakers with athetoid cerebral palsy.

Several attempts have been made to relate selected speech characteristics of overall speech intelligibility. Andrews, Platt, and Young (1977) found that specific features contribute to the intelligibility problem of adults with athetoid and spastic dysarthria, including reduced vowel target space, poor anterior lingual place accuracy for consonants, and reduced articulatory precision of fricative and affricate consonants. Subsequently, these authors suggested that both groups of speakers with cerebral palsy exhibited word-final consonant errors, devoicing of voiced consonants, and extensive within-manner errors. Ansel and Kent (1992) sought to identify the specific acoustic features that would predict speech intelligibility in groups of adult male speakers with cerebral palsy. These researchers concluded that the acoustic factors of vowel duration and F_1 and F_2 formant location and noise duration were major predictors of speech intelligibility scores. Thus, the physiological parameters of temporal control and tongue position appear to influence speech intelligibility. Obviously, the relationship between specific speech parameters and speech intelligibility is very complex. However, because improvement in speech intelligibility is a central focus of nearly all dysarthria intervention programs, further research in this area would be extremely beneficial.

LEVELS OF FUNCTIONAL LIMITATIONS IN CEREBRAL PALSY

The staging of speech intervention based on level of functional limitation has been described in populations with degenerative disease (Yorkston, Miller, & Strand, 1995). Other staging systems for recovering populations will be described in Chapter 3 of this text. In the area of developmental motor speech disorders, creating a staging system for functional limitation is difficult and perhaps inappropriate because it implies a progression from one stage or step to another. Instead of progressive staging, categorizing children into groupings based on level of function may be useful in conceptualizing overall intervention goals. The following groups have been described more completely by Beukelman and Mirenda (1998).

Group 1 contains individuals who are so severely impaired that they need augmentative communication to support communication of their wants and need, interaction, and language development. In this case, the speech work focuses on the development of the physiologic building blocks of speech. Because this preparatory work may not lead to immediate changes in functional use of natural speech, augmentative communication intervention is critical for individuals in this group.

Group 2 is composed of individuals who need augmentative communication for interaction and to support language learning. However, these children or adults are able to vocalize and speak well enough to meet basic needs.

Group 3 is composed of individuals who speak well enough to handle much of their basic communication of wants or needs and a fair amount of their interaction. These children need backup for communication breakdown resolution and often need augmentative communication to support their language learning as they are required to learn new words and to combine words into grammatical utterances.

Group 4 comprises individuals who tend to communicate everything verbally, despite obvious dysarthria. They may have augmentative communication systems to back up their writing, as well as some breakdown resolution. In this group a physiologic approach to improving speech production is often beneficial. Readers are referred to Chapters 7 through 12 for detailed discussions of other topics.

Question: In addition to dysarthria associated with cerebral palsy, are there other congential causes of dysarthria?

Yes. Let us describe two—*Moebius syndrome*, a rare disorder associated with facial paralysis, and *Down syndrome*, a much more common disorder in which dysarthria is complicated by a combination of intellectual deficits and language delays.

Moebius syndrome is a rare congenital bilateral paralysis affecting Cranial Nerves VI and VII (facial and abducent nerves). A number of additional characteristics are also described in some cases, including involvement of other cranial nerves, musculoskeletal deformities, reduced muscle mass in the extremities, ocular ptosis, and ear deformities (Merz & Wojtowicz, 1967). Occurrence of the disorder is sporadic, with the male-to-female ratio being equal (Gorlin, Pindborg, & Cohen, 1976). The pathology of the disorder is unclear. Speculations are available, including theories suggesting either nuclear or nerve agenesis or underlying muscular deficits (Meyerson & Foushee, 1978). A variety of surgical intervention strategies have been reported for Moebius syndrome. These include repair of maxillary or mandibular deformities, correction of limb anomalies, and muscle/tendon transplants to correct focial weakness (Edgerton, Tuerck, & Fisher, 1975; Federman & Stoopack, 1975).

Characteristic speech and hearing problems in children with Moebius syndrome have been described (Kahane, 1979). Most of these children exhibit flaccid dysarthria (Meyerson & Foushee, 1978). Characteristics include limited strength, range, and speed of movement of the articulators, and inaccurate consonant production. The dysarthria ranges in severity from mild distortion of phonemes requiring bilabial closure or lingual elevation to unintelligible speech. Small mouth opening and micrognathia (unusual smallness of the jaw) contribute to a "muffled" quality in some of the subjects. Over half of the children in Meyerson and Foushee's study also reported feeding problems. Other problems occurring in this population were cleft palate, hearing loss, mental retardation, and delayed language development.

The compensatory efforts of children with Moebious syndrome are interesting (DeFeo & Schaefer, 1983). For example, they may approximate their tongue tip and upper lip to produce the /p/ and /b/ sounds. In their case report, DeFeo and Schaefer reported that listeners sometimes comprehended the child's compensated sounds more accurately when they did not view the speaker. In the example of /p/, the tongue tip move-

(continues)

ment pattern may influence the listener to perceive a /t/ sound instead of a compensatory /p/ sound.

Down syndrome is a genetic condition causing some degree of cognitive impairment and other developmental delays. Common physical characteristics include epicanthal folds over the eyes, flattened bridge of the nose, a single palmar crease, and decreased muscle tone. It is the decreased muscle tone or hypotonicity that may cause dysarthria and feeding problems in infants. Significant hearing impairments occur in many children with Down syndrome (Dahle & McCollister, 1988; Marcel & Cohen, 1992). Down syndrome occurs in all races, with an overall incidence of approximately 1 in 800 births. Most cases are associated with extra chromosomal material from the mother causing a trisomy 21, with unbalanced translocation of chromosome 21. Excellent general sources of information are available in published form (Cooley & Graham, 1991; Rogers & Coleman, 1992) or on the Internet, including the following:

- Cohen, W. I. *Health Care Guidelines for Individuals with Down Syndrome* (July 7, 1997).
  http://www.denison.edu/dsq/health96.html

- *Questions About Down's Syndrome* (July 7, 1997).
  http://www.nas.com/downsyn/faq1.html

- Trumble, S. *How to Treat People with Down Syndrome* (July 7, 1997).
  http://www.nas.com/downsyn/trumble.html

Communication disorders associated with Down syndrome have been studied extensively, including language development (R. S. Chapman, Schwartz, & Bird, 1991; Pruess, Vadasy, & Fewell, 1987), phonologic development (Kumin, Councill, & Goodman, 1994; Van Borsel, 1996), oral praxis (Elliott, Weeks, & Gray, 1990), fluency (Devenny, Silverman, Bigley, & Wall, 1990), and voice quality (Montague & Hollien, 1973). There is consensus that children and adolescents with Down syndrome frequently exhibit deficits in expressive language development, which would be expected based on cognitive delay in nonverbal domains or comprehension skills (R. S. Chapman et al., 1991). Results of these research studies are confirmed by parent reports that suggest poor communication skills relative to daily living and socialization skills (Dykens, Hodapp, & Evans, 1994). Parents also report that reduction in intelligibility is a widespread

(continues)

problem influenced by a variety of factors, including familiarity with the listeners, communication setting, and message (single words vs. sentences) (Kumin, 1994). Although treatment studies specifically focusing on dysarthria in Down syndrome are not available, reports of augmentative communication techniques supplementing natural speech are promising (Hunt, 1991; Iacono & Duncum, 1995; Kouri, 1988).

DEVELOPMENTAL APRAXIA OF SPEECH

Nature of the Disorder

Developmental apraxia of speech (DAS) or developmental verbal apraxia is the term used by many speech–language pathologists to describe those children who exhibit severe articulatory output problems due to difficulty formulating and executing motor plans for speech. Most definitions of developmental apraxia of speech focus on the difficulty or inability to carry out purposeful voluntary movements for speech, in the absence of paralysis or weakness of the speech musculature (Chappell, 1973; Crary, 1984; Edwards, 1973; Hayden, 1994; Haynes, 1985; Morley, 1965; Robin, 1992; Rosenbek & Wertz, 1972; Yoss & Darley, 1974). Children with developmental apraxia will have difficulty with the complex motor activity involved in speech production because they have difficulty with sequential ordering of *movements* in the correct spatial and temporal relationship to each other.

Question: I am confused by some of the terminology. What is the difference between developmental apraxia of speech *and* developmental verbal apraxia? *Also, why do some people use the term* apraxia *and others use* dyspraxia? *Which is right?*

The term verbal apraxia came into use in the early 1980s by researchers who posited that children with developmental apraxia of speech experience language deficits as well as articulatory problems (Aram & Horwitz, 1983; Ekelman & Aram, 1983). Because these children exhibit both language and motor speech problems, the nature of the disorder is not solely motoric. Today, the terms are often used interchangeably by clinicians. Apraxia and dyspraxia are also used interchangeably. The prefix *a*, however, means not or without, whereas the prefix *dys* means abnormal or difficult. Therefore, it is probably more precise to use the word dyspraxia

(continues)

in that most children have some ability to plan movement for speech. In this chapter we use the term developmental apraxia of speech because it is the term most commonly used by practicing speech–language pathologists.

Aram and colleagues (Aram & Nation, 1982; Ekelman & Aram, 1983) provided evidence that not only did children with developmental apraxia exhibit articulatory error, but they also exhibited difficulty with the selection and sequencing of lexical and syntactic units during the production of speech. Their work led to the suggestion that the disorder encompasses both language and articulatory deficits. There is also evidence to suggest that some children with developmental apraxia have auditory perceptual problems as well (Jaffe, 1980). The linguistic components of developmental apraxia have been described within the context of development (Crary, 1984, 1993). Crary suggested that, for some children who exhibit a particular set of articulatory speech characteristics, the term developmental apraxia of speech might be used to represent the developmental counterpart of the acquired apraxia seen in adults. Because children are still acquiring language, however, the speech disorder "has a more widespread linguistic effect" (p. 33).

It is logical to assume that deficits in motor planning could affect acquisition of language. It is helpful to consider a developmental model that takes into account the interactive influences of cognitive, linguistic, and motor skill acquisition (R. S. Chapman et al., 1992; Strand, 1992). This model suggests that any problem with motor planning and programming during the early stages of language and speech acquisition will necessarily affect the development of phonology and other language processes. That is, these children will usually exhibit delays and deviancies in articulation, phonology, and expressive language skills. Consequently, it is sometimes difficult to determine how much of a severe delay or deviancy in articulation skill is due to motor planning problems versus delays or deviancy in phonological processing. Procedures for determining whether motor planning problems are contributing to delays or deviancy in speech development will be discussed in detail in Chapter 5.

Question: What is praxis? Why isn't the presence of apraxia of speech easier to identify in children?

Praxis is the term used to indicate difficulty with the conception and planning of a volitional, versus reflexive, motor act. Interestingly, much controversy exists as to whether there really is a deficit in processing that

(continues)

should be called "developmental apraxia." Further, even those who posit that praxis exists during movement for speech do not have a clear understanding of the nature of the disorder. It is difficult to determine praxis in speech motor control because speech is a complicated, fine motor activity that is continuously interactive with cognitive and linguistic processing. There is much that is not understood about how spoken language is produced. For example, the relationship between the linguistic processes (retrieving a word and mapping the phonology of the word) and generating the sequences of movements to produce the word is still unclear. While the construct of motor planning is well accepted, how and when movement parameters are planned or programmed is still unclear. In other words, we do not understand the process by which speakers "decide" how far, how fast, or in what direction to move the muscles of speech production.

"Subtle" or "soft" signs may (but not always) appear as an associated characteristic of developmental apraxia. A wide pattern of neurological signs has been reported across subjects (Crary, 1984; Yoss & Darley, 1974). These include fine and gross motor incoordination, difficulties with gait, and problems with alternating and repetitive movements. Studies fail, however, to find a consistent neurological correlate that would localize the neuroanatomical site of lesion in developmental apraxia. It is improbable that a biochemical or neurotransmitter deficit is responsible for developmental apraxia of speech. A particular focal deficit in anatomical, physiological, or biochemical function has yet to be determined.

There is no evidence to suggest that reductions in tactile sensation are associated with DAS. However, one type of sensory deficit often associated with DAS is decreased proprioception. Proprioception is the perception (at unconscious levels) of the movements and positions of structures of the body, independent of vision. Proprioception occurs partly due to the role of proprioceptive receptors (i.e., muscle spindles, golgi tendon organs) in combination with the cerebellum and vestibular system. The difficulty with achieving specific spatial targets is sometimes thought to be due to decreased proprioception. Although this seems intuitive, we do not have diagnostic procedures that allow confirmation of this.

Question: Why is so much attention paid to this linguistic versus motor controversy?

Because the "level" of deficit determines how we plan treatment. For example, if the speech disorder we call developmental apraxia of speech is

(continues)

linguistically based, we would use a treatment approach based on rules of language, primarily phonological rules. If, on the other hand, one believes that the nature of the disorder has to do with a disorder of planning and executing sequential movements, one would focus treatment on movements, specifically movements during speech. This type of treatment would emphasize principles important to motor learning, such as frequent and repetitive practice, feedback, and varying rate. As speech–language pathologists, we need to be sensitive to the nature of the deficit so that we may make reasonable decisions as to the relative contribution of linguistic versus motor deficits to the child's overall speech performance. Most important, paying attention to the possible motor contributions helps to plan a treatment approach that takes this level of deficit into account. Details of planning speech intervention can be found in Chapter 13.

Characteristics of Developmental Apraxia of Speech

One of the primary explanations for the persistence of controversy regarding developmental apraxia is that researchers are not consistent in describing the articulatory errors or behavioral characteristics necessary for diagnosis. In their cogent review of the literature, Shriberg, Aram, and Kwiatkowski (1997a, 1997b, 1997c) also point out the lack of a diagnostic marker for developmental apraxia of speech. Some even argue against use of the term developmental apraxia of speech because no specific set of characteristic symptoms has been identified (Guyette & Diedrich, 1981). Therefore, it is necessary to review those specific articulatory and behavioral characteristics most frequently associated with motor planning problems (or developmental apraxia). Although the literature presents sometimes conflicting descriptions of these characteristics, a few categories are frequently noted, including specific articulatory characteristics, particular movement characteristics, prosodic characteristics, and the influence of context on performance. Those characteristics most frequently cited as characteristic of DAS are listed in Table 2.2. Note that not all children with developmental apraxia will exhibit all these characteristics. On the other hand, many children who exhibit little or no difficulty with motor planning will exhibit some of these characteristics. In some cases, clinical diagnosis of DAS is relatively straightforward. However, because of the complex interaction between linguistic and motor development, diagnosis, at other times, can be controversial. Currently, no single feature or combination of features definitely confirms the diagnosis of developmental apraxia.

Table 2.2
Speech and Behavioral Characteristics
Frequently Associated with Developmental Apraxia of Speech

Articulatory Characteristics

Multiple Speech Sound Errors
Omissions—most common
Substitutions
Distortions
Additions
Greater difficulty with phonetically more complex sounds such as fricatives and affricates

Difficulties with Sound Sequencing
Metathetic errors
Difficulty with a particular sequence of sounds, even when the individual sounds are correct in isolation or CV combinations (Sounds produced correctly in some sequences will be in error in other sequences of sounds)
Consonant clusters more difficult to produce than singletons
Transposition of sounds and syllables

Movement Characteristics

Difficulty imitating articulatory configurations, especially for initial sounds
Difficulty making movement transitions in and out of spatial targets
Difficulty maintaining articulatory configurations
Frequent groping
Trial-and-error movement behavior

Disturbances in Prosody

Slower rate
Inappropriate or longer pauses
Reduced stress variation
Errors in syllabic stress

Contextual Changes in Articulatory Proficiency

Errors increase with increasing length of word or utterance
Repetition elicits better articulatory performance than spontaneous production
Sounds are more easily produced in single-word production than in conversation
Errors vary with the phonetic complexity of the utterance
Errors are inconsistently produced

Other Factors

Receptive language performance superior to expressive language performance
Presence of oral apraxia

ARTICULATORY CHARACTERISTICS

Children with developmental apraxia exhibit numerous articulatory errors. In severe cases, omissions are the most common error type. It is probable that the child attempts to compensate by reducing the number of phonemes attempted, thereby reducing demands to "create" a complex program of movement sequences. Substitutions are also common, and usually involve substituting an easier phoneme for a more phonetically complex one. Distortions, including vowel distortions, are common. Difficulty achieving specific spatial targets may result in deviancies in vocal tract shape and length as the child works to achieve a specific articulatory configuration. Additions are also present, often as an additional schwa. This may be a compensatory effort to achieve particular spatial configurations, thus reducing the need for complex transitions from movement to movement.

Question: What do you mean by compensation? How do you decide which behaviors are compensatory and which are a primary part of the disorder?

The primary problem may be thought of as the deficit. In the case of developmental apraxia of speech, the deficit is in motor planning. A direct consequence of the primary deficit is the inability to achieve particular spatial and temporal movement targets. The compensation is a response to a primary deficit. This response may not be conscious. Although it is often difficult to disambiguate the primary problem from the compensations, it is not a trivial issue when it comes to choosing treatment goals, such as for a child who has difficulty achieving articulatory configurations due to weakness (as in some types of dysarthria) or due to a motor planning deficit (as in developmental apraxia). In either case, the child may compensate by slowing his or her rate of speech. Choosing to increase speaking rate as a treatment target may not be appropriate in either case, because it is not the cause of the primary problem, but a response to it. See Chapter 13 for more detail regarding specific treatment approaches for developmental apraxia.

Difficulty with sound production in developmental apraxia may be made worse or better depending on the context in which the sounds are produced. If the target sound is surrounded by difficult sounds, then the movement transitions required to produce that sequence will be difficult. Therefore, difficulties with sound sequencing are often seen in children with developmental apraxia. Sometimes the difficulty is seen consistently for a particular sequence of sounds.

At other times, sounds produced correctly in some sequences will be in error in other sequences. In addition, children with developmental apraxia may exhibit sequencing errors that are seen in all children (e.g., common metathetic errors such as "cast" for "cats"). For some children, these sequencing errors may be due to higher level planning or phoneme selection errors. For others, they may be due to attempts at simplification because motor demands are too difficult.

MOVEMENT CHARACTERISTICS

As noted in the previous section, children with developmental apraxia have difficulties with producing individual sounds and especially sequences of sounds. This difficulty with producing sounds is due to difficulty with movement more than phonology. These children have difficulty imitating articulatory configurations and transitions into and out of spatial targets for phonetic strings, even in the absence of structural or functional abnormalities of the tongue, lips, jaw, or velum. They have particular difficulty achieving articulatory configurations for initial sounds. Observations of their repeated attempts to do so lead to the inference that they are attempting the movement for specific sounds, but cannot achieve or stay at the spatial target. Certainly, children with developmental apraxia are frequently observed to have difficulty achieving and maintaining articulatory configurations. In severe cases, children exhibit frequent groping for articulatory configurations and/or trial-and-error behavior.

DISTURBANCES IN PROSODY

Prosody involves rhythm and intonation patterns, speech rate or timing, and syllabic stress patterns. Clinicians observe a variety of prosodic differences in the speech of children with developmental apraxia, especially slower rate, inappropriate or lengthy pauses, and reduced stress variation. These clinical observations have been confirmed in a number of research reports (Rosenbek & Wertz, 1972; Yoss & Darley, 1974). In fact, recent reports have suggested that inappropriate stress patterning may differentiate children with suspected DAS from those with speech delay (Shriberg et al., 1997a). Thus, a deficit in phrasal stress may be a diagnostic marker for at least one subtype of DAS (Shriberg et al., 1997b).

CONTEXTUAL CHANGES IN ARTICULATORY PROFICIENCY

One of the characteristics most commonly mentioned as differentiating developmental apraxia from other causes of articulatory disorder is the observation that errors are more frequent with increasing phonetic complexity and increasing length of the word or utterance. If the word contains phonemes such as sibilants, affricates, or blends, articulatory errors will increase. Increasing the length of the utterance will also have a significant effect on articulatory accuracy. For example, if a child is asked to say "Mom," he or she may do so quite easily. If then asked to say, "Hi Mom," the child may not be able to produce the movement pattern for lip closure that he or she just did in the isolated word.

Repetition elicits better articulatory performance than spontaneous production of utterances, especially if the child is attending to the clinician's face. This is true especially for novel movement patterns. Such novel utterances are new and therefore have not been practiced. Temporal relationships are also important. The more time between the clinician's model of the utterance and the child's repetition, the more difficulty the child with developmental apraxia will have in producing the movement pattern for the sound sequence.

Error inconsistency is another frequently observed attribute in DAS. Much of this inconsistency in sound production can be attributed to context (i.e., the longer, more phonetically complex utterances will elicit errors on sounds that are produced quite easily in shorter, less complex utterances). Even within similar contexts, however, it is common for children with developmental apraxia to be inconsistent in the accuracy with which they produce sequences of movement for utterances.

Question: In your discussion of cerebral palsy, you suggest that children could be placed into one of four groups based on severity of functional limitations and their dependence on augmentative communication approaches. Do children with developmental apraxia fall into similar groups?

Yes, the general framework is similiar. Some children with DAS have such severe functional limitations that all communication must depend on augmentative approaches. For others, natural speech is useful for some or nearly all of their communication needs. Because children with developmental apraxia usually walk without difficulty and are able to produce gestures with their hands, the types of augmentative communication approaches may differ from those used for individuals with cerebral palsy. The relationship between DAS and augmentative communication has been described by Culp (1989) and Mirenda and Mathy-Laikko (1989).

REFERENCES

Achilles, R. (1955). Communication anomalies of individuals with cerebral palsy: I. Analysis of communication processes in 151 cases of cerebral palsy. *Cerebral Palsy Review, 16,* 15–24.

American Academy of Pediatrics Committee on Drugs. (1995). Behavioral and cognitive effects of anticonvulsant therapy. *Pediatrics, 96*(3 Pt. 1), 538–540.

Andrews, G., Platt, L. J., & Young, M. (1977). Factors affecting intelligibility of cerebral palsied speech to the average listener. *Folia Phoniatrica, 29*, 292–301.

Ansel, B. M., & Kent, R. D. (1992). Ascoustic–phonetic contrasts and intelligibility in dysarthria associated with mixed cerebral palsy. *Journal of Speech and Hearing Research, 35*, 296–308.

Aram, D. M., & Horwitz, S. J. (1983). Sequential and non-speech praxic abilities in developmental verbal apraxia. *Developmental Medicine and Child Neurology, 25*, 197–206.

Aram, D. M., & Nation, J. E. (1982). *Child language disorders*. St. Louis: Mosby.

Arvedson, J. C., & Brodsky, L. (1993). *Pediatric swallowing and feeding*. San Diego: Singular Press.

Berry, M., & Eisenson, J. (1956). *Speech disorders*. New York: Appleton-Century-Crofts.

Beukelman, D. R., & Mirenda, P. (1998). *Augmentative and alternative communication: Management of severe communication disorders in children and adults* (2nd ed.). Baltimore: Brookes.

Blasco, P. A., & Stansbury, J. C. (1996). Glycopyrrolate treatment of chronic drooling. *Archives of Pediatrics and Adolescent Medicine, 150*, 932–935.

Bleck, E. E. (1984). Where have all the CP children gone? The need of adults. *Developmental Medicine and Child Neurology, 26*, 674–676.

Blumberg, M. (1955). Respiration and speech in the cerebral palsied child. *American Journal of Disabled Children, 89*, 48–53.

Bourgeois, B. F. D. (1996). New antiepileptic drugs. *Current Opinion in Pediatrics, 8*, 543–548.

Byrne, M. (1959). Speech and language development of athetoid and spastic children. *Journal of Speech and Hearing Disorders, 24*, 231–240.

Casas, M. J., Kenny, D. J., & McPherson, K. A. (1994). Swallowing/ventilation interactions during oral swallow in normal children and children with cerebral palsy. *Dysphagia, 9*(1), 40–46.

Casas, M. J., McPherson, K. A., & Kenny, D. J. (1995). Durational aspects of oral swallow in neurologically normal children and children with cerebral palsy: An ultrasound investigation. *Dysphagia, 10*(3), 155–159.

Chapman, R. S., Crais, E., Solomon, D., Strand, E., & Nigri, N. (1992). Child talk: Assumptions of a developmental process model for early language learning. In R. Chapman (Ed.), *Processes in Language Acquisition and Disorders* (pp. 3–19). St. Louis: Mosby Yearbook.

Chapman, R. S., Schwartz, S. E., & Bird, E. K. (1991). Language skills of children and adolescents with Down syndrome: I. Comprehension. *Journal of Speech and Hearing Research, 34*(5), 1106–1120.

Chapman, S. B., Culhane, K. A., Levin, H. S., Harward, H., Mendelsohn, D., Ewing-Cobbs, L., & Fletcher, J. M. (1992). Narrative discourse after closed head injury in children and adolescents. *Brain and Language, 43*(2), 42–65.

Chappell, G. E. (1973). Childhood verbal apraxia and its treatment. *Journal of Speech and Hearing Disorders, 38*, 362–368.

Clement, M., & Twitchell, T. (1959). Dysarthria in cerebral palsy. *Journal of Speech and Hearing Disorders, 4*, 118–122.

Cooley, W. C., & Graham, J. M. (1991). Down syndrome: An update and review for the primary pediatrician. *Clinical Pediatrics, 30*(4), 233–253.

Crary, M. (1984). Phonological characteristics of developmental verbal apraxia. *Seminars in Speech and Language, 5*, 71–83.

Crary, M. A. (1993). *Developmental motor speech disorders*. San Diego: Singular.

Culp, D. M. (1989). Developmental apraxia and augmentative or alternative communication: A case example. *Augmentative and Alternative Communication, 5*(1), 27–34.

Dabney, K. W., Lyston, G. E., & Miller, F. (1997). Cerebral palsy. *Current Opinion in Pediatrics, 9*, 81–88.

Dahl, M., Thommeseen, M., Rasmussen, M., & Selberg, T. (1996). Feeding and nutritional characteristics in children with moderate or severe cerebral palsy. *Acta Paediatrica, 85*(6), 697–701.

Dahle, A. J., & McCollister, F. P. (1988). Hearing and otologic disorders in children with Down syndrome. *Journal of Mental Deficiency Research, 32*, 333–336.

DeFeo, A. B., & Schaefer, C. M. (1983). Bilateral facial paralysis in a preschool child: Oral-facial and articulatory characteristics: A case study. In W. Berry (Ed.), *Clinical dysarthria* (pp. 165–190). Austin, TX: PRO-ED.

DeLuca, P. A. (1996). The musculoskeletal management of children with cerebral palsy. *Pediatric Clinics of North America, 43*(5), 1135–1149.

Denhoff, E. (1976). Medical aspects. In W. M. Cruickshank (Ed.), *Cerebral palsy: A developmental disability* (pp. 29–71). Syracuse, NY: Syracuse University Press.

Devenny, D. A., Silverman, W., Bigley, H., & Wall, M. J. (1990). Specific motor abilities associated with speech fluency. *Journal of Mental Deficiency Research, 34*, 437–443.

Dykens, E. M., Hodapp, R. M., & Evans, D. M. (1994). Profiles and development of adaptive behavior in childen with Down syndrome. *American Journal of Mental Retardation, 98*, 580–587.

Edgerton, M. T., Tuerck, D. B., & Fisher, J. C. (1975). Surgical treatment of Moebius syndrome by platysma and temporalis muscle transfers. *Plastic and Reconstructive Surgery, 77*, 305–311.

Edwards, M. (1973). Developmental verbal dyspraxia. *British Journal of Disorders of Communication, 8*, 64–70.

Eicher, P. S., & Batshaw, M. L. (1993). Cerebral palsy. *Pediatric Clinics of North America, 40*(3), 537–551.

Ekelman, B. L., & Aram, D. M. (1983). Syntactic findings in developmental verbal apraxia. *Journal of Communication Disorders, 16*, 237–250.

Elliott, D., Weeks, D. J., & Gray, S. (1990). Manual and oral praxis in adults with Down's syndrome. *Neuropsychologia, 28*, 1307–1315.

Erenberg, G. (1984). Cerebral palsy. *Postgraduate Medicine, 75*, 87–93.

Evans, P. M., Evans, S. J., & Alberman, E. (1990). Cerebral palsy: Why we must plan for survival. *Archives of Disease in Childhood, 65*, 1329–1333.

Federman, R., & Stoopack, J. C. (1975). Moebius syndrome. *Journal of Oral Surgery, 33*, 676–678.

Gisel, E. G. (1994). Oral-motor skills following sensorimotor intervention in the moderately eating-impaired child with cerebral palsy. *Dysphagia, 9*, 180–192.

Gisel, E. G., & Alphonce, E. (1995). Classification of eating impairments based on eating efficiency in children with cerebral palsy. *Dysphagia, 10*, 268–274.

Gisel, E. G., Applegate-Ferrante, T., Benson, J. E., & Bosma, J. F. (1995). Effect of oral sensorimotor treatment on measures of growth, eating efficiency and aspiration in the dysphagic child with cerebral palsy. *Developmental Medicine and Child Neurology, 37*, 528–543.

Gorlin, R. J., Pindborg, J. J., & Cohen, M. M. (1976). *Syndromes of the face and neck* (2nd ed.). New York: McGraw-Hill.

Guyette, T. W., & Diedrich, W. M. (1981). A critical review of developmental apraxia of speech. In N. Lass (Ed.), *Speech and language: Advances in basic research and practice* (pp. 1–48). New York: Academic Press.

Hardy, J. (1961). Intraoral breath pressure in cerebral palsy. *Journal of Speech and Hearing Disorders, 26*, 310–319.

Hardy, J. (1964). Lung function of athetoid and spastic quadriplegic children. *Developmental and Child Neurology, 6*, 378–388.

Hardy, J. (1967). Suggestions for physiologic research in dysarthria. *Cortex, 3*, 128–156.

Hardy, J. C. (1983). *Cerebral palsy.* Englewood Cliffs, NJ: Prentice–Hall.

Hayden, D. A. (1994). Differential diagnosis of motor speech dysfunction in children. *Clinics in Communication Disorders, 4*, 119–141.

Haynes, S. (1985). Developmental apraxia of speech: Symptoms and treatment. In D. Johns (Ed.), *Clinical management of neurogenic communication disorders* (pp. 259–266). Boston: Little, Brown.

Hixon, T., & Hardy, J. (1964). Restricted motility of speech articulators in cerebral palsy. *Journal of Speech and Hearing Research, 29*, 293–306.

Hunt, P. (1991). Interacting with peers through conversation turntaking with a communication book adaptation. *Augmentative and Alternative Communication, 7*(2), 117–126.

Iacono, T. A., & Duncum, J. E. (1995). Comparison of sign alone and in combination with an electronic communication device in early language. *Augmentative and Alternative Communication, 11*(4), 249–254.

Ingram, T., & Barn, J. (1961). A description and classification of common speech disorders associated with cerebral palsy. *Cerebral Palsy Bulletin, 2*, 254–277.

Irwin, J. (1955). Phonetic equipment of spastic and athetoid children. *Journal of Speech and Hearing Disorders, 20*, 54–67.

Jaffe, M. B. (1980, November). *An investigation of perceptual abilities in developmental apraxia of speech and comparison with functional articulation disorders.* Paper presented at the Annual Convention of the American Speech-language-Hearing Association, Detroit.

Kahane, J. (1979). Pathophysiological effects of Moebius syndrome on speech and hearing. *Archives of Otolaryngology, 105*, 29–34.

Kent, R. D. (1997). *The speech sciences.* San Diego: Singular.

Kent, R., & Netsell, R. (1978). Articulatory abnormalities in athetoid cerebral palsy. *Journal of Speech and Hearing Disorders, 43*, 353–373.

Koheil, R., Sochaniwskyj, A. E., Bablich, K., Kenny, D. J., & Milner, M. (1987). Biofeedback techniques and behaviour modification in the conservative remediation of drooling by children with cerebral palsy. *Developmental Medicine and Child Neurology, 29*(1), 19–26.

Kouri, T. A. (1988). Effects of simultaneous communication in a child-directed treatment approach with preschoolers with severe disabilities. *Augmentative and Alternative Communication, 4*, 222–232.

Kramer, S. S. (1988). Radiologic examination of swallowing impairment in children. *Dysphagia, 3*, 117–125.

Kumin, L. (1994). Intelligibility of speech in children with Down syndrome in natural settings: Parents' perspective. *Perceptual and Motor Skills, 78*(1), 307–313.

Kumin, L., Councill, C., & Goodman, M. (1994). A longitudinal study of the emergence of phonemes in children with Down syndrome. *Journal of Communication Disorders, 27*, 293–303.

Larnert, G., & Bkberg, O. (1995). Positioning improves the oral and pharyngeal swallowing function in children with cerebral palsy. *Acta Paediatrica, 84*, 689–692.

Lespargot, A., Langevin, M. F., Muller, S., & Guillemont, S. (1993). Swallowing distribution associated with drooling in cerebral-palsied children. *Developmental Medicine and Child Neurology, 35*, 298–304.

Lord, J. (1984). Cerebral palsy: A clinical approach. *Archives of Physical Medicine and Rehabilitation, 65,* 542–548.

Love, R. J., & Webb, W. G. (1986). *Neurology for the speech–language pathologist.* Stoneham, MA: Butterworth.

Marcel, M. M., & Cohen, S. (1992). Hearing abilities of Down syndrome and other mentally handicapped adolescents. *Research in Developmental Disabilities, 13,* 533–551.

McDonald, E., & Chance, B. (1964). *Cerebral palsy.* Englewood Cliffs, NJ: Prentice-Hall.

McGrath, S. J., Splaingard, M. L., Alba, H. M., Kaufman, B. H., & Glicklick, M. (1992). Survival and functional outcome of children with severe cerebral palsy folowing gastrostomy. *Archives of Physical Medicine and Rehabilitation, 73,* 133–137.

Meek, M. (1991). Alternate feeding methods. In M. B. Langley & L. J. Lombardino (Eds.), *Neurodevelopmental strategies for managing communication disorders in children with severe motor dysfunction* (pp. 81–112). Austin, TX: PRO-ED.

Merz, M., & Wojtowicz, S. (1967). The Moebius syndrome. *American Journal of Ophthalmology, 63,* 837–840.

Meyerson, M., & Foushee, D. (1978). Speech, language and hearing in Moebius syndrome. *Developmental Medicine and Child Neurology, 20,* 357–365.

Mirenda, P., & Mathy-Laikko, P. (1989). Augmentative and alternative communication applications for persons with severe congenital communication disorders: An introduction. *Augmentative and Alternative Communication, 5,* 3–13.

Montague, J. C., & Hollien, H. (1973). Perceived voice quality disorders in Down's syndrome children. *Journal of Communication Disorders, 6*(2), 76–87.

Morley, M. (1965). *Developmental and disorders of speech in childhood.* Baltimore: Williams & Wilkins.

Netsell, R. (1969). Changes in oropharyngeal cavity size of dysarthric children. *Journal of Speech and Hearing Research, 12,* 646–649.

Platt, L., Andrews, G., & Howie, P. M. (1980). Dysarthria of adult cerebral palsy: II. Phonemic analysis of articulation errors. *Journal of Speech and Hearing Disorders, 23,* 41–55.

Platt, L., Andrews, G., Young, M., & Quinn, P. T. (1980). Dysarthria of adult cerebral palsy: I. Intelligibility and articulatory impairment. *Journal of Speech and Hearing Disorders, 23,* 28.

Pruess, J. B., Vadasy, P. F., & Fewell, R. R. (1987). Language development in children with Down syndrome: An overview of recent research. *Education and Training in Mental Retardation, 22*(1), 44–55.

Reilly, S., Skuse, D., & Poblete, X. (1996). Prevalence of feeding problems and oral motor dysfunction in children with cerebral palsy: A community survey. *Journal of Pediatrics, 126,* 877–882.

Robin, D. (1992). Developmental apraxia of speech: Just another motor problem. *American Journal of Speech–Language Pathology, 1*(3), 19–22.

Rogers, B., Arvedson, J., Buck, G., Smart, P., & Msall, M. (1994). Characteristics of dysphagia in children with cerebral palsy. *Dysphagia, 9*(1), 69–73.

Rogers, P. T., & Coleman, M. (1992). *Medical care in Down syndrome.* New York: Marcel Dekker.

Rosenbek, J. C., & Wertz, R. T. (1972). A review of 50 cases of developmental apraxia of speech. *Language, Speech and Hearing Services in Schools, 3,* 23–33.

Rutherford, B. (1944). A comparative study of loudness, pitch rate, rhythm, and quality of speech of children handicapped by cerebral palsy. *Journal of Speech and Hearing Disorders, 9,* 262–271.

Shriberg, L. D., Aram, D. M., & Kwiatkowski, J. (1997a). Developmental apraxia of speech: I. Descriptive and theoretical perspectives. *Journal of Speech, Language and Hearing Research, 40,* 273–285.

Shriberg, L. D., Aram, D. M., & Kwiatkowski, J. (1997b). Developmental apraxia of speech: II. Toward a diagnostic marker. *Journal of Speech, Language and Hearing Research, 40*, 286–312.

Shriberg, L. D., Aram, D. M., & Kwiatkowski, J. (1997c). Developmental apraxia of speech: III. A subtype marked by inappropriate stress. *Journal of Speech, Language and Hearing Research, 40*, 313–337.

Sochaniwskyj, A. E., Koheil, R. M., Bablich, K., Milner, M., & Kenny, D. J. (1986). Oral motor functioning, frequency of swallowing and drooling in normal children and in children with cerebral palsy. *Archives of Physical Medicine and Rehabilitation, 67*, 866–874.

Stalling, V. A., Zemel, B. S., Davies, J. C., Cronk, C. E., & Charney, E. B. (1996). Energy expenditure of children and adolescents with severe disabilitites: A cerebral palsy model. *American Journal of Clinical Nutrition, 64*, 627–634.

Stempien, L. M., & Gaebler-Spira, D. (1996). Rehabilitation of children and adults with cerebral palsy. In R. L. Braddon (Ed.), *Physical medicine and rehabilitation* (pp. 1113–1132). Philadelphia: Saunders.

Strand, E. A. (1992). The integration of speech motor control and language formulation in process models of acquisition. In R. Chapman (Ed.), *Processes in language acquisition and disorders* (pp. 86–107). St. Louis: Mosby–Yearbook.

Towbin, A. (1960). *The pathology of cerebral palsy.* Springfield, IL: Charles C Thomas.

Van Borsel, J. (1996). Articulation in Down syndrome adolescents and adults. *European Journal of Disorders of Communication, 31*, 415–444.

Waterman, E. T., Koltai, P. J., Downey, J. C., & Cacace, A. T. (1992). Swallowing disorders in a population of children with cerebral palsy. *International Journal of Pediatric Otorhinolaryngology, 24*(1), 63–71.

Wolfe, W. (1950). A comprehensive evaluation of fifty cases of cerebral palsy. *Journal of Speech and Hearing Disorders, 15*, 234–251.

Workinger, M. S., & Kent, R. D. (1991). Perceptual analysis of the dysarthria in children with athetoid and spastic cerebral palsy. In C. A. Moore, K. M. Yorkston, & D. R. Beukelman (Eds.), *Dysarthria and apraxia of speech: Perspectives on management* (pp. 109–126). Baltimore: Brookes.

Yorkston, K. M., Miller, R. M., & Strand, E. A. (1995). *Management of speech and swallowing disorders in degenerative disease.* Tucson, AZ: Communication Skill Builders.

Yoss, K. A., & Darley, F. (1974). Developmental apraxia of speech in children with defective articulation. *Journal of Speech and Hearing Research, 17*, 399–416.

C H A P T E R

ADULT-ONSET, NONPROGRESSIVE DYSARTHRIA AND APRAXIA OF SPEECH

For some motor speech disorders, onset occurs in adulthood. The typical course of these disorders involves a sudden onset, followed by a period of neurologic recovery and later stabilization. Etiologies of these dysarthrias include stroke and traumatic brain injury. The type and characteristics of the speech problems vary considerably and are dependent on the site and extent of the neurologic damage. In addition, some adult-onset dysarthrias have a progressive course. These are discussed in Chapter 4.

STROKE

Pathology–Medical Aspects

POPULATION

Stroke is responsible for almost 10% of deaths in the United States; each year there are 500,000 new cases. Most strokes occur in people over age 55; the average age is 70. Seventy to 80% survive their first episode, and the 10-year survival rate is about 50%. Risk factors are those conditions or behaviors that occur more frequently in those who have or will get the disease. The medical risk factors include arterial hypertension (both ischemic and hemorrhagic types), diabetes mellitus, hyperlipidemia, oral contraceptive use in women over the age of 35 who smoke, and cardiac disease. Other factors implicated in association with stroke are obesity, cigarette smoking, and life stresses. Any patient with a history of transient neurologic deficits and the previously listed factors is at extremely high risk for developing a stroke (Goldstein, Bolis, Fieschi, Gorini, & Millikan, 1979; Meyer & Shaw, 1982). Information about risk factors is important because many are treatable. A number of general sources of information about stroke rehabilitation are available (e.g., Brandstater & Basmajian, 1987; Garrison & Rolak, 1993).

There are two types of stroke, ischemic and hemorrhagic. Ischemic strokes result from (a) a sudden blockage of a major blood vessel supplying the brain (internal carotid, vertebrobasilar artery, or their branches); (b) a blood or air embolus that lodges in a vessel, causing complete occlusion; or (c) a microinfarct or "lacune," which results from the effects of chronic hypertension. Hemorrhagic infarcts are caused by (a) subarachnoid hemorrhage due to a congenital defect, hypertension, or infection; (b) intracerebral hemorrhage; or (c) arteriovenous malformations (Meyer & Shaw, 1982).

Question: I've recently heard the term "brain attack." Is that synonymous with cerebrovascular accident (CVA) or stroke? If so, why is the term used?

The terms are being used synonymously and extensively in public information campaigns in an effort to make people aware that they should seek immediate medical attention for the following warning signs:

- Sudden weakness or numbness of the face, arm, or leg on one side of the body
- Sudden dimness or loss of vision, particularly in one eye
- Sudden difficulty speaking or trouble understanding speech
- Sudden severe headache with no known cause
- Unexplained dizziness, unsteadiness, or sudden falls, especially with any of the other signs

The term brain attack is used because of its parallelism with the term heart attack. Recently clot-dissolving drugs have become available for the treatment of acute ischemic stroke. Studies have shown them to be effective if they are used within 3 hours of the initial stroke symptoms. Therefore, immediate attention to stroke symptoms is urgent.

SYNDROMES AND SITE OF LESION

In stroke, damage to certain areas of the brain causes a unique constellation of symptoms. These collections of symptoms, called *syndromes*, are determined by the arterial system that is affected. Certain syndromes are quite common or distinctive. Table 3.1 contains a summary of common syndromes that are associated with communication disorders.

DIAGNOSIS OF STROKE

The history of onset and the clinical appearance of the patient can be helpful in both localizing the lesion and determining the etiology. Thrombotic or atherosclerotic strokes tend to be stepwise in progression, whereas embolic strokes tend to occur suddenly and completely; hemorrhage often is associated with severe headache and nausea. Beyond this, computerized tomography (CT scan) is commonly used to differentiate between the two types of stroke. An ischemic infarct is seen as a hypodense area against normal brain tissue; hemorrhage is seen as a hyperdense area that enhances when contrast material is injected. Magnetic resonance imaging (MRI) has also been used to visualize the brain anatomy after cerebral damage.

Some tests may be used to identify the cause of the stroke or to evaluate the patient for possible surgical treatment, rather than strictly for diagnosis of the presence or absence of stroke. Echocardiography is useful in embolic stroke to

Table 3.1
Stroke Syndromes Frequently Associated with Communication Disorders

Syndrome	Common Causes	Symptoms
Middle cerebral artery syndrome	Unilateral carotid artery disease involving stenosis of the artery, ulceration, or occlusion by an atheromatous plaque	Contralateral hemiplegia and hemisensory defect, aphasia if the lesion is on the dominant side, and visual–perceptual deficits if the lesion is on the nondominant side
Anterior cerebral artery syndrome	Same as middle cerebral artery syndrome	Paralysis of the contralateral leg with sensory loss and occasional bowel and bladder incontinence
Vertebrobasilar artery syndrome	Trauma, atherosclerosis, or arthritic compression of the vessels	Quadriplegia with dysarthria
Posterior inferior cerebellar artery (PICA) syndrome (Wallenberg's or lateral medullary syndromes)		Vertigo, dysphagia, ataxia, nausea and vomiting, and ipsilateral loss of facial sensation with contralateral sensory loss over the body

localize the source of the embolus, often the left ventricle of the heart. Cerebral angiography may be used to better identify the anatomy of an arteriovenous malformation or aneurysm in a hemorrhagic stroke. Ultrasound studies of the carotid arteries can be used to determine if there is a surgically correctable obstruction. Electroencephalography (EEG) is used to distinguish seizure activity from possible recurrence or enlargement of a stroke (Meyer & Shaw, 1982).

NATURAL COURSE

As mentioned before, a stroke may be heralded by a transient loss of neurologic function, called a transient ischemic attack (TIA) or reversible ischemic neurologic defect (RIND). Fifteen to 40% of these patients will have a cerebral infarct within 5 years (Goldstein et al., 1979). After a stroke, there will generally be a period of hypotonicity for 4 to 48 hours, with depressed deep tendon reflexes, a lack of voluntary movement, and possible urinary retention. Following this, there is a return of muscle tone and the onset of spasticity. Most motor recovery takes place within the first 3 to 6 weeks; upper extremity function may continue to improve over the first 6 months, especially in those patients most severely affected at the outset. Motor return usually occurs in a proximal to distal sequence (Kaplan & Cerullo, 1986). The return of language function may continue at a slow rate for an even longer time. Positive prognostic indicators for overall recovery include strong family support, preservation of visuoperceptual abilities, early return of voluntary movement, and good trunk control. Negative factors include prolonged coma, incontinence past the first 48 hours, presence of unilateral neglect, and profound aphasia.

The long-term prognosis for recurrence of stroke varies according to the type of lesion. It is difficult to identify clearly what percentage of patients experience recurrence because "silent strokes," or TIAs, may confuse the picture. In about 80% of strokes with embolic origins, a second episode will occur if the patient is untreated; up to 20% of these may occur within 10 days of the initial episode. Patients with hemorrhagic strokes also have a varied outcome. Those with an intracerebral hemorrhage have little chance of rebleeding from the same site. However, among patients with untreated aneurysms, almost half will rebleed and 78% of these recurrences are fatal (Adams & Victor, 1985; Gordon, Drenth, Jarvis, Johnson, & Wright, 1978; Henley, Pettit, Todd-Pakropek, & Tupper, 1985).

Certain complications occur frequently enough after a CVA to merit comment. Spasticity with resulting joint contractures is common. Clonus associated with leg spasticity may interfere with independent ambulation and may require bracing or other intervention. Depression may be significant and occurs more commonly than generally acknowledged; evidence of vegetative symptoms such as a loss of appetite, disturbed sleep patterns, and loss of enjoyment indicate the need for antidepressant medications.

MEDICAL TREATMENT

The most effective treatment of stroke is prevention. Since hypertension and cardiac disease are the most strongly linked precursors of cerebrovascular disease, good control of these disorders will be the most effective means of prevention. Other factors such as smoking, diet, and stress are not as directly associated with cerebrovascular disease but should also be addressed (Meyer & Shaw, 1982).

TIAs should be treated aggressively because of the high percentage of persons who go on to complete a stroke. Standard medical treatment consists of the use of antiplatelet drugs, such as aspirin, ticlopidine, or clopidogrel. If the patient with TIAs has evidence of significant narrowing of the carotid arteries and his or her transient symptoms are reflective of ischemia in cortical areas supplied by branches of the carotid arteries, then surgical endarterectomy of the carotid arteries may be done.

Certain patients who are seen in emergency rooms within 3 hours after the stroke are candidates for thrombolysis with tissue plasminigin activator. Others may be treated with an anticoagulant (Heparin) to halt further thrombosis. If a stroke is thought to be embolic and the patient has an identifiable source of such emboli or cardiac arrhythmias such as atrial fibrillations, then he or she may receive long-term oral anticoagulation (Coumadin). Neuroprotection agents are presently being evaluated for use in stroke.

Although many patients with completed strokes are treated with antiplatelet drugs to prevent recurrences, there is no treatment that can reverse the neurological deficits. However, function can be considerably improved by providing the patient with physical and cognitive retraining. Recent studies are available that examine the effectiveness of rehabilitation services (Evans, Connis, Hendricks, & Haselkorn, 1995). Their results suggest that patients who participate in inpatient rehabilitation do better than others on a number of measures, including function at the time of discharge, short-term survival, and chances of returning home.

A number of types of therapy are useful. Physical therapy can improve the patients' independence with mobility skills (transfer skills, wheelchair usage, and ambulation). Some physical therapists use neuromuscular facilitation programs to encourage resumption of normal movement patterns and muscle tone. Excessive spasticity can be treated with a number of drugs, including diazepam (Valium), baclofen (Lioresal), and dantrolene sodium (Dantrium). The major side effects of all these drugs include central nervous system sedation and possible weakness of nonparetic muscles. Other treatments such as nerve blocks and botulinum toxin blocks may be directed at specific muscle groups that are interfering with independence. The patient may require lower extremity bracing to provide instruction in performing basic and advanced levels of daily living activities, evaluate the need for environmental adaptation and equipment, and retrain the patient in perceptual and fine motor skills. Recreation therapists may offer patients some insight into new or old leisure skills that are available to them despite neurologic deficits. Resocialization and community reintegration are also important components of rehabilitation. It is common for the elderly after stroke to be receiving one or more medications. Although most agents are well tolerated, the use of multiple drugs may result in adverse effects, including confusion and sedation.

SWALLOWING DISORDERS

Swallowing disorders are common especially early postonset of stroke. In rare cases of discrete brain stem lesions, dysphagia can be the only manifestation of the stroke (Buchholz, 1993). Researchers have reported on the prevalence of dysphagia following stroke. Approximately one third of patients with single-hemisphere strokes initially exhibited dysphagia, with most deficits resolving by the end of the first week (Barer, 1989). Aspiration occurred most frequently in patients with combined cerebral–brain stem stroke with bilateral cranial nerve signs, but also occurred within the context of unilateral stroke (Horner, Massey, Riski, Lathrop, & Chase, 1988). In a group of patients in whom clinical concerns of aspiration were present and videofluoroscopic modified barium swallow studies were performed, presence of aspiration varied with site of lesion, with the lowest prevalence in unilateral right hemispheric strokes (9.9%), followed by unilateral left hemispheric strokes (12.1%), bilateral hemispheric strokes (24%), and brain stem stroke (39.5%) (Teasell, Bach, & McRae, 1994). Aspiration in brain stem stroke has been associated with Cranial Nerve IX and X abnormality, vocal fold weakness, and severe dysarthria (Horner, Buoyer, Alberts, & Helms, 1991). Despite the initial severity and high prevalence of dysphagia in brain stem stroke, recovery is reported to be good, with 80% of patients resuming full oral feeding (Horner et al., 1991). Prevalence of dysphagia also varied with the size of lesion. In a study of 38 patients with acute stroke, those with infarcts restricted only to small vessels exhibited aspiration less frequently (21%) than did those with both large and small vessel infarcts (75%) (Alberts, Horner, Gray, & Brazer, 1992).

Descriptions of the nature of dysphagia in stroke are also available. Most frequently, disorders occurred during the pharyngeal phases of swallowing, with a delayed triggering of the swallow reflex occurring in approximately one third of patients (Veis & Logemann, 1985). Pharyngeal transit times in stroke patients with dysphagia are longer than normal (Johnson, McKenzie, Rosenquist, Lieberman, & Sievers, 1992; Robbins, Levine, Maser, Rosenbek, & Kempster, 1993). A large proportion of stroke patients with severe dysphagia were found to have sensory impairment in the laryngopharynx that may have contributed to the development of aspiration (Aviv et al., 1996).

Recently considerable attention has been paid to swallowing disorders because they place individuals at risk for malnutrition, pneumonia, and other medical complications (Finestone, Greene-Finestone, Wilson, & Teasell, 1995; Smithard et al., 1996; Young & Durant-Jones, 1990). The relative risk of developing pneumonia was nearly seven times greater for those patients who aspirated compared with those who did not and over eight times greater for those who aspirated 10% or greater on one or more barium test swallows (Holas, DePippor, & Reding, 1994). The risk for developing pneumonia was 5.6 times greater for those who aspirated thickened liquids or more solid consistencies compared with those who did not aspirate or who aspirated thin liquids only (Schmidt, Holas, Halvorson, & Reding, 1994). The early presence of dysphagia may be predictive of overall rehabilitation outcomes. In a study of 124 patients with acute nonhemorrhagic stroke tracked through an inpatient rehabilitation unit, patients with dysphagia had lower functional levels (Functional Independence Measure [FIM] scores) than those who passed the dysphagia screening (Odderson, Keaton, & McKenna, 1995). At discharge, patients with dysphagia were less likely to go home than those without dysphagia.

Although reports of intervention for dysphagia have appeared in the literature for many years, there has been a substantial increase in the number of these reports recently (Langmore & Miller, 1994). General guidelines for feeding patients with dysphagia include topics such as positioning, feeding environment, compensation for cognitive issues, diet quality, and so on (Langmore & Miller, 1994). Generally, these interventions can be categorized as (a) maneuvers, such as supraglottic swallow, the Mendelsohn maneuver, and so on; (b) postural adjustments, such as chin-tuck, head rotation, and so on; and (c) facilitation techniques, such as strengthening exercises and thermal stimulation (Miller & Langmore, 1994).

Speech Characteristics

The speech characteristics associated with stroke vary widely depending on site and extent of lesion. The two main categories of motor speech disorder, dysarthria and apraxia of speech, are both seen in individuals following stroke.

Acquired apraxia of speech is a term used to refer to a speech disorder, resulting from brain injury, that is characterized primarily by articulatory and prosodic symptoms. Most definitions of the term imply deficits in the planning or programming of movement for speech, although movement of the same musculature for nonspeech tasks is normal. Although many clinical researchers believe that apraxia of speech is a motor disorder, others argue that the impairment is linguistic in nature. This controversy exists, at least in part, because models and theories of speech production in general, as well as specific issues related to speech motor control, are still debated. Also, apraxia rarely occurs without concomitant aphasia or other neurologic deficits. Thus, description, differential diagnosis, and treatment planning often become complicated. In this section, we present several definitions of apraxia of speech, illustrating how research has shaped current opinion regarding the nature of the disorder. We then describe behavioral and speech characteristics associated with apraxia, and point out which characteristics differentiate it from aphasia and dysarthria.

An Evolving Definition

A variety of terms historically have been applied to the articulatory disorders now called apraxia of speech, including Broca's aphasia, anterior aphasia, motor aphasia, aphemia, speech apraxia, and verbal apraxia. A review of the evolution of the definition of apraxia of speech is useful in providing a perspective about the disorder as research and experience in treating individuals with apraxia of speech have progressed. In 1969, Fred Darley presented a session titled "The Classification of Output Disturbances in Neurologic Communication Disorders" at the American Speech and Hearing Association convention. In this presentation, he argued for distinguishing apraxia from other disorders, such as aphasia. He did so because of evidence that, in speakers with apraxia, the impairment was restricted to speech and did not cross into other modalities such as comprehension, gesture, and perhaps writing. He labeled this specific modality-bound impairment as verbal apraxia, and noted that the disorder represented difficulty positioning and sequencing movements of muscles specifically for speech. He also noted that prosodic alterations were associated with the articulation disorder, but may be due to compensation. Later, Wertz, LaPointe, and Rosenbek (1984) referred to apraxia of speech as a "phonologic disorder" that results from sensorimotor impairment, and described the impairment to be one of motor planning or programming. They noted that the individual with apraxia has a deficit in the ability to "select, program, and/or execute" (p. 4) movement for the positioning of the speech musculature in a coordinated and well-timed manner. They also specified that this is the case only for "volitional production of speech sounds" (p. 4). McNeil, Robin, and Schmidt (1997) recently proposed a definition of apraxia of speech that encompasses concepts related to the nature of the disorder as well as the characteristics of the disorder. They suggested that apraxia of speech is a "phonetic–motoric" disorder in which speech production is impaired by "inefficiencies in the translation of a well-formed and filled phonologic frame to previously learned kinematic parameters assembled for carrying out the intended movement, resulting in intra and interarticulator temporal and spatial segmental and prosodic distortions" (p. 329).

There are similarities in these definitions. First, they all refer to an impairment in the performance in planning, programming, and executing sequences of intentional movement for speech production. They all emphasize that the disruption is specific to volitional movement for speech; that is, the problem occurs when a person intends to say a specific utterance. All definitions refer to some disruption in prosody, although it is not clear whether that disruption is primary to the disorder or a consequence of the impairment. In addition, all definitions make the distinction that the difficulty in movement for volitional speech production is not seen in reflexive movement, or in volitional nonspeech movement such as in chewing or swallowing. Darley's (1969) contribution was to distinguish apraxia as a distinct level of impairment different from aphasia or dysarthria. Although Wertz and colleagues (1984) used the term neurogenic phonologic disorder in their definition, they also suggested that the difficulty with phonologic rules alone could not explain the characteristics of the disorder. McNeil and colleagues' (1997) definition emphasizes the nature of the disorder from the motor control perspective. Although most definitions have suggested the impairment in apraxia of speech to be one of planning or programming, there is still debate about what that really means.

Question: What are motor planning and programming, and why are these concepts so important in understanding apraxia of speech?

For movement to occur, neural mechanisms must establish a set of commands to muscles so that structures move in a particular direction and with a particular speed and range of motion. In movement for speech, this planning or programming involves the rapid, finely coordinated movement of a variety of structures so that each will arrive in a particular configuration to produce the intended acoustic target. In addition, speech motor control involves the interaction of motor systems with the ongoing linguistic formulation.

(continues)

It is likely that the planning and programming occur in stages. First, one has to conceptually plan the movement so that specific goals can be reached. That is, one needs a strategy to reach a particular movement goal given all the conditions under which the movement will be made. For example, if one is reaching for a cup of coffee, the person plans a strategy for the movement. The individual conceptualizes what type of movement (up, down, near, far, etc.) will help to reach the goal. In speech, one might plan a strategy for yelling to a friend across the street, keeping in mind the extra breath support needed for the louder acoustic goal.

In addition to the more conceptual level of planning movement, programming of specific parameters of movement must be accomplished. Some process must select the specific muscle(s) involved in the intended movement, and tell that muscle or set of muscles when to start contracting, how much, and how long. In that way, the structures that need to move will move with the right range of motion, in the right direction, with the right speed, and with the right amount of muscle tension to achieve the desired movement result. Because this happens very rapidly, it is likely that one uses stored commands for particular movements. These stored "motor tapes" can be retrieved and "played out," and integrated with more novel movement patterns fairly automatically when needed. Apraxia of speech is thought to be due to deficits in those processes involved in motor planning and in determining movement specification for sequences of movement for volitional speech production. Some have posited that there may be subtypes of apraxia of speech, as different stages of this planning and programming may be affected. For clinicians, it is important to understand that those individuals with apraxia of speech have a motor level of impairment and that treatment should take that into account.

Paradigms for Studying Apraxia of Speech

Any brief overview of the apraxia literature reveals that a variety of paradigms have been used to study this disorder. Placing these studies in a historical perspective points out how differences in opinion about the nature of the disorder may have evolved. Comprehensive reviews of apraxia of speech are available (Duffy, 1995; McNeil, 1997; Rosenbek, McNeil, & Aronson, 1984; Wertz et al., 1984).

Perceptual Studies. Early work in the 1960s and 1970s consisted of perceptually based descriptions of articulatory error patterns in speakers with apraxia (see

McNeil et al., 1997, for a detailed discussion). Primarily through the use of broad phonetic transcription, researchers provided a wide base of descriptive data regarding the articulatory characteristics. These studies were limited, however, in that all perceptions of articulatory events were forced into a relatively few phonologic categories. Thus, attempts to interpret the data in order to explain the nature of apraxia of speech were constrained. Then, the theoretical approach to studying the disorder shifted. Later studies examined patterns of articulatory errors, but did so in contexts designed to relate analyses to linguistic theory. They used distinctive feature analyses, and interpreted data to suggest that apraxia of speech is primarily a phonologic disorder. Findings of frequent substitution errors that often closely approximated the target phonemes led researchers to suggest that these errors were "rule governed," and therefore that the level of impairment was linguistic. This implied a reduction in the discriminative selection needed for motor speech encoding rather than a problem with the encoding process itself.

The early perceptual studies provided a broad and fairly consistent description of articulatory error patterns exhibited by speakers with apraxia. Studies then began to examine which linguistic and situational variables would influence apraxic error patterns, including phoneme difficulty, grammatical class, type of instruction noise, and visual monitoring. Although interpretation of the data was less consistent than the body of literature describing the articulatory characteristics, results indicate that (a) subjects with apraxia make more errors as grammatical class, difficulty of initial phoneme, and sentence or word length increase or are more complex; (b) errors increase when speakers repeat nonsense as opposed to real words; and (c) situational stress and fast rate conditions have no significant effect on articulatory performance, but articulation errors in polysyllabic words are more variable in those conditions. Some researchers argued against the concept of apraxia of speech as a phenomenon separate from aphasia. The majority, however, were suggesting that apraxic speakers demonstrate difficulty planning or executing the sequential motor organization necessary for speech production.

Acoustic Studies. Repeated observations of difficulty in initiation, slow rate, and prosodic or temporal abnormalities next led researchers to investigate apraxia of speech through specific acoustic measures. These studies demonstrated that some articulatory errors, including both substitution and distortion errors, are actually phonetic errors rather than phonemic selection errors. Acoustic studies demonstrated that vowel and consonant durations were longer for individuals with apraxia, although results were inconsistent from study to study. Some suggest that slow rate in apraxia of speech is due both to articulatory prolongation (lengthening of the steady state segments and the intervening transitions) and syllable segregation (intervals between lengthened syllables) (Kent & Rosenbek, 1983). Although vowel durations were longer overall in individuals with apraxia, these speakers still followed normal "rules" for changes in the segment duration by shortening the vowel length as words increased in length (Collins, Rosenbek, & Wertz, 1983).

> *Question: I am confused by the terms* phonologic *and* phonetic. *How are they different? What is the difference between a* phonologic error *and a* phonetic error*?*
>
> *Phonology* concerns the patterns of sounds in a language and the rules that guide how the sounds can be combined. The term *phonologic* refers to this rule-governed linguistic system of phonology. A *phoneme* is the smallest linguistic unit (or segment of sound) that can be distinguished within words (e.g., the "t" in "sit"). In contrast, the term *phonetic* is often used to denote the articulatory representation of the phoneme, or the observable elements of speech (what we hear). Whereas the phoneme can be thought of as a mental linguistic unit, a phonetic unit is at a physical level, in that it is the acoustic result of a specific sequence of movements. Many people are familiar with the term *phonetic transcription*, which involves writing down each phonetic unit as it is heard (e.g., /sɪt/). Therefore, a phonologic error refers to a linguistic error in the ability to retrieve a particular phoneme (or set of phonemes) and a phonetic error refers to inaccuracy in the acoustic representation of that phoneme. This acoustic error is usually caused by inaccuracy in achieving specific spatial configurations of the vocal tract.

Voice onset time, or VOT (the interval between the articulatory burst release of a stop consonant and the beginning of the periodic vocal fold activity associated with the vowel), can be measured acoustically and has been used to determine if there is a distinction between phonetic and phonemic disorders. It can be argued that where the VOT values are within the normal range of the perceptual category for the voiced–voiceless distinction, errors are phonemic. Errors in which VOT values are *between* the range of VOT values for voiced and voiceless sounds provide evidence for phonetic errors. Because several studies have illustrated overlapping VOT profiles for apraxic speakers, researchers have suggested that speakers with apraxia experience difficulty with timing of laryngeal and supralaryngeal events (McNeil, Liss, Tseng, & Kent, 1990). These studies have added to our understanding of the nature of apraxia of speech by demonstrating that some instances of apraxic errors, which, although perceived to be phoneme selection errors, may really be errors in mistiming between laryngeal and supralaryngeal gestures.

Physiologic Studies. Physiologic measures of movement have also provided more specific descriptions of perceived articulatory errors in apraxia of speech. Fiberscopic studies illustrate mistiming between the lowering of the velum and tongue-tip movement during word production in speakers with apraxia (Itoh, Sasanuma, & Ushijima, 1979). Coarticulatory effects are deviant and variability is noted in velar height and segment duration. These studies indicate motor impairment in programming the positioning and timing of the speech movement (McNeil et al., 1997). Technology involving X-ray microbeam allows observations of the movements of the mandible, lower lip, tongue, and velum. Disorganization of timing among the several articulators in microbeam studies also suggests impairment in motor programming. Simultaneous physiologic and perceptual measures (including measures of lip and jaw movement, electromyography [EMG], and accelerometry to measure onset of voicing) show antagonistic muscle co-contraction, continuous undifferentiated EMG, muscle activity shutdown, movement without voice, movement discoordination, and groping (Forrest, Adams, McNeil, & Southwood, 1991). Because most substitution and distortion errors are produced with one or more accompanying neuromuscular abnormalities, it can be argued that these segment errors are due to difficulty in neuromotor execution and programming rather than phonologic selection errors.

Neuroanatomical Sites of Lesion Associated with Apraxia of Speech

Apraxia of speech is most frequently due to a stroke in the hemisphere dominant for language, usually the left hemisphere. The area most frequently cited as being associated with apraxia has been Brodman's area 44 (third frontal convolution). Other sites of lesion have also been noted to be frequently associated with apraxia of speech, including the parietal lobe, subcortical structures such as the thalamus and the basal ganglia, and the insula (Duffy, 1995). Advances in brain imaging have contributed to professionals' understanding of site of lesion in apraxia of speech. For example, brain lesions of groups of speakers with deficits in motor planning of articulatory movements have been compared with those without such deficits (Dronker, 1996). All individuals with apraxia showed lesions in a discrete region of the left precentral gyrus of the insula, a cortical area beneath the frontal and temporal lobes. None of the speakers without apraxia showed lesions in this area. Because the sites of lesion causing apraxia of speech are also associated with language functioning, individuals with apraxia will usually also exhibit aphasia. Apraxia of speech is also seen with other types of neurologic disease or injury, such as traumatic brain injury, anoxia, and tumors. The more diffuse the damage (especially with head injury and anoxia), the more likely other cognitive and linguistic disorders will occur along with the apraxia.

Speech and Behavioral Characteristics

Most researchers and clinicians who observe apraxic speech production mention articulatory and prosodic errors that become more numerous and more severe with increases in the length and/or phonetic complexity of the intended utterance. The clinical characteristics of apraxic speech have been summarized as (a) effortful trial-and-error groping of articulatory movement with attempts to self-correct, (b) dysprosody in which there are no extended periods of normal rhythm or stress, (c) articulatory inconsistency on repeated productions of the same utterance, and (d) difficulty initiating utterances (Wertz et al., 1984). The following sections provide brief descriptions of the major categories of characteristics that have been noted to be associated with apraxia of speech. Specifying speech and behavioral characteristics associated with apraxia of speech is difficult because these characteristics are not all observed in all apraxic speakers. Further, the degree to which concomitant aphasia or dysarthria is present may confound one's ability to interpret error types. Individuals will vary in the number and severity of the characteristics they exhibit. Note that these categories and many of the specific characteristics overlap those noted in Chapter 2 for children with developmental apraxia of speech. They cannot be directly compared, however, as those characteristics exhibited by the child are confounded by the fact that the motor planning impairment is influencing the development of stored motor schemas or plans, the development of phonologic rule use, and probably the development of other linguistic skills such as morphology and syntax.

Level of Severity of Apraxia of Speech. With the caution that aphasia most frequently co-occurs with apraxia of speech and thus complicates assessment, the following discussion describes speakers with apraxia along a continuum of severity of their motor speech disorders. The speaker with severe apraxia may produce no speech or perhaps a few stereotypical utterances that may or may not be meaningful. Initially, some speakers will not be able to produce voice, even though their vocal folds may function well for reflexive cough or laughter. These speakers may also exhibit extensive groping in an apparent attempt to achieve articulatory targets. Imitation of even very phonetically simple utterances (e.g., "me," "no," "bye") will probably be very difficult. Individuals with severe apraxia will usually exhibit much frustration. Some individuals will respond to this by repeated phonation and groping movements accompanied by gestures. Others may give up and not want to initiate any attempts at speech.

Question: What is meant by "stereotypic" utterances?

Individuals with severe apraxia may not be able to generate and execute movement patterns even for very simple intended utterances, yet they may have two or three utterances that they say with almost every attempt to communicate. Sometimes these utterances may be quite phonetically complex, given the severity of their apraxia. One example comes from a 47-year-old man who had a left hemisphere thrombotic stroke, leaving him with good auditory comprehension and excellent gestural communication, but severe apraxia of speech. Whenever he was greeted or asked a question, he would say, "You betcha; gettin better and better." This phrase was always produced with exactly the same stress and intonation pattern, and was used even in response to questions such as "What's your name?" and "What day is it today?" He knew what he was saying and also knew what he intended to say, but the stereotypic utterance would always be produced. Another example is a 67-year-old woman who had moderate aphasia and severe apraxia of speech. She would consistently say "because," often repeatedly, when attempting to verbally communicate. She would use it in response to any question, such as "Are you hungry?" She also used it in all attempts to initiate speech. It was, in fact, the only word she said. Repeated attempts to imitate even simple utterances such as "oh" or "no" took much time and effort. Yet, she produced the word *because* effortlessly and with articulatory precision. The mechanisms for stereotypical utterances is unclear. The individuals seem able to retrieve stored plans and programs for movement for those particular words, but no others.

Moderate apraxia of speech is characterized by numerous articulatory errors and dysprosody. Individuals also exhibit trial-and-error behavior and occasional groping, but not on every utterance. Occasional phrases are produced with near-normal articulatory precision and prosody. Because many individuals with moderate apraxia of speech will also have a coexisting Broca's aphasia, utterances may be telegraphic, lacking functor words. Individuals with mild apraxia of speech may exhibit minor and inconsistent articulatory errors. Their speech will be more accurate if they go slowly and, as a result, may sound less natural. Much of what has been written about the speech characteristics associated with apraxia of speech are from observations of speakers with moderate and mild apraxia.

Articulatory Characteristics. As mentioned previously, early research in apraxia of speech focused on articulatory error patterns. Descriptions of apraxia of speech since that time have emphasized the type and severity of these articulation errors. The following summary of articulatory characteristics has been compiled from a number of sources (Darley, Aronson, & Brown, 1975; Duffy, 1995; Johns & Darley, 1970; LaPointe & Johns, 1975; Shankweiler & Harris, 1966; Trost & Canter, 1974; Wertz et al., 1984).

Substitution, often similar to metathetic errors seen in speech of individuals without neurologic impairment, is the most common type of error in apraxia of speech. However, recent acoustic and physiologic work that argues for distortion may also be important because distortions are often perceived by a listener as substitutions. Although substitutions are common in speakers with moderate and mild apraxia, fewer substitutions are noted in speakers with very severe apraxia, for whom distortions and omissions are most frequent. Errors occur on both consonants and vowels, especially diphthongs. Other articulatory error types include omissions and additions. Omissions are likely due to attempts to simplify the phonetic string, and are seen frequently in speakers with moderate to severe apraxia of speech. Additions are often in the form of a schwa, perhaps reflecting the difficulty with moving from one articulatory configuration to the next or providing the speaker more time to plan the next movement sequence. See Table 3.2 for a summary of characteristics in apraxia of speech.

Generally, the more difficult the phonetic unit, the more articulatory errors will occur in apraxia. Fricatives, affricates, and blends, therefore, are more often in error than are stops or nasals. More frequent errors are noted in the initial position of words, especially by individuals with moderate to severe apraxia who have difficulty achieving initial articulatory configurations. Speakers with apraxia are typically aware of their errors. They may also anticipate errors perhaps because they know what target utterances will give them difficulty. They also may make repeated attempts to self-correct that at times seem similar to the repetition observed in speakers who stutter. However, there is less consistency in the repeated productions of speakers with apraxia than of those who stutter.

Contextual Influences on Speech Characteristics. Unlike speakers with dysarthria who tend to be somewhat consistent in the type and severity of their articulatory, phonatory, and prosodic speech characteristics, speakers with apraxia tend to show considerable variability. Some of this variability is due to the context in which the utterance is produced. The two most salient contextual influences are (1) the degree to which the utterance is "habituated" or well practiced and (2) the length and phonetic complexity of the utterance.

Table 3.2
Characteristics Frequently Associated with Apraxia of Speech

Articulatory Characteristics

Multiple speech sound errors
    Perceived substitutions most common
    Distortions and additions also common
Transposition of sounds and syllables
Perceived voicing errors (may be due to mistiming)
Affricates and fricatives more likely to be in error than stops or nasals
Consonant clusters more difficult to produce than singletons
Errors inconsistently produced

Movement Characteristics

Groping
Silent posturing
Difficulty imitating and maintaining articulatory configurations, especially for initial sounds
Difficulty making movement transitions in and out of spatial targets
Trial-and-error movement behavior

Disturbances in Prosody

Slower rate
Reduced use of word and sentence stress patterns
Inappropriate or longer pauses
Longer duration of both vowels and consonants

Contextual Influences

Length and Phonetic Complexity

Errors increase with increasing length of word or utterance
Repetition (if the individual is paying attention, and watching the clinician) elicits better
    articulatory performance than spontaneous production
Sounds are more easily produced in single-word production than in sentences or
    conversation
Errors increase as the phonetic complexity of the utterance increases
Difficulty with a particular sequence of movement for sequences of sounds, even when the
    individual sounds are correct in isolation or consonant–vowel combinations

Automatic Versus Novel Utterances

Novel, or less practiced, utterances will be more difficult than well-practiced utterances
More errors on nonsense words than real words

The more times an utterance has been produced, the more "automatic" it is said to be. In other words, less conscious attention and effort are involved in its production. For example, if you count to 10, little conscious effort or attention has to be paid. On the other hand, if you are asked to give a guest lecture to speech pathology interns and want to describe homonymous hemianopsia, you will probably need to pay more attention and maybe even slow down a little as you say that word. Individuals with apraxia of speech may be able to count to 10 easily but have great difficulty saying the word "three" in any other context. Similarly, if you ask an individual with apraxia to repeat the phrase, "Hi, how are you?" he or she will likely have less difficulty than if you ask the person to produce a novel utterance. Therefore, the individual will say novel or less practiced utterances with more articulatory error and more dysprosody than utterances that he or she has said frequently, such as "How are you?" or "I'm fine." This notion is consistent with reports that frequently occurring sounds are more likely to be correct, and that articulatory error is more likely for nonsense words than real words.

Studies have shown that if the length and/or linguistic complexity of an utterance increases, so will articulatory and prosodic errors (Johns & Darley, 1970). For example, it would be much easier for an individual with apraxia to produce the movement sequence for the word *top* than the same movement sequence as part of the word *topographical*. Likewise, the speaker asked to repeat the word *help* will do so with more ease than if asked to repeat the same word in the phrase "Please help me with this." Prosodic changes also occur if the utterance becomes longer or phonetically more complex. For example, segmental durations, including vowel and interword interval durations, have been shown to be longer in sentences than when the same words are produced in isolation (Strand & McNeil, 1996).

The speaking task itself also influences articulatory and prosodic errors. For example, the speaker with apraxia will perform differently depending on whether he or she is asked to produce a phrase in imitation, to describe a picture or read an utterance, or to speak spontaneously. Although individuals vary, most speakers with apraxia will benefit greatly from watching and listening to someone model the utterance they are imitating.

Movement Characteristics. Most descriptions of apraxia of speech include these characteristics: groping, silent posturing, and difficulty achieving articulatory configurations. These characteristics all point to difficulty producing sequential movement. When planning treatment, it may be helpful to think in terms of movement, rather than sound production. Speech–language pathologists are typically very well trained in phonology, but have little or no training in how motor skill occurs or is learned; very few were required to take courses in kinesiology or cognitive motor learning. Yet, highly skilled and rapid movement is necessary for phonemes to be realized as acoustic events.

Speakers with apraxia have difficulty imitating articulatory configurations and transitions into and out of spatial targets for phonetic strings. This is true even when the individual has no weakness or other abnormalities of movement in the tongue, lips, jaw, or velum for nonspeech movement. In fact, physiologic studies have shown that speakers with apraxia were able to achieve peak velocities in the lip and jaw that were similar to normal speakers, even though overall movement time was slower (McNeil, Caligiuri, & Rosenbek, 1989; Robin, Bean, & Folkins, 1989). These data suggest that the oral articulatory structures have the ability to move with normal speed, but that movement gestures toward a particular configuration take longer. This may be due to the speakers' difficulty achieving the right spatial target, the extra movement that occurs in attempts to reach that target, or the inability to maintain the target once it is achieved. Articulatory configurations are particularly hard to achieve for initial sounds.

Prosodic Characteristics: Rate and Speech Timing. Prosodic disturbance has always been included as a primary and salient characteristic of apraxia of speech. These deficits include slow rate, reduced stress patterning for words and sentences, reduced variability in intonational contours, longer or inappropriate intersyllabic or interword pauses, and increased length of segmental durations. Prosodic deficits may be primary to the disorder of apraxia, a compensatory mechanism employed by speakers who are having difficulty with achieving specific movement patterns, or both. Slow rate is due both to articulatory prolongation (increased duration of vowels and consonants) and increased pause time between syllables (Kent & Rosenbek, 1983). Increased consonant and vowel durations are particularly apparent in multisyllabic words and in sentences (McNeil et al., 1990; Ryalls, 1981; Strand & McNeil, 1996). Interestingly, individuals with apraxia will follow linguistic rules for changes in vowel duration similarly to normal speakers. For example, they will reduce vowel duration as root words increase in length (e.g., zip, zipper, and zippering), although absolute durations are always longer (Collins et al., 1983).

Associated Deficits

In addition to aphasia, a variety of neurologic deficits co-occur with apraxia of speech, including oral apraxia, limb apraxia, and apraxia for phonation. These associated deficits are due to damage in the left hemisphere, especially the frontal or parietal lobes and left subcortical structures or pathways. Many individuals with apraxia of speech also exhibit right hemiparesis due to involvement in the left descending pathways that cross to the right side of the body.

This hemiparesis can vary from mild to severe and may be accompanied by some sensory deficits.

Oral apraxia, sometimes called nonverbal apraxia, refers to difficulty performing specific movements of the oral articulatory structures on command or in imitation. For example, if the clinician asks an individual with oral apraxia to "round your lips" or "raise your tongue to your top teeth," the individual will often attempt the movement. Frequently, he or she will move the lips or the tongue in a groping manner, but not be able to achieve the same movement even as an imitative response. Oral apraxia is not due to weakness, or decreased range of motion. Therefore, to identify oral apraxia, the clinician should observe the target movement in a reflexive task, such as blowing, or licking the top lip during eating. Similarly, one must determine that the inability to imitate the movement is due to a comprehension problem. The individual with oral apraxia understands what to do, and has the appropriate strength, range of motion, and coordination to perform the movement, but cannot do so volitionally. Although oral apraxia does not always accompany apraxia of speech, it occurs frequently especially early following stroke.

Limb apraxia is the term used to indicate difficulty performing arm movements even though there is no reduction in strength or reduced range of motion. Individuals will attempt to imitate arm positions or movements, but not be able to do so; however, the same or similar movement may be made easily in a non-imitative context. For example, the clinician may model moving the hand to touch the nose. The individual may attempt the movement but not be able to achieve it, yet a few minutes later will do so easily when needing to scratch his or her nose. Limb apraxia may not be evident unless specific testing is done to determine its presence. The clinician should be aware of the presence of a limb apraxia so that these deficits can be taken into account when planning gestural treatment or when making clinical decisions about augmentative communication.

Apraxia for phonation is sometimes seen immediately after the stroke and may last 2 to 3 weeks. It is characterized by the individual's inability to produce voice, even for a short sustained phonation or for a syllable, even though the vocal folds adduct adequately during reflexive cough and laughter. Individuals will often attempt to phonate, and will usually be very frustrated and frightened by their inability to produce a voice.

Differentiating Apraxia from Other Communication Disorders

Differentiation from Aphasia. The definitions presented in Chapter 1 of this text state that apraxia of speech is a motor planning deficit, that aphasia is a language deficit, and that dysarthria is a movement execution deficit. Despite these differing underlying impairments, some of the perceptual characteristics, such as incoordination, sound substitutions or distortions, and dysprosody, overlap. This overlap can be somewhat confusing. Several sources have detailed discussions differentiating specific behaviors among these disorders (Duffy, 1995; McNeil, 1997; Wertz et al., 1984). Even with such cogent descriptions, however, it can still be difficult to determine if the error in "I want a piece of bie" is a paraphasia due to aphasia or a mistiming error due to apraxia. The fact that individuals often have coexisting disorders, such as Broca's aphasia and apraxia of speech, further complicates the issue.

Whether sound level errors (especially sound substitutions) are linguistically based errors due to aphasia or phonetic errors due to apraxia is one of the most common questions discussed with regard to differential diagnosis. One way of distinguishing the two problems is by site of lesion. Apraxia of speech often results from damage to the frontal lobe and literal paraphasias from damage to the temporal and/or parietal lobes. However, because apraxia of speech can also occur following lesions to the dominant temporal and/or parietal lobes, the neuroanatomical lesion site alone does not always differentiate the two error types.

Other factors distinguish apraxic sound errors from literal paraphasias, including the following: (a) apraxic errors are more predictable than aphasic errors, (b) prosody is more interrupted in apraxia than in aphasia, (c) apraxic errors are less "off target" in place and manner than aphasic errors, and (d) speakers with apraxia may produce sounds that are perceived to be non-English, whereas literal paraphasias are always real English phonemes (Wertz et al., 1984). Although many similarities exist in descriptions of sound errors for individuals with aphasia and for those with apraxia of speech (McNeil, 1997), clinicians usually note that individuals for whom apraxia of speech contributes to the overall communication disorder will have difficulty initiating utterances, will attempt to correct articulatory errors, may grope toward articulatory configurations, will exhibit sound distortions, and will have more dysprosody than individuals with aphasia but no apraxia of speech.

Question: Since it seems common for apraxia of speech and aphasia to occur together, why is it so important to determine differential diagnosis? If an individual has both, why does it matter?

It is important to be able to differentiate the relative contribution of each of these disorders to an individual's communication deficit because it is necessary for devising an appropriate treatment approach, that is, one that focuses on the nature of the impairment. For example, if language deficits, such as difficulty retrieving words, making paraphasic errors, and

(continues)

so on, contribute more to the individual's inability to complete communicative intent, it would be important to devise treatment strategies designed to improve these linguistic skills. On the other hand, if motor planning is impaired so that the apraxia contributes substantially to the communication disorder, one would need to provide intervention that focused on motor learning. Readers will find in Chapter 13 that these approaches to intervention are quite different. In order to provide the most efficient and efficacious treatment, the clinician should focus on remediation of the impairment that most interferes with communication.

Although much has been written about the importance of differential diagnosis, it is also critical to remember that it is okay not to be sure. Apraxic individuals will present with a huge variety of presenting symptoms. It is not necessary that the individual display a particular specific set of symptoms that fits a certain diagnostic label in order for you to plan treatment. It is necessary that you look at the individual's *pattern* of errors in a variety of contexts, make a reasonable judgment as to the relative contribution of linguistic versus motoric deficits, and plan treatment taking both into account.

Differentiation from Dysarthria. Differentiating apraxia of speech from dysarthria seems more straightforward than distinguishing aphasic from apraxic errors. However, there are similarities between the two disorders. First, both are disorders of speech, not language. Recently, researchers have emphasized that the distinction between errors of planning and programming movement may not be easily distinguished from errors in execution of that movement (McNeil et al., 1997; Rosenbek & McNeil, 1991). Because of the complex interaction of central and peripheral motor control systems, as well as the important role of afferent information, differentiating among levels of motor impairment can be difficult, especially for speech. Perhaps because of this complicated interaction of motor systems, both dysarthria and apraxia are characterized by symptoms that overlap each other. For example, dysprosody, articulatory distortion, and slow rate are common symptoms found in both disorders.

Although some symptoms occur in each of the disorders, there are also factors that differentiate the two. First, individuals with apraxia of speech typically do not exhibit paralysis, weakness, or incoordination of movement due to problems with innervation of the muscles themselves (e.g., peripheral nerve damage). Therefore, there is no problem with chewing, swallowing, or coughing, as is commonly associated with dysarthria. Individuals with apraxia of speech typically perform oral articulatory movement for nonspeech tasks with correct range of motion, speed, and strength.

Another factor frequently differentiating the two motor speech disorders is that in dysarthria, one often sees impairment in all speech subsystems, including respiration, phonation, resonance, articulation, and prosody. In apraxia of speech, the primary impairment is specifically articulatory with prosodic alterations that may be compensatory. One does see laryngeal involvement in individuals who are apraxic for phonation, but in this case one would hear phonation for reflexive acts like coughing and laughter. In dysarthria, movement of the vocal folds for reflexive action will usually be similar to movement of the vocal folds during phonation.

Speakers with apraxia are more affected by the context in which an utterance is produced than are speakers with dysarthria. Individuals with apraxia will have more difficulty with novel or unpracticed utterances than with those that they have said often. Speakers with dysarthria will exhibit motor speech performance that is quite similar, no matter how well practiced the utterance. In general, individuals with dysarthria will also exhibit error patterns such as hypernasality, sound distortions, and weak articulatory contacts consistently, even as the phonetic complexity is increased.

UNILATERAL UPPER MOTOR NEURON LESIONS—FLACCID DYSARTHRIA

Although the communication disorders of aphasia and apraxia of speech are common in stroke, dysarthria may also occur. The features of dysarthria associated with stroke are dependent upon the size and site of the vascular lesion. In unilateral upper motor neuron (UUMN) lesions, the clinical features of the dysarthria include weakness and in some cases incoordination of the face and tongue on the side opposite the lesion (Hartman & Abbs, 1992). Dysarthria in unilateral stroke is typically mild and temporary and may coexist with and be masked by other neurologic communication disorders such as apraxia of speech or aphasia (Duffy, 1995). In a retrospective study of 56 individuals with UUMN dysarthria at the Mayo Clinic, imprecise consonant production was by far the most common deviant speech feature. Slow speaking and reduced oral movement rates were also found. These changes in articulation are consistent with the physical findings of unilateral lower facial weakness and unilateral lingual weakness. Although much less common than changes in articulation, changes in phonation (vocal harshness) and velopharyngeal function (hypernasality) were also noted on occasion. The neurologic bases of the phonatory and velopharyngeal features are unclear.

Question: What is a lacunar stroke and why is the disorder important in the discussion of UUMN dysarthria?

A *lacune* is a small cavity. Thus, the term *lacunar infarct* arises because of the small cavity left as the lesion heals. Lacunar infarcts are small strokes usually associated with hypertension. There are at least 20 different lacunar syndromes (Fisher, 1982; Huang & Broe, 1984; Urban, Hopf, Zorowka, Fleischer, & Andreas, 1996). A number of these have dysarthria as one of their defining characteristics (Duffy, 1995):

- *Pure motor hemiparesis:* Symptoms are isolated to motor function of the face, arm, and leg on one side. Lesions may be in the corona radiata, internal capsule, cerebral peduncle, or pons.

- *Ataxic hemiparesis:* Symptoms include motor hemiparesis and cerebellar dysmetria. Lesions may be in the pons or corona radiata.

- *Dysarthria clumsy hand syndrome:* Symptoms include dysarthria, dysphagia, and slight weakness or clumsiness of the hand. Lesions are usually in the genu or posterior limb of the internal capsule or the adjacent corona radiata, and sometimes in the pons (Spertell & Ransom, 1979).

- *Pure dysarthria:* The symptom is dysarthria with no other signs. Lesions are usually in the genu of the internal capsule or the adjacent corona radiata (Ichikawa & Kageyame, 1991; Kim, 1994).

For background information regarding neurology and neurophysiology, readers are encouraged to access the World Wide Web site maintained by the authors:

http://www.skyport.com/ticetech/

BILATERAL CORTICAL LESIONS—SPASTIC DYSARTHRIA

Bilateral lesions of the corticobulbar fibers are much more likely than unilateral lesions to produce chronic dysarthria. Bilateral cortical lesions produce a pseudobulbar palsy and associated spastic dysarthria in approximately 4% of patients with cerebrovascular disease (Loeb, Gandolfo, Caponnetto, & Del-Sette, 1990). Cerebral palsy, severe brain injuries, multiple sclerosis, progressive degeneration of the brain, encephalitis, and extensive brain tumors may also cause spastic dysarthria.

The perceptual characteristics of speakers with pseudobulbar dysarthria were studied as part of the classical Mayo Clinic study (Darley et al., 1975).

Bilateral upper motor neuron lesions result in a number of motor problems, including spasticity, weakness, reduced range of movement, and slowness of movement. These motor problems can affect all components of speech production. The strained–strangled voice quality is associated with hyperadduction of the true and false vocal cords and is characterized aerodynamically by elevated laryngeal airway resistance and subglottal pressure, and by reduced laryngeal airflow (Murdoch, Thompson, & Stokes, 1994). Velopharyngeal dysfunction includes increased pharyngeal constriction; slow, sluggish velopharyngeal movement; and incomplete velopharyngeal closure (Aten, 1983). Hypernasality was perceived in many subjects with stroke (Darley et al., 1975); hyponasality and normal nasal resonance are also apparent (Thompson & Murdoch, 1995). Speakers with upper motor neuron lesions exhibit reductions in maximum lip force, endurance of lip strength, and rate of lip movements (Thompson, Murdoch, & Stokes, 1995b). Although the correlation between physiologic deficit and the perceptual characteristics of speech is far from perfect (Thompson et al., 1995a, 1995b), such articulatory impairments may result in imprecise consonant production and slowed speaking rates.

LESIONS IN THE AREA OF VERTEBROBASILAR CIRCULATION—FLACCID DYSARTHRIA

The vertebral arteries and the basilar artery, and their branches, supply blood to a number of areas, including the upper cervical spinal cord, the cerebellum, the medulla oblongata, the pons, and most of the remaining mesencephalon. Infarcts in these areas are less common than cortical infarcts, accounting for 15% of all CVAs. Brainstem strokes may result in a flaccid paralysis of the speech muscles. The two major muscular abnormalities are weakness and hypotonia. These abnormalities are seen in all movements of affected muscles, including those movements that are reflexive, automatic, or voluntary in origin. The salient perceptual speech characteristics of a group of 30 individuals with bulbar palsy included marked hypernasality often coupled with nasal emission of air, continuous breathiness during phonation, and audible inspiration (stridor on inhalation) (Darley et al., 1975).

Locked-in syndrome (LIS) is a term applied to a complex of symptoms with particularly profound effects on communication. Individuals with LIS have severe movement problems that affect the speech musculature, as well as limbs; however, language and cognition do not limit function. Early medical complications also include pulmonary, visual, and swallowing problems. The most common etiology, vascular occlusion of the basilar artery, affects the ventral aspects of the pons and descending motor pathways. Damage in this area results in the inability to control muscles voluntarily or reflexively. The nerve tracts that activate the trunk and limbs via the spinal nerves also pass through the brain stem. Therefore, severe damage to this area may impair motor control of the limbs as well as the oral structures. The dysarthria experienced by these individuals is usually of the predominantly flaccid type, but a marked spastic component may also be present in addition to the flaccidity.

Three levels of severity have been proposed for LIS (Bauer, Gerstenbrand, & Rumpl, 1979): a *complete form* in which individuals are immobile and unable to communicate but EEGs do not reflect abnormalities, a *classical form* in which individuals are conscious but mute with preservation of voluntary vertical eye movements, and an *incomplete form* in which individuals have limited voluntary movement in addition to eye movements. Although many individuals with LIS survive, the prognosis for good recovery of motor function is poor (Haig, Katz, & Sahgal, 1987; McCusker, Rudick, Honch, & Griggs, 1982; Patterson & Grabois, 1986). Early recovery of horizontal eye movements may be a good prognostic indicator (Yang, Lieberman, & Hong, 1989).

Reports of long-term follow-up studies of individuals with LIS and severe dysarthria are available (Culp & Ladtkow, 1992; McGann & Paslawski, 1991; Simpson, Till, & Goff, 1988). Culp and Ladtkow followed 16 individuals for at least 1 year. Outcomes in terms of general medical characteristics suggested that all remained nonambulatory, and many continued to experience visual impairment (44%) and swallowing difficulties (19%). Only 12% continued to need ventilatory assistance. Outcomes for communication suggested that functional natural speech returned in one quarter of the cases, and one half of the cases were able to operate augmentative communication systems by direct selection and the others used scanning strategies.

Question: Is the term locked-in syndrome synonymous with other terms associated with severe communication problems, such as akinetic mutism or persistent vegetable state?

No, these terms are not synonymous. Although they share the common symptom of mutism or speechlessness, they differ in underlying pathophysiology and other clinical features. An excellent review of the various types of acquired mutism can be found elsewhere (Turkstra & Bayles, 1992). *Locked-in syndrome* is the result of bilateral corticospinal and bulbar lesions. Individuals with LIS are alert but, because of profound movement problems, may be able to communicate only through eye movements. *Persistent vegetative state* is the result of widespread neocortical damage frequently associated with traumatic brain injury. Individuals in this state may have sleep–wake cycles but are not responsive to external stimulation and do not visually track objects. Their muteness is consistent with severe reduction in arousal and cognition. *Akinetic mutism* is

(continues)

the result of frontal lobe–limbic system pathology and is characterized by a profound motor initiation problem in the absence of paralysis or sensory deficits. These individuals may have a damaged drive mechanism for actions and emotions (Sapir & Aronson, 1985).

The patterns of augmentative communication intervention have been presented in five stages (Beukelman & Mirenda, 1998). The following sections describe these stages as they relate to the recovery of motor speech function.

Stage 1: No Useful Speech

During the acute stages of locked-in syndrome, individuals are typically left with no useful speech and may be ventilator dependent. The goals during this stage include providing the patient and family with information and establishing basic communication (Culp & Ladtkow, 1992). Establishing communication involves assessing basic comprehension skills, identifying reliable motor responses, and faciliting a simple yes/no response. Unfortunately some individuals remain at this stage for prolonged periods of time. For these individuals, more complex augmentative communication techniques are developed, including choice making, pointing, and use of multipurpose electronic devices (Beukelman & Mirenda, 1998).

After medical stabilization and establishment of a simple means of communication, attention may turn to establishing the physiologic building blocks for natural speech. Frequently this involves exercises and posture adjustments designed to increase respiratory support. These techniques are reviewed in Chapter 7. Oral and lingual exercises to increase the rate, range, and precision of articulatory movements may also be used.

J. H. Montgomery (1991) wrote about his experience with early speech therapy following his brain stem stroke:

> I well remember hearing those first useful vowel sounds I made. They were music to my ears. Mind you, the quality was poor, but Pam [the Speech–Language Pathologist] was getting the chords to work. Someone told me that my lack of speech etc., would create a "locked-in" syndrome. Believe me, I was "locked-in" my body all right, but those first sounds were as a key rattling in the lock. (p. 88)

Stage 2: Natural Speech Supplemented by Augmentative Communication

During this stage some natural speech may begin to emerge. This is often characterized by the ability to produce voluntary phonation, that is, to interrupt the vegetative respiratory cycle and coordinate the respiration with vocal fold adduction. Phonation may first be apparent when the speaker is in the supine position where gravity is of assistance in generating a forceful exhalation. Velopharyngeal and oral articulatory function are typically so compromised that vowels are undifferentiated and consonants are not understandable. Speakers at this stage need to rely on augmentative communication approaches (often alphabet and word boards) for most of their novel messages. They may be able to respond verbally to some questions in which the set of possible responses is small or may point to the first letter of words they are producing. See Chapter 12 for a detailed discussion of the integration of augmentative communication approaches and natural speech.

In the previous stage, speech treatment usually focuses on strengthening of specific components of speech production, for example, respiratory or tongue movement. This type of treatment often involves nonspeech exercises, such as the blow-bottle activities described in Chapter 7. During Stage 2, treatment usually shifts to speech activities. Intelligibility drills in which the speaker produces one word from a small set of options is one such activity. These drills are described in Chapter 11 and can be constructed so that they focus on vowel differentiation (*hill, hole, who'll*), final consonants (*mad, man, map*), and so on. Prosthetic devices such as palatal lifts or respiratory paddles may also be considered at this stage.

Stage 3: Reduction in Speech Intelligibility

At this stage, natural speech may be the primary means of communication. Although not completely understandable in all situations, speech has gone beyond a one-word-at-a-time effort to the ability to produce multiple syllables or words on a single breath. Augmentative communication approaches are used only in specific situations, such as resolving a communication breakdown or communicating in a very noisy environment. Prosthetic devices, such as palatal lifts, continue to be helpful. Other devices such as voice amplifiers may help some speakers reduce respiratory fatigue. Speech treatment focuses on those aspects of speech that appear to be interfering with intelligibility, naturalness, or ease of production.

Stage 4: Obvious Disorder with Intelligible Speech

During this stage, speech rate and naturalness may be affected but intelligibility is good. Therefore, treatment focuses on producing natural sounding speech in a manner that is nonfatiguing. Pausing at appropriate grammatical boundaries, signaling prominence of stressed words, and other techniques that focus on the prosodic aspects of speech may be employed.

When recovery of speech occurs during this stage, it is typically over a long period of time. Excellent case reports are available that describe the chronology of recovery and sequence of treatment for individuals with brain stem stroke (Simpson et al., 1988). The case described by Simpson and her colleagues extended over a 42-month period. Obviously, there are many challenges involved in managing such cases. Typically, more than one service unit and thus more than one clinician is involved. The continuity of information needed for treatment planning is difficult, especially when one considers the variety of different types of intervention that may be appropriate at different stages of recovery.

Stage 5: No Detectable Motor Speech Disorder

It is rare in cases of severe brain stem stroke that individuals regain speech that is normal in terms of rate and articulatory precision.

TRAUMATIC BRAIN INJURY
Pathology–Medical Aspects

EPIDEMIOLOGY

Injuries to the head resulting in either temporary or permanent brain damage are, unfortunately, common. However, the actual number of head injuries is difficult to estimate for at least two reasons. First, head injuries frequently go unreported because they may not require hospitalization. Second, no consistent definition of such an injury has been used across studies. For example, diagnoses such as facial lacerations, skull fractures, or brain contusions may be reported as head injuries. For purposes of this text, the discussion will be restricted to traumatic brain injury (TBI). Based on vehicle registration data, hospital records, trauma registries, and personal interview surveys, the Centers for Disease Control and Prevention estimated roughly 2 million cases of traumatic brain injury in 1990. Of these injuries, 20% to 30% are severe enough to result in chronic disability (Waxweiler, Thurman, Sniezek, Sosin, & O'Neil, 1995).

The occurrence of brain injury is two to three times higher in men than in women for all ages. However, the greatest difference in incidence between the sexes occurs in the group between 15 and 24 years of age. Other high-risk groups include the elderly over age 75 years and infants. Road crashes (including motorcycle, bicycle, other vehicles, and pedestrians) account for the majority of traumatic brain injuries. National trends in TBI deaths from 1979 through 1992 suggest a 25% decline in motor vehicle–related rates but a 13% increase in firearm-related rates (Sosin, Sniezek, & Waxweiler, 1995). Among children, falls constitute another major cause of head injuries. Both chronic and acute types of brain injuries can be attributed to some sports (American Academy of Neurology, 1997; Sandel, Bell, & Michaud, in press). Although some advances have been made in modifying sports equipment and practices and in mandating the use of safety equipment on motor vehicles, recent trends to repeal such safety and speed laws and increasing use of firearms may impact the future statistics regarding TBI.

CLASSIFICATION OF BRAIN INJURY

Brain injuries can be classified as either *penetrating* or *closed*. Penetrating injuries include bullet or knife wounds, or wounds from other sharp instruments seen in pediatric cases, such as pencils and knitting needles. On the whole, penetrating injuries are less frequent in the civilian population than in the military and often manifest more focal neurologic findings than closed head injuries. The biomechanics of closed head injury are important in understanding the resultant neuropathology. With a blow to the head or a simple fall, a compression injury may result in a local indentation of the skull, with the lesion appearing directly below the site of impact (the coup lesion). With acceleration injuries, a number of different mechanisms may occur singly or in combination. A simple linear translation motion of the brain substance may occur and result in lesions distal or opposite to the site of impact (the contrecoup lesion). When a rotational force occurs, shear strains are applied to the brain substance, resulting in more diffuse injuries. Any combination of these forces may occur with multiple sites and types of injuries (Shapiro, 1983).

The actual pathologic findings may include a skull fracture, found frequently in fatal injuries. However, the presence of a skull fracture by itself does not indicate a significant traumatic brain injury, nor is it necessarily present in severe TBI. Brain lesions may be focal, for example, in extradural or subdural hematomas or intracerebral contusions. These contusions are frequently found on the undersurface of the temporal and frontal lobes and at the anterior poles of the temporal lobe, regardless of the actual site of impact. This is probably due to the bony structure of the skull. Diffuse white matter lesions may also occur, especially in the corpus callosum and the superior cerebellar peduncles (Grossman & Gildenberg, 1982; Jennett & Teasdale, 1981).

A further distinction can be made between the primary damage due to the impact and secondary damage, which occurs in response to injury. The secondary processes include edema (tissue swelling), hypoxia (low level of oxygen), hypotension (low blood pressure level), and vasospasm (constriction of blood vessels resulting in deficient blood supply). Tissue injury also produces free radicals, molecules that cause a flood of excitatory amino acids resulting in axonal injury.

Other injuries, including *mild traumatic brain injury* and *chronic brain injury*, fall under the general category of closed head injury. Although terminological confusion exists in the area of mild TBI, classification of mild traumatic brain injury may be made on the basis of the presence or absence of mental status changes, amnesia, loss of consciousness, anatomical lesion, or neurologic deficit (Cattelani, Gugliotta, Maravita, & Mazzucchi, 1996; Esselman & Uomoto, 1995; Kibby & Long, 1996). In chronic traumatic brain injury or posttraumatic dementia ("Boxer's Brain"), lesions are often found in deep central structures of the brain such as the thalamus and basal ganglia. These lesions result in a parkinsonian-type neurologic picture, as well as dementia.

COURSE OF RECOVERY

In general, rapid recovery after traumatic brain injury probably occurs on a biochemical basis; restoration of neurotransmitter function, oxygenation, and perfusion to brain tissue may also play a part (Jennett & Teasdale, 1981; Rosenthal, Griffith, Bond, & Miller, 1983). Recovery occurring over hours to days indicates that the neural system is likely to be still intact, although damaged. Restoration of function may be seen even after months or perhaps years; the reason for this recovery is not yet understood. For motor activity, it appears that therapy encourages a reorganization of the motor cortex that preserves or redirects neural activity (Nudo, Wise, SiFuentes, & Milliken, 1996).

In individuals with severe brain injuries, roving eye movement and spontaneous eye opening are usually the first functions to appear; they may appear deceptively purposeful even in unresponsive patients. The motor response is the best indicator of recovery in these patients and usually occurs in the sequence listed in the *Glasgow Coma Scale* (Teasdale & Jennett, 1972). Improving motor abilities may be accompanied by emerging movement disorders, such as tremors or dystonic movements. These movement disorders generally improve over time. The verbal response also improves along the same scale: Initially, the person may be noisy and disinhibited; this is usually followed by a period of confusion, disorientation, and possible delusional or hallucinatory behavior. Verbal ability may be difficult to evaluate in critically injured persons who may be intubated or otherwise unable to produce audible speech.

The end of coma is usually marked by the patient's ability to follow one-stage commands and to communicate in some manner with others. However, posttraumatic amnesia (the length of time from the point of injury to return of continuous memory) may persist beyond the end of coma by weeks. The end of posttraumatic amnesia is often described by the patient as "waking up." At this time, other, more subtle, behavior abnormalities may manifest themselves.

PHYSICAL AND NEUROLOGIC COMPLICATIONS AND SEQUELAE

The patient with TBI acquired in a vehicular accident is likely to have other injuries in such areas as the thoracic, abdominal, and skeletal systems. Of particular consequence to future communication abilities are craniofacial fractures and cervical spine fracture/dislocations. Long-term musculoskeletal problems may include the formation of heterotopic bone in limbs where spasticity and paresis occur, especially at the hip, shoulder, and elbow. Untreated, this may significantly decrease functional range of motion at the involved joint and compromise seating, mobility, and hand use. Treatment consists of the administration of etidronates or radiation and surgical resection of the abnormal bone (Buschbacher, 1992).

Permanent neurologic sequelae and complications are common. Cranial nerve deficits are observed in about 32% of persons with severe head injuries (Jennett & Teasdale, 1981). Some of these cranial nerve injuries impact motor speech production. Visual disturbances are common and may include disorders of eye movement and gaze fusion, visual field deficits, or acuity defects. The most common disorders include mild exotropia, accommodative dysfunction, convergence insufficiency, poor fixation and pursuits, and diplopia, resulting in blurred vision, difficulty in reading or using a computer monitor, and headaches (Schlageter, Gray, Hall, Shaw, & Sammet, 1993). The facial nerve is second only to the olfactory nerve in frequency of involvement. Signs of recovery should be present within 8 weeks of injury if recovery is to occur; nerve conduction and electromyographic studies may assist in assessing prognosis. Vestibular dysfunction may be the basis for dizziness or vertigo in some patients. Auditory loss may be frequent but often goes undetected; of those tested, greater than 50% of individuals with TBI are abnormal, especially with high-frequency losses. Tinnitus is often present without any objective eighth-nerve findings on auditory or vestibular testing (Gizzi, 1995).

Disorders of movement are also quite common in individuals with TBI. Hemiparesis is present in 49% of individuals with severe brain injuries. The other most frequently encountered disorders include spasticity, bradykinesia, ataxia, tremors, rigidity, and apraxia. Sensory impairment may occur from decreased cortical function, such as deficits in graphesthesia, stereognosis, two-point discrimination, simultaneous tactile discrimination, and deep pain. Disorders of peripheral nerve function, especially at the brachial plexus in motorcycle injuries, may result in local paralysis or causalgia (Jennett & Teasdale, 1981; Rosenthal et al., 1995).

Epileptic seizures occurring early in the first week following TBI are not indicators of later epilepsy. Seizures occur commonly immediately after injury and during the first week after injury. Anticonvulsant medication is used during this time. The use of anticonvulsant medications (e.g., phenytoin, carbamazepine, valproic acid) for prophylaxis after the first week has not been shown to be effective to prevent the onset of later epilepsy. Posttraumatic seizures may occur in 10% to 40% of those with moderate to severe injuries, usually within the first 2 years postinjury. All anticonvulsants can cause some degree of psychomotor slowing (Massagli, 1991; Temkin et al., 1990; Yablon, 1993).

COGNITIVE AND BEHAVIORAL SEQUELAE

The cognitive impairment that remains after severe or even mild brain injury may frequently persist despite the resolution of motor or sensory deficits. Several comprehensive sources of information regarding cognition and communication are available (Coelho, DeRuyter, & Stein, 1996; Gillis, 1996; Hartley, 1995; Sohlberg & Mateer, 1989; Yorkston & Kennedy, in press). Cognitive and behavioral deficits have a greater impact on the resumption of normal occupation than do neurologic sequelae. The areas most affected appear to be initiative and activity level, attention and concentration, memory, language and thinking, problem solving, judgment, and pragmatic skills. Persons often demonstrate decreased drive and stamina, as well as a slowness of movement or reaction after TBI. Studies have indicated that, even in individuals with good recovery, significant reductions in attention and concentration, rapid processing of information, and endurance in problem solving may exist (Stuss et al., 1985). Memory in all areas can be affected, but especially in complex new learning situations. The recovery of memory and learning is much slower than other functions. Treatments for cognitive disorders may include attentional training, incorporation of implicit memory strategies into task structures, or the use of medications including methylphenidate, pemoline, dextroamphetamine, piracetam, selegiline, and selective serotonin reuptake inhibitors such as fluoxetine.

The behavior of the individual with brain injury may be attributable to the premorbid personality, organic damage sustained during the injury, and reaction to the injury itself. Frontal lobe lesions are manifested by decreased drive, apathy, lethargy, social disinhibition, poor judgment, inappropriate sexual and aggressive behavior, dull affect, and denial of deficits. Depression occurs in about 26% of persons with TBI and may adversely affect cognitive function (Fedoroff et al., 1992; Rosenthal, Christensen, & Ross, 1998; Sandel & Zwil, 1997). Anger management and episodic lack of control are frequent behavioral issues, sometimes complicated by alcohol use (Corrigan, Smith-Knapp, & Granger, 1998; Wiercisiewski & McDeavitt, 1997). Treatment for these syndromes includes counseling, behavioral strategies, and the use of psychoactive medications. Families must contend with altered family roles as well as adjusting to their family member's cognitive, behavioral, and physical challenges (Kreutzer, Marwitz, & Depler, 1992).

Outcome and Prognosis

At least two premorbid factors—psychosocial status and age—have a bearing on overall recovery from traumatic brain injury. Patients with premorbid job stability and higher education are more likely to return to work after traumatic brain injury (Dikmen et al., 1994). Persons under 20 years of age are more likely to achieve a good outcome. Morbidity increases with increasing age. This may be due to the medical consequences accompanying severe brain injury rather than to the injury itself (Rosenthal et al., 1983).

The type of injury will also have an effect on survival and recovery. The presence of coma after injury is a negative prognostic factor, particularly when one looks at the duration and depth of coma, as measured by the *Glasgow Coma Scale*. The motor response is the most powerful predictor of global outcome. The duration of posttraumatic amnesia is another powerful predictor of outcome (Katz & Alexander, 1994).

Although there may be individual exceptions, the statistics on overall outcome indicate that the major part of recovery is accomplished by 3 to 6 months after injury. Of those who have a good recovery by 12 months, about two thirds have done so by 3 months and fully 90% by 6 months (Rosenthal et al., 1983). Of all patients with severe brain injury, about half are dead within 6 months. Between 12% and 26% will achieve a good recovery. The rest will be significantly disabled, and about half will remain dependent on others for activities of daily living (Jennett & Teasdale, 1981).

The situation for children is quite different. However, what may initially appear to be a good outcome for a child may still represent a loss because mental and physical development may not reach the child's true potential. Children under age 15 are rarely in a vegetative state or severely disabled (totally dependent for all activities of daily living, but conscious). Ninety percent or more are moderately disabled or better at 3 years after their injuries. In fact, independent ambulation can be expected in 70% to 80% of children in a coma for up to 3 months. However, cognitive impairment commonly persists despite physical recovery and, as noted, may be even more disabling to children who must accomplish so much new learning (Shapiro, 1983). Studies of the long-term recovery of children with TBI are available (Fay et al., 1993; Fay et al., 1994; Jaffe et al., 1992; Jaffe et al., 1993; Jaffe, Polissar, Fay, & Liao, 1995).

Swallowing Disorders

Like swallowing disorders associated with stroke, prevalence of dysphagia in TBI is initially high but decreases as time goes by. In a study of the prevalence of swallowing problems in three clinical settings, acute medical wards, acute rehabilitation units, and an outpatient rehabilitation program, prevalence declined from a high of nearly 80% on acute medical wards to approximately 10% later in recovery when patients were participating in outpatient services (Yorkston, Honsinger, Mitsuda, & Hammen, 1989). In another long-term follow-up study, over 90% of individuals with TBI and swallowing or oral motor problems on admission eventually successfully ate by mouth (Winstein, 1983). The average time from injury to the first oral meal in this group was 3 months. The simultaneous clearing of cognition and resolution of primitive oral motor reflexes may contribute to these positive changes in swallowing.

Descriptions of the nature of dysphagia in TBI are also available. Most frequently, disorders include delayed or absent swallowing reflex, reduced tongue control, and reduced peristalsis (Lazarus, 1991; Lazarus & Logemann, 1987). In this study of 53 individuals with head trauma, most of the time multiple swallowing problems were apparent and individuals frequently did not cough reflexively during or after episodes of aspiration. Detailed description of assessment and management of swallowing disorders in TBI, including such topics as tracheostomy tubes and hyperreflexia–hypersensitivity are available elsewhere (Lazarus, 1991).

Careful management of swallowing disorders in individuals with TBI is particularly critical because hypermetabolism in this population may require increased nutritional support (Godbole, Berbiglia, & Baddard, 1991). In a study of nonsedated, nonparalyzed patients with severe head injuries, mean rest metabolic rates were approximately 140% of normal. Thus, patients with head injuries have a metabolic response similar to that reported for patients with severe burns.

Speech Characteristics

OCCURRENCE OF DYSARTHRIA

The neuropathology associated with TBI is diffuse and variable. Therefore, a number of communication problems are common. Language is frequently disrupted as part of a complex constellation of memory and cognitive deficits. Reviews of these communication problems can be found elsewhere (Gillis, 1996; Kennedy & DeRuyter, 1991; Yorkston & Kennedy, in press). The focus of the remainder of this section will not be on the cognitive–communication problems but rather on the dysarthria, one of the motor speech disorders commonly associated with TBI. Overall dysarthria is present as a sequelae to TBI in approximately one third of the population (Sarno, Buonaguro, & Levita, 1986). However, the prevalence varies depending on the time postonset, with estimates of 60% of individuals acutely exhibiting dysarthria and 10% exhibiting the disorder at long-term follow-up (Yorkston et al., 1989).

CHARACTERISTICS OF THE DYSARTHRIA

Dysarthria associated with TBI may be temporary or persistent, mild or severe, compatible with deficits or disproportionately severe, and accompanied or not by other language and cognitive disorders (Yorkston & Beukelman, 1991). A growing number of case reports document the diversity in the pattern of dysarthria associated with TBI. Most dysarthrias are characterized as mixed (i.e., spastic–ataxic or flaccid–spastic); however, case reports also exist of predominately ataxic and predominately flaccid types (Yorkston & Beukelman, 1991). Variability in the site of the lesion and the nature and severity of the physiologic impairment necessitates the development of individualized treatment programs based on a thorough understanding of the disorder (Theodoros, Murdoch, & Stokes, 1995). Multiple examples of speech intervention programs for individuals with TBI can be found in Chapters 7 through 12 of this text.

The physiologic impairment associated with dysarthria in TBI is not restricted to a single subsystem; rather multiple aspects of speech production are impaired, including the prosodic, resonance, articulatory, respiratory, and phonatory aspects of speech (Theodoros, Murdoch, & Chenery, 1994). Group studies of speech breathing suggest that individuals with TBI have lower vital capacities and lower forced expiratory volumes than nondisabled speakers (Murdoch, Theodoros, Stokes, & Chenery, 1993). Kinematic analysis of the same groups indicated that speakers with TBI had problems coordinating the action of the rib cage and abdomen during speech. Individuals with dysarthria also may differ from controls in that they tend to pause to breathe at ungrammatical locations (Hammen & Yorkston, 1994). Differences between speakers with TBI and control speakers have also been found in the laryngeal (Theodoros & Murdoch, 1994), velopharyngeal (Theodoros, Murdoch, Stokes, & Chenery, 1993; Ziegler & von Cramon, 1983a, 1983b), and articulation (Barlow & Burton, 1990; Theodoros et al., 1994) systems.

COURSE OF RECOVERY

Long-term studies of dysarthria associated with TBI are becoming available for both children and adults. Although dysarthria may resolve during the early and middle stages of recovery, severe motor speech deficits may persist (Dongilli, Hakel, & Beukelman, 1992). In the case of severe dysarthria, a strong trend emerging from the literature is the idea that important changes in speech can be obtained many years postonset of TBI (Enderby & Crow, 1990; Harris & Murry, 1984; Jordan & Murdoch, 1990; Jordan, Ozanne, & Murdoch, 1988; Keatley & Wirz, 1994; Light, Beesley, & Collier, 1988; Najensen, Sazbon, Feiselzon, Becker, & Schechter, 1978; Workinger & Netsell, 1992). See Table 3.3 for a summary of selected studies that report long-term follow-up or treatment after the acute recovery phase. For example, in a long-term study of four indi-

Table 3.3

Speech Follow-up and/or Treatment After the Acute Recovery Period

Reference	Case(s)	Symptoms	Time Frame	Outcomes
Enderby & Crow (1990)	4 young adults	Severe bulbar dysfunction	7 years	Changes in bulbar function began to improve as late as 24 to 30 months postonset
Harris & Murry (1984)	44-year-old man	Flaccid dysarthria, left facial paresis, left vocal fold paralysis	7 years	After 9 weeks of intensive practice, gains were noted in strength and movement of the tongue, velum, and larynx.
Jordan & Murdoch (1990, 1994)	7-year-old female	Mutism	10 months	Rapid recovery of communication skills with persistent higher level language deficits
Light, Beesley, & Collier (1988)	13-year-old female	Severe motor involvement with strong jaw extension flex	44 months	Used a series of augmentative communication systems, and finally used natural speech supplemented with augmentative techniques
McHenry, Wilson, & Minton (1994)	18-year-old woman	Inefficient speech breathing strategies, weak vocal fold adduction, open velopharyngeal port, and reduced articulatory muscle strength	21 months	Moderate improvement was noted in all of the speech subsystems treated
Netsell & Daniel (1979)	20-year-old man	Uniform weakness of speech components	7 months	With treatment, speech intelligibility improved from 5–10% to 95%, after other types of treatment had not resulted in change
Workinger & Netsell (1992)	16-year-old male	Spastic hemiplegia, cognitive deficits, and severe dysarthria	13 years	After 9 months of treatment, used natural speech as a functional means of communication

viduals with head injury and severe bulbar dysfunction, few gains were made within the first 18 months and substantial changes in function were noted for as long as 48 months postonset (Enderby & Crow, 1990). The implication of these findings is that the majority of recovery may not occur within the first year following injury. In order to exploit and extend return of motor speech function, long-term follow-up is necessary.

UNIQUE MANAGEMENT ISSUES

Individuals with TBI are becoming increasingly important in the caseloads of many speech–language pathologists who work in rehabilitation settings. Management of dysarthria in this population offers a number of unique challenges (Yorkston & Beukelman, 1991). First, clinicians are faced with dual challenges of a large population and a relatively meager fund of past experience and expertise. Unlike other populations associated with dysarthria, such as cerebral palsy, clinicians cannot rely on decades of clinical practice as the basis of their intervention. Second, changes in speech can be expected to occur over long periods of time. This, combined with the young age of many individuals with TBI and the diversity of their disorders, suggests that long-term planning and individual intervention are necessary. Delivery of such services may be difficult. Finally, individuals with TBI and dysarthria are particularly challenging because their cognitive deficits interact the motor speech disorders in ways that are both complex and poorly understood.

SCALES OF RECOVERY

Scales are available for describing recovery from TBI. For example, the *Glasgow Outcome Scale* (Jennett & Bond, 1975) was an early attempt to categorize individuals with TBI within one of five general outcomes: good recovery (resumption of normal life), moderate disability (disability is present but the individual is independent), severe disability (the individual is conscious but disabled and dependent), persistent vegetative state (the individual is unresponsive and speechless but has some wakefulness or eye opening), and death.

Another commonly used scale, often simply called the *Ranchos Scale*, is the *Levels of Cognitive Function* (LOCF) *Scale* developed at Ranchos Los Amigos Hospital (Hagen, 1984; Hagen, Malkmus, & Durham, 1979). This scale is commonly used to track individuals as they emerge from coma in the acute and middle stages of recovery. It contains the following eight levels:

I. No Response: The individual appears to be in a deep sleep and is completely unresponsive to any stimuli

II. Generalized Response: The individual reacts consistently and nonpurposefully to stimuli in a nonspecific manner.

III. Localized Response: The individual reacts specifically but inconsistently to stimuli.

IV. Confused–Agitated: The individual's behavior is bizarre and non-purposeful relative to the immediate environment.

V. Confused, Inappropriate, Nonagitated: The individual is able to respond to simple commands fairly consistently; however, with increased complexity of commands, responses are nonpurposeful, random, or fragmented.

VI. Confused–Appropriate: The individual shows goal-directed behavior but depends on external input for direction.

VII. Automatic Appropriate: The individual appears appropriate and oriented within hospital and home setting, goes through daily routine automatically, but is frequently robotlike; has shallow recall of activities; shows carryover for new learning but at a decreased rate; and continues to demonstrate impaired judgment.

VIII. Purposeful and Appropriate: The individual is able to recall and integrate past and recent events and is aware of and responsive to the environment, shows carryover for new learning and needs no supervision once activities are learned; and may continue to show a decreased ability relative to premorbid abilities.

Language behaviors (Kennedy & DeRuyter, 1991) and augmentative communication intervention (Ladtkow & Culp, 1992) for each of these levels has been described elsewhere.

STAGES OF FUNCTIONAL LIMITATIONS IN DYSARTHRIA

Dysarthria associated with TBI varies considerably both in type and severity. The following section summarizes five stages of intervention for motor speech disorders in TBI. At each stage, the features of functional limitation in dysarthria are described, along with some common augmentative communication and speech treatment approaches. Because the speakers' levels of awareness and cognition play an important role in this intervention, issues related to cognitive function are also described at each stage.

Stage 1: No Useful Speech

Some individuals with TBI produce no useful speech. The absence of useful speech may be the result of a number of factors, including poor cognition or arousal, severe motor deficits, or severe language deficits. Many individuals who came into rehabilitation during this stage regained speech once they reached Rancho Levels V and VI (Dongilli et al., 1992). For these individuals, the primary factors involved in their lack of speech were arousal deficits or severe cognitive limitation. For other nonspeaking individuals who may have progressed beyond cognitive levels V or VI, the underlying cause of speechlessness may be severe motor speech impairments or, more rarely, severe language impairment similar to a speaker with classic aphasia. The early prediction of later severe and persistent motor speech problems is very difficult. Factors such as primitive oral reflexes have been investigated and found to have a limited long-term predictive capability for persistent severe motor speech disorder. Many individuals who exhibit primitive oral reflexes at Levels III or IV later develop speech (Dongilli et al., 1992). When studying the prevalence of severe motor speech disorder, the greatest proportion occurred early postonset in the acute medical units, less occurred in the stage of acute rehabilitation, and the fewest occurred when individuals with TBI were in the outpatient phase (Yorkston et al., 1989).

Augmentative communication intervention at this stage depends on the level of cognitive function (DeRuyter & Kennedy, 1991; DeRuyter & Lafontaine, 1987). Three phases of intervention have been proposed for individuals in the early, middle, and late stages of cognitive recovery (Ladtkow & Culp, 1992): (1) initial choice making, which may involve establishing a consistent yes/no system; (2) pointing to simple alphabet board or common messages; and (3) multiple-purpose augmentative communication devices that allow for the production of unique messages. Table 3.4 lists the progress of augmentative

Table 3.4
Principal Goals of Intervention with a 13-Year-Old Girl over a 3-Year Period

Phase One: 6–9 months posttrauma
1. To establish consistent and reliable yes/no responses.
2. To develop a preliminary communication display as a means to indicate basic needs and wants.

Phase Two: 13–16 months posttrauma
1. To provide a means to request attention.
2. To encourage more explicit "yes" responses.
3. To develop a communication display as a means to share information and express needs and wants.

Phase Three: 22–23 months posttrauma
1. To provide access to a microcomputer for written communication.
2. To establish more explicit "no" responses for unfamiliar listeners.
3. To develop strategies to share information and generate novel vocabulary.

(continues)

Table 3.4 (*continued*)

Phase Four: 36 months posttrauma
1. To develop breath control, articulation skills, and voicing.
2. To develop strategies to interact effectively with unfamiliar partners and in group activities.
3. To develop conversational skills around a range of topics.
4. To enhance rate of written communication.

Phase Five: 40–44 months posttrauma
1. To continue to develop breath control, articulation skills, and voicing.
2. To recognize breakdowns in communication.
3. To use clarification strategies to repair conversation.

Note. From "Transition Through Multiple Augmentative and Alternative Communication Systems: A Three-Year Case Study of a Head Injury Adolescent," by J. Light, M. Beesley, and B. Collier, 1988, *Augmentative and Alternative Communication*, 4, p. 3. Copyright 1988 by AAC. Reprinted with permission.

communication approaches employed with an adolescent girl who experienced a severe brain injury.

Speech intervention during this stage focuses on establishing the physiologic support for speech. Typically this involves work with the various speech subsystems in nonspeech tasks. For example, blow-bottle tasks to establish adequate respiratory support for speech are reviewed in Chapter 7. Working with the speaker to achieve respiratory control, establishing phonation, palatal lift fitting, and so on, are described in Chapters 7 through 11.

Stage 2: Natural Speech Supplemented by Augmentative Communication

During Stage 2, natural speech can be used to carry part of the communicative load; however, communication is often easier if speech is supplemented with alphabet supplementation or other techniques, such as establishing the context or topics. See Chapter 12 for a more complete discussion of these techniques. Depending on the level of cognitive function, communication partners may need to take more or less responsibility for managing the interaction. At this stage, individuals may be taught to use *expectation dictionaries*, in which are listed a number of phrases that the individual with dysarthria is likely to say. When the individual with TBI says something that listeners do not understand, the listener says, "Is it in the dictionary?" If it is there, listeners request a repetition and attempt to respond to the verbal communication. If the utterance is not in the expectation dictionary, then the listener requests use of a different communication strategy, such as pointing to letters on an alphabet board.

Many augmentative communication techniques are designed to assist the speaker in using natural speech before his or her level of intelligibility would otherwise allow. This provides the speaker with early practice beyond what could be accomplished in the therapy room alone. During this stage, speech intervention activities move from nonspeech to speech tasks. For example, once an individual is able to achieve minimal competencies (i.e., a performance of 5 cm of water for 5 seconds on the blow bottle), respiratory–phonatory exercises shift to more speechlike tasks, such as sustained phonation, or consistently achieving good phonation on one- and two-syllable words. See Chapters 7 through 11 for details of these activities.

Stage 3: Reduction in Speech Intelligibility

At Stage 3, natural speech may be the primary means of communication, although dysarthria is obvious and communication breakdowns may need to be resolved with augmentative techniques. Speakers at this stage must learn to optimize their situation and manage their listeners well. Some speakers are able to do this easily and others are not. Intervention involves listener training to help them structure the communication exchange.

Speech treatment during this stage involves speech production rather than extensive use of nonspeech or speechlike activities. Treatment targets the specific aspects of speech that appear to be interfering with intelligibility. For example, if the speaker has not adopted the proper speaking rate, then treatment may focus on rate control. If the speaker has adopted some maladaptive behaviors, such as inappropriate breath groupings, then elimination of these behaviors may be the focus of work.

Stage 4: Obvious Disorder with Intelligible Speech

During Stage 4, dysarthria may persist but it does not impact speech intelligibility, although rate and naturalness are typically affected. Intervention may focus on improving speech naturalness. Because naturalness, or lack of it, does not usually involve a single speech subsystem, treatment usually focuses on some simple, overall aspect of speech that will impact a variety of symptoms. This approach to treatment can best be illustrated with a case. A 25-year-old man was several years postonset of TBI when he was evaluated through a job reentry program. For many months, he had independently practiced a list, given to him by a previous speech–language pathologist, of about a dozen "things to remember when talking." They included items such as "keep the volume up," "speak slowly," and "remember to enunciate all the sounds." As he talked about each of the items, he was successful in accomplishing the task. For example, when talking about the item "keep the volume up," he spoke quite loudly; when talking about the item "produce all speech sounds carefully," his articulation became very precise; and when talking about the item "speak slowly," he did so. When the conversation reverted to other things, he did none of the things on his list. He was probably being asked to do too much, to integrate too many separate actions. Depending on each client's cognitive level, the clinician needs to manage the complexity of the speech change assignment.

Stage 5: No Detectable Motor Speech Disorder

Although individuals with TBI at Stage 5 may not have a detectable motor speech disorder, they may still have considerable residual communication disorders that are reflected mostly in the areas of discourse and pragmatics. Here again, the cognitive issues are pertinent. During this stage, there is probably no detectable motor speech disorder, if the speaker is asked to perform a very controlled set of tasks. Such structured tasks involve few cognitive demands, such as those involved in generating novel discourse or interacting with a conversational partner. Speech may become more unusual (e.g., in intonation or pausal structure) in cognitively demanding situations. The absence of frank motor speech disorders does not suggest the absence of other cognitively based communication problems. At this point, motor speech intervention may well be over, but much work may remain in the areas of discourse and pragmatics.

REFERENCES

Adams, R. D., & Victor, M. (1985). *Principles of neurology*. New York: McGraw-Hill.

Alberts, M. J., Horner, J., Gray, L., & Brazer, S. R. (1992). Aspiration after stroke: Lesion analysis by brain MRI. *Dysphagia, 7*(3), 170–173.

American Academy of Neurology. (1997). Practice parameters: The management of concussion in sports. *Neurology, 48*, 581–585.

Aten, J. L. (1983). Treatment of spastic dysarthria. In W. H. Perkins (Ed.), *Dysarthria and apraxia*. New York: Thieme-Stratton.

Aviv, J. E., Martin, J. H., Sacco, R. L., Zagar, D., Diamond, B., Keen, M. S., & Blitzer, A. (1996). Supraglottic and pharyngeal sensory abnormalities in stroke patients with dysphagia. *Annals of Otology, Rhinology and Laryngology, 105*(2), 92–97.

Barer, D. H. (1989). The natural history and functional consequences of dysphagia after hemispheric stroke. *Journal of Neurology, Neurosurgery and Psychiatry, 52*, 236–241.

Barlow, S. M., & Burton, M. S. (1990). Ramp-and-hold force control in the upper and lower lips: Developing new neuromotor assessment applications in traumatic brain injured adults. *Journal of Speech and Hearing Research, 33*, 660–675.

Bauer, G., Gerstenbrand, F., & Rumpl, E. (1979). Varieties of the locked-in syndrome. *Journal of Neurology, 221*, 77–91.

Beukelman, D. R., & Mirenda, P. (1998). *Augmentative and alternative communication: Management of severe communication disorders in children and adults* (2nd ed.). Baltimore: Brookes.

Brandstater, M., & Basmajian, J. (1987). *Stroke rehabilitation.* Baltimore: Williams & Wilkins.

Buchholz, D. W. (1993). Clinically probable brainstem stroke presenting primarily as dysphagia and nonvisualized by MRI. *Dysphagia, 8,* 235–238.

Buschbacher, R. (1992). Heterotopic ossification: A review. *Critical Reviews in Physical Medicine & Rehabilitation, 4,* 199–213.

Cattelani, R., Gugliotta, M., Maravita, A., & Mazzucchi, A. (1996). Post-concussive syndrome: Para-clinical signs, subjective symptoms, congitive functions and MMPI profiles. *Brain Injury, 10*(3), 187–195.

Coelho, C. A., DeRuyter, F., & Stein, M. (1996). Treatment efficacy: Cognitive–communication disorders resulting from traumatic brain injury. *Journal of Speech and Hearing Research, 39*(5), S5–S17.

Collins, M. J., Rosenbek, J. C., & Wertz, R. T. (1983). Spectrographic analysis of vowel and word duration in apraxia of speech. *Journal of Speech and Hearing Research, 26,* 244.

Corrigan, J. D., Smith-Knapp, K., & Granger, C. V. (1998). Outcomes in the first 5 years after traumatic brain injury. *Archives of Physical Medicine and Rehabilitation, 79*(3), 298–305.

Culp, D., & Ladtkow, M. C. (1992). Locked-in syndrome and augmentative communication. In K. M. Yorkston (Ed.), *Augmentative communication in the medical setting* (pp. 59–138). Tucson, AZ: Communication Skill Builders.

Darley, F. (1969, November). *The classification of output disturbances in neurologic communication disorders.* A presentation at the American Speech and Hearing Association convention, Chicago.

Darley, F. L., Aronson, A. E., & Brown, J. R. (1975). *Motor speech disorders.* Philadelphia: Saunders.

DeRuyter, F., & Kennedy, M. R. (1991). Augmentative communication following traumatic brain injury. In D. R. Beukelman & K. M. Yorkston (Eds.), *Communication disorders following traumatic brain injury: Management of cognitive, language, and motor impairments* (pp. 317–365). Austin, TX: PRO-ED.

DeRuyter, F., & Lafontaine, L. M. (1987). The nonspeaking brain injured: A clinical and demographic database report. *Augmentative and Alternative Communication, 3,* 18–25.

Dikmen, S., Temkin, N. R., Machamer, J., Holubkor, A. L., Fraser, R., & Winn, H. R. (1994). Employment following traumatic head injuries. *Archives of Neurology, 51,* 177–186.

Dongilli, J. P., Hakel, M., & Beukelman, D. (1992). Recovery of functional speech following traumatic brain injury. *Journal of Head Trauma Rehabilitation, 7,* 91–101.

Dronker, N. F. (1996). A new brain region for coordinating speech articulation. *Nature, 384*(6605), 159–161.

Duffy, J. R. (1995). *Motor speech disorders: Substrates, differential diagnosis, and management.* St. Louis: Mosby.

Enderby, P., & Crow, E. (1990). Long-term recovery patterns of severe dysarthria following head injury. *British Journal of Disorders of Communication, 25,* 341–354.

Esselman, P. C., & Uomoto, J. M. (1995). Classification of the spectrum of mild traumatic brain injury. *Brain Injury, 9,* 417–424.

Evans, R. L., Connis, R. T., Hendricks, R. D., & Haselkorn, J. K. (1995). Multidisciplinary rehabilitation versus medical care: A meta-analysis. *Social Science and Medicine, 40,* 1699–1706.

Fay, G. C., Jaffe, K. M., Polissar, N. L., Liao, S., Martin, K. M., Shurtleff, H. A., Rivara, J. B., & Winn, H. R. (1993). Mild pediatric traumatic brain injury: A cohort study. *Archives of Physical Medicine and Rehabilitation, 74,* 895–901.

Fay, G. C., Jaffe, K. M., Polissar, N. L., Liao, S., Rivara, J. B., & Martin, K. M. (1994). Outcome of pediatric traumatic brain injury at three years: A cohort study. *Archives of Physical Medicine and Rehabilitation, 75*, 733–741.

Fedoroff, J. P., Starkstein, S. E., Forrester, A. W., Geisler, F., Jorge, R. E., Arndt, S. V., & Robinson, R. G. (1992). Depression in patients with acute traumatic brain injury. *American Journal of Psychiatry, 149*, 918–923.

Finestone, H. M., Greene-Finestone, L. S., Wilson, E. S., & Teasell, R. W. (1995). Malnutrition in stroke patients on the rehabilitation service and at follow-up: Prevalence and predictors. *Archives of Physical Medicine and Rehabilitation, 76*, 310–316.

Fisher, C. M. (1982). Lacunar strokes and infarcts: A review. *Neurology, 32*, 871–876.

Forrest, K., Adams, S., McNeil, M. R., & Southwood, H. (1991). Kinematic, electromyographic, and perceptual evaluation of speech apraxia, conduction aphasia, ataxic dysarthria, and normal speech production. In C. A. Moore, K. M. Yorkston, & D. R. Beukelman (Eds.), *Dysarthria and apraxia of speech: Perspective on management* (pp. 147–172). Baltimore: Brookes.

Garrison, S. J., & Rolak, L. A. (1993). Rehabilitation of the stroke patient. In J. A. DeLisa (Ed.), *Rehabilitation medicine: Principles and practice* (2nd ed., pp. 801–824). Philadelphia: Lippincott.

Gillis, R. J. (1996). *Traumatic brain injury rehabilitation for speech–language pathologists.* Boston: Butterworth-Heinemann.

Gizzi, M. (1995). The efficacy of vestibular rehabilitation for patients with head trauma. *Journal of Heady Injury Rehabilitation, 10*, 60–77.

Godbole, K. B., Berbiglia, V. A., & Baddard, L. (1991). A head-injured patient: Caloric needs, clinical progress and nursing care priorities. *Journal of Neuroscience Nursing, 23*(5), 290–294.

Goldstein, M., Bolis, L., Fieschi, C., Gorini, S., & Millikan, C. H. (Eds.). (1979). *Cerebrovascular disorders and strokes: Advances in neurology* (Vol. 25). New York: Raven Press.

Gordon, E. E., Drenth, V., Jarvis, L., Johnson, J., & Wright, V. (1978). Neurophysiologic syndromes in stroke as predictors of outcome. *Archives of Physical Medicine and Rehabilitation, 59*, 399.

Grossman, R. G., & Gildenberg, P. L. (1982). *Head injury: Basic and clinical concepts.* New York: Raven Press.

Hagen, C. (1984). Language disorders in head trauma. In A. Holland (Ed.), *Language disorders in adults: Recent advances* (pp. 245–282). Austin, TX: PRO-ED.

Hagen, C., Malkmus, D., & Durham, P. (1979). Levels of cognitive functions. In *Rehabilitation of head injured adults: Comprehensive physical management.* Downey, CA: Professional Staff Association of Ranchos Los Amigos Hospital.

Haig, A. J., Katz, R. T., & Sahgal, V. (1987). Mortality and complications of the locked-in syndrome. *Archives of Physical Medicine and Rehabilitation, 68*, 24–27.

Hammen, V. L., & Yorkston, K. M. (1994). Respiratory patterning and variability in dysarthric speech. *Journal of Medical Speech–Language Pathology, 2*, 253–262.

Harris, B., & Murry, T. (1984). Dysarthria and aphagia: A case study of neuromuscular treatment. *Archives of Physical Medicine and Rehabilitation, 65*, 408–412.

Hartley, L. L. (1995). *Cognitive–communicative abilities following brain injury.* San Diego: Singular.

Hartman, D. E., & Abbs, J. H. (1992). Dysarthria associated with focal unilateral upper motor neuron lesion. *European Journal of Disorders of Communication, 27*, 187–196.

Henley, S. H., Pettit, S., Todd-Pakropek, A., & Tupper, A. (1985). Who goes home? Prediction factors in stroke recovery. *Journal of Neurology, Neurosurgery and Psychiatry, 48*(1), 1–6.

Holas, M. A., DePippor, K. L., & Reding, M. J. (1994). Aspiration and relative risk of medical complications following stroke. *Archives of Neurology, 51*, 1051–1053.

Horner, J., Buoyer, F. G., Alberts, M. J., & Helms, M. J. (1991). Dysphagia following brain-stem stroke. Clinical correlations and outcome. *Archives of Neurology, 48,* 1170–1173.

Horner, J., Massey, E., Riski, J., Lathrop, D., & Chase, K. (1988). Aspiration following stroke: Clinical correlates and outcome. *Neurology, 38,* 1359–1362.

Huang, C. Y., & Broe, G. (1984). Isolated facial palsy: A new lacunar syndrome. *Journal of Neurology, Neurosurgery and Psychiatry, 47,* 84–86.

Ichikawa, K., & Kageyame, Y. (1991). Clinical anatomic study of pure dysarthria. *Stroke, 22,* 809–812.

Itoh, M., Sasanuma, S., & Ushijima, T. (1979). Velar movement during speech in a patient with apraxia of speech. *Brain and Language, 7,* 227–239.

Jaffe, K. M., Fay, G. C., Polissar, N. L., Martin, K. M., Shurtleff, H., Rivara, J., & Winn, H. R. (1992). Severity of pediatric traumatic brain injury and early neurobehavioral outcome—A cohort study. *Archives of Physical Medicine and Rehabilitation, 74,* 540–547.

Jaffe, K. M., Fay, G. C., Polissar, N. L., Martin, K. M., Shurtleff, H., Rivara, J., & Winn, H. R. (1993). Severity of pediatric traumatic brain injury and neurobehavioral recovery at one year—A cohort study. *Archives of Physical Medicine and Rehabilitation, 74,* 587–595.

Jaffe, K. M., Polissar, N. L., Fay, G. C., & Liao, S. (1995). Recovery trends over three years following pediatric traumatic brain injury. *Archives of Physical Medicine and Rehabilitation, 76*(1), 17–26.

Jennett, W. B., & Bond, M. (1975). Assessment of outcome after severe brain damage. *Lancet, 1,* 480.

Jennett, W. B., & Teasdale, G. (1981). *Management of head injuries.* Philadelphia: F. A. Davis.

Johns, D. F., & Darley, F. L. (1970). Phonemic variability in apraxia of speech. *Journal of Speech and Hearing Research, 13,* 556.

Johnson, E. R., McKenzie, S. W., Rosenquist, C. J., Lieberman, J. S., & Sievers, A. E. (1992). Dysphagia following stroke: Quantitative evaluation of pharyngeal transit times. *Archives of Physical Medicine and Rehabilitation, 73,* 419–423.

Jordan, F. M., & Murdoch, B. E. (1990). Unexpected recovery of functional communication following a prolonged period of mutism post–head injury. *Brain Injury, 4*(1), 101–108.

Jordan, F. M., & Murdoch, B. E. (1994). Severe closed-head injury in childhood: Linguistic outcomes into adulthood. *Brain Injury, 8*(6), 501–508.

Jordan, F. M., Ozanne, A. E., & Murdoch, B. E. (1988). Long term speech and language disorders subsequent to closed head injury in children. *Brain Injury, 2,* 179–185.

Kaplan, P. E., & Cerullo, L. J. (1986). *Stoke rehabilitation.* Boston: Butterworth.

Katz, D. I., & Alexander, M. P. (1994). Traumatic brain injury: Predicting course of recovery and outcomes for patients admitted to rehabilitation. *Archives of Neurology, 51,* 661–670.

Keatley, A., & Wirz, S. (1994). Is 20 years too long? Improving intelligibility in longstanding dysarthria—A single case treatment study. *European Journal of Disorders of Communication, 29,* 183–201.

Kennedy, M. R. T., & DeRuyter, F. (1991). Cognitive and language bases for communication disorders. In D. R. Beukelman & K. M. Yorkston (Eds.), *Communication disorders following traumatic brain injury: Management of cognitive, language, and motor impairment* (pp. 123–190). Austin, TX: PRO-ED.

Kent, R. D., & Rosenbek, J. C. (1983). Acoustic patterns of apraxia of speech. *Journal of Speech and Hearing Research, 26,* 231.

Kibby, M. Y., & Long, C. J. (1996). Minor head injury: Attempts at clarifying the confusion. *Brain Injury, 10*(3), 159–186.

Kim, J. S. (1994). Pure dysarthria, isolated facial paresis, or dysarthria–facial paresis syndrome. *Stroke*, *25*, 1994–1998.

Kreutzer, J. S., Marwitz, J. H., & Depler, K. (1992). Traumatic brain injury: Family response and outcome. *Archives of Physical Medicine and Rehabilitation*, *73*, 771–778.

Ladtkow, M. C., & Culp, D. (1992). Augmentative communication with the traumatic brain-injured population. In K. M. Yorkston (Ed.), *Augmentative communication in the medical setting* (pp. 139–213). Tucson, AZ: Communication Skill Builders.

Langmore, S. E., & Miller, R. M. (1994). Behavioral treatment for adults with oropharyngeal dysphagia. *Archives of Physical Medicine and Rehabilitation*, *75*, 1154–1160.

LaPointe, L. L., & Johns, D. F. (1975). Some phonemic characteristics of apraxia in speech. *Journal of Communication Disorders*, *8*, 259.

Lazarus, C. L. (1991). Diagnosis and management of swallowing disorders in traumatic brain injury. In D. R. Beukelman & K. M. Yorkston (Eds.), *Communication disorders following traumatic brain injury: Management of cognitive, language, and motor impairments* (pp. 367–418). Austin, TX: PRO-ED.

Lazarus, C., & Logemann, J. A. (1987). Swallowing disorders in closed head trauma. *Archives of Physical Medicine and Rehabilitation*, *68*, 79–84.

Light, J., Beesley, M., & Collier, B. (1988). Transition through multiple augmentative and alternative communication systems: A three-year case study of a head injury adolescent. *Augmentative and Alternative Communication*, *4*, 2–14.

Loeb, C., Gandolfo, C., Caponnetto, C., & Del-Sette, M. (1990). Pseudobulbar palsy: A clinical computed tomography study. *European Neurology*, *30*, 42–46.

Massagli, T. L. (1991). Neurobehavioral effect of phenytoin, carbamazepine, and valproic acid: Implications for use in traumatic brain injury. *Archives of Physical Medicine and Rehabilitation*, *72*, 219–226.

McCusker, E. A., Rudick, R. A., Honch, G. W., & Griggs, R. C. (1982). Recovery from the "locked-in" syndrome. *Archives of Neurology*, *39*, 145–147.

McGann, W. M., & Paslawski, T. M. (1991). Incomplete locked-in syndrome: Two cases with successful communication outcomes. *American Journal of Speech–Language Pathology*, *1*, 32–37.

McHenry, M. A., Wilson, R. L., & Minton, J. T. (1994). Management of multiple physiological deficits following traumatic brain injury. *Journal of Medical Speech–Language Pathology*, *2*, 58–74.

McNeil, M. R. (Ed.). (1997). *Clinical management of sensorimotor speech disorders*. New York: Thieme.

McNeil, M. R., Caligiuri, M. A., & Rosenbek, J. C. (1989). A comparison of labio-mandibular kinematic durations, displacement, velocities and dysmetrias in apraxic and normal adults. In T. E. Prescott (Ed.), *Clinical aphasiology* (pp. 173–193). Austin, TX: PRO-ED.

McNeil, M. R., Liss, J., Tseng, C.-H., & Kent, R. D. (1990). Effects of speech rate on the absolute and relative timing of apraxic and conduction aphasic sentence production. *Brain and Language*, *38*, 135–158.

McNeil, M. R., Robin, D. A., & Schmidt, R. A. (1997). Apraxia of speech: Definition, differentiation, and treatment. In M. R. McNeil (Ed.), *Clinical management of sensorimotor speech disorders* (pp. 311–344). New York: Thieme.

Meyer, J. S., & Shaw, T. (Eds.). (1982). *Diagnosis and management of strokes and TIA's*. Menlo Park, CA: Addison-Wesley.

Miller, R. M., & Langmore, S. E. (1994). Treatment efficacy for adults with oropharyngeal dysphagia. *Archives of Physical Medicine and Rehabilitation*, *75*, 1256–1262.

Montgomery, J. H. (1991). *To the edge and back.* Edmonton, Alberta: Glenrose Rehabilitation Hospital.

Murdoch, B. E., Theodoros, D. G., Stokes, P. D., & Chenery, H. J. (1993). Abnormal patterns of speech breathing in dysarthric speakers following severe closed head injury. *Brain Injury, 7,* 295–308.

Murdoch, B. E., Thompson, E. C., & Stokes, P. D. (1994). Phonatory and laryngeal dysfunction following upper motor neuron vascular lesions. *Journal of Medical Speech–Language Pathology, 2,* 177–190.

Najensen, T., Sazbon, L., Feiselzon, J., Becker, E., & Schechter, I. (1978). Recovery of communicative functions after prolonged traumatic coma. *Scandinavian Journal of Rehabilitation Medicine, 10,* 15–21.

Netsell, R., & Daniel, B. (1979). Dysarthria in adults: Physiologic approach to rehabilitation. *Archives of Physical Medicine and Rehabilitation, 60,* 502.

Nudo, R. J., Wise, B. M., SiFuentes, F., & Milliken, G. W. (1996). Neural stustrates for the effects of rehabilitation training on motor recovery after ischemic infarct. *Science, 272,* 1791–1795.

Odderson, I. R., Keaton, J. C., & McKenna, B. S. (1995). Swallow management in patients on an acute stroke pathway: Quality is cost effective. *Archives of Physical Medicine and Rehabilitation, 76,* 1130–1133.

Patterson, J. R., & Grabois, M. (1986). Locked-in syndrome: A review of 139 cases. *Stroke, 17,* 758–764.

Robbins, J., Levine, R. L., Maser, A., Rosenbek, J. C., & Kempster, G. B. (1993). Swallowing after unilateral stroke of the cerebral cortex. *Archives of Physical Medicine and Rehabilitation, 74,* 1293–1300.

Robin, D. A., Bean, C., & Folkins, J. W. (1989). Lip movement in apraxia of speech. *Journal of Speech and Hearing Research, 32,* 512–523.

Rosenbek, J. C., & McNeil, M. R. (1991). A discussion of classification in motor speech disorders: Dysarthria and apraxia of speech. In C. A. Moore, K. M. Yorkston, & D. R. Beukelman (Eds.), *Dysarthria and apraxia of speech: Perspectives on management* (pp. 289–296). Baltimore: Brookes.

Rosenbek, J. C., McNeil, M. R., & Aronson, A. E. (Eds.). (1984). *Apraxia of speech: Physiology, acoustics, linguistics, management.* Austin, TX: PRO-ED.

Rosenthal, M., Christensen, B. K., & Ross, T. P. (1998). Depression following traumatic brain injury. *Archives of Physical Medicine and Rehabilitation, 79*(1), 90–103.

Rosenthal, M., Griffith, E. R., Bond, M. R., & Miller, J. D. (Eds.). (1983). *Rehabilitation of the head injured adult.* Philadelphia: F. A. Davis.

Ryalls, J. H. (1981). Motor aphasia: Acoustic correlates of phonetic disintegration in vowels. *Neuropsychologia, 19,* 365–374.

Sandel, M. E., Bell, K. R., & Michaud, L. J. (1998). Brain injury rehabilitation—I. Traumatic brain injury: Prevention, pathophysiology and outcome predictions. *Archives of Physical Medicine and Rehabilitation, 79*(3), 3–9.

Sandel, M. E., & Zwil, A. S. (1997). Psychopharmacologic treatment for affective disorders after traumatic brain injury. *Physical Medicine and Rehabilitation Clinics of North America, 8*(4), 743–762.

Sapir, S., & Aronson, A. E. (1985). Aphonia after closed head injury: Aetiologic considerations. *British Journal of Disorders of Communication, 20,* 289–296.

Sarno, M. T., Buonaguro, A., & Levita, E. (1986). Characteristics of verbal impairment in closed head injured patients. *Archives of Physical Medicine and Rehabilitation, 67,* 400–405.

Schlageter, K., Gray, B., Hall, K., Shaw, R., & Sammet, R. (1993). Incidence and treatment of visual dysfunction in traumatic brain injury. *Brain Injury, 7,* 439–448.

Schmidt, J., Holas, M., Halvorson, K., & Reding, M. (1994). Videofluoroscopic evidence of aspiration predicts pneumonia and death but not dehydration following stroke. *Dysphagia, 9*, 7–11.

Shankweiler, D., & Harris, K. (1966). An experimental approach to the problem of articulation in aphasia. *Cortex, 2*, 277.

Shapiro, K. (1983). *Pediatric head trauma.* Mount Kisco, NY: Futura.

Simpson, M. B., Till, J. A., & Goff, A. M. (1988). Long-term treatment of severe dysarthria: A case study. *Journal of Speech and Hearing Disorders, 53*, 433–440.

Smithard, D. G., O'Neill, P. A., Park, C., Morris, J., Wyatt, R., England, R., & Martin, D. F. (1996). Complications and outcome after acute stroke: Does dysphagia matter? *Stroke, 27*(7), 1200–1204.

Sohlberg, M. M., & Mateer, C. A. (Eds.). (1989). *Introduction to cognitive rehabilitation: Theory and practice.* New York: Guilford Press.

Sosin, D. M., Sniezek, J. E., & Waxweiler, R. J. (1995). Trends in death associated with traumatic brain injury, 1972 through 1992: Success and failure. *JAMA, 273*(22), 1778–1889.

Spertell, R. B., & Ransom, B. R. (1979). Dysarthria—Clumsy hand syndrome produced by capsular infarct. *Annals of Neurology, 6*, 263–265.

Strand, E. A., & McNeil, M. R. (1996). Effects of length and linguistic complexity on temporal acoustic measures in apraxia of speech. *Journal of Speech and Hearing Research, 39*(5), 1018–1034.

Stuss, D. T., Ely, P., Hugenholtz, H., Richard, M. T., LaRochelle, S., Poirier, C. A., & Bell, I. (1985). Subtle neuropsychological deficits in patients with good recovery after closed head injury. *Neurosurgery, 17*, 41.

Teasdale, G., & Jennett, W. B. (1974). Assessment of coma and impaired consciousness. *Lancet, 2*, 81–84.

Teasell, R. W., Bach, D., & McRae, M. (1994). Prevalence and recovery of aspiration poststroke: A retrospective analysis. *Dysphagia, 9*(1), 35–39.

Temkin, N. R., Dikmen, S. S., Wilensky, A. J., Keihm, J., Chabal, S., & Winn, H. R. (1990). A randomized double-blind study of phenytoin for prevention of post-traumatic seizures. *New England Journal of Medicine, 323*, 497–502.

Theodoros, D. G., & Murdoch, B. E. (1994). Laryngeal dysfunction in dysarthric speakers following severe closed-head injury. *Brain Injury, 8*, 667–684.

Theodoros, D. G., Murdoch, B. E., & Chenery, H. J. (1994). Perceptual speech characteristics of dysarthric speakers. *Brain Injury, 8*, 101–124.

Theodoros, D. G., Murdoch, B. E., & Stokes, P. D. (1995). Variability in the perceptual and physiological features of dysarthria following severe closed head injury: An examination of five cases. *Brain Injury, 9*, 671–696.

Theodoros, D., Murdoch, B. E., Stokes, P. D., & Chenery, H. J. (1993). Hypernasality in dysarthric speakers following severe closed head injury: A perceptual and instrumental analysis. *Brain Injury, 7*(1), 59–69.

Thompson, E. C., & Murdoch, B. E. (1995). Disorders of nasality in subjects with upper motor neuron type dysarthria following cerebrovascular accident. *Journal of Communication Disorders, 28*, 261–276.

Thompson, E. C., Murdoch, B. E., & Stokes, P. D. (1995a). Lip function in subjects with upper motor neuron type dysarthria following cerebrovascular accidents. *European Journal of Disorders of Communication, 30*, 451–466.

Thompson, E. C., Murdoch, B. E., & Stokes, P. D. (1995b). Tongue function in subjects with upper motor neuron type dysarthria following cerebrovascular accident. *Journal of Medical Speech–Language Pathology, 3*(1), 27–40.

Trost, J. E., & Canter, G. J. (1974). Apraxia of speech in patients with Broca's aphasia: A study of phoneme production accuracy and error pattern. *Brain and Language, 1,* 63.

Turkstra, L. S., & Bayles, K. A. (1992). Acquired mutism: Physiopathy and assessment. *Archives of Physical Medicine and Rehabilitation, 73,* 138–144.

Urban, P. P., Hopf, H. C., Zorowka, P. G., Fleischer, S., & Andreas, J. (1996). Dysarthria and lacunar stroke: Pathophysiologic aspects. *Neurology, 47,* 1135–1141.

Veis, S. L., & Logemann, J. A. (1985). Swallowing disorders in persons with cerebrovascular accident. *Archives of Physical Medicine and Rehabilitation, 66,* 372–375.

Waxweiler, R. J., Thurman, D., Sniezek, J., Sosin, D., & O'Neil, J. (1995). Monitoring the impact of traumatic brain injury: A review and update. *Journal of Neurotrauma, 12,* 509–516.

Wertz, R. T., LaPointe, L., & Rosenbek, J. (1984). *Apraxia of speech in adults: The disorder and its management.* Orlando, FL: Grune & Stratton.

Wiercisiewski, D. R., & McDeavitt, D. (1997). Drugs for management of acute and chronic behavioral disorders. *Physical Medicine and Rehabilitation Clinics of North America, 8*(4), 763–780.

Winstein, C. (1983). Neurogenic dysphagia: Frequency, progression, outcome in adults following head injury. *Physical Therapy, 63,* 1992–1997.

Workinger, M. S., & Netsell, R. (1992). Restoration of intelligible speech 13 years post–head injury. *Brain Injury, 6,* 183–187.

Yablon, S. A. (1993). Posttraumatic seizures. *Archives of Physical Medicine and Rehabilitation, 74*(9), 983–1001.

Yang, C. C., Lieberman, J. S., & Hong, C. Z. (1989). Early smooth horizontal eye movement: A favorable prognostic sign in patients with locked-in syndrome. *Archives of Physical Medicine and Rehabilitation, 70,* 230–232.

Yorkston, K. M., & Beukelman, D. R. (1991). Motor speech disorders. In D. R. Beukelman & K. M. Yorkston (Eds.), *Communication disorders following traumatic brain injury: Management of cognitive, language, and motor impairment* (pp. 251–316). Boston: College-Hill.

Yorkston, K. M., Honsinger, M. J., Mitsuda, P. M., & Hammen, V. (1989). The relationship between speech and swallowing disorders in head-injured patients. *Journal of Head Trauma Rehabilitation, 4*(4), 1–16.

Yorkston, K. M., & Kennedy, M. R. T. (in press). Treatment approaches for communication disorders. In M. Rosenthal (Ed.), *Rehabilitation of the adult and child with traumatic brain injury* (2nd ed.). Philadelphia: F.A. Davis.

Young, E. C., & Durant-Jones, L. (1990). Developing a dysphagia program in an acute care hospital: A needs assessment. *Dysphagia, 5,* 159–165.

Ziegler, W., & von Cramon, D. (1983a). Vowel distortion in traumatic dysarthria: Lip rounding versus tongue advancement. *Phonetica, 40,* 312–322.

Ziegler, W., & von Cramon, D. (1983b). Vowel distortion in traumatic dysarthria: A formant study. *Phonetica, 40,* 63–78.

CHAPTER

DYSARTHRIA IN
DEGENERATIVE DISEASE

This chapter contains a review of the pathology–medical aspects, speech characteristics, and stages of functional limitations in dysarthria for a diverse group of neurologic disorders with a degenerative natural course. Onset of these disorders occurs after childhood, and in most cases the disorders are insidious, with signs and symptoms appearing gradually. Although many progressive neuromotor disorders may result in dysarthria, we have selected those disorders that occur frequently in a clinical caseload of speech–language pathologists, together with those disorders that are uncommon but whose speech characteristics have been studied carefully and are reported in the literature. See Table 4.1 for a brief summary of pathology, symptoms, medical management, and dysarthria characteristics of each of the diseases reviewed here.

Many advances are currently being made in both the basic understanding of these diseases and their effective medical management. Through this chapter, the reader will find World Wide Web site locations that provide brief reviews of current advances for a variety of neurologic diseases.

Table 4.1
Summary of Degenerative Diseases Associated with Dysarthria

Disease	Pathology	Primary Symptoms	Medical Management	Type of Dysarthria	Occurrence of Dysarthria
Parkinson's disease	Loss of dopaminergic neurons in basal ganglia	Resting tremor, rigidity, bradykinesis, postural instability	Pharmacologic	Hypokinetic	Rare as initial symptom, common in later stages
Progressive supranuclear palsy	Many neural structures may be involved	Ophthalmoplegia, dystonic rigidity, pseudobulbar palsy, dementia, and dysarthria	Symptomatic	Mixed with components of spasticity, hypokinesia, and ataxia	Common and may be one of the initial symptoms
Shy-Drager syndrome	Many neural structures may be involved	Rigidity, tremor, poor balance with orthostatic hypotension	Symptomatic	Mixed with components of spasticity, hypokinesia, and ataxia	Common
Striatonigral degeneration	Basal ganglia involvement with striatal degeneration	Rigidity, akinesia, postural instability, increased tendon reflexes, and dysarthria	Symptomatic	Mixed with components of hypokinesia, hyperkinesia, and spasticity	Common and may be one of the initial symptoms
Olivopontocerebellar degeneration	Cerebellum, pons, inferior olives, and basal ganglia	Ataxia, tremor, and rigidity	Symptomatic	Mixed spastic–ataxic or flaccid–hypokinetic	Common
Wilson's disease	Excessive accumulation of copper in the brain and other tissue	Incoordination, tremor, dysarthria, drooling, dysphagia, and masklike face	Pharmacologic and dietary	Mixed with components of ataxic, spastic, and hypokinetic	Occurs in nearly all cases and may be initial symptom

(continues)

Table 4.1 (*continued*)

Disease	Pathology	Primary Symptoms	Medical Management	Type of Dysarthria	Occurrence of Dysarthria
Friedreich's ataxia	Spinocerebellar degeneration	Ataxia with skeletal deformities and sensory changes	Symptomatic	Ataxia but spasticity also possible	Common
Dystonia	Extrapyramidal	Abnormal, involuntary movements and postures	Symptomatic; when localized botulinum toxin	Hyperkinetic	Depends on the distribution of disorder
Huntington's disease	Extrapyramidal	Chorea, dementia, and emotional instability	Symptomatic	Hyperkinetic	Common especially in late stages
Amyotrophic lateral sclerosis	Upper and lower motor neuron degeneration	Weakness and spasticity	Symptomatic	Mixed spastic–flaccid	Initial symptom in 30%; common in later stages
Multiple sclerosis	Plaques in the white matter	Balance abnormalities, impaired sensation, paraparesis optic neuritis	Interferon for preventing relapses	Mixed ataxic–spastic	Approximately 40% of cases

Question: Many of the diseases in this chapter are uncommon. Are there organizations that provide information about the diseases?

Yes, many of the diseases discussed in this chapter have national organizations that provide information to the public. Another excellent source of information is The National Organization for Rare Diseases (NORD, P.O. Box 8923, New Fairfield, CT 06812-8923). NORD is a federation of more than 140 not-for-profit voluntary health organizations serving people with rare disorders and disabilities. The following is a sampling of member organizations: Amyotrophic Lateral Sclerosis Association, Dystonic Medical Research Foundation, Guillain-Barré Syndrome Foundation International, Huntington's Disease Society of America, Myasthenia Gravis Foundation, National Multiple Sclerosis Society, Parkinson's Disease Foundation, and Wilson's Disease Association. Web site for The National Organization for Rare Disorders (June 20, 1997):

http://www.pcnet.com/~orphan

Parkinsonism

Pathology–Medical Aspects

Parkinsonism is a general syndrome that encompasses the symptoms of "resting" tremor, rigidity, akinesia (paucity of movement), and postural instability. The acronym TRAP (Tremor, Rigidity, Akinesia, and Postural instability) is used as a mnemonic device. Communication disorders are common, often beginning with a decrease in vocal loudness and at times progressing to more severe functional limitations characterized by changes in speaking rate, articulatory precision, and speech intelligibility. The pathology of Parkinsonism is associated with the loss of dopaminergic neurons in the basal ganglia (especially the substantia nigra) and brain stem. It can be divided into subgroups depending upon its etiology and associated signs and symptoms. *Idiopathic or primary Parkinson's disease* (also known as paralysis agitans) is the term applied when the cause of the syndrome is unknown. *Secondary parkinsonism*, which includes a number of disorders with extrapyramidal features that have an identifiable causal agent, some of which would include toxins (e.g., derivative of meperidine, MPTP), infections, drugs (neuroleptics), and repeated trauma or multiple strokes. Another group of syndromes, known as *parkinsonism-plus*, refers to heterogeneous system degeneration, such as progressive supranuclear palsy, striatonigral degeneration, Shy-Drager syndrome, or olivopontocerebellar degeneration (Marttila, 1983; Marttila & Rinne, 1981). Because these syndromes are associated with damage to multiple neural systems, the type of dysarthria associated with them may be different from that associated with parkinsonism. Therefore, these syndromes will be described separately in the next section.

More information about parkinsonism-plus syndromes can be found at the National Institute of Neurology Disorders and Stroke Web site (May 22, 1997):

http://www.ninds.nih.gov/healinfo/nindspub.htm

Question: Do the terms parkinsonism and Parkinson's disease refer to the same disorder?

No, there is a subtle distinction. The term Parkinson's disease is most often used to describe a constellation of symptoms with an unknown cause (i.e., idiopathic). The term parkinsonism is a more general term to include a syndrome where the symptoms are similar to Parkinson's disease but the cause is known. For example, parkinsonism may be drug induced or caused by multiple strokes or repeated trauma.

DIAGNOSIS

To be diagnosed with Parkinson's disease, an individual must demonstrate at least two of the four classic signs: tremor-at-rest, rigidity, akinesia/bradykinesia, or loss of postural reflexes. However, before the diagnosis of Parkinson's disease can be made, other types of parkinsonism must be ruled out. Because most of the parkinsonism-plus syndromes also have the classic symptoms (particularly rigidity and bradykinesia), a search must be made for signs and symptoms that are not typically seen in Parkinson's disease. Some of these signs are pyramidal tract signs (exaggerated reflexes, extensor plantar response), intention tremor, ataxia, or other evidence of cerebellar dysfunction, or profound early dementia (Fahn, 1988; Marttila, 1983). The diagnosis of Parkinson's disease is made on clinical grounds. In the patient who does not show the classic signs of tremor, rigidity, and akinesia, computerized tomography (CT scan) may be helpful in the differential diagnosis.

POPULATION CHARACTERISTICS

About 1.5 million people in the United States have a form of Parkinson's disease. This affects one of every 100 persons over the age of 60 years. There is no significant difference between men and women. The incidence increases sharply above the age of 64 and the peak of incidence is between 75 and 84 years of age. There has been a trend toward increased age at the time of diagnosis; in 1967, the diagnosis was 10 years earlier than it was made in 1984 (Hoehn & Yahr, 1967; Rajput, Offord, Beard, & Kurland, 1984).

CAUSES

Three areas are presently being investigated as possible etiologies for parkinsonism: genetic, age related, and environmental. In terms of genetics, there have been two familial subgroups identified with variants of parkinsonism, demonstrating different symptoms. Twin studies have not shown any genetic transmission of typical idiopathic Parkinson's disease. It has been argued by some that Parkinson's disease is an accelerated form of normal aging with a loss of substantia nigra neurons. Again, however, twin studies do not support this. Another argument against the aging theory is that "parkinsonian" traits of normal elderly people do not respond to treatment with levodopa. Another possibility, that of an environmental toxin, has received some support by the development of a severe form of parkinsonism in a number of drug abusers. A derivative of meperidine, MPTP, has been shown to cause a severe loss of dopaminergic substantia nigra neurons. Although the pathology found after the use of this drug is not identical to that of Parkinson's disease (which includes other regions of the brain), it is the best model available. Other studies have suggested common exposures among patients from similar geographic areas that trigger eventual cell death (Lang & Blair, 1984).

NATURAL COURSE

The most common assessment scale rating Parkinson's disease is the Unified Parkinson's Disease Rating Scale (Fahn, Elton, & Members of the UPDRS Development Committee, 1987). This measures behavior, mood, activities of daily living, motor status, and complications of therapy. It also contains an indication of the overall stage of disability (Hoehn & Yahr, 1967). Parkinson's disease typically has an insidious onset; in retrospect, individuals recall increasing difficulty with "stiffness" and "muscle aches" that they had attributed to the normal course of aging. Changes in speech are typically not among the first symptoms of Parkinson's disease; they typically do not occur until Stages III through V of Hoehn and Yahr's scale. The problem that initiates the first visit to a physician is most commonly tremor. The tremor of Parkinson's disease is of the distal extremities and occurs at rest (the pill-rolling phenomenon). Individuals who initially show symptoms of tremor apparently have a slower progression of the disease, at least in the first 10 years (Hoehn & Yahr, 1967).

Early in the disease, individuals might notice increasing difficulty in repetitive or alternating movements such as walking. When a joint is passively moved through its range, a "catch" can be felt; this phenomenon is known as cogwheeling. This rigidity affects all striated muscles, causing difficulties in respiration, facial expression, swallowing, mastication, and speech. Progression of rigidity can lead to flexion contractures of the fingers, elbows, cervical spine, hips, and knees, with ensuing loss of movement.

Bradykinesia (or akinesia, in its most extreme form) is a slowness or decrease in spontaneous movements. Often the earliest manifestation of this is a decrease in the frequency of eye blinking (normal range is 14 to 17 per minute). Paucity of facial movement leads to a masklike appearance. Thus, bradykinesia may have a broad effect on interactive communication because of the associated lack of facial expression, reduction in spontaneous smiling, and, when severe, decreased initiation of speech movements. With progression of the disease, individuals with parkinsonism may not be able to perform simple volitional acts, such as initiating ambulation or arising from a chair. These episodes (called freezing) may at times be overcome by diverting attention from the desired act or by an emotional response. Loss of postural reflexes, shuffling gait, retropulsion (the tendency to fall backward), and festination (progressive rapidity of forward movement with a loss of control) all severely affect safe ambulation. In some individuals, rapid rushes of speech are similar to the festinating gait patterns. Prior to treatment with levodopa, over one quarter of patients were dead or severely disabled within 5 years of their diagnosis. Modern medical treatment has extended the life expectancy considerably. Given the rather severe communication disorders of some individuals with Parkinson's disease, increased life expectancy means that many live in a number of types of facilities (retirement centers, nursing homes, etc.) and their communication needs must be met in those contexts.

MEDICAL MANAGEMENT

The major method of treatment is pharmacological; the discovery that levodopa (L-dopa) could cross the blood–brain barrier and be metabolized to dopamine in the brain revolutionized the treatment of Parkinson's disease. L-dopa most effectively treats akinesia and rigidity but is less effective in treating balance, speech, and cognitive impairments. There are many fluctuations in the clinical response to levodopa, even within the individual (known as the on–off response), probably due to differences in absorption and dopamine receptor responsivity. Levodopa is usually combined with a dopamine decarboxylase inhibitor (carbidopa), which decreases the inactivation of levodopa in the peripheral tissues and decreases the dosage required (Bianchine, 1976). Unfortunately, it has become apparent that there are a number of therapeutic problems with levodopa usage, including the failure to respond, the loss of response with prolonged treatment, the occurrence of involuntary movements with long-standing therapy, and the previously mentioned fluctuations in response (Playfer, 1997). The other drugs used in treatment are the anticholinergic agents for younger patients early in disease (primarily for tremor), the dopamine agonist-ergot derivative (e.g., bromocriptine, pergolide, and lisuride), MOA-B inhibitors (selegiline), and amantadine hydrochloride. Excellent sources of information about the drug treatment of Parkinson's disease can be found in Duvoisin (1991) and Nutt (1995).

Rigrodsky and Morrison (1970) studied the speech of 21 speakers with parkinsonism under various conditions of L-dopa therapy. They reported,

> Although statistical significance was obtained for only one aspect (time factor—overall rate of speaking, appropriateness of phrasing and pauses, and rhythmic and fluency of speech) of speech in favor of improvement during maximal dosages (4–8 gm daily), there appeared to be a trend in the direction of improved speech during L-dopa therapy. These findings are not nearly as dramatic as the improvement in physical symptoms observed in the same patients. However, the speech changes all occurred within less than one month; greater changes might have been observed had the patients been followed for a longer period with maximal dosage. (p. 150)

Pharmacological or surgical treatment improving akinesia, rigidity, and tremor are not always successful in speech (Gentil & Pollak, 1995).

Stereotactic thalamotomy is more effective than levodopa in alleviating the tremor of Parkinson's disease, and is usually considered for the individual with an incapacitating tremor that is unresponsive to other forms of therapy (Narabayashi, 1991). Recently posteroventral pallidotomy has demonstrated significant therapeutic effects for akinesia resistant to medication (Iacono et al., 1995). In a study of fine motor control of the speech mechanism in patients with posteroventral pallidotomy, results suggest reduction in certain forms of muscle instability in the oral system (Barlow, Iacono, Paseman, Biswas, & D'Antonio, 1998). Stimulation of the ventral intermedialis nuclei is presently being explored as another method to treat dyskinesia (Nutt, 1995; Playfer, 1997).

Physical therapy does not contribute to halting the progression of the disease; however, it can be very useful in preventing secondary complications due to rigidity and problems with balance. Patients and their families should be trained in the use of walkers or wheelchairs, if necessary. Range-of-motion exercises can prevent unnecessary contractures that would further hinder mobility and care. Proper positioning in bed and while working can ameliorate the cervical flexion that can affect vision and mobility. Occupational therapists can assist families in evaluating the home for safety and can prolong patients' independence through the use of assistive devices for dressing and eating.

COGNITIVE AND LANGUAGE DEFICITS

Because cognitive and language deficits influence a speaker's ability to compensate for motor speech disorders, speech–language pathologists who manage the communication needs of individuals with parkinsonism must be aware of potential deficits in these areas. Controversy exists as to whether dementia is a feature of Parkinson's disease. For some, specific memory deficits are present on testing, and individuals may complain of slowness in problem solving. However, objective testing of these individuals is difficult because of the extreme slowness of motor responses, poor handwriting, and dysarthria. Agreement certainly exists that if dementia is prominent and occurs before major motoric disability, a diagnosis other than Parkinson's disease (e.g., Alzheimer's disease or progressive supranuclear palsy) should be considered (Morris, 1982). Conservative estimates suggest that about 15% of individuals with Parkinson's disease meet a strict criterion for dementia (Levin, Tomer, & Rey, 1992). Some evidence suggests that individuals with Parkinson's disease experience changes in cognitive function more frequently than matched controls (Bayles et al., 1996).

Language use in Parkinson's disease is complicated by a number of potentially coexisting factors, such as cognitive changes, depression, and motor disorders including slowness of movement initiation. Despite these difficulties, a number of studies are available (Bayles, 1990; Cooper, Sagar, Jordan, Harvey, & Sullivan, 1991; Illes, 1989; Illes, Metter, Hanson, & Iritani, 1988; Lieberman, Friedman, & Feldman, 1990; Lieberman et al., 1992). These studies suggest that individuals with Parkinson's disease differ from nondisabled peers on a number of language-related measures, including comprehension of complex commands, processing of sentences, and syntactic complexity of spontaneous speech.

SWALLOWING PROBLEMS

Speech–language pathologists who treat individuals with dysarthria are usually called on also to deal with their swallowing problems. The incidence of changes in swallowing in individuals with Parkinson's disease is high (Leopold & Kagel, 1996). Although quantitative studies of swallowing (suction pressure, bolus volume, and timing of important events in the swallowing cycle) suggest abnormality in over 90% of individuals with moderate to severe parkinsonism (Nilsson, Ekberg, Olsson, & Hindfelt, 1996), a much smaller proportion of the population recognizes that the problem exists (Bushman, Bomeyer, Leeker, & Perlmutter, 1989; Robbins, Logemann, & Kirschner, 1986). In a study conducted in Sweden, less than half of the individuals surveyed regarding speech and swallowing problems reported that their ability to chew and swallow was worse than prior to the onset of the disease (Hartelius & Svensson, 1994). Caution is warranted because self-reports of swallowing difficulty may underestimate the problem. Clinical and radiographic studies in elderly individuals with Parkinson's disease who did not have symptoms of dysphagia suggest the presence of at least some abnormalities. Included among these abnormalities are aspiration and vallecular residue which are considered to create greater risk for aspiration (Bird, Woodward, Gibson, Phyland, & Fonda, 1994).

The swallowing disorders in people with Parkinson's disease may be only partially accounted for by the primary pathology in the basal ganglia. The dysphagia appears to be related to changes in both the striated musculature under dopaminergic control and the smooth musculature under autonomic control (Morrell, 1992). Symptoms may occur in the oral, pharyngeal, or esophageal stages. For example, repetitive tongue pumping, difficulty with bolus formation, and hesitancy in initiating the swallow may occur in the oral phase. Other prepharyngeal abnormalities include jaw rigidity, impaired head and neck posture during meals, impulsive feeding behavior, and impaired amount of regulation (Leopold & Kagel, 1996). Once a bolus is propelled into the pharyngeal cavity, there may be a delay in triggering pharyngeal contractions. In a radiographic study of 71 individuals with Parkinson's disease ranging from mild to advanced, the most common pharyngeal abnormalities were impaired motility, vallecular and pyriform sinus stasis, supraglottal and glottal aspiration, and deficient epiglottis positioning and range of motion (Leopold & Kagel, 1997). Once the bolus passes through the upper esophageal sphincter, the transit continues to be slow due to reduced esophageal peristalsis. The most common problems include delayed transport, stasis, bolus reduction, and tertiary contractions. The rate of spontaneous swallows is lower in a group of individuals with Parkinson's disease than in normal controls (Pehlivan et al., 1996).

Rating scales for the severity of dysphagia are available for Parkinson's disease. One such scale (Waxman, Durfee, Moore, & Morantz, 1990) grades swallowing performance based on the patient's report, observations of family members, and results of a radiographic examination. A note of caution may be appropriate here because performance on the swallowing scales may not correspond closely with the overall severity of the disease. Studies suggest that the clinical severity of disease predicted neither the presence nor the severity of the dysphagia (Ali et al., 1996).

Swallowing intervention in this population has been described in three stages: early, moderate, and severe problems (Yorkston, Miller, & Strand, 1995). The presenting features in the early stage include reduction in pharyngeal peristalsis, and repetitive rocking motion of the tongue. During this stage, intervention may involve providing counseling to bring swallowing under voluntary control, monitoring weight, and coordinating eating with the drug cycle. Presenting features of moderate swallowing problems include, in addition to those seen in the early stage, delay in swallowing reflex, cricopharyngeal dysfunction, and incomplete laryngeal closure during swallowing. During this stage, intervention may include the introduction of aid to promote independence, teaching double swallow techniques, and recommending small, frequent, highly nutritious meals. Presenting features of the severe stage also include aspiration both during and after swallowing. At this point, dietary changes such as switching to a soft diet and techniques such as the chin tuck may be appropriate. If aspiration remains a critical issue, alternative means of feeding may be needed.

Speech Characteristics

Extensive research has been focused on the description of the speech patterns of individuals with Parkinson's disease. The prevalence of speech disorder in the parkinsonian population is high. Logemann and colleagues studied 200 speakers with parkinsonism and reported that 89% exhibited laryngeal-related problems and 45% demonstrated articulatory problems (Logemann, Fischer, Boshes, & Blonsky, 1978). A study of 65 speakers with parkinsonism reported that 37% had normal speech or were mildly involved, 22% had a moderate degree of speech involvement, and 29% had severely impaired speech (Buck & Cooper, 1956). In self-reports, individuals with Parkinson's disease also note a high incidence of dysarthria. In a survey of 230 people with Parkinson's disease, 70% reported that their speech or voice was worse than prior to disease onset (Hartelius & Svensson, 1994). Several of the most common problems these individuals reported were related to the voice: weak voice (61% reporting this problem), hoarse voice (32%), and monotonous voice (17%). Other common problems were imprecise articulation (36%) and difficulties getting started (27%).

The perceptual features of speech in Parkinson's disease are distinctive. Perhaps the most complete overview of hypokinetic dysarthria associated with parkinsonism comes from the Mayo Clinic studies (Darley, Aronson, & Brown, 1975). These researchers recorded 32 speakers and rated the speech samples on 38 perceptual dimensions. They concluded,

> reduced variability in pitch and loudness, reduced loudness level overall, and decreased use of all vocal parameters for achieving stress and emphasis. Markedly imprecise articulation is generated at variable rates in short bursts of speech punctuated by illogical pauses and often by inappropriate silences. Voice quality is sometimes harsh, sometimes breathy. (p. 195)

The perceptual features of dysarthria in Parkinson's disease are consistent with the underlying pathophysiology. Reduced ranges of movement may be reflected in the features of monopitch, monoloudness, reduced stress, and short phrases. Variable rate, short rushes of speech, and imprecise consonants may also be related to the reduced range of speech movements. Inappropriate silences may be the result of bradykinesia and its associated difficulty in initiating movement. The deviant voice dimensions (breathiness, voice harshness, and low pitch) may be the result of rigidity of the laryngeal musculature. The perceptual features of hypokinetic dysarthria associated with Parkinson's disease have been documented with a growing body of acoustic evidence (Forrest, Weismer, & Turner, 1989; Ludlow, Connor, & Bassich, 1987; Metter & Hanson, 1986). The acoustic features of parkinsonian dysarthria include reduced duration of vocalic segments, reduced formant transitions, and increased voice onset time compared with typically aging controls (Forrest et al., 1989).

SPEECH COMPONENTS

Respiratory Function

Because reduced loudness level is a consistent perceptual feature of hypokinetic dysarthria, one could speculate that the respiratory system may be an important contributor to the overall problem. With few exceptions, researchers have supported the conclusion that for speakers with parkinsonism, respiratory function is reduced compared with that of normal speakers (Murdoch, Chenery, Bowler, & Ingram, 1989; Solomon & Hixon, 1993). Several investigators instructed their subjects to sustain phonation as a measure of respiratory support. Although some reported a reduction of sustained phonation time in subjects with parkinsonism (Boshes, 1966; Canter, 1965a), other investigators did not (Kruel, 1972). The differences in these results are probably related to the severity of the parkinsonism. Speakers with parkinsonism may have "inflexible" respiratory patterns for speech. In part, this inflexibility may be reflected in reduction of lung volume excursions or restricted use of chest wall movements to achieve lung volume displacements. The stooped posture that is characteristic of many people with parkinsonism may also interfere with adequate respiratory support for speech.

Phonation

Impairment of phonatory performance has been measured in numerous studies that consistently report an important reduction in laryngeal function for individuals with Parkinson's disease. Many of the perceptually deviant speech features identified by the Mayo Clinic studies are associated with pitch, loudness, or changes in voice quality (Darley et al., 1975). Physical examination of the vocal folds suggests that adductor and abductor movements are bilaterally symmetrical, but there may be incomplete closure of the vocal folds, which may account for the breathy voice quality (Aronson, 1985). There may be a direct relationship between the perceptual symptoms (breathiness and reduced loudness) and physiologic impairment (glottic gap and bowing of the vocal folds) (Hanson, Gerratt, & Ward, 1984). The perceptual features of hoarseness, breathiness, and roughness may be associated with the acoustic features of cycle-to-cycle shifts in intensity and frequency and of increased spectral noise (Ramig & Gould, 1986). Breakdowns in the coordination of voicing with other aspects of speech may account for some of the other features of parkinsonian speech, including difficulty initiating voicing, voiceless transitions, abnormal control of fundamental frequency contours, and voice timing deficits.

Velopharyngeal Function

Velopharyngeal dysfunction is not a major aspect of dysarthria associated with Parkinson's disease. Some abnormal airflow may occur as the disorder progresses because the velopharyngeal port does not close completely (Hoodin & Gilbert, 1989). Darley and colleagues (1975) reported that only 8 of 32 subjects demonstrated hypernasality to a minor degree. No subject was judged to display nasal emission during speech.

Oral Articulation

The primary articulatory characteristics of parkinsonism result from inadequate articulatory valving during production of plosives and breakdowns in the coordination of laryngeal and oral activity (Canter, 1965b). Perceptually, imprecise consonant production is a common feature of dysarthria in Parkinson's disease. Consonants that require the most constriction tend to be produced with the least accuracy (Logemann & Fischer, 1981). Spirantization of stops (the tendency of stops to be fricated) is characteristic of these patterns because of undershoots of the structures needed to create an oral obstruction for these sounds. Speakers with Parkinson's disease have reduced articulatory displacement as compared to normal speakers and incoordination of agonist and antagonist muscle groups (Hirose, Kiritani, & Sawashima, 1982; Hirose, Kiritani, Ushijama, Yoshioka, & Sawashima, 1981; Hunker, Abbs, & Barlow, 1982; Leanderson, Meyerson, & Persson, 1972).

Speaking Rate

There is considerable variation in speaking rate among individuals with parkin-sonism. Some exhibit a slower than normal rate, whereas others exhibit a rate much more rapid than normal. Studies report a large range of speaking rate, from 70 to 250 words per minute (Canter, 1965b). The underlying mechanism for these rate alterations is a topic for speculation. The "rushes of speech" that occur in some individuals with Parkinson's disease exceed a rate of 13 syllables per minute, suggesting that these movements may not be under voluntary con-trol (Netsell, Daniel, & Celesia, 1975). Hunker and Abbs (1984) found that a phase relationship exists between the onset of voluntary movement and the resting tremor cycle, and that this phase relationship is responsible for delays in movement. In other words, some of the delay in initiating movements by speakers with tremor at rest may be the result of "waiting" to get into the appro-priate phase of the tremor cycle. The support for this conclusion was the obser-vation that "voluntary movements of symptomatic structures were executed in-phase with the ongoing resting tremor oscillations" (p. 96). Inferiorly and superiorly directed movement trajectories were initiated during the appropriate negative or positive phases of the resting tremor cycle.

STAGES OF FUNCTIONAL LIMITATIONS IN DYSARTHRIA

Dysarthria associated with Parkinson's disease may vary from absence, through mild and moderate, to severe. Because the focus of intervention, at least in part, depends on the severity of the functional limitation, this section is organized by stage based on these limitations. In each section, the features of the speech are described, along with some common treatment approaches. These treatment approaches will be discussed in detail in Chapters 7 through 12.

Stage 1: No Detectable Speech Disorder

Individuals with the early stage of Parkinson's disease have received the diag-nosis but often do not yet exhibit speech symptoms. During this stage, individ-uals with Parkinson's disease and their family members may engage in educa-tional activities, from which they attempt to learn as much about the condition as they can. Although many individuals with Parkinson's disease do not approach a speech–language pathologist until they are experiencing difficulty with their speech, some may wish to have additional information about communication disorders and what can be done about them. Individuals who participate in highly demanding communication activities, such as trial attorneys, ministers, and teachers, may seek early speech treatment in order to prevent even the mildest of speech disorders. Speakers participating in these demanding roles should be made aware that they may not personally be as sensitive to the onset of speech problems as are others around them. These individuals may need to seek the feedback of others closely associated with them to monitor the appearance of mild symptoms. Some speakers with parkinsonism may complain of increased effort even though they do not have detectable speech symptoms.

Speech–language pathologists involved with Parkinson support groups or in multidisciplinary neurology clinics may be involved in the education of newly diagnosed individuals who are not yet experiencing speech difficulty. During this stage, intervention involves confirmation that speech is normal and provision of information about the types of intervention that are appropriate and available. For individuals who live in rural areas or long distances from speech pathology resources, careful early education about access to services is important. Depending on the natural course and medical management of the disease, this stage with no detectable speech disorders may go on for many years.

Stage 2: Obvious Speech Disorder with Intelligible Speech

Changes in the voice are typically the first speech features to be observed in individuals with Parkinson's disease. In fact, nearly half of the individuals in a large study of prevalence of speech problems in Parkinson's disease exhibited only changes in voice without other features of dysarthria (Logemann et al., 1978). The vocal features associated with this stage of parkinsonian dysarthria include reduced loudness; breathy or weak voice; reduced pitch variability; and an unsteady, hoarse, or rough voice (Ramig, 1992).

Treatment approaches at this stage include techniques to increase vocal fold adduction, to maximize duration of phonation, and to increase respiratory support (Yorkston et al., 1995). As with all stages of dysarthria associated with Parkinson's disease, client and family education is critical. Often, the Lee Silverman Voice Treatment (Ramig, Pawlas, & Countryman, 1995) or similar approaches are implemented in Stage 2. These techniques will be discussed in Chapter 8. Ideal candidates for this type of treatment are individuals with hypoadduction of the vocal folds due to Parkinson's disease. These individuals are highly motivated because oral communication is an important aspect of daily living. The best candidates are able to produce louder phonation when asked to do so. When the voice problems preclude participation in specific communication contexts, such as those involving noise, electronic amplification may be considered.

Stage 3: Reduction in Speech Intelligibility

A reduction in speech intelligibility in certain situations is a key feature distinguishing this stage from the previous one. Frequent communication partners may complain that they need to ask the speaker with Parkinson's disease to repeat or to "speak up." Speaking in groups may be difficult for these individuals. In addition to the voice changes mentioned earlier, dysarthria in this stage is typically characterized by imprecise oral articulation. The range of oral movements may be limited and speakers may fail to reach articulatory targets. Some speakers may pause longer than normal or may pause at unusual locations within an utterance. Other speakers may begin to use excessively rapid rates or rushes of rapid speech.

Treatment approaches at this stage may include many of the techniques used earlier, that is, those that focus on increasing respiratory–phonatory effort. If speakers have received this type of treatment during Stage 2, they may be engaged in an ongoing practice program that appears to be important for maintaining motor learning. They may also need to engage periodically in a maintenance period of therapy to preserve speech gains.

Depending on the individual, a variety of techniques may be effective in slowing speaking rate. Although these techniques are discussed in Chapter 10, the goal is to use the least intrusive rate control technique that provides adequate rate control and optimizes speech naturalness. For some speakers, slowing speech alone appears to be a major factor in maintaining speech intelligibility. Some of these individuals may be speaking at excessive rates, more rapid than normal speakers. Others have an overall speech rate that is nearly normal but appear to speak rapidly. These speakers are typically producing utterances in rapid rushes separated by inappropriately long pauses. As was apparent in Stages 1 and 2, there is a continuing need to "calibrate" for perception of speech effectiveness in individuals with parkinsonism. Speakers may be taught to consider speech as a "performance" whereby they are no longer regular speakers but are "public" speakers (Sullivan, Brune, & Beukelman, 1996). Behavioral rate control techniques and those involving prosthetic devices such as delayed auditory feedback units and voice amplifiers are described in Chapters 8 and 10.

Stage 4: Natural Speech Supplemented by Augmentative Techniques

In Stage 4, natural speech is no longer a functional means of communication for individuals with Parkinson's disease. Speech features may include difficulty initiating voicing and short rushes of poorly articulated speech. Once speech is initiated, the speaker may freeze in mid-utterance and be unable to continue.

Language production may be sparse, perhaps because of associated cognitive problems. Speech performance may noticeably worsen in "off" periods as compared with "on" periods.

During this stage, treatment may focus on supplementing natural speech with augmentative communication approaches such as alphabet supplementation. In this procedure, the speaker points to the first letter of each word as the word is spoken. This technique controls speaking rate as well as providing the listener with additional information.

Because of the reduced intelligibility of their natural speech, these individuals may experience frequent communication breakdowns. Typically, they are taught to resolve these communication breakdowns by spelling words on their alphabet board or by using a portable typing system to clarify their messages. Techniques to assist their partners in assuming more responsibility for communication exchanges will be reviewed in Chapter 12.

Stage 5: No Functional Speech

A small percentage of individuals with Parkinson's disease lose all functional speech. When such a severe speech disorder is present, augmentative communication intervention is required. Given the overall motor control impairment and the relatively frequent cognitive impairments late in the disease, complex augmentative communication interventions are very difficult to institute and must be individualized. Typically, these individuals do not use multifunctional augmentative communication devices, but rather use systems that require letter-by-letter typing with print or speech output.

Web site for a Parkinson glossary (April 23, 1997):

http://www.cfn.cs.dal.ca/Health/NSPF/glossary.html

Acetylcholine: A chemical messenger released by cholinergic nerves. Normally in many parts of the body, including the brain, and necessary to normal body functioning. There appears to be a reciprocal seesaw relationship between acetylcholine and dopamine and their respective nerve cell systems.

Agonist: A chemical or drug that mimics neurotransmitter activity.

Akinesia: Absence of body movements.

Amantadine: A drug that stimulates the release of available dopamine in the brain.

(continues)

Anticholinergic Parkinson's Drugs (Artane, Cogentin): The group of drugs that decreases the action of acetylcholine. The specified drugs may help reduce rigidity, tremor, and drooling in Parkinson's disease.

Basal Ganglia or Nuclei: Deeper structures in the brain, concerned with normal movement and walking. The caudate nucleus, putamen, and substantia nigra are basal ganglia affected in Parkinson's disease.

Benign Essential Tremor: A condition characterized by tremor of the hands, head, voice, and sometimes other parts of the body. Essential tremor often runs in families and is sometimes called familial tremor. It is sometimes mistaken for a symptom of Parkinson's disease. However, this is an action tremor and there is no rigidity or bradykinesia.

Bradykinesia: Slowing down of a movement. Bradykinesia involves slowness of initiating and executing gross and fine motor movements and difficulty in performing repetitive movements. It is a major symptom of Parkinson's disease.

Carbidopa: The ingredient in Sinemet that prevents the breakdown of the levodopa in the body before it can reach the brain.

Cogwheel Rigidity: Stiffness in the muscles, with a jerky quality when arm and leg joints are repeatedly moved.

Deprenyl (Eldepryl, Selegiline, Jumex): A drug that slows the breakdown of chemicals like dopamine by inhibiting the action of certain enzymes. It increases effects of dopamine in the brain.

Dopa Decarboxylase Inhibitors: Drugs that block the conversion of levodopa to dopamine outside the brain. These include carbidopa and benserazide.

Dopamine: A chemical produced by the brain that assists in the effective transmission of electrochemical messages from one nerve cell to the next. It is deficient in the basal ganglia and substantia nigra of a person with Parkinson's disease. It governs actions of movement, balance, and walking.

Dopamine Agonist: Drugs that mimic the effects of dopamine and stimulate the dopamine receptors.

Festination: Walking in rapid, short, shuffling steps.

Freezing: Temporary, involuntary inability to move.

Idiopathic: An adjective meaning "of unknown cause." The usual form of Parkinson's disease is idiopathic.

(continues)

Levodopa-Induced Dyskinesias: A side effect of medication that may occur with prolonged use. These abnormal, involuntary movements may be alleviated by reducing the amount of medication.

Micrographia: The tendency to have very small handwriting due to difficulty with fine motor movements in Parkinson's disease.

MPTP: A toxic chemical exposure that can lead to Parkinson's disease.

Neurotransmitter: A specialized chemical produced in nerve cells that permits the transmission of information between nerve cells.

Nigrostriatal Degeneration: Degeneration of the nerve pathways from substantia nigra to the striatum. These pathways are normally rich in dopamine and are those affected in parkinsonism.

On–Off Fluctuations: Fluctuations that occur in response to levodopa therapy in which the person's mobility changes suddenly and unpredictably from a good response (on) to a poor response (off).

Palilalia: A symptom of parkinsonism, especially the postencephalitic form, in which a word or syllable is repeated and the flow of speech is interrupted.

Pallidectomy: Excision or destruction of the globus pallidus, which is part of the lenticular nucleus, which is part of the striatum.

Paralysis agitans: The Latin form of the older, popular term "shaking palsy," which was used to designate Parkinson's disease before James Parkinson named it.

Parlodel (Bromocriptine): A dopamine agonist useful in treating all of the primary symptoms of Parkinson's disease. It may be used alone or with other antiparkinson medications.

Permax (Pergolide): A drug similar in action to Parlodel but more potent.

Postural Instability: Difficulty with balance.

Propulsive Gait: Disturbance of gait typical of parkinsonism in which, during walking, steps become faster and faster with progressively shorter steps that pass from a walking to a running pace and may precipitate falling forward.

Resting Tremor: Shaking that occurs in a relaxed and supported limb.

Rigidity: Refers in medical usage to a type of muscular stiffness encountered when examining people with Parkinson's disease. It is characterized by a constant, even resistance to passive manipulation of the limbs.

(continues)

Sialorrhea: Drooling of saliva.

Sinemet: Trade name for the antiparkinson drug that is a mixture of levodopa and carbidopa. This drug combination contains a ratio of levodopa 4 mg or 10 mg to carbidopa 1 mg (Sinemet 100/25, Sinemet 250/25).

Sinemet CR: Controlled-release Sinemet. 200 mg Levodopa with 50 mg Carbidopa in a capsule contained in a matrix (outer layer) releasing the drug more slowly in the body. These capsules are not to be taken all at once, but rather in separate doses over the course of a day.

Stereotactic Surgery: Surgical technique that involves placing a small electrode in an area of the brain to destroy a tiny amount of brain tissue.

Substantia Nigra: Black pigmented area of the midbrain where cells manufacture the neurotransmitter dopamine.

Symmetrel (Amantadine): A drug that releases dopamine and is useful in parkinsonism.

Tremor: Rhythmic shaking and involuntary movement of part(s) of the body as a result of sequential muscle contractions.

Note. Modified from the glossary published by The Parkinson's Society of Southern Alberta.

PARKINSONISM-PLUS SYNDROMES

Progressive Supranuclear Palsy

PATHOLOGY–MEDICAL ASPECTS

Clinical Features

Progressive supranuclear palsy is an extrapyramidal syndrome first described in the mid-1960s (Steele, Richardson, & Olszewski, 1964). It is one of the disorders included under the category of parkinsonism-plus syndromes. Symptoms include ophthalmoplegia (mainly of vertical gaze), dystonic rigidity of the neck, pseudobulbar palsy, mild dementia, and spastic dysarthria. The following parkinsonian symptoms have been cited in subsequent reports: akinesia, lack of facial expression, poor postural reflexes, and hypokinetic dysarthria (Behrman, Carroll, Janota, & Matthews, 1969; Blumenthal & Miller, 1969; Hanson & Metter, 1980; Klawans & Ringel, 1971; Verny et al., 1996). Neuropathological alterations are found in many neural structures, including subthalamic nucleus, red nucleus, substantia nigra, superior colliculus, periaqueductal gray matter, globus pallidus, and dentate nucleus of the cerebellum. The disease has an onset in middle and later life, with a mean age of onset of approximately 60 years (Kristensen, 1985). Life expectancy after diagnosis averages 5 to 7 years. This relatively uncommon disease is more frequent in men than women (Steele, 1972). Studies of the natural course of the disease suggest that on average gait assistance is needed 3.1 years after onset, dysarthria is present 3.4 years after onset, visual symptoms 3.9 years after onset, and dysphagia 4.4 years after onset (Golbe, Davis, Schoenberg, & Duvoisin, 1988).

More information about progressive supranuclear palsy can be found at the National Institute of Neurology Disorders and Stroke Web site (June 20, 1997):

http://www.ninds.nih.gov/healinfo/disorder/psp/psp.htm

Diagnosis

Progressive supranuclear palsy can be distinguished from Parkinson's disease in several ways (Cummings & Benson, 1983). In progressive supranuclear palsy, the posture is extended rather than bowed as in Parkinson's disease. In progressive supranuclear palsy, rigidity primarily affects the trunk, whereas in Parkinson's disease, the limbs are primarily affected. Also, tremor is unusual in progressive supranuclear palsy.

Medical Treatment

Currently, there is no generally effective medical treatment for progressive supranuclear palsy. Although reports vary, most suggest that the remarkable response to levodopa seen in Parkinson's disease does not occur in progressive supranuclear palsy. Akinesia improves in some patients treated with levodopa, rigidity and extraocular movements improve in a few patients, and dementia is consistently unaffected (Cummings & Benson, 1983). Preliminary reports of successful rehabilitation programs are available, which include exercise to improve strength and coordination, static and dynamic balance training, and cognitive and speech training (Sosner, Gayten, & Sznajder, 1993).

SPEECH CHARACTERISTICS AND INTERVENTION

Dysarthria may occur early in the course of progressive supranuclear palsy. Dysarthria may be severe even in the early stages, and individuals may exhibit anarthria or mutism in the later stages of the disorder. Palilalia (the compulsive repetition of utterances, often in a context of increasing rate and decreasing loudness) is also a prevalent symptom (LaPointe & Horner, 1981; Metter & Hanson, 1991). The dysarthria associated with progressive supranuclear palsy is a mixed type, including components of spasticity, hypokinesia, and ataxia. Approximately 40% of speakers with progressive supranuclear palsy exhibit two of the three components, and the remainder exhibit all three (Kluin, Foster, Berent, & Gilman, 1993).

Speech and language symptoms vary considerably across individuals (Lebrun, Devreux, & Rousseau, 1986). Although dysarthria is the most common communication problem in progressive supranuclear palsy, language and cognitive deficits (the latter associated with frontal lobe function) have also been reported (Capitani, Laiacona, & Barbarotto, 1993; Esmonde, Giles, Xuereb, & Hodges, 1996; Grafman, Litvan, Gomez, & Chase, 1990; Maher, Smith, & Lees, 1985; Podoll, Schwarz, & Noth, 1991). The most common cognitive problems include slowed information processing and motor execution, rapid forgetting, problems in orienting attentional resources, and difficulty in planning and shifting conceptual sets (Grafman, Litvan, & Stark, 1995). Other neuropsychiatric problems, such as apathy and disinhibition, may also be present (Litvan, Mega, Cummings, & Fairbanks, 1996).

With a few exceptions (Countryman, Ramig, & Pawlas, 1994), reports of successful speech intervention for individuals with progressive supranuclear palsy are rare. However, the effects of delayed auditory feedback (DAF) intervention have been reported with an individual with progressive supranuclear palsy (Hanson & Metter, 1980). See Chapter 10 for a more detailed description of DAF application for individuals with dysarthria. Perhaps one reason for the lack of intervention in this population is the pervasive cognitive problems that place considerable burden on the spouse and the relatively rapid progression of the disease. Beyond brief references in the literature to speech intervention for progressive supranuclear palsy, there is not sufficient information at this time to stage the functional limitation and speech interventions as we have done with other etiologies.

Question: How can you distinguish progressive supranuclear palsy from Parkinson's disease in terms of speech characteristics?

First, dysarthria is frequently one of the earliest symptoms in progressive supranuclear palsy, whereas it is not in Parkinson's disease. Second, in progressive supranuclear palsy, hypokinetic dysarthria is typically accom-
(continues)

panied by some other type of dysarthria (i.e., ataxic or spastic), whereas in Parkinson's disease, hypokinetic dysarthria predominates. The following comparison of speech characteristics is derived from a retrospective review of records of individuals with progressive supranuclear palsy (PSP) and Parkinson's disease (PD) (Duffy, 1995).

More frequent in PSP than PD	More frequent in PD than PSP
Monopitch	Vocal flutter
Hoarseness	Reduced loudness
Nasal emission	Reduced stress
Excess and equal stress	Tremor
Hypernasality	Breathiness
Imprecise articulation	Rapid rate
Slow rate	

Multiple System Atrophy

A number of degenerative neurologic diseases involve multiple areas of the brain. However, the term *multiple system atrophy* has been applied to a specific group of disorders, including Shy-Drager syndrome, olivopontocerebellar atrophy, and striatonigral degeneration (Quinn & Wenning, 1995). Because each of these disorders may be associated with dysarthria, we review each briefly in this text.

SHY-DRAGER SYNDROME

Pathology–Medical Aspects

Shy-Drager syndrome is a progressive disorder of multiple system atrophy with autonomic failure. Individuals with the disorder experience orthostatic hypotension, which is an excessive drop in blood pressure causing dizziness or momentary blackouts when standing or sitting up. Three types of the disorder have been described: (1) a parkinsonian type, which includes slow movement, stiff muscles, and mild tremors; (2) a cerebellar type, which includes problems with loss of balance, stiff muscles, and mild tremors; and (3) a mixed type, which includes a combination of parkinsonian and ataxic features. Both speech and swallowing problems are common. The prognosis for the syndrome is poor, with death occurring from 7 to 10 years after the onset of symptoms.

Speech Characteristics

The type of dysarthria associated with Shy-Drager syndrome is a mixed type (hypokinetic–ataxic, ataxic–spastic, or spastic–ataxic–hypokinetic) (Kluin, Gilman, Lohman, & Junck, 1996; Linebaugh, 1979). The hypokinetic component predominates in approximately half of the cases, the ataxic in approximately a third, and the spastic in approximately 10% of cases. In addition, vocal characteristics associated with paralysis may be present (Bawa, Ramadan, & Wetmore, 1993; Isozaki et al., 1995; Williams, Hanson, & Calne, 1979).

Question: How can the dysarthria associated with Shy-Drager syndrome be differentiated from the dysarthria associated with Parkinson's disease?

Perceptual analysis of the type of dysarthria is useful in making this distinction. The dysarthria in Shy-Drager syndrome is frequently a mixed dysarthria associated with involvement of multiple neural systems. Inspiratory stridor (laryngeal stridor on inhalation) may also occur in Shy-Drager syndrome. Thus, the combination of a mixed dysarthria of the hypokinetic–ataxic–spastic type with inhalatory stridor may raise suspicions about the presence of Shy-Drager syndrome (Duffy, 1995). In comparison with speakers with Parkinson's disease, speakers with Shy-Drager syndrome may have excess vocal hoarseness, intermittent glottal fry, and a slow and deliberate speaking rate (D. G. Hanson, Ludlow, & Bassich, 1983).

STRIATONIGRAL DEGENERATION

Striatonigral degeneration is closely related to Parkinson's disease, but, unlike idiopathic Parkinson's disease where the striatum is normal, striatal degeneration occurs in this disorder. Response to levodopa is usually transient, poor, or absent. The disorder is usually associated with unilateral rigidity, stiffness, and akinesia, which may progress to the other side. Autonomic disorders may also be present. Early appearance of the following signs and symptoms is helpful in distinguishing striatonigral degeneration and Parkinson's disease: severe and atypical progression of bradykinesia and rigidity, slowness of gait, postural instability and increased tendon reflexes, severe dysarthria, and less consistently, dysphagia, stridor, and stimulus-sensitive myoclonus (Gouider-Khouja, Vidailhet, Bonnet, Pichon, & Agid, 1995). Although dysarthria occurs, specifics of the type and severity have not been investigated. Based on underlying neuropathology, a mixed dysarthria with components of hypokinetic, hyperkinetic, and spasticity might be possible (Duffy, 1995).

Medical Aspects

Olivopontocerebellar atrophy refers to a group of inherited and sporadic ataxias characterized by a progressive neurologic degeneration affecting the cerebellum, pons, and inferior olives, as well as the basal ganglia and spinal cord. One of the five clinical types is associated with dementia and extrapyramidal signs. The disorder is associated with ataxia, tremor, and rigidity, and is slowly progressive, with death usually occurring approximately 20 years after onset.

Dementia in the mid to late stages of disease may occur in 30% to 50% of cases (Berciano, 1982). A pattern of cognitive deficits typical of those associated with frontal lobe function may be present. The frontal system deficits include damage to the cerebello-cerebral cortical pathways, and a cholinergic deficit affecting the frontal cortex or caudate (Cohen & Freedman, 1995).

Speech Characteristics

The dysarthria associated with olivopontocerebellar atrophy is mixed and varies depending on which neurologic systems are involved. Spasticity and ataxia are frequently present, but flaccidity and hypokinesia are also possible (Duffy, 1995). The mixed spastic–ataxia dysarthria in olivopontocerebellar atrophy is characterized by continuously reduced pitch, monotony of pitch, monotony of loudness, and strained–strangled phonation (Gilman & Kluin, 1984). Case reports are available describing the medical diagnosis and progression of speech and swallowing disorders associated with olivopontocerebellar atrophy (Hartman & O'Neill, 1989).

HEREDITARY DISEASES
Wilson's Disease

MEDICAL ASPECTS

Wilson's disease is a rare, hereditary disorder caused by inadequate processing of the dietary intake of copper. Because it is an autosomal recessive trait, the affected individual must receive the abnormal gene from both parents. Pathological changes occur in the liver, the brain, and the cornea of the eye as a result of excessive accumulation of copper in the tissue over a period of years. The first signs of the disease usually appear between the ages of 6 and 40. Neurological abnormalities include incoordination, tremor, dysarthria, drooling, dysphagia, and masklike face. Wilson's disease may present as a neurologic syndrome, a psychiatric disturbance, or a hepatic disorder (Cartwright, 1978). Dysarthria is an important symptom in Wilson's disease because it occurs in nearly all cases (Starosta-Rubinstein et al., 1987), it is often the initial symptom of the disorder (Shimizu et al., 1996; Walshe & Yealland, 1992), and it may be the only symptom (Liao, Wang, Kwan, Kong, & Wu, 1992; Topaloglu, Gucuyener, Orkun, & Renda, 1990).

Timely diagnosis is critical because early treatment may lead to complete symptomatic recovery, but it is difficult because of the varied clinical presentations of the disease. If treatment is begun too late, recovery will be only partial. Although there is no method for reversing the metabolic deficit, the destructive effects of copper deposition in tissue can be prevented by appropriate treatment. The current drugs of choice for removing tissue copper and preventing its deposition are a chelating agent, D-penicillamine (S. E. Woods & Colon, 1989), and zinc. Although lifelong treatment is necessary, in most cases penicillamine will eventually reverse many of the neurologic manifestations (Cummings & Benson, 1983). Unfortunately, advanced cases may fail to improve. Foods high in copper, such as shellfish, nuts, liver, chocolate, and mushrooms, should be avoided by individuals with Wilson's disease (Brewer, 1995).

SPEECH CHARACTERISTICS

Dysarthria was recognized as a prominent neurologic feature in Wilson's disease when the disorder was first described by Wilson in 1912. Slowed rates of maximum syllable production rates have been reported (Hefter, Arendt, Stremmel, & Freund, 1993). The speech of 20 individuals with Wilson's disease was studied perceptually (Berry, Darley, Aronson, & Goldstein, 1974). The data suggested the presence of a mixed dysarthria with prominent ataxic, spastic, and hypokinetic features. Cases of pure forms of each type of dysarthria were also reported by Berry and colleagues. Further, speech samples were obtained at two points of medical treatment for 10 of the 20 individuals. Their findings indicated that a regimen of D-penicillamine and a low copper diet produces a significant remission of dysarthria. Long-term treatment for dysarthria has been reported to be helpful in maintaining speech intelligibility in Wilson's disease (Day & Parnell, 1987).

Friedreich's Ataxia

MEDICAL ASPECTS

Friedreich's ataxia is one of a heterogeneous group of degenerative spinocerebellar disorders (Johnson, 1995). The most common type of Friedreich's ataxia is the result of an autosomal recessive trait. Males and females are affected in equal proportions, with age of onset between 11 and 12 years. Most patients die within 20 years of the onset of symptoms. The disorder is usually first observed as it affects the lower extremities with gait disturbance. Dysmetria of the upper extremities and dysarthria occur later. A number of abnormalities frequently occur as part of this syndrome, including skeletal deformities, loss of vibration and position sense, absent muscle stretch reflexes in the lower extremities, nystagmus, limb weakness, optic atrophy, pigmentary retinal degeneration, vestibular involvement, and myocardial degeneration (Brain & Walton, 1969; Menkes, 1974). A constant feature of the neuropathology of Friedreich's ataxia is the degeneration of the large myelinated sensory fibers, posterior roots, and dorsal root ganglion cells. Currently, there is no medical treatment that changes the progressive course of the disorder. However, supportive measures to maximize mobility and other aspects of daily function are important.

SPEECH CHARACTERISTICS

Dysarthria has long been recognized as a symptom of Friedreich's ataxia. In 1877, Charcot described it as a disease in which the tongue became too "thick." The speech disorder is a common finding in Friedreich's ataxia, with an estimated incidence of 63% to 93% (Heck, 1964). Although ataxic dysarthria is the most common type, other types including spasticity also occur (Duffy, 1995). Numerous attempts have been made to describe precisely the characteristics of the dysarthria associated with Friedreich's ataxia, including acoustic analysis (Ackermann, Hertrich, & Hehr, 1995; Cisneros & Braun, 1995; Gentil, 1990; Ouellon, Ryalls, Lebeuf, & Joanette, 1991), kinematics (Devanne, Gentil, & Maton, 1995), and perceptual studies (Gilman & Kluin, 1984). The dysarthric speech resulting from Friedreich's ataxia has been described as either a *general dysarthria,* including reduced intelligibility, monoloudness, prolonged phonemes, inappropriate silences, imprecise consonants, and distorted vowels, or a *vocal stenosis type,* including harshness, pitch breaks, and pitch level (Joanette & Dudley, 1980).

Question: Both Wilson's disease and Friedreich's ataxia have onset of symptoms after childhood. Are there hereditary diseases of childhood in which dysarthria is an important symptom?

Yes, one such disease is ataxia telangiectasia (AT), in which symptoms appear during the second year of life with cerebellar symptoms. In addition to the neurologic problems, the disorder is characterized by an immunodeficiency that results in recurrent respiratory infections. Children

(continues)

with AT are also predisposed to develop malignancies of the blood system. Common neurologic symptoms include ataxia, dysarthria, ocular motor apraxia, an impassive face, chorea, dystonia, and peripheral neuropathy (C. G. Woods & Taylor, 1992).

Dystonia

Pathology–Medical Aspects

The dystonias are a group of motor disorders characterized by abnormal, involuntary movements and postures. The term *dystonia* was coined by Oppenheim, who described individuals with sustained posturing and also tonic and clonic spasms of muscles in different parts of the body (Fahn, 1984). These spasms are typically activated with voluntary motor activity. There is neither weakness nor wasting of muscle. Sensory, sphincter, and reflex alternations do not occur. The severity of dystonia may vary from a mild nuisance to a catastrophic condition. Generally, the most rapid, progressive, and severe symptomatology is seen in individuals with onset before the age of 8 years (Cooper, Cullinan, & Riklan, 1976).

Although dystonia is attributed to disturbances of the extrapyramidal system, the underlying neuropathology and mechanisms have not yet been fully described (Berardelli, Curra, & Manfredi, 1996; Marsden & Harrison, 1974). Certain familial forms of dystonia suggest a heterogeneous genetic component to disease occurrence. Cortical excitability is altered, as is the basal ganglia input to the cortex. A deficit in the body's ability to process a group of chemicals called neurotransmitters is suspected. These neural transmitters include GABA (an inhibitory substance that helps the brain maintain muscle control), dopamine (an inhibitory chemical that influences the brain's control of complex movement), acetylcholine (an excitatory chemical that in the brain helps regulate dopamine and in the body released at nerve endings causes muscle contractions), and norepinephrine and serotonin (inhibitory chemicals that help regulate acetylcholine). In electromyographic studies of dystonia, several abnormalities of motor control have been identified including abnormal input from muscle afferents and disturbed segmental spinal cord control especially of reciprocal inhibition of neurons (Berardelli et al., 1996; Kaji, Ikeda, et al., 1995a; Kaji, Rothwell, et al., 1995b; Priori, Berardelli, Mercuri, & Manfredi, 1995; Ridding, Sheean, Rothwell, Inzelberg, & Kujirai, 1995).

CLASSIFICATIONS

The dystonias may be classified in a number of ways, including age of onset, etiology, and distribution of symptoms. See Table 4.2.

Age of Onset

In the study by Marsden, Harrison, and Bundy (1976), generalized dystonia developed in 85% of those with onset at or before age 10, in 60% of those with onset between ages 11 and 20, and in only 4% of those with onset after age 20. The initial patterns for the three groups are as follows (I. Cooper, 1969):

Table 4.2
Classification of Dystonia

Age of Onset

Infantile
Childhood
Adolescent
Adult

Etiology

Primary
   Inherited
   Sporadic
Secondary
   Associated with hereditary neurologic disease (e.g., Wilson's disease)
   Environmental (e.g., drug exposure)
   Associated with parkinsonism
   Psychogenic

Distribution

Focal
Segmental (e.g., cranial)
Multifocal
Generalized

Note. Adapted from "Movement Disorders of the Larynx," by M. F. Brin, S. Fahn, A. Blitzer, L. O. Ramig, and C. Stewart, 1992, in *Neurologic Disorders of the Larynx* (pp. 248–278), by A. Blitzer, M. F. Brin, C. T. Sasaki, S. Fahn, and K. S. Harris (Eds.), New York: Thieme Medical Publishers.

- *Childhood form*—Onset occurs at 4 to 6 years of age. The initial symptom nearly always is flexion inversion of the foot, with progression to generalized dystonia within 4 to 6 years of onset.

- *Adolescent form*—Onset occurs at 8 to 13 years of age. The initial symptom is usually in the foot, but sometimes in the arm; the rate of progression is slower than the childhood form.

- *Adult form*—Initial symptoms usually start in the arm; this form usually develops into axial (trunk) dystonia with relative sparing of the extremities.

Etiology

A number of etiologies exist for dystonia. Those that are idiopathic and inherited are considered primary, whereas those that are associated with other disorders (e.g., Wilson's disease or parkinsonism) or environmental agents (e.g., drug exposure or trauma) are considered secondary. The primary dystonias are slowly progressive disorders that can plateau anywhere in the course of the illness. They begin insidiously and almost always with action dystonia (Fahn, 1984).

In contrast to primary forms of dystonia, most secondary dystonias begin with dystonia at rest and even with sustained postures. Some secondary dystonias have an obvious sudden beginning, such as on recovery from an acute encephalopathic event. Secondary dystonias may also be associated with metabolic disease (e.g., Wilson's disease, Hallervorden-Spatz disease), and tend to have a more rapidly progressive course than do the primary dystonias. Some secondary dystonias are due to environmental causes, such as head trauma, encephalitis, and exposure to toxins, and tend to have a course that stabilizes and does not progress. Drugs that block the dopamine D2 receptor (antipsychotic and substituted benzamides, such as metoclopramide) can induce two types of dystonia: acute dystonic reaction and delayed persistent dystonia (tardive dystonia). Acute dystonic reaction can be reversed readily with administration of anticholinergics or diazepam. Tardive dystonia is not only persistent, but is also frequently unresponsive to therapeutic attempts.

Distribution

The distribution of signs and symptoms in dystonia is usually categorized as generalized (affecting many areas of the body), segmental (limited involvement, such as in the arm and neck, both arms, or neck and trunk but sparing the legs), focal (signs limited to a single arm or hand), or multifocal. The diagnosis of idiopathic torsion dystonia or generalized dystonia is based on the following criteria (Marsden et al., 1976):

- The presence of dystonic movements and postures (but arbitrarily excluding spasmodic torticollis)

- Normal prenatal history and early development

- No history of precipitating illness or exposure to drugs known to provoke torsion dystonia prior to the onset of the disease

- No evidence of intellectual, pyramidal, cerebellar, or sensory deficit on clinical examination

- Failure of laboratory investigations, including copper studies, to demonstrate any cause of the disease

The "typical" picture of segmental dystonia in adults is onset with dystonic postures and spasms affecting one arm, with subsequent spread to the other arm and neck or the neck alone (Marsden et al., 1976). Focal dystonia usually involves symptoms in one area of the body, such as the arm (writer's cramp) or the face (cranial dystonia). The syndrome of cranial dystonia, also known as blepharospasm-oromandibular dystonia, Breughel's syndrome, or Meige's syndrome, was described in 1910 by Henry Meige (Golper, Nutt, Rou, & Coleman, 1983). The hallmark features of this syndrome are blepharospasm, a prolonged tonic contraction of the orbicularis oculi muscles, and both fluctuating and sustained contractions of facial, lingual, and mandibular muscle groups (Golper et al., 1983). Dystonic spasms disappear during sleep and are triggered by initiation of speech or presentation of food or drink to the mouth. See Table 4.3 for a description of the focal dystonias that may affect speech.

MEDICAL MANAGEMENT

Usually the underlying disorder of dystonia is not treatable, except in some cases of secondary dystonia. For example, Wilson's disease can be treated with D-penicillamine. Drug-induced dystonia requires the elimination of the drug. Some patients with tardive dystonia have improved with anticholinergics (Burke, Fahn, & Gold, 1980). Symptomatic therapy is initiated when no specific therapy is available. Anticholinergics may have the highest percentage chance of benefit (Fahn & Jankowic, 1984; Vogels, Maassen, Rotteveel, & Merx, 1994). Some patients will benefit from diazepam, levodopa, or bromocriptine. Surgical approaches are considered when chemical therapies have failed; these may include lesioning peripheral nerves and unilateral or bilateral thalamotomies (Andrew, Fowler, & Harrison, 1983). Thalamotomy has been

Table 4.3
Types of Focal Dystonia

Type	Symptoms	Common Misdiagnoses
Spasmodic torticollis	Affects muscles in the head, neck, and spine, causing the head to assume unnatural postures and to turn uncontrollably. Often results in considerable pain.	Stiff neck, arthritis, stress, psychogenic disorder
Blepharospasm	Causes involuntary muscle contraction of the eyelids, holding them closed for increasing period of time. When muscles of the face are affected, grimacing occurs.	Dry eye syndrome, tic, stress, psychogenic disorder
Oromandibular dystonia	Jaw muscles, lips, and tongue are affected, causing the jaw to be held open or clamped shut. When severe, eating, swallowing, and speaking are difficult.	Temporomandibular joint syndrome, stress, psychogenic disorder
Meige's syndrome	A combination of blepharospasm and oromandibular dystonia	A combination of blepharospasm and oromandibular dystonia
Spasmodic dysphonia	Affects muscles that control the vocal cords resulting in speech that is strained–strangled, halting, or reduced to a whisper.	Laryngitis, vocal abuse, sore throat, stress, or psychogenic disorder
Writer's cramp	Triggered by writing or performing other fine hand functions, such as playing a musical instrument. The hand and finger muscles contract or extend, halting the action, or requiring an exaggerated posture to continue.	Carpel tunnel syndrome, tennis elbow, strain, stress, psychogenic disorder

Note. Adapted from *Dystonia Dialog* [Online], by Dystonia Medical Foundation, April 30, 1997. Available: http://www.ziplink.net/users/dystonia/

effective for contralateral limb dystonia in some patients, but has not been effective for axial dystonia (Fahn & Jankowic, 1984). Rehabilitation programs for individuals with generalized dystonia have been beneficial in improving function (McGuire, Palaganas-Tosco, & Redford, 1988).

Recently, the injection of botulinum toxin or Botox to paralyze the affected muscles has been the treatment of choice in focal dystonia (Tsui, 1996).

Botulinum toxin reduces muscle activity by temporarily blocking the release of acetylcholine at the neuromuscular junction. Muscle activity returns usually within 3 to 4 months with the sprouting of new terminals. Botulinum toxin has been used in the treatment of a number of the focal dystonias, including blepharospasm (Scott, 1980), writer's cramp (L. G. Cohen, Hallett, Geller, & Hochberg, 1989), spasmodic dysphonia (Blitzer & Brin, 1991; Ludlow, Naunton, Sedory, Schulz, & Hallett, 1988), hemifacial spasm (Brin et al., 1987; Tolosa, Marti, & Kulisevsky, 1988), spasmodic torticollis (Tsui & Calne, 1988), Meige syndrome (Mauriello, 1985), and orolingual mandibular dystonia (Blitzer, Greene, Brin, & Fahn, 1989; Schulz & Ludlow, 1991).

In 1990, the National Institutes of Health Consensus Panel published a statement about the clinical use of botulinum toxin injection. The panel, which comprised neurologists, ophthalmologists, otolaryngologists, and speech pathologists, recommended the following:

- Botulinum toxin therapy is safe and effective for treating strabismus, blepharospasm, hemifacial spasm, adductor spasmodic dysphonia, jaw-closing oromandibular dystonia, and cervical dystonia.

- Botulinum toxin is not curative in chronic neurologic disorders.

- The safety of botulinum toxin therapy during pregnancy and breast feeding, and chronic use during childhood is unknown.

- The long-term effect of chronic treatment with botulinum toxin remains unknown.

- Botulinum toxin should be administered by committed interdisciplinary teams of physicians and related heath care professionals with appropriate instrumentation.

Speech Characteristics

GENERALIZED DYSTONIA

Due to varying severity and symptom patterns, not all individuals with generalized dystonia exhibit dysarthria. However, severe generalized dystonia may be associated with severe communication and swallowing problems. Decreased speech intelligibility may be related to abnormal breathing patterns (LaBlance & Rutherford, 1991). Speakers with generalized dystonia showed a faster than normal breathing rate, less rhythmic breathing patterns, decreased lung volume, and apnea-like periods that were accompanied by decreased arterial blood oxygen saturation. At times, speech and writing problems necessitate the use of augmentative communication systems (Shahar, Nowaczyk, & Tervo, 1987).

FOCAL DYSTONIA

Spastic Torticollis

Spastic torticollis or cervical dystonia is one of the focal dystonias in which the abnormal postures and movements involve the strap muscles of the neck. It is one of the most common types of focal dystonia (McGeer & McGeer, 1988). The speech of 70 individuals with spastic torticollis has been studied. Detailed acoustic and perceptual analyses suggested that, although dysarthria is not severe, a number of abnormalities are apparent (LaPointe, Case, & Duane, 1994). The abnormalities are related to fundamental frequency, sequential and alternate movement rates, sibilant and vowel duration, and phonation reaction time.

Focal Cranial Dystonia

In the dystonias involving the mouth, face, and larynx, a variety of symptoms may be observed (Fahn, 1984). Lingual dystonia often accompanies other forms of oromandibular dystonias. Occasionally, however, it is an isolated phenomenon. It may be present at rest, with either a sustained protrusion of the tongue or an upward deflection, so that the tongue is curved and touches the hard palate. More often it occurs as an action dystonia. The tongue appears normal when not in use, but abnormal lingual movements appear when the patient begins to speak or bring food to the back of the pharynx for deglutition. Dystonic movements of the jaw indicate that the abnormal movements involve muscles innervated by Cranial Nerve V, termed oromandibular dystonia. The two most common manifestations of the mandibular dystonia are a pulling down or a pulling up of the jaw. The movements are often repetitive, in part because the patient is trying to overcome the involuntary pulling of the muscles. Commonly, lower facial muscles are involved in association with jaw dystonia.

Several researchers have studied groups of dystonic speakers. The Mayo Clinic studies of 30 patients with dystonia showed that in dystonia, phonation, articulation, and prosody were all significantly disturbed (Darley et al., 1975). For example, 27 or 30 patients displayed vocal harshness, 17 produced strained–strangled sound during speech, 9 demonstrated excessive loudness, and 11 exhibited voice stoppages. Slow speaking rate was observed in 23 of 30 dystonic speakers, and short phrases were demonstrated in 11 speakers. All 30 dystonic speakers demonstrated imprecise consonants, and 24 displayed disordered vowels and irregular articulatory breakdowns.

Golper and colleagues (1983) described the perceptual speech characteristics of 10 individuals with focal cranial dystonia. They summarized their findings as follows:

> Five subjects displayed abnormal contraction of cranial muscles which were to varying degrees exacerbated by speech initiation. The speech impairment varied depending upon the primary muscle groups affected. Speech intelligibility was decreased as a function of the severity of the dystonia and the location of involvement rather than the number of muscle groups affected. The most noticeable decreases in intelligibility were found in two subjects with severe oromandibular dystonia. Those subjects with relatively mild to moderate impairment across several muscle groups maintained remarkably intelligible speech. However, their speech was judged as sounding bizarre. . . . Although there were differences among the dysarthric subjects in loci and degree of dystonia, the prominent speech characteristics were similar to the dystonia patients of Darley et al. (1975). (pp. 132–133)

Spasmodic Dysphonia

Spasmodic dysphonia and laryngeal dystonia (formerly called spastic dysphonia) are terms used to describe an action-induced disorder of laryngeal movement. Two types of spasmodic dysphonia occur: adductor spasmodic dysphonia, involving irregular hyperadduction of the vocal folds, and abductor spasmodic dysphonia, involving intermittent abduction of the vocal folds (Aronson, 1985). The perceptual characteristics of each of these disorders are distinctive. In adductor spasmodic dysphonia, voice quality is strained–strangled, with abrupt initiation and termination of voicing resulting in short breaks in phonation. In abductor spasmodic dysphonia, on the other hand, voice quality may be breathy with abrupt termination of voicing resulting in whispered segments of speech.

With the increasing use of botulinum toxin injection for treatment of spasmodic dysphonia, a number of studies of the changes in speech associated with the procedure are becoming available (Adams, Hunt, Charles, & Lang, 1993; Ludlow et al., 1988; Ludlow, Naunton, Terada, & Anderson, 1991). Although injection may result in dramatic improvement in speech, adverse effects may include decreased loudness, breathiness, and difficulty swallowing liquids (Holzer & Ludlow, 1996).

HUNTINGTON'S DISEASE

Huntington's disease is a degenerative disorder of the nervous system characterized by clinical features including chorea (excessive, irregular, nonrepetitive, randomly distributed movements), dementia, emotional instability, and a history of familial occurrence. See Table 4.4 for a listing of the cardinal features. Inheritance is via an autosomal dominant trait with complete penetrance. Thus, half the offspring of an afflicted individual will develop the disease. Males and females are equally likely to have the disease. The abnormal Huntington gene has been located on the short arm of chromosome 4 using recombinant DNA technology. Average age of onset of symptoms is 35 to 40 years, although symptoms may appear as early as 2 years and as late as 70 years. The average course from onset to death is 14 years. Prevalence in the United States is 40 to 70 per 1 million population (Hogg, Massey, & Schoenberg, 1979). Huntington's disease directly affects about 25,000 individuals in the United States.

Table 4.4
Cardinal Features of Huntington's Disease

Motor signs and symptoms
  Chorea
  Clumsiness
  Motor impersistence
  Abnormal gait
  Loss of postural reflexes
Personality changes
  Inappropriate behavior
  Impetuousness
  Irritability with loss of social inhibitions
  Low threshold for frustration
Emotional disorders
  Depression
Lack of motivation
  Apathy
  Need to be reminded to perform daily chores
  Decreased initiation of conversation
Cognitive decline
Changes on neural imaging
  Caudate atrophy on computed tomography scan
  Decreased glucose metabolism in striatum on positron emission tomography scan
Progressive course

Note. Adapted from "Movement Disorders of the Larynx," by M. F. Brin, S. Fahn, A. Blitzer, L. O. Ramig, and C. Stewart, 1992, in *Neurologic Disorders of the Larynx*, New York: Thieme Medical.

At least 100,000 blood relatives of these individuals are at risk (National Institute of Neurological Disorders and Stroke, Huntington's Disease—Research Highlights, May 1997; available at:

http://www.ninds.nih.gov/healinfo/disorder/huntingt/hdreport.htm)

Question: I don't understand use of the term movement disorders. Aren't all dysarthrias movement disorders?

The term movement disorders has a specific meaning in the field of neurology to refer to a group of diseases of the extrapyramidal system that are associated with involuntary movement or abnormalities of skeletal muscle tone, posture, or both. Movement disorders can be classified as either hypokinesia (those demonstrating a poverty of movement, such as parkinsonism) or hyperkinesia (those displaying excessive abnormal involuntary movement, such as in dystonia or Huntington's disease). Detailed descriptions of the anatomy, physiology, and neuropharmacology of movement disorders are available (Jain & Kirshblum, 1993).

Pathology–Medical Aspects

NEUROPATHOLOGY

Huntington's disease is a disorder of the extrapyramidal system (those motor centers that are not part of the pyramidal cortex and tracts) that involves neurotransmitters. Neuropathologic findings consist of atrophy of the striatal bodies, which is associated with loss of small neurons. Cortical neurons may also degenerate. Frontotemporal atrophy has been identified using magnetic resonance imaging. The biochemistry of Huntington's disease involves a deficiency of the neurotransmitter, gamma-aminobutyric acid (GABA) and enkephalin in the basal ganglia. The lack of GABA inhibition may lead to a relative overactivity of the dopaminergic systems. Hypofunction of the cholinergic neurons has also been suggested (Chong et al., 1997).

NATURAL COURSE

An understanding of the natural course of a disease is critical for planning intervention with any progressive disorders. The impact of Huntington's disease is multidimensional, impairing such things as motor control, cognition, and personality. These in turn have consequences for the level of functional limitation experienced by the individual. A functional scale developed from review of questionnaire data is available for Huntington's disease (Shoulson &

Fahn, 1979); this scale rates the general areas of occupation, finances, domestic responsibilities, activities of daily living, and living situation, rather than motor or cognitive function per se. Personality changes usually occur before the onset of chorea. These alterations include irritability, untidiness, and loss of interest (Cummings & Benson, 1983). Transient facial grimacing, head nodding, and flexion–extension movement of the fingers may be the first manifestation of the choreic movements. In advanced stages of disease, the speed of movement slows and patients acquire an athetotic or dystonic character.

DIAGNOSIS

The diagnosis of Huntington's disease is made initially on the basis of clinical findings of choreiform movement disorder and dementia occurring on a familial basis. There is now a laboratory test utilizing polymerase chain reactions in any DNA containing samples that confirm the diagnosis of Huntington's disease (Chong et al., 1997). Huntington's disease may be distinguished from other types of chorea, including Sydenham's chorea (a self-limited disease of children usually associated with episodes of inflammatory or infectious processes), tardive dyskinesia (a movement disorder developed in individuals who are chronically exposed to neuroleptic drugs), and other inherited or familial choreas (benign hereditary chorea).

Question: If presymptomatic testing is available for individuals with Huntington's disease, why doesn't everyone take advantage of this technology?

The decision to undergo or not to undergo genetic testing is a complex one. At-risk individuals who had chosen not to undergo testing were surveyed (Quaid & Morris, 1993). The reasons they gave for their decision included the following:

- Increased risk to children if one is a gene carrier
- Absence of an effective cure
- Potential loss of health insurance
- Financial cost of testing
- Inability to "undo" the knowledge

MEDICAL TREATMENT

No medical treatment changes the course of Huntington's disease for afflicted individuals. Phenothiazines and other dopamine antagonists, such as tetrabecazine, have been used to control the choreiform movements (Swash, Roberts, Zakko, & Heathfield, 1972). Depression, psychosis, and anxiety are treated with standard agents.

COGNITIVE CHANGES

Understanding of the cognitive changes associated with Huntington's disease is critical not only because they are a hallmark of the disease but also because the constraints imposed by cognitive limitations dictate both the timing and the strategies for communication training. Cognitive changes may occur early in the disease; in fact, individuals who carry the Huntington's disease gene perform more poorly than noncarriers on tests of intellectual function such as the *Wechsler Adult Intelligence Scale–Revised* (Foroud et al., 1995). Intellectual impairment is a major factor in reducing a person's functional capacity in the early stages of the disease (Mayeux, Stern, Herman, Greenbaum, & Fahn, 1986). Early changes have been found in cognitive efficiency, memory, and sensorimotor function (Lundervold & Reinvang, 1991). With progression, a broader range of function becomes involved. Attentional deficits have also been implicated as a partial cause of other higher cognitive deficits (Sprengelmeyer, Lange, & Homberg, 1995) and early changes in daily function (Rothlind, Bylsma, Peyser, Folstein, & Brandt, 1993). The dementia associated with Huntington's disease is considered a subcortical type with disruption in concentration and acquisition of new information (Perry & Hodges, 1996; Pillon, Dubois, Ploska, & Agid, 1991).

SWALLOWING DISORDERS

Swallowing problems are common but not universal in Huntington's disease. The symptoms vary depending on underlying movement problems (Kagel & Leopold, 1992). Individuals with predominant hyperkinesia may exhibit uncontrolled tachyphagia, darting lingual chorea, uninhibited swallowing initiation, and impaired respiratory inhibition during swallowing. Individuals with rigid-bradykinetic symptoms share many features of parkinsonism, including mandibular rigidity, inefficient mastication, and slowed oral transit. Challenges involved in swallowing management include cognitive changes and the individual's reduced ability to accurately report problems. Approaches to management of swallowing disorders in Huntington's disease are reported elsewhere (Yorkston et al., 1995).

As readers review the literature related to swallowing disorders in Huntington's disease, a number of terms specific to this disorder may be used (Kagel & Leopold, 1992). The following swallowing disruptions characterize Huntington's disease:

- *Tachyphagia* is rapid uncontrolled swallowing that is common. This may be the result of impaired cognitive and intraoral

(continues)

sensory functions that disable a centrally mediated inhibitory process.

- *Respiratory chorea* is involuntary movement of the respiratory system that may interrupt the normal reciprocal respiration–deglutition cycle and places the individual at risk for aspiration.

- *Eructation* is excessive belching and is most likely associated with chorea.

- *Aerophagia* is swallowing of air that may result from lingual chorea and repetitive swallows.

Speech Characteristics

PERCEPTUAL CHARACTERISTICS

Chorea is associated with involuntary movements of muscle groups that the speaker cannot predict. Speech may be disrupted by sudden movements of the respiratory muscles, tongue, and face. Speech symptoms may range from little or no dysarthria in cases where choreic movements are restricted to the limbs and body, to speech that is so severely impaired that it is unintelligible. Darley and colleagues (1975) summarized the perceptual characteristics of 30 individuals with hyperkinetic dysarthria of chorea as follows:

> a highly variable pattern of interference with articulation; episodes of hypernasality, harshness, and breathiness; and unplanned variations in loudness. In the speaker's apparent attempt to avoid the inevitable interruptions and to compensate for them, his rate of speech is variably altered, phonemes and intervals between words are prolonged, stress is equalized and inappropriate silences appear. (p. 210)

Speech symptoms are so closely related to the underlying movement disorder that marked improvement in speech symptoms is dependent on modification of the severity of the movement disorders. In an acoustic analysis of phonation in individuals with Huntington's disease, Ramig (1986) found that abnormalities include low-frequency segments (abrupt drops in fundamental frequency of approximately one octave), vocal arrests, and reduced maximal vowel duration. Changes due to behavioral speech intervention have not been reported, although speech may improve coincident with medication management of the choreic movements (Beukelman, 1983).

STAGES OF FUNCTIONAL LIMITATIONS IN DYSARTHRIA

Stage 1: No Detectable Speech Disorder

In the presymptomatic phases of Huntington's disease, individuals who carry the gene do not exhibit change in speech. Because cognitive and personality changes may occur early in the disease, early speech intervention may involve helping individuals with the disorder to manage their communication environment, for example, to develop simple scripts for ordinary communication exchanges, maintaining a topic, and reducing perseveration.

Stage 2: Obvious Speech Disorder with Intelligible Speech

At Stage 2, changes in speech are obvious but intelligibility is not reduced. Frequently, mild dysarthria does not impose a functional limitation. Approaches to intervention at this stage may involve improving speech production (Yorkston et al., 1995); they include techniques to reduce phonatory stenosis (e.g., relaxation techniques such as chewing or yawning) and techniques to maintain appropriate speaking rate.

As in Stage 1, communication partners may need to take on some responsibility for maintaining efficient communication exchanges. For example, for some with hypokinetic symptoms, speech is unusual, perhaps because they are slow in starting. Partners need to learn to wait until the speaker is able to initiate a response. For those with more hyperkinetic symptoms, partners may need to learn to focus on the content of the utterance and not be distracted by the usual and excessive movements. Others with cognitive deficits may need extra time to understand a partner's question and to formulate and initiate a response. This delay may seem to be unnaturally long, and uninformed partners may be too quick to "jump in" before a response can be given.

Stage 3: Reduction in Speech Intelligibility

Because speech intelligibility may be compromised at Stage 3, behavioral training focusing of normalizing respiratory patterning for speech may be helpful, along with strategies for identifying and resolving communication breakdowns. During this stage, partner training continues to be important in order for the partner to take on increasing responsibility for communication. This may include structuring communication so that responses are simplified, such as asking questions that require only a brief response. Partners may also need to establish and maintain topics. Communication may also be facilitated if the partner modifies the environment by reducing such distractions as extraneous noise.

Stage 4: Natural Speech Supplemented with Augmentative Techniques

At Stage 4, natural speech is no longer functional without assistance or supple-mentation. Severe chorea may limit the ability to write, type, or directly select words or phrases, and cognitive decline may limit the ability to learn to use complex augmentative communication systems. At this stage, more of the responsibility for communication must be placed on the partner to assist in the use of alphabet boards, to assist in choice making, and to help reduce persever-ation and maintain conversational topics (Klasner, 1993). Speakers may be taught to spell words aloud when they are not understandable.

Stage 5: No Useful Speech

A variety of augmentative communication techniques used with other individ-uals with severe cognitive problems may also be appropriate in Stage 5 of Hunt-ington's disease (e.g., schedule boxes and boards, basic choice alternatives, viewing disruptive or challenging behaviors as potentially communicative). Because individuals with Huntington's disease retain literacy skills, an alphabet board may be useful for a period of time, until uncontrolled movement makes direct selection difficult. Alphabet supplementation is used with success only occasionally because of the cognitive demands of the task (inhibiting speech, locating first letter, pointing accurately, waiting for the partner's response, etc.).

AMYOTROPHIC LATERAL SCLEROSIS

Pathology–Medical Aspects

Amyotrophic lateral sclerosis (ALS) or Lou Gehrig's disease is a progressive degenerative disease involving the motor neurons of both the brain and the spinal cord in adults. Some motor neuron diseases, such as *spinal muscular atrophy*, involve primarily the lower motor neurons; others, such as *primary lateral sclerosis*, involve the upper motor neurons. Classical ALS involves both types of motor neurons. Upper motor neuron signs include muscle weakness, increased muscle tone (spasticity), hyperreflexia, extensor plantar reflexes, and pseudobulbar palsy (manifested by hypertonic bulbar muscles, increased perioral reflexes, and exaggerated emotional responses). Lower motor neuron signs include muscle weakness, muscular atrophy, and diminished or absent deep tendon reflexes.

Question: Are the terms motor neuron disease and ALS the same?

No, ALS is one of a number of motor neuron diseases. Others include progressive bulbar palsy, a degeneration of bulbar nuclei, resulting in flaccid weakness of the bulbar musculature; primary progressive muscular atrophy, a degeneration of ventral horn cells of the spinal cord, resulting in weakness and wasting of the extremities; and primary lateral sclerosis, degeneration of motor cells in the cortex and corticospinal tracts, resulting in spastic weakness of trunk and extremities.

POPULATION CHARACTERISTICS

The average worldwide incidence of ALS ranges between 1 and 2 per 100,000 population (Ross, 1997). Ninety-five percent of all cases are sporadic. However, there are two familial inherited types of ALS. The familial adult type is based on an autosomal dominant inheritance, whereas with juvenile onset, the inheritance mechanism may be autosomal dominant or recessive (Tandan & Bradley, 1985b). For sporadic ALS in the United States and Europe, the mean age at onset is 58 years with a male-to-female ratio of 1.5:1. Between 14% and 39% of individuals with ALS survive for 5 years, about 10% live up to 10 years, and a few live for 20 years. Several factors appear to determine the course and duration of the disease for the individual patient. The prognosis becomes less positive progressively with each of the following symptoms: musculature atrophy, upper motor neuron involvement, respiratory insufficiency, and predominant bulbar symptoms (Tandan & Bradley, 1985a, 1985b).

ETIOLOGY

Numerous possible causative mechanisms have been investigated without any being overwhelmingly convincing (Amico & Antil, 1981; Rowland, 1991; Tandan & Bradley, 1985b). Among other causes, ALS may be the "age-limited resultant of one or more exogenous agents," including heavy metal exposure; trauma; and physical activity (Kurtzke, 1991). The possibility of genetic factors at least contributing to the development of the full-blown disease seems tempting in view of the fact that familial forms do exist. Other general factors that have been mentioned are the aging phenomenon and the association of ALS with neoplasia. Some degree of loss of motor neuron cells does occur in normal aging; however, if ALS is a form of "premature aging," it is unclear as to what the mechanism would be. A viral theory of causation is attractive because of the existence of such viruses as the poliomyelitis virus, which selectively affects anterior horn cells. A slow, virus-type infection is most likely, although no viral particles have been identified and tissue transplantation in animals has not resulted in ALS. The pathophysiologic mechanism underlying ALS has been described as complex, multifactorial, and interrelated (Eisen & Krieger, 1993). One recent theory suggests that glutamate, the primary excitatory neurotransmitter in the central nervous system, accumulates to toxic concentrations at synapses and causes neurons to die (Bensimon, Lacomblez, & Meininger, 1994). Another theory links the cause of ALS to autoimmunity (Appel, Smith, Engelhardt, & Stefanni, 1993) and suggests that autoimmune disorders may induce an excitotoxic state (Appel, 1993). Despite important advances, no current theory adequately accounts for all the clinical and epidemiologic features of ALS.

SIGNS, SYMPTOMS, AND NATURAL COURSE

The symptoms characteristic of ALS are generally classified by site of involvement (i.e., upper motor neuron or lower motor neuron) and whether spinal nerves (those innervating the arms and legs) or bulbar nerves (those innervating the muscles of speech and swallowing) are involved. The most common presenting symptom is a focal or segmental weakness (63%); the most common form is a paraparesis (20%), but the weakness may be more focal at outset. About one third of all individuals with ALS complain of hand clumsiness, and another one third of leg weakness, which may be manifested as tripping over carpets or on steps. Twenty-two percent show bulbar symptoms (dysarthria in 45%, dysphagia in 42%, dysphonia in 12%, and dyspnea in 6%). Fasciculations are rarely the presenting complaints. It is not unusual for individuals to complain of muscle pain and cramping or paresthetic-like pains even though ALS is a disease of the motor neuron cells (Adam, 1986; Gubbay, Kahana, Zilber, & Cooper, 1985).

ALS is a progressive disease with a median survival of 3 years from the time of symptom onset (Tandan & Bradley, 1985a). Those showing bulbar symptoms tend to have a more rapid course (median of 2.2 years). A subgroup of individuals (perhaps up to 25%) have a prolonged course; some have been reported to survive more than 20 years (Ross, 1997). Increasing weakness of the extremities, inability to swallow without aspiration, and decreased ability to speak ensue. Death is usually on the basis of respiratory failure or infection. Extraocular muscle movements are usually spared, as is sphincter control.

NEUROPATHOLOGY

The motor neurons of the brain stem and spinal cord show simple atrophy, shrinkage, and cell loss (Hirano & Iwata, 1979). In individuals with extensive upper motor neuron signs, there is a depletion of Betz cells and large pyramidal neurons from the fifth layer of the motor cortex and widespread degeneration of the corticospinal tracts (Hughes, 1982). Studies have shown a reduction in the number of large motor neurons in the cervical and lumbar spinal cord (Tohgi, Tsukagnoshi, & Toyokura, 1997). In the peripheral nervous system, several studies have reported a marked reduction in the number of large myelinated fibers in the ventral roots (Hanyu, Oguchi, Yanagisawa, & Tsukagnoshi, 1981; Sobue, Matsouka, & Maukai, 1981). In addition, an accumulation of neurofilaments has been noted in motor neuron cell bodies and proximal axons (Hirano, 1996).

DIAGNOSTIC TESTING

Because of the serious implications associated with the diagnosis of ALS, it is essential to diagnose and manage potentially treatable disorders with symptoms similar to ALS. However, because there is no specific biochemical marker for ALS, definitive diagnosis is difficult early in the disease. Diagnosis is primarily clinical, with supportive evidence from electrophysiological testing. On electromyography, evidence of denervation (the presence of fibrillations) and reinnervation (large, polyphasic motor unit action potentials) from two or more extremities outside any peripheral nerve or root distribution supports the diagnosis of ALS. Other diseases to be excluded include multifocal motor neuropathy or other polyneuropathies (Ross, 1997).

MEDICAL MANAGEMENT

There is no known cure for ALS. The Food and Drug Administration has approved riluzole (Bensimon et al., 1994) as the first drug that has been shown to prolong the survival by several months of individuals with ALS. Gabapentia, an anticonvulsant, has shown some promise in retarding disease progression (Miller et al., 1996). Updates of recent research development can be found on a number of Web sites, including that of Amyotrophic Lateral Sclerosis, National Institute of Neurologic Disorders and Stroke (May 8, 1997):

http://www.ninds.nih.gov/healinfo/DISORDER/als/als.htm

Currently, the treatment of ALS relies on education of the patient and family and the alleviation of distressing or disabling symptoms with the ongoing evaluation and intervention of a multidisciplinary team (Adam, 1986; DeLisa, Mikulic, Miller, & Melnick, 1979; Ross, 1997). The early management of muscle weakness relies on the prevention of disuse weakness in unaffected muscles. The use of energy conservation techniques and work simplification, along with adaptive devices, is also helpful. Lightweight plastic orthoses may prolong a patient's ability to ambulate. Wheelchair seating systems with an eye toward adjustability in response to disease progression is an important component to preserving mobility. The use of static orthoses and exercise to maintain joint range of motion is important to prevent uncomfortable contractures. Medications for spasticity and musculoskeletal discomfort may be indicated.

Various types of adaptive equipment may address the problem of decreased mobility, including electric mobility devices with various means of control. A decreased ability to perform activities of daily living is expected; again, adaptive equipment for the patient's or caretaker's use may be helpful. Environmental control units can use sensitive switches to allow access to television, lights, and telephone.

Respiratory care is an important area for long-term management of the individual with ALS (Bach, 1993). Weakening of the respiratory muscles causes a number of complications, including respiratory muscle fatigue, respiratory failure, ineffective cough, and failure to protect the lungs from aspiration (Braun, 1987; Tidwell, 1993). The issue of ventilatory support at the time of respiratory failure is one that should be discussed with the patient and his or her family well before it becomes an issue. Home ventilation and use of a bimodal positive airway pressure (BIPAP) device are possibilities, albeit expensive and labor intensive. The quality of communication is a potentially important factor when individuals with ALS are making decisions about ventilation. Therefore, speech–language pathologists should be prepared to discuss issues, such as the rate of progression of speech symptoms and augmentative communication options, with these individuals.

The incidence of depression in ALS patients is similar to that of patients with other progressive chronic diseases. Sleep disorders and depression are responsive to usual medications. Patients and their families benefit from ongoing counseling regarding issues related to chronic illness and acceptance of death or grieving; hospice services are very helpful for those patients with a predicted survival of 6 months or less.

COGNITIVE AND LANGUAGE FUNCTION

Classically, the clinical features of ALS have included changes in motor function with preserved cognition. This traditional view has recently come under critical review (Iwasaki, Kinoshita, Ikeda, Takamiya, & Shiojima, 1990; Kew et al., 1993; Ludolph et al., 1992). Case reports of ALS dementia have been reported (Montgomery & Erickson, 1987). Deficits were most common in the areas of problem solving, attention/mental control, continuous visual recognition memory, word generation, and verbal free recall. Because some individuals with ALS demonstrate cognitive problems that interfere with communication and the learning of new communication techniques, speech–language pathologists should take care to understand the cognitive capability of these individuals before recommending complex communication systems.

Changes in language use in ALS are also receiving some current attention (Massman et al., 1996; Strong, Grace, Orange, & Leeper, 1996). Verbal language samples produced by speakers with moderate dysarthria were compared with those of gender- and age-matched controls (Wilkinson, Yorkston, Strand, & Rogers, 1995). Although the speakers with ALS generated the same number of concepts, they produced fewer words than did the controls. Three possible explanations for the "economy of wording" were offered: (1) response to increasingly effortful speech, (2) subtle language deficits, and (3) response to slowed speaking rates.

SWALLOWING PROBLEMS

Maintenance of adequate nutrition is a peculiar problem for many individuals with ALS. Progressive muscular atrophy will lead to cachexia (a profound state of illness and malnutrition), predisposing the patient to skin breakdown and continuing loss of protein stores. In addition, dysphagia will lead to decreased intake of calories and fluids with possible aspiration. When aspiration is not preventable, alternative feeding methods must be considered (Mathus-Viliegen, Louwerse, Merkus, Tytgat, & Vianney de Jong, 1994; Mazzini et al., 1995). A strong relationship exists between swallowing symptoms and other bulbar functions, including speech production (Strand, Miller, Yorkston, & Hillel, 1996). Unlike Parkinson's disease, where there is a lack of correspondence between the severity of speech and swallowing disorders, speech and swallowing in ALS tend to be similarly affected. In other words, if speech is mildly impaired, swallowing is the same; and if speech is severely impaired, one could predict severe swallowing impairment.

Respiratory status must be carefully monitored when swallowing problems occur in bulbar ALS. Because respiration is momentarily interrupted during the pharyngeal phase of swallowing, individuals with severely compromised respiratory support may experience fatigue with eating. Adequate respiratory support is also needed for a productive cough, one of the primary defense mechanisms against aspiration. Adequate respiratory status is critical when undergoing surgical interventions such as percutaneous endoscopic gastrostomies.

Related to swallowing are problems with saliva. The source of these secretions may not be only the oral salivary glands. The nose and lungs may also contribute a constant flow of serous and particularly mucoid fluids (Newall, Orser, & Hunt, 1996). Thick, viscous mucus may impede swallowing and must be liquefied. Measures include adequate fluid intake, the use of Papase tablets or meat tenderizer, or the use of a mechanical aspirator. Anticholinergic drugs to decrease oral secretions are not a long-term solution; an aspirator or surgery (salivary duct relocation) must be considered in extreme cases. Descriptions of interventions for swallowing and saliva management at various stages of this disease are found elsewhere (Yorkston et al., 1995).

Speech Characteristics

PERCEPTUAL CHARACTERISTICS

The characteristic speech of individuals with ALS has been classified as a mixed dysarthria (Darley et al., 1975; Duffy, 1995). Symptoms associated with both spastic and flaccid dysarthria are often present; however, as the disease progresses, the contributions of each type of dysarthria may change. As the individual becomes increasingly weaker, the symptoms associated with the flaccid dysarthria usually become more apparent. As the disease progresses, the spastic symptoms often are not as evident because of the profoundly weakened neuromuscular system.

Many of the perceptual features associated with dysarthria in ALS are present in both spastic and flaccid dysarthria. For example, imprecise consonants, hypernasality, and harsh voice quality are found in both types of dysarthria. Other features are found either in spastic or flaccid dysarthria. For example, low pitch, reduced stress, and strained–strangled voice quality are found in spastic dysarthria, and audible inspiration and nasal emission are found in flaccid dysarthria as well as ALS.

SPEECH COMPONENTS

A review of the description of speech characteristics reveals that, as in most dysarthrias, individuals with ALS demonstrate impairment in all components of the speech mechanism. A moderate to strong relationship between changes in speech impairment (changes in muscle tone, weakness, and range and rate of movement) and measures of functional limitations (changes in speech intelligibility and rate) has been found in a group of speakers with ALS (Yorkston, Strand, & Hume, 1998). A number of studies are also available that focus on impairment in each of the various components of speech production.

Respiratory Function

The abnormal speech breathing patterns of two individuals with ALS have been studied (Putnam & Hixon, 1984). These individuals used limited lung volume ranges for speech that may have resulted from reductions in vital capacity. Limitations in vital capacity have been associated with changes in maximum phonation time (Hillel, Yorkston, & Miller, 1989). Individuals with initial bulbar symptoms experience a decline in respiratory status earlier than those with initial spinal symptoms. Poor respiratory support exaggerates the oral movement problems of individuals with bulbar symptoms and contributes to vocal changes in individuals with spinal symptoms (Yorkston, Strand, &

Miller, 1996). For some individuals with ALS, respiratory impairment becomes so severe that they choose to be ventilated with a respirator.

Laryngeal Function

The phonatory subsystem may reveal a mixed dysarthria. This subsystem has been described as follows (Aronson, 1980, p. 220):

> If spasticity is predominant, hyperadduction of the true and false vocal folds, technically a pseudobulbar dysphonia, will require that the exhaled air be forced through a constricted glottis. Such elevated laryngeal resistance to the exhaled air stream, coupled with a reduced exhalatory force, decreases the volume of voice in addition to producing a strained hoarseness or harshness. . . . A greater flaccid (lower motor neuron) component produced adductor vocal-fold weakness . . . extreme breathiness and reduced loudness.

Acoustic analysis techniques have identified phonatory instability in speakers with ALS (Aronson, Ramig, Winholtz, & Silber, 1992; R. D. Kent et al., 1994; Ramig, Scherer, Klasner, Titze, & Horii, 1990). Phonatory characteristics are not consistent from one speaker to another (Strand, Buder, Yorkston, & Ramig, 1994). Variability across speakers, from breathy to strained–strangled, may be associated with differences in the relative contribution of vocal weakness and vocal spasticity. Reports are available suggesting that ALS can initially be misdiagnosed as spasmodic dysphonia because of predominately laryngeal involvement (Roth, Glaze, Goding, & David, 1996).

Velopharyngeal Function

Velopharyngeal incompetence with resulting hypernasality and nasal emission is commonly associated with ALS. Often the nasal emission is not easily perceived, because of the lack of respiratory support. Nevertheless, inadequate closure of the velopharyngeal port decreases the speaker's ability to impound air pressure in the oral cavity for pressure consonant production.

Oral Articulation

The tongue and the lips of speakers with ALS frequently exhibit excessive weakness. A variety of changes in tongue structure and function have been identified. Tongue atrophy is a prevalent neurologic sign in individuals with severely reduced speech intelligibility (Carrow, Rivera, Maulden, & Shamblin,

1974). Other changes in tongue function include reductions in range and velocity of movement (Hirose, Kiritani, Ushijima, & Sawashima, 1978); changes in tongue strength (Dworkin, Aronson, & Mulder, 1980; Dworkin & Hartman, 1979); and changes in size, shape, position, and histopathological characteristics (Cha & Patten, 1989; DePaul, Waclawik, Abbs, & Brooks, 1998). Studies suggest a strong relationship between tongue impairment and speech production, with increasing weakness associated with increasing severity of articulatory deficit (Dworkin & Aronson, 1986). Tongue involvement may be associated with impaired ability to regulate tongue height and thus may affect vowel production. Speakers with ALS exhibit smaller vowel space areas and less systematic changes in vowel space than do normal speakers as a function of speaking rate (Turner, Tjaden, & Weismer, 1995). A number of acoustic studies document changes in vowel formant trajectories, particularly a flattening of the slope of F_2 trajectories (J. F. Kent et al., 1992; R. D. Kent et al., 1990; Weismer, Kent, Hodge, & Martin, 1988; Weismer, Martin, Kent, & Kent, 1992).

STAGES OF FUNCTIONAL LIMITATIONS IN DYSARTHRIA

The speech characteristics associated with ALS vary, depending on the course of the disease. For individuals with initial symptoms appearing in areas served by the bulbar (lower cranial) nerves, motor speech and swallowing disorders occur quite precipitously. However, for individuals with initial symptoms in areas served by the spinal nerves, speech symptoms may occur late in the course of the disease. In either case, many individuals with ALS are severely dysarthric during the later stages of the disease and require an alternative communication system (Saunders, Walsh, & Smith, 1981).

Information about rate of symptom progression is critical in treatment planning. Results of a study that tracked the progression of dysarthria in 44 individuals with ALS (Yorkston, Strand, Miller, Hillel, & Smith, 1993) suggest that rapid decline of speech function is not inevitable. However, it occurs frequently enough that sound clinical management dictates early preparation for the potential loss of speech. Whereas some individuals progress slowly, others progress rapidly to the need for augmentative communication (Yorkston et al., 1995). The following stages describe a typical progression of the speech course in individuals with ALS.

Stage 1: No Detectable Speech Disorder

The speech of individuals with a spinal presentation of ALS may be normal; that is, the speaker has noticed no change in function and the examiner judges speech rate, precision, and loudness to be within normal limits. Normal speech and voice are uncommon, however, in bulbar ALS. The purpose of intervention at this stage is to confirm that speech is still normal and to answer questions. General information about the natural course of communication changes is usually welcome at this phase. Many individuals and their families are coping with the difficult nature of the diagnosis. Therefore, it is important for them to know that services and assistance are available when they are needed and that these services will allow them to maintain communication.

Question: How much information do you provide about severe dysarthria and augmentative communication approaches to individuals with early bulbar involvement?

Generally, we let the patient and family dictate the timing and pace of information that we provide. In our experience, the level of inquiry ranges from intense interest in possible course of dysarthria to limited desire to know possible future changes. There are two situations where we tend to provide extensive information early in the course of the disease. The first is with individuals who live in rural areas where services are at times difficult to obtain. We provide these patients with enough information so that they can return at appropriate intervals for intervention. If this information is not provided, many individuals will wait until speech is completely unintelligible before considering augmentative communication approaches, thus making prompt intervention difficult. The other individuals with normal speech to whom we provide extensive early information are those with a spinal presentation and severe respiratory compromise who are already in the process of making decisions about ventilation and need to ask questions about progression changes in natural speech and management of speech on ventilation.

Stage 2: Obvious Speech Disorder with Intelligible Speech

At Stage 2, both the speaker and the listener notice changes. These changes may be particularly apparent during stress or fatigue. As articulatory and respiratory impairments increase, most speakers with ALS compensate unconsciously by decreasing their speaking rate and decreasing the length of their breath groups. Speech at this stage remains easy to understand. Perhaps the most common early perceptual change is in voice quality. Vocal fold spasticity can cause the voice to become harsh and flaccidity can cause it to be weak. In our experience, if voice change is the presenting symptom, it is characterized by harshness. Intervention for speakers at this stage may include minimizing environmental adversity, establishing the context of the message, maximizing the hearing of frequent communication partners, and teaching strategies for coping with communication in groups (Yorkston et al., 1995). These strategies will be reviewed in Chapter 12. In Stage 2, most individuals with ALS begin to reduce their speaking rates to minimize the speech disturbance and maintain speech intelligibility. When speaking rate is 50% of normal, augmentative communication assessment and intervention should be initiated.

Stage 3: Reduction in Speech Intelligibility

Because speaking rate, articulation, and resonance are all impaired, conscious behavioral modifications are needed at Stage 3. Modifications include simply needing to repeat on occasion when speech is not understood or when the environment is noisy. Speech production may be both fatiguing and frustrating. While most individuals with ALS decrease their speaking rate without instruction, some individuals with cognitive impairment require instruction to make these changes. Individuals at this stage can and do modify their speech production (Kennedy, Strand, & Yorkston, 1994). Intervention activities that require a great deal of exercise and repetition of movement at maximum effort levels should be used only with great caution, because it is our goal not to exercise patients to the point of fatigue. Intervention for speakers at this stage may include maintaining a slow speaking rate, conserving energy, increasing the precision of speech production, and developing strategies to resolve communication breakdowns (Yorkston et al., 1995). Some speakers may begin to use "translators" to assist them or to limit the complexity and length of the message.

Stage 4: Natural Speech Supplemented
with Augmentative Communication Approaches

Stage 4 requires combining speech with augmentative communication approaches (Beukelman & Mirenda, 1992; Kazandjian, 1997). Natural speech may be limited to highly predictable messages, such as responses to questions or greetings. The speaker with ALS may supplement natural speech by writing key words or by pointing to the first letter of each word as he or she speaks. Communication breakdowns need to be resolved by spelling out the word or using a spokesperson as translator. Intervention for speakers at this stage may include alphabet supplementation, changing communication modes for different situations, an alerting system, augmented telephone communication, and portable writing systems (Yorkston et al., 1995). These strategies will be discussed in detail in Chapter 12.

Stage 5: No Useful Speech

Speakers with advanced bulbar ALS have lost functional speech. Speakers with spinal symptoms may retain their useful speech throughout the disease. Some individuals at Stage 5 may vocalize for emotional expression or with extreme effort, but cannot produce understandable speech. Intervention for speakers at this stage may include establishing a reliable yes/no system, eye-gaze system, and communication system for a speaker dependent on ventilators (Yorkston et al., 1995).

MULTIPLE SCLEROSIS

Multiple sclerosis (MS), a disease of the white matter of the central nervous system, is characterized by progressive neurologic deficits and, most commonly, a remitting–relapsing course. The scattered lesions or plaques produce varying combinations of motor, sensory, or cognitive impairments. Although not universal, dysarthria is common and is positively related to the severity of neurologic involvement.

Pathology–Medical Aspects

CHANGES IN NEURAL TISSUE

The macroscopic lesions of MS are multiple plaques that are scattered throughout the nervous system, predominantly in the white matter. These are commonly seen in the periventricular area and tend to be symmetrical (McFarlin & McFarland, 1982). Commonly affected sites are the optic nerves, brain stem, cerebellum, and spinal cord. Microscopically, the lesion is shown to cause destruction of the myelin sheath with preservation of the axon, except in chronic cases. In an "acute" plaque, edema is seen in the vicinity of the affected nerve fiber. Resolution of this edema may be an explanation for the early reversal of some neurologic deficits after an exacerbation. The persistent neurologic signs are thought to be due to impaired conduction along the nerve axon (Hallpike, Adams, & Tourtelotte, 1983).

ETIOLOGY

Although not completely understood, the etiology of MS is thought to be the result of multiple factors. Current opinion holds that an environmental influence interacts with a certain genetic predisposition to result in clinical sclerosis (Hogancamp, Rodriguez, & Weinshenker, 1997). Geographic studies indicate that the disease is most prevalent in northern Europeans. Migrants from northern Europe to a lower prevalence area may have a decreased prevalence rate (Poser, 1992; Weinshenker, 1996). There is a higher risk of disease in the relatives of affected persons. The critical age of exposure appears to be about 15 years, which may also indicate some genetic predisposition to the disease. Because of the similarities between MS and other demyelinating diseases that are caused by viruses, and because of its similar onset to slow viral disease (e.g., Creutzfeldt-Jacob disease), a search for a viral cause has been made. No viral components have yet been identified; however, new nucleic acid hybridization techniques may prove fruitful in future identification. The presence of lymphocytes and macrophages in MS lesions and of elevated levels of certain components in the cerebrospinal fluid has led to the consideration of a malfunctioning immune system. Again, however, there has been no evidence of cross-reactivity between patients; it seems more likely that the immune response is a reaction to an environmental agent (Ellison, Wisscher, Graves, & Fahey, 1984).

Question: I understand that autoimmune diseases are those in which the body's immune system mistakenly attacks and destroys its own tissue. In the case of MS, myelin in the central and peripheral nervous system is affected. Are there other autoimmune diseases that affect the nervous system and cause dysarthria?

Yes, myasthenia gravis and Guillain-Barré syndrome are autoimmune diseases that may result in flaccid dysarthria. We will briefly review the characteristics of each and describe the role of the speech–language pathologist in management.

Myasthenia gravis is characterized by abnormal fatiguability and weakness of skeletal muscles. The cause of this weakness is a defect in neuromuscular transmission. Different muscle groups are affected in different people. Involvement of muscles of the eye and eyelid is common, as is involvement of the muscles of speech and swallowing. Weakness of bulbar musculature is usually reflected in increasing hypernasality, deterioration of articulation, increasing dysphonia, and reduction of loudness level. After prolonged periods of talking, speech may become unintelligible (Darley, Aronson, & Brown, 1969). The mainstay of therapy is the use of anticholinesterase drugs, which boost the body's neuromuscular transmitter acetylcholine by blocking the enzyme that breaks it down. Medical management often leads to good relief from symptoms (Sanders & Scoppetta, 1994). However, life-threatening respiratory muscle involvement (myasthenic crisis) occurs in some people. This may be preceded by increasing dysarthria and dysphagia. The speech–language pathologist is

(continues)

typically involved in two aspects of management. The first is contributing diagnosis information (Khan & Campbell, 1994). Speech stress testing, or speaking for prolonged periods to induce fatigue, is frequently part of the diagnostic procedures in which the effects of Tensilon injections are evaluated. The second role is to provide augmentative communication approaches and dysphagia management techniques when bulbar symptoms become severe during myasthenic crises.

Guillain-Barré syndrome is an autoimmune disorder in which the myelin sheath surrounding the axons of many nerve cells is affected. Because it is frequently preceded by a viral infection, it is thought that the virus has changed the nature of cells in the nervous system so that the immune system treats them as foreign cells. The first symptoms are usually weakness or tingling sensations in the legs. Over a period of 3 to 4 weeks, symptoms may increase in intensity and spread through the body, causing total paralysis. Because weakness progresses upward, speech symptoms typically occur after the diagnosis has been made. Recovery is not necessarily quick. It may occur in as little time as a few weeks or as long as years. About 30% of individuals with Guillain-Barré syndrome still feel a residual weakness after 3 years. Four stages of speech intervention have been described (Beukelman & Mirenda, 1998). The first is deterioration of speech in which the progression of speech symptoms is monitored. The next stage is loss of speech, during which the speaker is frequently supported on a ventilator and may use some simple communication boards and a reliable yes/no system. The third stage is prolonged speechlessness in which high-technology augmentative communication systems may be implemented. The last stage is the gradual recovery of speech, during which time natural speech is supplemented by devices such a mouth-type electrolarynx or augmentative and alternative communication system to resolve communication breakdowns.

For more information, see Guillain-Barré Syndrome Fact Sheet, National Institute of Neurology Disorders and Stroke Web site (June 19, 1997):

http://www.ninds.nih.gov/healinfo/disorder/guillain/guillain.htm

POPULATION CHARACTERISTICS

In the northern part of the United States, the prevalence of MS is about 1 in 1,000 of the population; it is one third to one half that in the southern states. About 95% of cases begin between the ages of 10 and 50 years, with a median onset age of 27 years. Although it is a disease of younger people, it is not unusual to be first diagnosed at 50 to 60 years; in these patients, there are usually signs of chronicity. The female-to-male ratio is 1.5:1 (Arnason, 1982).

SIGNS, SYMPTOMS, AND NATURAL COURSE

Charcot first comprehensively described MS in 1877 with his triad of nystagmus, scanning speech, and intention tremor. The most common symptoms in the population with MS are balance abnormalities (70%), impaired sensation (71%), paraparesis (62%), difficulty with micturition (62%), optic neuritis (55%), and impotence (5% to 80%) (Hallpike et al., 1983). Optic neuritis is the acute or subacute loss of central vision with peripheral sparing in one eye; it is the first symptom of MS in 16% to 30% of patients. A young adult with isolated optic neuritis has a 17% to 65% risk of developing MS in later life. Other reliable symptoms of MS are intranuclear ophthalmoplegia or bilateral ocular paresis, tic douloureuz or trigeminal neuralgia in a young adult, Lhermitte's symptom (an electric shock–like sensation down the spine and into the legs), acute transverse myelitis, and a "sensory useless" hand. Fatigue for which no objective explanation can be found is both a common and quite disabling complaint. On physical examination, vibration and position sense are frequently decreased or absent. Intention tremor, ataxia, and hyperreflexia are common (Poser, 1984). Vision and hearing are commonly ignored in evaluation, but cranial nerve dysfunction, scotomas, and decreased visual and auditory acuity are not uncommonly present.

The clinical course of multiple sclerosis varies widely. About 20% of people with multiple sclerosis have relatively mild disability even 10 years after diagnosis. In about 60%, the disease is manifested by a relapsing–remitting course which eventually becomes chronically progressive. The most favorable profile for onset of disability is early age at onset, female gender, initial relapsing–remitting course, and relatively few attacks during the initial years (Weinshenker, 1996).

The median survival from the onset of disease is 28 to 33 years (Bronnum-Hensen, Koch-Henriksen, & Hyllested, 1994). A number of studies have shown that disability scores calculated 5 years after onset correlate well with disability at 10 and 15 years; careful evaluation of function, therefore, can be of prognostic value (Hallpike et al., 1983). Other negative prognostic indicators include a high rate of relapses per year, incomplete recovery from the first attack, and a short interval between the first and second attacks.

DIAGNOSTIC TESTING

Many tests exist that are useful in the diagnosis of MS, but none is sufficient for diagnosis. The laboratory examination of cerebrospinal fluid reveals the presence of abnormal clusters of immunoglobulins. Myelin basic protein, which is a breakdown product of myelin and may be an indicator of disease activity, also can be found in the cerebrospinal fluid.

Magnetic resonance imaging (MRI) uses a property of atomic nuclei called spin to visualize changes in the hydrogen in brain tissue. A strong magnetic field is applied to the area to be studied, causing an alignment of the nuclei of the tissue; when this field is removed, the nuclei "spin," producing a radio frequency signal that matches the secondary spin frequency of the nucleus. These signals are processed into anatomical images. Evoked potentials measured over the cortex can be elicited with limb electrical stimulation or auditory or visual stimuli and can be helpful as adjuncts in the diagnosis of MS.

To be used in the diagnosis of multiple sclerosis, neurologic deficits should be present in different anatomical locations and should be present for at least 24 hours per episode at separate points in time. Clinical and laboratory criteria have been used to form the following diagnostic classifications: clinically definite MS, laboratory supported definite MS, and laboratory supported probable MS (Poser et al., 1983).

MEDICAL MANAGEMENT

The history of MS is one of a long and continuing series of false claims of cure for this disease. It is difficult to ascribe a therapeutic effect in many studies because of the differing course of MS patients and the remitting–relapsing nature of the disease.

The treatment of individuals with MS has changed in important ways in the last decade. Because new treatment regimes continue to be on the horizon, readers should be aware that excellent sources of current information are available. One such source is a Web site produced by the School of Medicine, University of Utah:

http://www-medlib.med.utah.edu/kw/ms/

This site is designed as an introduction to multiple sclerosis for medical students and students in training.

Treatment of MS focuses on three different goals: treatment of relapses, prevention of relapses, and treatment of symptoms. Methylprednisolene, a steroid intraveneously administed, followed by an oral prednisone taper, is used to treat optic neuritis and relapses.

Recently, drugs with antiviral action have become available that may prevent the occurrence of relapses. Two recombinant interferon-β's have been approved for treatment of patients with MS who have a relapsing–remitting course: Interferon β-1b (Betaseron) and Interferon β-1a (Avonex). Research with Interferon β-1a is positive and suggests that this treatment is associated with fewer exacerbations and a decrease in enhancing MRI lesions and MRI plaque load (Jacobs & Johnson, 1994; Jacobs et al., 1996). There is no clear effect on eventual level of disability (Jacobs, Goodkin, Rudick, & Herndon, 1994), but disability may be delayed (Munschauer & Stuart, 1997). Other agents being investigated include copolyner 1 for relapses and methatrexate and cyclophosphamid for progressive disease (Jacobs et al., 1994).

Many approaches to the treatment of MS focus on minimizing symptoms and preventing complications. The care of the MS patient requires the expertise of a wide variety of practitioners: neurologists, physiatrists, physical and occupational therapists, speech pathologists, community nursing personnel, vocational counselors, psychologists, and social workers (DeLisa, Miller, Mikulic, & Hammond, 1985; Cobble, Dietz, Grigsby, & Kennedy, 1993). The education of the patient and his or her family and friends and their active participation in the health care process may be the single most effective treatment.

Drug therapy is used to treat spasticity that interferes with daily functioning. Common drugs include baclofen, diazepam, dantrolene, and tizanidine (Young & Delwaide, 1981a, 1981b). Botulinum toxin or phenal blocks or baclafen pumps may also be used to treat spasticity. Drugs may also be used to treat bladder incontinence or retention. Bethanechol acts to increase the tone of the detrusor muscle and aid urination; its side effects include flushing, salivation, and abdominal discomfort. Propantheline and oxybutynin inhibit detrusor action; their side effects include all those of anticholinergics—dry mouth, blurred vision, tachycardia, confusion, and constipation. Antibiotics and urinary antispeptics are frequently used. Occasionally, tricyclic antidepressants and anticonvulsants may be prescribed for the paresthesias associated with MS.

Physical therapy, or at least a regular program of stretching and exercise, is necessary for almost all patients to prevent worsening of spasticity, contractures, and the cardiovascular deconditioning and osteopenia associated with inactivity. There is no evidence that exercise in moderation has any deleterious effects on the disease process and much evidence that it enhances the general condition and well-being of the patient. Various mobility devices, including bracing, supports, and manual and electric wheelchairs, can assist in maintaining ambulation or independence in mobility. Occupational therapists can provide advice on structuring activities of daily living to minimize fatigue and can supply assistive devices as needed. Driving aids such as hand controls can help to prolong independence in these areas.

OTHER COGNITIVE AND COMMUNICATION PROBLEMS

Intellectual function declines over time in MS. The cognitive impairment in MS varies greatly and depends on the location, number, and activity of lesions. These impairments are correlated with increasing lesion load on MRI (Rao, 1995). Accurate appreciation of the extent of cognitive change is important because even mild changes may be distressing to individuals with MS and their families. Changes in cognitive status may affect quality of life. Studies suggest that individuals with cognitive impairment engaged in fewer social and avocational activities, were less likely to be working, and exhibited more psychopathology than those without cognitive change (Reischies, Baum, Brau, & Hedde, 1988). Cognitive impairment has been associated with depression, perhaps because cognitive deficits caused problems with occupational performance and influenced close personal relationships (Gilchrist & Creed, 1994).

Generally, visuospatial processes are felt to be more vulnerable than linguistic processes (Rao, 1986). Memory changes and impairments in executive function are among the most consistently reported findings. Estimates of the proportion of individuals with MS experiencing cognitive problems vary depending on how the estimates are made. Estimates of cognitive deficits that are based on unstructured conversation or simple screening examinations are not sensitive to subtle changes and thus may underestimate occurrence. Self-reports of a large group of individuals with MS indicate that 38% reported significant cognitive problems (Sullivan, Edgley, & Dehoux, 1990). When neuropsychological testing is used to estimate the occurrence of cognitive changes, prevalence rates increase from 50% to 70% (Heaton, Nelson, Thompson, Burks, & Franklin, 1985; Rao, Leo, Bernardin, & Unverzagt, 1991).

Although dysarthria is the most common communication problem observed in individuals with MS, impaired language performance has been attributed to mild cognitive deterioration rather than to sensory or motor factors (Kujala, Portin, & Ruutiainen, 1996; Lethlean & Murdoch, 1993; Wallace & Holmes, 1993). Focal aphasia has also been reported in rare cases (Olmas-Lau, Ginsberg, & Geller, 1977). Changes in sentence comprehension have been reported in a subgroup of individuals with MS and have been associated with selectively compromised mental information processing speed (Grossman et al., 1995). Affective disorders related to emotion or feelings such as euphoria, pathological laughing or weeping, depression, and bipolar disorders are common in MS (Minden & Schiffer, 1990). These may be responsive to medication or behavioral intervention (White, Catanzaro, & Kraft, 1993).

Speech Characteristics

Speech symptomatology played an important role in the early description of MS. In 1877, Charcot described a characteristic triad of signs—nystagmus, intention tremor, and scanning speech—which he termed "disseminated sclerosis," today called multiple sclerosis. Scanning speech referred to the prolonged phonation of words with slow and slurred articulation. However, as large groups of individuals with MS were studied, it became apparent that dysarthria was not a universal characteristic of MS. Dysarthria is reported in approximately one fifth of cases and was the presenting symptom in only 2% of cases (Ivers & Goldstein, 1963). The Mayo Clinic studies suggested that approximately 40% of their cases demonstrated some changes in speech. In self-reports, also, approximately 25% to 45% of patients reported a "speech and/or communication disorder" (Beukelman, Kraft, & Freal, 1985; Hartelius & Svensson, 1994). Prevalence of dysarthria increases as the disease progresses, with approximately 70% of individuals with ambulation problem, weakness, and lack of arm or hand control also reporting changes in speech.

PERCEPTUAL CHARACTERISTICS

Although "scanning speech" was included as an early symptom of MS in early literature, modern studies suggest that speech symptoms are not restricted to those associated with cerebellar involvement. Rather, speech symptoms may be related to changes in multiple neural systems. Characteristics have been described as contributing to the dysarthric pattern: nasal voice quality, weak phonation, poor respiratory cycle, changes in pitch, slow rate, intellectual deterioration, and emotional lability. In the Mayo Clinic studies, the perceptual speech patterns were consistent with a mixed dysarthria with both ataxic and spastic components (Darley et al., 1975). Darley et al. summarized the speech characteristics as follows: "The most prominent speech deviations in MS are impaired control of loudness, harshness, and defective articulation. Impaired use of vocal variability for emphasis, impaired pitch control, hypernasality, inappropriate pitch level, and breathiness are observed with less degrees of frequency" (pp. 242–243).

STAGES OF FUNCTIONAL LIMITATION IN DYSARTHRIA

Stage 1: No Detectable Speech Disorder

Normal speech and voice occur in approximately 40% of individuals with MS. As with other degenerative diseases, intervention at Stage 1 focuses on confirmation that speech is normal and answering questions related to the possible impact of the disease on speech and voice. Because fatigue is a common complaint of individuals with MS, energy conservation techniques may be introduced even before speech changes are obvious.

Stage 2: Obvious Speech Disorder with Intelligible Speech

Although changes at Stage 2 may not interfere with speech intelligibility, speech rate may be slow, prosody may be disturbed, and vocal quality changes may be present. At this stage, vocal instability may be more obvious on sustained phonation than in connected speech. Techniques both to conserve energy and to regulate loudness level may be appropriate (see Chapter 7). These techniques share a common focus on respiratory control and may be useful both for individuals who are weak and have difficulty achieving the steady subglottal air pressure needed for speech production and for individuals with ataxia who are quite strong but uncoordinated. Successful speech treatment of individuals with MS has been reported (Hartelius, Wising, & Nord, 1997). This treatment focuses on a number of areas, including vocal efficiency (the production of relaxed and coordinated phonation), contrastive stress (in an effort to enhance linguistic prominence and reduce speech monotony), and verbal repairs (to improve production of an utterance that has been misunderstood).

Stage 3: Reduction in Speech Intelligibility

Individuals with motor speech impairment so severe that intelligibility is compromised tend to exhibit involvement of multiple neural systems. When examining the relationship of neural system involvement and speech adequacy, Darley et al. (1975) found those speakers with a combined cerebral, brain stem, and cerebellar involvement to have the most severely dysarthric speech. Those with combined cerebral–cerebellar or brain stem–cerebellar involvement exhibited slightly less severe dysarthria. Those with single system involvement exhibited still less severe dysarthria. The implication of this finding is that speakers at this stage are dealing with multiple problems, which may include respiratory impairment (incoordination and/or weakness), laryngeal impairment (commonly spasticity), and oral articulatory impairment characterized by weakness, slowness, and poor coordination.

Treatment may involve maintaining an appropriate speaking rate (see Chapter 10 for specific techniques) and techniques to resolve communication breakdown. As with speakers at earlier stages, exercises focusing on achieving good respiratory support and control may also be appropriate. Chunking utterances into small syntactic units separated by pauses may enhance speech intelligibility for some speakers.

Stage 4: Natural Speech Supplemented by Augmentative Techniques

At Stage 4, natural speech is so severely impaired that it must be supplemented by other information. For example, techniques where the speaker points to the first letter of each word slows speech and provides the listener with extra information. Candidates for this technique need to have sufficient hand function to point to letters on a board. Intention tremor and visual problems may make this difficult for some individuals with MS. Other breakdown resolution strategies may also be taught at this point. Because of the potential for cognitive problems that limit new learning, it may be appropriate to provide training before it is urgently needed. By anticipating change, practice can occur at a pace at which it is likely to succeed.

Stage 5: No Functional Speech

Providing augmentative communication systems for individuals with MS and profound dysarthria is particularly challenging. Hand function may be limited by spasticity, ataxia, or intention tremor. Visual problems may also limit use of a system that depends on reading. Although bold print and proper positioning of material in the visual field may be helpful, it is appropriate to assume that a visual problem will continue to progress. Augmentative communication systems for individuals with MS and no functional speech have been reported (Honsinger, 1989; Porter, 1989).

REFERENCES

Ackermann, H., Hertrich, I., & Hehr, T. (1995). Oral diadochokinesis in neurological dysarthrias. *Folia Phoniatrica et Logopedica, 47*(1), 15–23.

Adam, M. (Ed.). (1986). *Amyotrophic lateral sclerosis: A teaching manual for health professionals.* Kirkland, WA: ALS Health Support Services.

Adams, S. G., Hunt, E. J., Charles, D. A., & Lang, A. E. (1993). Unilateral versus bilateral botulinum toxin injections in spasmodic dysphonia: Acoustic and perceptual results. *Journal of Otolaryngology, 22*, 171–175.

Ali, G. N., Wallace, K. L., Schwartz, R., DeCarle, D. J., Zagami, A. S., & Cook, I. J. (1996). Mechanism of oral–pharyngeal dysphagia in patients with Parkinson's disease. *Gastroenterology, 110*, 383–392.

Allen, I., & Brankin, B. (1993). Pathogenesis of multiple sclerosis: The immune diathesis and the role of viruses. *Journal of Neuropathology and Experimental Neurology, 52*, 95–105.

Amico, L. L., & Antil, J. P. (1981). Amyotrophic lateral sclerosis. *Postgraduate Medicine, 70*, 50–61.

Andrew, J., Fowler, C. J., & Harrison, M. J. (1983). Stereotaxic thalamotomy in 55 cases of dystonia. *Brain, 106*, 981–1000.

Appel, S. H. (1993). Excitotoxic neuronal cell death in amyotrophic lateral sclerosis. *Trends in Neurosciences, 16*, 3–5.

Appel, S. H., Smith, R. G., Engelhardt, J. I., & Stefanni, E. (1993). Evidence for autoimmunity in amyotrophic lateral sclerosis. *Journal of Neurological Sciences, 118*, 169–174.

Arnason, B. G. W. (1982). Multiple sclerosis: Current concepts and management. *Hospital Practice, 17*, 81–89.

Aronson, A. (1980). Definition and scope of communication disorders. In D. Mulder (Ed.), *The diagnosis and treatment of amyotrophic lateral sclerosis* (pp. 217–224). Boston: Houghton Mifflin.

Aronson, A. E. (1985). *Clinical voice disorders: An interdisciplinary approach* (2nd ed.). New York: Thieme.

Aronson, A. E., Ramig, L. O., Winholtz, W. S., & Silber, S. R. (1992). Rapid voice tremor, or "flutter," in amyotrophic lateral sclerosis. *Annals of Otology, Rhinology and Laryngology, 101,* 511–518.

Bach, J. R. (1993). Amyotrophic lateral sclerosis: Communication status and survival with ventilatory support. *American Journal of Physical Medicine & Rehabilitation, 72*(6), 343–349.

Barlow, S. M., Iacono, R. P., Paseman, L. A., Biswas, A., & D'Antonio, L. (1998). The effects of posteroventral pallidotomy on force and speech aerodynamics in Parkinson's disease. In M. Cannito, K. M. Yorkston, & D. R. Beukelman (Eds.), *Neuromotor speech disorders: Nature, assessment, and management* (pp. 117–156). Baltimore: Brookes.

Bawa, R., Ramadan, H. H., & Wetmore, S. J. (1993). Bilateral vocal cord paralysis with Shy-Drager syndrome. *Otolaryngology—Head and Neck Surgery, 109,* 911–914.

Bayles, K. A. (1990). Language and Parkinson disease. *Alzheimer Disease and Associated Disorders, 4*(3), 171–180.

Bayles, K. A., Tomoeda, C. K., Wood, J. A., Montgomery, E. B., Cruz, R. F., Azuma, T., & McGeagh, A. (1996). Change in cognitive function in idiopathic Parkinson disease. *Archives of Neurology, 53,* 1140–1146.

Behrman, S., Carroll, J. D., Janota, A., & Matthews, W. B. (1969). Progressive supranuclear palsy: Clinico-pathological study of four cases. *Brain, 92,* 663–678.

Bensimon, G., Lacomblez, L., & Meininger, V. (1994). A controlled trial of riluzole in amyotrophic lateral sclerosis. *New England Journal of Medicine, 330*(9), 585–591.

Berardelli, A., Curra, A., & Manfredi, M. (1996). Torsion dystonia. *Current Opinion in Neurology, 9,* 317–320.

Berciano, J. (1982). Olivopontocerebellar atrophy: A review of 117 cases. *Journal of the Neurological Sciences, 53,* 253–272.

Berry, W. R., Darley, F. L., Aronson, A. E., & Goldstein, N. P. (1974). Dysarthria in Wilson's disease. *Journal of Speech and Hearing Research, 49,* 405–408.

Beukelman, D. R. (1983). Treatment of hyperkinetic dysarthria. In W. H. Perkins (Ed.), *Dysarthria and apraxia* (pp. 105–114). New York: Thieme-Stratton.

Beukelman, D. R., Kraft, G. H., & Freal, J. (1985). Expressive communication disorders in persons with multiple sclerosis. *Archives of Physical Medicine and Rehabilitation, 66,* 675–677.

Beukelman, D. R., & Mirenda, P. (1992). *Augmentative and alternative communication: Management of severe communication disorders in children and adults.* Baltimore: Brookes.

Beukelman, D. R., & Mirenda, P. (1998). *Augmentative and alternative communication: Management of severe communication disorders in children and adults* (2nd ed.). Baltimore: Brookes.

Bianchine, J. R. (1976). Drug therapy of parkinsonism. *New England Journal of Medicine, 295,* 814–818.

Bird, M. R., Woodward, M. C., Gibson, E. M., Phyland, D. J., & Fonda, D. (1994). Asymptomatic swallowing disorders in elderly patients with Parkinson's disease: A description of findings on clinical examination and videofluoroscopy in sixteen patients. *Age and Aging, 23,* 251–254.

Blitzer, A., & Brin, M. F. (1991). Laryngeal dystonia: A series of botulinum toxin therapy. *Annals of Otology, Rhinology and Laryngology, 100,* 85–89.

Blitzer, A., Greene, P. E., Brin, M. F., & Fahn, S. (1989). Botulinum toxin injection for the treatment of oromandibular dystonia. *Annals of Otology, Rhinology and Laryngology, 98,* 93–97.

Blumenthal, H., & Miller, C. (1969). Motor nuclear involvement in progressive supranuclear palsy. *Archives of Neurology, 20,* 362–367.

Boshes, B. (1966). Voice changes in parkinsonism. *Journal of Neurosurgery, 24,* 286–288.

Brain, W., & Walton, J. (1969). *Brain's diseases of the nervous system.* London: Oxford University Press.

Braun, S. R. (1987). Respiratory systems in amyotrophic lateral sclerosis. *Neurologic Clinics, 5*(1), 9–31.

Brewer, G. J. (1995). Practical recommendations and new therapies for Wilson's disease. *Drugs, 50,* 240–249.

Brin, M. F., Fahn, S., Blitzer, A., Ramig, L. O., & Stewart, C. (1992). Movement disorders of the larynx. In A. Blitzer, M. F. Brin, C. T. Sasaki, S. Fahn, & K. S. Harris (Eds.), *Neurologic disorders of the larynx* (pp. 248–278). New York: Thieme Medical.

Brin, M. F., Fahn, S., Moskowitz, C., Friedman, A., Shale, H. M., Greene, P. E., Blitzer, A., List, T., Lange, D., Lovelace, R. E., & McMahon, D. (1987). Localized injections of botulinum toxin for the treatment of focal dystonia and hemifacial spasm. *Movement Disorders, 2,* 237–254.

Bronnum-Hensen, H., Koch-Henriksen, N., & Hyllested, K. (1994). Survival of patients with multiple sclerosis in Denmark: A nationwide, long-term epidemiologic survey. *Neurology, 44,* 1901–1907.

Brooke, M. H., Florence, J. M., Heller, S. L., Kaiser, K. K., Phillips, D., Gruber, A., Babcock, D., & Miller, J. P. (1986). Controlled trial of Thyrotropic Releasing Hormone in amyotrophic lateral sclerosis. *Neurology, 36,* 146–151.

Buck, J. F., & Cooper, I. S. (1956). Speech problems in parkinsonian patients undergoing anterior choroidal artery occlusion or chemopallidectomy. *Journal of the American Geriatric Society, 4,* 1285–1290.

Burke, B., Fahn, S., & Gold, A. (1980). Delayed-onset dystonia in patients with "static" encephalopathy. *Journal of Neurology, Neurosurgery, Psychiatry, 43,* 789–797.

Bushman, M., Bomeyer, S. M., Leeker, L., & Perlmutter, J. S. (1989). Swallowing abnormalities and their response to treatment in Parkinson's disease. *Neurology, 39,* 1309–1314.

Canter, G. C. (1965a). Speech characteristics of patients with Parkinson's disease: II. Physiological support for speech. *Journal of Speech and Hearing Disorders, 30,* 44–49.

Canter, G. C. (1965b). Speech characteristics of patients with Parkinson's disease: III. Articulation, diadochokinesis, and overall adequacy. *Journal of Speech and Hearing Disorders, 30,* 217–224.

Capitani, E., Laiacona, M., & Barbarotto, R. (1993). Progressive neuropsychological and extrapyramidal deterioration resembling progressive supranuclear palsy: Is aphasia relevant for correct diagnosis? *European Archives of Psychiatry and Clinical Neuroscience, 242,* 347–351.

Carrow, E., Rivera, V., Maulden, M., & Shamblin, L. (1974). Deviant speech characteristics in motor neuron disease. *Archives of Otolaryngology, 100,* 212–219.

Cartwright, G. E. (1978). Diagnosis of treatable Wilson's disease. *New England Journal of Medicine, 298,* 1347–1350.

Cha, C. H., & Patten, B. M. (1989). Amyotrophic lateral sclerosis: Abnormalities of the tongue on magnetic resonance imaging. *Annuals of Neurology, 25,* 468–472.

Charcot, J. M. (1877). *Lectures on the disease of the nervous system* (Vol. 1). London: New Sydenham Society.

Chong, S. S., Almqvist, E., Telenius, H., LaTray, L., Nichol, K., Bourdelat-Parks, B., Geldbeg, Y. P., Haddad, B. R., Richards, F., Sillence, D., Greenberg, C. R., Ives, E., Van den Engh, G., Hughes, M. R., & Hayden, M. R. (1997). Contribution of DNA sequence and CAG size to mutation frequencies of intermediate alleles for Huntington disease: Evidence from single sperm analyses. *Human Molecular Genetics, 6,* 301–309.

Cisneros, E., & Braun, C. M. (1995). Vocal and respiratory diadochokinesia in Friedreich's ataxia. *Revue Neurologique, 151,* 113–123.

Cobble, N. D., Dietz, M. A., Grigsby, J., & Kennedy, P. M. (1993). Rehabilitation of the patient with multiple sclerosis. In J. A. DeLisa (Ed.), *Rehabilitation medicine: Principles and practice* (2nd ed., pp. 861–885). Philadelphia: Lippincott.

Cohen, L. G., Hallett, M., Geller, B. D., & Hochberg, F. (1989). Treatment of focal dystonias of the hand with botulinum toxin injections. *Journal of Neurology, Neurosurgery and Psychiatry, 52,* 355–363.

Cohen, S., & Freedman, M. (1995). Cognitive and behavioral changes in the Parkinson-plus syndromes. *Advance in Neurology, 65,* 139–157.

Cooper, I. (1969). *Involuntary movement disorders.* New York: Harper & Row.

Cooper, I. S., Cullinan, T., & Riklan, M. (1976). The natural history of dystonia. *Advances in Neurology, 14,* 157–169.

Cooper, J., Sagar, H., Jordan, N., Harvey, N., & Sullivan, E. (1991). Cognitive impairment in early, untreated Parkinson's disease and its relationship to motor disability. *Brain, 114,* 2095–2122.

Countryman, S., Ramig, L. O., & Pawlas, A. A. (1994). Speech and voice deficits in parkinsonism plus syndromes: Can they be treated? *Journal of Medical Speech–Language Pathology, 2*(3), 211–226.

Cummings, J. L., & Benson, D. F. (1983). *Dementia: A clinical approach.* Boston: Butterworth.

Darley, F., Aronson, A., & Brown, J. (1969). Differential diagnostics patterns of dysarthria. *Journal of Speech and Hearing Research, 12,* 224.

Darley, F. L., Aronson, A. E., & Brown, J. R. (1975). *Motor speech disorders.* Philadelphia: Saunders.

Day, L. S., & Parnell, M. M. (1987). Ten-year study of a Wilson's disease dysarthric. *Journal of Communication Disorders, 20*(3), 207–218.

DeLisa, J. A., Mikulic, M. A., Miller, R. M., & Melnick, R. R. (1979). Amyotrophic lateral sclerosis: Comprehensive management. *American Family Physician, 19*(3), 137–142.

DeLisa, J. A., Miller, R. M., Mikulic, M. A., & Hammond, M. C. (1985). Multiple sclerosis: Part II. Common functional problems and rehabilitation. *American Family Physician, 32*(5), 127–132.

DePaul, R., Waclawik, A. J., Abbs, J. H., & Brooks, B. R. (1998). Histopathological characteristics in lingual muscle tissue in ALS: Perspectives on the natural history of the disease. In M. Cannito, K. M. Yorkston, & D. R. Beukelman (Eds.), *Neuromotor speech disorders: Nature, assessment, and management* (pp. 69–84). Baltimore: Brookes.

Devanne, H., Gentil, M., & Maton, B. (1995). Biomechanical analysis of simple jaw movements in Friedreich's ataxia. *Electroencephalograph and Clinical Neurophysiology, 97*(1), 29–35.

Duffy, J. R. (1995). *Motor speech disorders: Substrates, differential diagnosis, and management.* St. Louis: Mosby.

Duvoisin, R. C. (1991). *Parkinson's disease: A guide for patient and family* (3rd ed.). New York: Raven Press.

Dworkin, J., & Aronson, A. (1986). Tongue strength and alternate motion rates in normal and dysarthric subjects. *Journal of Communication Disorders, 19,* 115–132.

Dworkin, J., Aronson, A., & Mulder, D. (1980). Tongue force in normals and in dysarthric patients with amyotrophic lateral sclerosis. *Journal of Speech and Hearing Research, 23,* 828–837.

Dworkin, J. P., & Hartman, D. E. (1979). Progressive speech deterioration and dysphagia in amyotrophic lateral sclerosis: Case report. *Archives of Physical Medicine and Rehabilitation, 60,* 423–425.

Eisen, A., & Krieger, C. (1993). Pathogenic mechanism in sporadic amyotrophic lateral sclerosis. *Canadian Journal of Neurologic Sciences, 20*(4), 286–296.

Ellison, G. W., Wisscher, B. R., Graves, M. C., & Fahey, J. L. (1984). Multiple sclerosis. *Annals of Internal Medicine, 101,* 514–526.

Emery, A., & Holloway, S. (1982). Familial motor neuron diseases. In L. Rowland (Ed.), *Human motor neuron diseases* (pp. 139–148). New York: Raven.

Esmonde, T., Giles, E., Xuereb, J., & Hodges, J. (1996). Progressive supranuclear palsy presenting with dynamic aphasia. *Journal of Neurology, Neurosurgery and Psychiatry, 60*, 403–410.

Fahn, S. (1984). The varied clinical expression dystonia. *Neurologic Clinics, 2*, 541–553.

Fahn, S. (1988). Disorders with parkinsonism features. In J. W. Hurst (Ed.), *Medicine for the practicing physician* (2nd ed., pp. 1522–1525). Boston: Butterworths.

Fahn, S., Elton, R. I., & Members of the UPDRS Development Committee. (1987). Unified Parkinson's Disease Rating Scale. In S. Fahn, C. D. Marsden, D. B. Calne, & M. Goldstein (Eds.), *Recent developments in Parkinson's disease* (pp. 153–304). New York: Macmillan.

Fahn, S., & Jankowic, J. (1984). Practical management of dystonia. *Neurologic Clinics, 2*, 555–569.

Foroud, T., Siemers, E., Kleindorfer, D., Bill, D. J., Hodes, M. E., Norton, J. A., Conneally, P. M., & Christian, J. C. (1995). Cognitive scores in carriers of Huntington's disease gene compared to noncarriers. *Annals of Neurology, 37*, 657–664.

Forrest, K., Weismer, G., & Turner, G. S. (1989). Kinematic, acoustic, and perceptual analyses of connected speech produced by Parkinsonian and normal geriatric adults. *Journal of the Acoustic Society of America, 85*(6), 2608–2622.

Gentil, M. (1990). Dysarthria in Friedreich's disease. *Brain and Language, 38*, 438–448.

Gentil, M., & Pollak, P. P. J. (1995). Parkinsonian dysarthria. *Revue Neurologique, 151*(2), 105–112.

Gilchrist, A. C., & Creed, F. H. (1994). Depression, cognitive impairment and social stress in multiple sclerosis. *Journal of Psychosomatic Research, 38*, 193–201.

Gilman, S., & Kluin, K. (1984). Perceptual analyses of speech disorders in Friedreich disease and olivopontocerebellar atrophy. In J. R. Bloedel, J. Dichgans, & W. Precht (Eds.), *Cerebellar functions* (pp. 148–163). Heidelberg: Springer-Verlag.

Golbe, L. I., Davis, P. H., Schoenberg, B. S., & Duvoisin, R. C. (1988). Prevalence and natural history of progressive supranuclear palsy. *Neurology, 38*, 1031–1034.

Golper, L. H., Nutt, J. G., Rou, M. T., & Coleman, R. O. (1983). Focal cranial dystonia. *Journal of Speech and Hearing Disorders, 2*, 128–134.

Gouider-Khouja, N., Vidailhet, M., Bonnet, A. M., Pichon, J., & Agid, Y. (1995). "Pure" striatonigral degeneration and Parkinson's disease: A comparative clinical study. *Movement Disorders, 10*, 288–294.

Grafman, J., Litvan, I., Gomez, C., & Chase, T. N. (1990). Frontal lobe function in progressive supranuclear palsy. *Archives of Neurology, 47*, 553–558.

Grafman, J., Litvan, I., & Stark, M. (1995). Neuropsychological features of progressive supranuclear palsy. *Brain and Cognition, 28*, 311–320.

Grossman, M., Robinson, K. M., Onishi, K., Thompson, H., Cohen, J., & D'Esposito, M. (1995). Sentence comprehension in multiple sclerosis. *Acta Neurologica Scandinavica, 92*, 324–331.

Gubbay, S. S., Kahana, E., Zilber, N., & Cooper, G. (1985). Amyotrophic lateral sclerosis: A study of its presentation and prognosis. *Journal of Neurology, 232*, 295–300.

Hallpike, J. F., Adams, C. W. M., & Tourtelotte, W. W. (Eds.). (1983). *Multiple sclerosis: Pathology, diagnosis and management.* Baltimore: Williams & Wilkins.

Hanson, D., Gerratt, B. R., & Ward, P. H. (1984). Cinegraphic observations of laryngeal function in Parkinson's disease. *Laryngoscope, 94*, 348–353.

Hanson, D. G., Ludlow, C. L., & Bassich, C. J. (1983). Vocal fold paresis in Shy-Drager syndrome. *Annals of Otology, Rhinology and Laryngology, 92*, 85–90.

Hanson, W., & Metter, E. J. (1980). DAF as instrumental treatment for dysarthria in progressive supranuclear palsy: A case report. *Journal of Speech and Hearing Disorders, 45*, 268–276.

Hanyu, N., Oguchi, K., Yanagisawa, N., & Tsukagnoshi, H. (1981). Degeneration and regeneration of ventral root motor fibers in amyotrophic lateral sclerosis. *Journal of Neurological Sciences, 55*, 99–115.

Hartelius, L., & Svensson, P. (1994). Speech and swallowing symptoms associated with Parkinson's disease and multiple sclerosis: A survey. *Phoniatrica et Logopaedica, 46*, 9–17.

Hartelius, L., Wising, C., & Nord, L. (1997). Speech modification in dysarthria associated with multiple sclerosis: An intervention based on vocal efficiency, contrastive stress, and verbal repair strategies. *Journal of Medical Speech–Language Pathology, 5*(2), 113–140.

Hartman, D. E., & O'Neill, B. P. (1989). Progressive dysfluency, dysphagia, dysarthria: A case of olivo-pontocerebellar atrophy. In K. M. Yorkston & D. R. Beukelman (Eds.), *Recent advances in clinical dysarthria* (pp. 119–128). Austin, TX: PRO-ED.

Hauser, S. L., Sawson, D. M., Lehich, J. R., Beal, M. F., Kevy, S. B., Propper, R. D., Mills, J. A., & Weiner, H. L. (1983). Intensive immunosuppression in progressive multiple sclerosis. *New England Journal of Medicine, 308*, 173–180.

Heaton, R. K., Nelson, L. M., Thompson, D. S., Burks, J. S., & Franklin, G. M. (1985). Neuropsychological findings in relapsing–remitting and chronic progressive multiple sclerosis. *Journal of Consulting and Clinical Psychology, 53*, 103–110.

Heck, A. (1964). A study of neural and extra neural findings in a large family with Friedreich's ataxia. *Journal of Neurological Sciences, 1*, 226–255.

Hefter, H., Arendt, G., Stremmel, W., & Freund, H. J. (1993). Motor impairment in Wilson's disease: II. Slowness of speech. *Acta Neurologica Scandinavica, 87*, 148–160.

Hillel, A. D., Yorkston, K. M., & Miller, R. M. (1989). Use of phonation time to estimate vital capacity in amyotrophic lateral sclerosis. *Archives of Physical Medicine and Rehabilitation, 70*, 618–620.

Hirano, A. (1996). Neuropathology of ALS: An overview. *Neurology, 47*(Suppl. 2), S63–66.

Hirano, A., & Iwata, M. (1979). Pathology of motor neurons with special reference to amyotrophic lateral sclerosis and related diseases. In T. Tsubaki & Y. Toyokura (Eds.), *Amyotrophic lateral sclerosis*. Baltimore: University Park Press.

Hirose, H., Kiritani, S., & Sawashima, M. (1982). Velocity of articulatory movements in normal and dysarthric subjects. *Folia Phoniatrica, 34*, 210–215.

Hirose, H., Kiritani, S., Ushijima, T., & Sawashima, M. (1978). Analysis of abnormal articulatory dynamics in two dysarthric patients. *Journal of Speech and Hearing Disorders, 43*(1), 96–105.

Hirose, H., Kiritani, S., Ushijima, T., Yoshioka, H., & Sawashima, M. (1981). Pattern of dysarthric movements in patients with Parkinsonism. *Folia Phoniatrica, 34*, 203–215.

Hoehn, M. M., & Yahr, M. D. (1967). Parkinsonism: Onset, progression and mortality. *Neurology, 17*, 427–442.

Hogancamp, W. E., Rodriguez, M., & Weinshenker, B. G. (1997). The epidemiology of multiple sclerosis. *Mayo Clinic Proceedings, 72*, 871–878.

Hogg, J. E., Massey, E. W., & Schoenberg, B. S. (1979). Mortality from Huntington's disease in the United States. *Advanced Neurology, 23*, 27–35.

Holzer, S. E., & Ludlow, C. L. (1996). The swallowing side effects of botulinum toxin type A injection in spasmodic dysphonia. *Laryngoscope, 106*, 86–92.

Honsinger, M. J. (1989). Midcourse intervention in multiple sclerosis: An inpatient model. *Augmentative and Alternative Communication, 5*(1), 103–110.

Hoodin, R. B., & Gilbert, H. R. (1989). Nasal airflows in parkinsonian speakers. *Journal of Communication Disorders, 22,* 169–180.

Hughes, J. T. (1982). Pathology of amyotrophic lateral sclerosis. *Advances in Neurology, 36,* 61.

Hunker, C. J., & Abbs, J. H. (1984). Physiological analyses of parkinsonian tremors in the orofacial system. In M. R. McNeil, J. C. Rosenbek, & A. E. Aronson (Eds.), *The dysarthrias* (pp. 69–100). Austin, TX: PRO-ED.

Hunker, C. J., Abbs, J. H., & Barlow, S. M. (1982). The relationship between parkinsonism rigidity and hypokinesia in the orofacial system: A quantitative analysis. *Neurology, 32,* 749–754.

Iacono, R. P., Shima, F., Lonser, R. R., Kuniyoshi, S., Maeda, G., & Yamada, S. (1995). The results, indications, and physiology of posteroventral pallidotomy for patients with Parkinson's disease. *Neurosurgery, 36*(6), 1118–1127.

Illes, J. (1989). Neurolinguistic features of spontaneous language production dissociate three forms of neurodegenerative disease: Alzheimer's, Huntington's, and Parkinson's. *Brain and Language, 37*(4), 628–642.

Illes, J., Metter, E. J., Hanson, W. R., & Iritani, S. (1988). Language production in Parkinson's disease: Acoustic and linguistic considerations. *Brain and Language, 33,* 146–160.

Isozaki, E., Shimizu, T., Takamoto, K., Horiguchi, S., Hayashida, T., Oda, M., & Tanabe, H. (1995). Vocal cord abductor paralysis (VCAP) in Parkinson's disease: Difference from VCAP in multiple system atrophy. *Journal of the Neurological Sciences, 130,* 197–202.

Ivers, R., & Goldstein, N. (1963). Multiple sclerosis: A current appraisal of symptoms and signs. *Proceedings of the Staff Meeting of the Mayo Clinic, 38,* 457–466.

Iwasaki, Y., Kinoshita, M., Ikeda, K., Takamiya, K., & Shiojima, T. (1990). Neuropsychological dysfunction in amyotrophic lateral sclerosis: Relation to motor abilities. *International Journal of Neuroscience, 54,* 191–195.

Jacobs, L., Goodkin, D. E., Rudick, R. A., & Herndon, R. (1994). Advances in specific therapy for multiple sclerosis. *Current Opinion in Neurology, 7,* 250–254.

Jacobs, L., & Johnson, K. P. (1994). A brief history of the use of interferons as treatment of multiple sclerosis. *Archives of Neurology, 51,* 1245–1252.

Jacobs, L. D., Cookfair, D. L., Rudick, R. A., Herndon, R. M., Richert, J. R., Salazar, A. M., Fischer, J. S., Goodkin, D. E., Granger, C. V., Simon, J. H., Alam, J. J., Bartoszak, D. M., Bourdette, D. N., Braiman, J., Brownscheidle, C. M., Coats, M. E., Cohan, S. L., Dougherty, D. S., Kinkel, R. P., Mass, M. K., Munschauer, F. E., Priore, R. L., Pullicino, P. M., Scherokman, B. J., & Whitham, R. H. (1996). Intramuscular interferon beta-1a for disease progression in relapsing multiple sclerosis. The Multiple Sclerosis Collaborative Research Group. *Annals of Neurology, 39,* 285–294.

Jain, S. S., & Kirshblum, S. C. (1993). Movement disorders, including tremors. In J. A. DeLisa & B. M. Gans (Eds.), *Rehabilitation medicine: Principles and practices* (2nd ed., pp. 700–715). Philadelphia: Lippincott.

Joanette, Y., & Dudley, J. (1980). Dysarthria symptomatology of Friedreich's ataxia. *Brain and Language, 10,* 39–50.

Johnson, W. G. (1995). Friedreich's ataxia. *Clinical Neuroscience, 3,* 33–38.

Kagel, M. C., & Leopold, N. A. (1992). Dysphagia in Huntington's disease: A 16-year retrospective. *Dysphagia, 7,* 106–114.

Kaji, R., Ikeda, A., Ikeda, T., Kubori, T., Mazaki, T., Kohara, N., Kanada, M., Nagamine, T., Honda, M., Rothwell, J. C., et al. (1995). Physiological study of cervical dystonia. *Brain, 118,* 511–522.

Kaji, R., Rothwell, J. C., Katayama, M., Ikeda, T., Kubori, T., Kohara, N., Mezaki, T., Shibasaki, H., & Kimura, J. (1995). Tonic vibration reflex and muscle afferent block in writer's cramp. *Annals of Neurology, 38,* 155–162.

Kazandjian, M. S. (1997). *Communication and swallowing solutions for the ALS/MND community.* San Diego: Singular.

Kennedy, M. R. T., Strand, E. A., & Yorkston, K. M. (1994). Selected acoustic changes in the verbal repairs of dysarthric speakers. *Journal of Medical Speech–Language Pathology, 2*(4), 263–280.

Kent, J. F., Kent, R. D., Rosenbek, J. C., Weismer, G., Martin, R., Sufit, R., & Brooks, B. R. (1992). Quantitative description of the dysarthria in women with amyotrophic lateral sclerosis. *Journal of Speech and Hearing Research, 35,* 723–733.

Kent, R. D., Hyang-Hee, K., Weismer, G., Kent, J. F., Rosenbek, J. C., Brooks, B. R., & Workinger, M. (1994). Laryngeal dysfunction in neurological disease: Amyotrophic lateral sclerosis, Parkinson disease, and stroke. *Journal of Medical Speech–Language Pathology, 2*(3), 157–176.

Kent, R. D., Kent, J. F., Weismer, G., Sufit, R. L., Rosenbek, J. C., Martin, R. E., & Brooks, B. R. (1990). Impairment of speech intelligibility in men with amyotrophic lateral sclerosis. *Journal of Speech and Hearing Disorders, 55*(4), 721–728.

Kew, J. J., Goldstein, L. H., Leigh, P. N., Abrahams, S., Cograve, N., Passingham, R. E., Frackowiak, R. S., & Brooks, D. J. (1993). The relationship between abnormalities of cognitive function and cerebral activation in amyotrophic lateral sclerosis: A neuropsychological and positron emission tomography study. *Brain, 116,* 1399–1423.

Khan, O. A., & Campbell, W. W. (1994). Myasthenia gravis presenting as dysphagia: Clinical considerations. *American Journal of Gastroenterology, 89,* 1083–1085.

Klasner, E. (1993). *Communication strategies for people with Huntington's disease* [Video tape]. Toronto: Huntington's Society of Canada.

Klawans, H. L., & Ringel, S. P. (1971). Observations on the efficacy of L-DOPA in progressive supranuclear palsy. *European Neurology, 5,* 115–129.

Kluin, K. J., Foster, N. L., Berent, S., & Gilman, S. (1993). Perceptual analysis of speech disorders in progressive supranuclear palsy. *Neurology, 43,* 563–566.

Kluin, K. J., Gilman, S., Lohman, M., & Junck, L. (1996). Characteristics of the dysarthria of multiple system atrophy. *Archives of Neurology, 53,* 545–548.

Kristensen, M. O. (1985). Progressive supranuclear palsy—20 years later. *Acta Neurologica Scandinavica, 71,* 177–189.

Kruel, E. J. (1972). Neuromuscular control examination (NMC) for parkinsonism: Vowel prolongations and diadochokinetic and reading rates. *Journal of Speech and Hearing Disorders, 15,* 72–83.

Kujala, P., Portin, R., & Ruutiainen, J. (1996). Language functions in incipient cognitive decline in multiple sclerosis. *Journal of the Neurological Sciences, 141,* 79–86.

Kurtzke, J. F. (1991). Risk factors in amyotrophic lateral sclerosis. *Advances in Neurology, 56,* 245–270.

LaBlance, G. R., & Rutherford, D. R. (1991). Respiratory dynamics and speech intelligibility in speakers with generalized dystonia. *Journal of Communication Disorders, 24*(2), 141–156.

Lang, A. E., & Blair, R. D. G. (1984). Parkinson's disease in 1984: An update. *Canadian Medical Association Journal, 131,* 1031–1037.

LaPointe, L. L., Case, J. L., & Duane, D. D. (1994). Perceptual–acoustic speech and voice characteristics of subjects with spasmodic torticollis. In J. A. Till, K. M. Yorkston, & D. R. Beukelman (Eds.), *Motor speech disorders: Advances in assessment and treatment* (pp. 57–64). Baltimore: Brookes.

LaPointe, L. L., & Horner, J. (1981). Palilalia: A descriptive study of pathological reiterative utterances. *Journal of Speech and Hearing Research, 46*(1), 34–38.

Leanderson, R., Meyerson, B. A., & Persson, A. (1972). Lip muscle function in parkinsonian dysarthria. *Acta Otolaryngologica, 74,* 350–357.

Lebrun, Y., Devreux, F., & Rousseau, J. J. (1986). Language and speech in a patient with a clinical diagnosis of progressive supranuclear palsy. *Brain and Language, 27*(2), 247–256.

Leopold, N. A., & Kagel, M. C. (1996). Prepharyngeal dysphagia in Parkinson's disease. *Dysphagia, 11,* 14–22.

Leopold, N. A., & Kagel, M. C. (1997). Pharyngo–esophageal dysphagia in Parkinson's disease. *Dysphagia, 12,* 11–18.

Lethlean, J. B., & Murdoch, B. E. (1993). Language problems in multiple sclerosis. *Journal of Medical Speech/Language Pathology, 1*(1), 47–59.

Levin, B. E., Tomer, R., & Rey, G. J. (1992). Cognitive impairments in Parkinson's disease. *Neurologic Clinics, 10*(2), 471–481.

Liao, K. K., Wang, S. J., Kwan, S. Y., Kong, K. W., & Wu, Z. A. (1992). Tongue dyskinesia as an early manifestation of Wilson disease. *Brain and Development, 13,* 451–453.

Lieberman, P., Friedman, J., & Feldman, L. (1990). Syntax comprehension deficits in Parkinson's disease. *Journal of Nervous and Mental Disorders, 178,* 360–365.

Lieberman, P., Kako, E., Friedman, J., Tajchman, G., Feldman, L. S., & Jiminez, E. B. (1992). Speech production, syntax comprehension, and cognitive deficits in Parkinson's disease. *Brain and Language, 43,* 169–189.

Linebaugh, C. (1979). The dysarthrias of Shy-Drager syndrome. *Journal of Speech and Hearing Disorders, 44,* 55–60.

Litvan, I., Mega, M. S., Cummings, J. L., & Fairbanks, L. (1996). Neuropsychiatric aspects of progressive supranuclear palsy. *Neurology, 47,* 1184–1189.

Logemann, J., & Fischer, H. (1981). Vocal tract control in Parkinson's disease: Phonetic feature analyses of misarticulations. *Journal of Speech and Hearing Disorders, 46,* 348.

Logemann, J. A., Fischer, H. B., Boshes, B., & Blonsky, E. (1978). Frequency and cooccurrence of vocal tract dysfunction in the speech of a large sample of Parkinson patients. *Journal of Speech and Hearing Disorders, 43,* 47–57.

Ludlow, C. L., Connor, N. P., & Bassich, C. J. (1987). Speech timing in Parkinson's and Huntington's disease. *Brain and Language, 32,* 195–214.

Ludlow, C. L., Naunton, R. F., Sedory, S. E., Schulz, G. M., & Hallett, M. (1988). Effects of botulinum toxin injections on speech in adductor spasmodic dysphonia. *Neurology, 38,* 1220–1225.

Ludlow, C. L., Naunton, R. F., Terada, S., & Anderson, B. J. (1991). Successful treatment of selected cases of abductor spasmodic dysphonia using botulinum toxin injection. *Otolaryngology—Head and Neck Surgery, 104,* 849–855.

Ludolph, A. C., Langen, K. J., Regard, M., Herzog, H., Kemper, B., Kuwert, T., Bottger, I. G., & Feinendegen, L. (1992). Frontal lobe function in amyotrophic lateral sclerosis: A neuropsychologic and positron emission tomography study. *Acta Neurologica Scandinavica, 85*(2), 81–89.

Lundervold, A. J., & Reinvang, I. (1991). Neuropsychological findings and depressive symptoms in patients with Huntington's disease. *Scandinavian Journal of Psychology, 32,* 275–283.

Maher, E. R., Smith, E. M., & Lees, A. J. (1985). Cognitive deficits in the Steele-Richardson-Olszewski syndrome (progressive supranuclear palsy). *Journal of Neurology, Neurosurgery and Psychiatry, 48,* 1234–1239.

Marsden, C., & Harrison, M. (1974). Idiopathic torsion dystonia (dystonia musculorum deformans): A review of 42 patients. *Brain, 97,* 793–810.

Marsden, C., Harrison, M., & Bundy, S. (1976). Natural history of idiopathic torsion dystonia. *Advances in Neurology, 14,* 177–187.

Marttila, R. J. (1983). Diagnosis and epidemiology of Parkinson's disease. *Acta Neurologica Scandinavica. Supplementum, 95*, 9–17.

Marttila, R. J., & Rinne, U. K. (1981). Epidemiology of Parkinson's disease—An overview. *Journal of Neural Transmission, 51*, 135–148.

Massman, P. J., Sims, J., Cook, N., Haverkamp, L. J., Appel, V., & Appel, S. H. (1996). Prevalence and correlates of neuropsychological deficits in amyotrophic lateral sclerosis. *Journal of Neurology, Neurosurgery and Psychiatry, 61*, 450–455.

Mathus-Viliegen, L. M., Louwerse, L. S., Merkus, M. P., Tytgat, G. N., & Vianney de Jong, J. M. (1994). Percutaneous endoscopic gastrostomy in patients with amyotrophic lateral sclerosis and impaired pulmonary function. *Gastrointestinal Endoscopy, 40*, 463–469.

Mauriello, J. A. (1985). Blepharospasm, Meige syndrome, and hemifacial spasm: Treatment with botulinum toxin. *Neurology, 35*, 1499–1500.

Mayeux, R., Stern, Y., Herman, A., Greenbaum, L., & Fahn, S. (1986). Correlates of early disability in Huntington's disease. *Annals of Neurology, 20*, 727–731.

Mazzini, L., Corra, T., Zaccala, M., Mora, G., Del Piano, M., & Galante, M. (1995). Percutaneous endoscopic gastrostomy and enteral nutrition in amyotrophic lateral sclerosis. *Journal of Neurology, 242*, 695–698.

McFarlin, D., & McFarland, H. F. (1982). Multiple sclerosis, Part I. *New England Journal of Medicine, 307*, 1183–1188.

McGeer, E., & McGeer, P. (1988). The dystonias. *Canadian Journal of Neurologic Sciences, 15*, 447–483.

McGuire, T. J., Palaganas-Tosco, A., & Redford, J. B. (1988). Dystonia musculorum deformans: Three cases treated on a rehabilitation unit. *Archives of Physical Medicine and Rehabilitation, 69*, 373–376.

Menkes, J. H. (1974). *Textbook of child neurology*. Philadelphia: Lea & Febiger.

Metter, E. J., & Hanson, W. R. (1986). Clinical and acoustical variability in hypokinetic dysarthria. *Journal of Communication Disorders, 19*, 347–366.

Metter, E. J., & Hanson, W. R. (1991). Dysarthria in progressive supranuclear palsy. In C. A. Moore, K. M. Yorkston, & D. R. Beukelman (Eds.), *Dysarthria and apraxia of speech: Perspectives on management* (pp. 127–136). Baltimore: Brookes.

Miller, R. G., Moore, D., Young, L. A., Armon, C., Barohn, R. J., Bromberg, M. B., Bryan, W. W., Gelinas, D. F., Mandoza, M. C., Neville, H. E., Parry, G. J., Petajan, J. H., Ravits, J. M., Ringel, S. P., & Ross, M. A. (1996). Placebo-controlled trail of gabapentin in patients with amyotrophic lateral sclerosis: Western Amyotrophic Lateral Sclerosis Study Group. *Neurology, 47*, 1383–1388.

Minden, S. L., & Schiffer, R. B. (1990). Affective disorders in multiple sclerosis: Review and recommendations for clinical research. *Archives of Neurology, 47*, 98–104.

Montgomery, G. K., & Erickson, L. M. (1987). Neuropsychological perspectives in amyotrophic lateral sclerosis. *Neurologic Clinics, 5*(1), 61–81.

Morrell, R. M. (1992). Neurologic disorders of swallowing. In M. E. Groher (Ed.), *Dysphagia: Diagnosis and management* (pp. 37–60). Stoneham, MA: Butterworth-Heinemann.

Morris, J. G. L. (1982). The manager of Parkinson's disease. *Australian–New Zealand Journal of Medicine, 12*, 195–205.

Munschauer, F. E., & Stuart, W. H. (1997). Rationale for early treatment with interferon beta-1a in relapsing–remitting multiple sclerosis. *Clinical Therapeutics, 19*, 868–882.

Murdoch, B. E., Chenery, H. J., Bowler, S., & Ingram, J. C. L. (1989). Respiratory function in Parkinson's subjects exhibiting a perceptible speech deficit: A kinematic and spirometric analysis. *Journal of Speech and Hearing Disorders, 54*, 610–626.

Narabayashi, H. (1991). Surgical treatment in the levodopa era. In G. Stern (Ed.), *Parkinson's disease* (pp. 597–646). London: Chapman & Hall.

National Institutes of Health Consensus Panel. (1990). Botulinum toxin. *National Institute of Health Consensus Statement, 8*, 1–20.

Netsell, R., Daniel, B., & Celesia, G. G. (1975). Acceleration and weakness in parkinsonian dysarthria. *Journal of Speech and Hearing Disorders, 40*, 170–178.

Newall, A. R., Orser, R., & Hunt, M. (1996). The control or oral secretions in bulbar ALS/MND. *Journal of the Neurological Sciences, 139*(Suppl.), 43–44.

Nilsson, H., Ekberg, O., Olsson, R., & Hindfelt, B. (1996). Quantitative assessment of oral and pharyngeal function in Parkinson's disease. *Dysphagia, 11*, 144–150.

Nutt, J. G. (1995). Management of parkinsonism and treatment of associated complications. *Current Opinion in Neurology, 8*, 327–330.

Olmas-Lau, N., Ginsberg, M., & Geller, G. (1977). Aphasia in multiple sclerosis. *Neurology, 27*, 623–626.

Ouellon, M., Ryalls, J., Lebeuf, J., & Joanette, Y. (1991). Voice onset time in Friedreich dysarthria. *Folia Phoniatrica, 43*, 295–303.

Pehlivan, M., Yuceyar, N., Ertekin, C., Celebi, G., Ertas, M., Kalayci, T., & Aydogdu, I. (1996). An electronic device measuring the frequency of spontaneous swallowing: Digital phagometer. *Dysphagia, 11*, 259–264.

Perry, R. J., & Hodges, J. R. (1996). Spectrum of memory dysfunction in degenerative disease. *Current Opinion in Neurology, 9*, 281–285.

Pillon, B., Dubois, B., Ploska, A., & Agid, Y. (1991). Severity and specificity of cognitive impairment in Alzheimer's, Huntington's, and Parkinson's disease and progressive supranuclear palsy. *Neurology, 41*, 634–643.

Playfer, J. P. (1997). Parkinson's disease. *Postgraduate Medicine, 73*, 257–284.

Podoll, K., Schwarz, M., & Noth, J. (1991). Language functions in progressive supranuclear palsy. *Brain, 114*(3), 1457–1472.

Porter, P. B. (1989). Intervention in end stage of multiple sclerosis: A case study. *Augmentative and Alternative Communication, 5*(2), 125–127.

Poser, C. M. (1984). *The diagnosis of multiple sclerosis*. New York: Thieme-Stratton.

Poser, C. M. (1992). Multiple sclerosis. Observations and reflections: A personal memoir. *Journal of Neurologic Sciences, 107*, 127–140.

Poser, C., Paty, D., Scheinberg, M., McDonald, W., Davis, F., Ebers, G., Johnson, K., Sibley, W., Silberg, D., & Tourtellotte, W. (1983). New diagnostic criteria for multiple sclerosis: Guidelines for research protocols. *Annals of Neurology, 13*, 227–231.

Priori, A., Berardelli, A., Mercuri, B., & Manfredi, M. (1995). Physiological effects produced by Botulinum toxin treatment of upper limb dystonia. *Brain, 118*, 801–807.

Putnam, A. H. B., & Hixon, T. (1984). Respiratory kinematics in speakers with motor neuron disease. In M. R. McNeil, J. C. Rosenbek, & A. E. Aronson (Eds.), *The dysarthrias: Physiology, acoustics, perception, management* (pp. 37–68). San Diego: College-Hill.

Quaid, K. A., & Morris, M. (1993). Reluctance to undergo predictive testing: The case of Huntington's disease. *American Journal of Medical Genetics, 45*, 41–45.

Quinn, N., & Wenning, G. (1995). Multiple system atrophy. *Current Opinion in Neurology, 8,* 323–326.

Rajput, A. H., Offord, K. P., Beard, C. M., & Kurland, L. T. (1984). Epidemiology of parkinsonism: Incidence, classification, and mortality. *Annual of Neurology, 16,* 278–282.

Ramig, L. A. (1986). Acoustic analyses of phonation in patients with Huntington's disease. *Annals of Otology, Rhinology and Laryngology, 95,* 288–293.

Ramig, L. (1992). The role of phonation in speech intelligibility: A review and preliminary data from patients with Parkinson's disease. In R. D. Kent (Ed.), *Intelligibility in speech disorders* (pp. 119–156). Philadelphia: John Benjamins.

Ramig, L. A., & Gould, W. J. (1986). Speech characteristics in Parkinson's disease. *Neurological Consultant, 4,* 1–6.

Ramig, L. O., Pawlas, A. A., & Countryman, S. (1995). *The Lee Silverman voice treatment.* Iowa City, IA: National Center for Voice and Speech.

Ramig, L. O., Scherer, R. C., Klasner, E. R., Titze, I. R., & Horii, Y. (1990). Acoustic analysis of voice in amyotrophic lateral sclerosis: A longitudinal case study. *Journal of Speech and Hearing Disorders, 55,* 2–14.

Rao, S. M. (1986). Neuropsychology of multiple sclerosis: A critical review. *Journal of Clinical and Experimental Neuropsychology, 8,* 503–542.

Rao, S. M. (1995). Neuropsychology of multiple sclerosis. *Current Opinion in Neurology, 8,* 216–220.

Rao, S. M., Leo, G. J., Bernardin, L., & Unverzagt, F. (1991). Cognitive dysfunction in multiple sclerosis: I. Frequency, patterns and predictions. *Neurology, 41,* 658–691.

Reischies, F. M., Baum, K., Brau, H., & Hedde, J. P. (1988). Cerebral magnetic resonance imaging findings in multiple sclerosis: Relation to disturbance of affect, drive, and cognition. *Archives of Neurology, 45,* 1114–1116.

Ridding, M. C., Sheean, G., Rothwell, J. C., Inzelberg, R., & Kujirai, T. (1995). Changes in the balance between motor cortical excitation and inhibition in focal, task specific dystonia. *Journal of Neurology, Neurosurgery & Psychiatry, 53,* 493–498.

Rigrodsky, S., & Morrison, E. (1970). Speech changes in parkinsonism during L-dopa therapy: Preliminary findings. *Journal of the American Geriatric Society, 18,* 142–151.

Robbins, J. A., Logemann, J. A., & Kirschner, H. S. (1986). Swallowing and speech production in Parkinson's disease. *Annals of Neurology, 19,* 283–287.

Ross, M. A. (1997). Acquired motor neuron disorders. *Neurologic Clinics, 15,* 481–500.

Roth, C. R., Glaze, L. E., Goding, G. S., & David, W. S. (1996). Spasmodic dysphonia symptoms as initial presentation of amyotrophic lateral sclerosis. *Journal of Voice, 10,* 362–367.

Rothlind, J. C., Bylsma, F. W., Peyser, C., Folstein, S. E., & Brandt, J. (1993). Cognitive and motor correlates of everyday functioning in early Huntington's disease. *Journal of Nervous and Mental Disease, 181,* 194–199.

Rowland, L. P. (1991). Ten central themes in a decade of ALS research. *Advances in Neurology, 56,* 3–23.

Sanders, D. B., & Scoppetta, C. (1994). The treatment of patients with myasthenia gravis. *Neurologic Clinics, 12,* 343–368.

Saunders, C., Walsh, T., & Smith, M. (1981). Hospice care in the motor neuron diseases. In C. Saunders & J. Teller (Eds.), *Hospice: The living idea* (pp. 223–235). London: Edward Arnold.

Schulz, G. M., & Ludlow, C. L. (1991). Botulinum treatment for orolingual–mandibular dystonia: Speech effects. In C. A. Moore, K. M. Yorkston, & D. R. Beukelman (Eds.), *Dysarthria and apraxia of speech: Perspectives on management* (pp. 227–242). Baltimore: Brookes.

Scott, A. B. (1980). Botulinum toxin injection into extraocular muscles as an alternative to strabismus surgery. *Ophthalmology, 87*, 1044–1047.

Shahar, E., Nowaczyk, M., & Tervo, R. C. (1987). Rehabilitation of communication impairment in dystonia musculorum deformans. *Pediatric Neurology, 3*, 97–100.

Shimizu, N., Suzuki, M., Yamaguchi, Y., Aoki, T., Matsuda, I., & Arima, M. (1996). A nation-wide survey for neurologic and hepato-neurologic type of Wilson disease: Clinical features and hepatic copper content. *No To Hattatsu [Brain and Development], 28*, 391–397.

Shoulson, I., & Fahn, S. (1979). Huntington's disease: Clinical care and evaluation. *Neurology, 29*, 1–3.

Sobue, G., Matsouka, Y., & Maukai, E. (1981). Pathology of myelinated fibers in cervical and lumbar ventral spinal roots in amyotrophic lateral sclerosis. *Journal of Neurological Sciences, 50*, 413–421.

Solomon, N. P., & Hixon, T. J. (1993). Speech breathing in Parkinson's disease. *Journal of Speech and Hearing Research, 36*, 294–310.

Sosner, J., Gayten, C. W., & Sznajder, J. (1993). Progressive supranuclear palsy: Clinical presentation and rehabilitation of two patients. *Archives of Physical Medicine and Rehabilitation, 74*, 537–539.

Sprengelmeyer, R., Lange, H., & Homberg, V. (1995). The pattern of attentional deficits in Huntington's disease. *Brain, 118*, 145–152.

Starosta-Rubinstein, S., Young, A. B., Kluin, K., Hill, G., Aisen, A. M., Gabrielson, T., & Brewer, G. J. (1987). Clinical assessment of 31 patients with Wilson's disease. Correlations with structural changes on magnetic resonance. *Archives of Neurology, 44*, 365–370.

Steele, J. C. (1972). Progressive supranuclear palsy. *Brain, 95*, 693–704.

Steele, J. C., Richardson, J. D., & Olszewski, J. (1964). Progressive supranuclear palsy. *Archives of Neurology, 10*, 333–359.

Strand, E. A., Buder, E. H., Yorkston, K. M., & Ramig, L. O. (1994). Differential phonatory characteristics of four women with amyotrophic lateral sclerosis. *Journal of Voice, 8*, 327–339.

Strand, E. A., Miller, R. M., Yorkston, K. M., & Hillel, A. D. (1996). Management of oral–pharyngeal dysphagia symptoms in amyotrophic lateral sclerosis. *Dysphagia, 11*, 129–139.

Strong, M. J., Grace, G. M., Orange, J. B., & Leeper, H. A. (1996). Cognition, language and speech in ALS: A review. *Journal of Clinical and Experimental Neuropsychology, 18*, 291–303.

Sullivan, M. D., Brune, P. J., & Beukelman, D. R. (1996). Maintenance of speech changes following group treatment for hypokinetic dysarthria of Parkinson's disease. In D. A. Robin, K. M. Yorkston, & D. R. Beukelman (Eds.), *Disorders of motor speech: Assessment, treatment and clinical characterization* (pp. 287–310). Baltimore: Brookes.

Sullivan, M. J., Edgley, K., & Dehoux, E. (1990). A survey of multiple sclerosis. Part I: Perceived cognitive problems and compensatory strategies use. *Canadian Journal of Rehabilitation, 4*(2), 99–105.

Swash, M., Roberts, A. H., Zakko, H., & Heathfield, K. W. G. (1972). Treatment of involuntary movement disorders with tetrabenzine. *Journal of Neurology, Neurosurgery and Psychiatry, 35*, 186–191.

Tandan, R., & Bradley, W. G. (1985a). Amyotrophic lateral sclerosis: Part 1. Clinical features, pathology, and ethical issues in management. *Annals of Neurology, 18*, 271–280.

Tandan, R., & Bradley, W. G. (1985b). Amyotrophic lateral sclerosis: Part 2. Etiopathogenesis. *Annals of Neurology, 18*, 419–431.

Temlett, J. A. (1996). Parkinson's disease: Biology and aetiology. *Current Opinion in Neurology, 9*, 303–307.

Tidwell, J. (1993). Pulmonary management of the ALS patient. *Journal of Neurologic Nursing, 25*(6), 337–342.

Tohgi, H., Tsukagnoshi, H., & Toyokura, Y. (1997). Quantitative changes of nerves in various neurological diseases. *Acta Neuropathologica, 38*, 95–101.

Tolosa, E., Marti, M. J., & Kulisevsky, J. (1988). Botulinum toxin injection therapy for hemifacial spasm. In J. Jankovic & E. Tolosa (Eds.), *Advances in neurology: Vol. 49. Facial dyskinesia* (pp. 479–491). New York: Raven Press.

Topaloglu, H., Gucuyener, K., Orkun, C., & Renda, Y. (1990). Tremor of tongue and dysarthria as the sole manifestation of Wilson's disease. *Clinical Neurology and Neurosurgery, 92*, 295–296.

Tsui, J. K. C. (1996). Botulinum toxin as a therapeutic agent. *Pharmacology and Therapeutics, 72*, 13–24.

Tsui, J. K., & Calne, D. B. (1988). Botulinum toxin in cervical dystonia. In J. Jankovic & E. Tolosa (Eds.), *Advances in neurology: Vol. 49. Facial dyskinesias* (pp. 473–486). New York: Raven Press.

Turner, G. S., Tjaden, K., & Weismer, G. (1995). The influence of speaking rate on vowel space and speech intelligibility for individuals with amyotrophic lateral sclerosis. *Journal of Speech and Hearing Research, 38*(5), 1001–1013.

Utz, U., & McFarland, H. F. (1994). The role of T cells in multiple sclerosis: Implications for therapies targeting the T cell receptor. *Journal of Neuropathology and Experimental Neurology, 53*, 351–358.

Verny, M., Jellinger, K. A., Hauw, J. J., Bancher, C., Litvan, I., & Agid, Y. (1996). Progressive supranuclear palsy: A clinicopathological study of 21 cases. *Acta Neuropathologica, 91*, 427–431.

Vogels, O. J., Maassen, B., Rotteveel, J. J., & Merx, J. L. (1994). Focal dystonia and speech impairment responding to anticholinergic therapy. *Pediatric Neurology, 11*, 346–348.

Wallace, G. L., & Holmes, S. (1993). Cognitive–linguistic assessment of individuals with multiple sclerosis. *Archives of Physical Medicine and Rehabilitation, 74*, 637–643.

Walshe, J. M., & Yealland, M. (1992). Wilson's disease: The problem of delayed diagnosis. *Journal of Neurology, Neurosurgery and Psychiatry, 55*, 692–696.

Waxman, M. J., Durfee, D., Moore, M., & Morantz, R. A. (1990). Nutritional aspects and swallowing function of patients with Parkinson's disease. *Nutrition in Clinical Practice, 5*(5), 196–199.

Weinshenker, B. G. (1996). Epidemiology of multiple sclerosis. *Neurologic Clinics, 14*, 291–308.

Weismer, G., Kent, R. D., Hodge, M., & Martin, R. (1988). The acoustic signature for intelligibility test words. *Journal of the Acoustic Society of America, 84*(4), 1281–1291.

Weismer, G., Martin, R., Kent, R. D., & Kent, J. F. (1992). Formant trajectory characteristics of males with amyotrophic lateral sclerosis. *Journal of the Acoustics Society of America, 91*(2), 1058–1098.

White, D. M., Catanzaro, M. L., & Kraft, G. H. (1993). An approach to the psychological aspects of multiple sclerosis: A coping guide for healthcare providers and families. *Journal of Neurologic Rehabilitation, 7*, 43–52.

Wilkinson, C., Yorkston, K. M., Strand, E. A., & Rogers, M. (1995). Features of spontaneous language in speakers with amyotrophic lateral sclerosis and dysarthria. *American Journal of Speech–Language Pathology, 4*(4), 139–142.

Williams, A., Hanson, D., & Calne, D. B. (1979). Vocal cord paralysis in the Shy-Drager syndrome. *Journal of Neurology, Neurosurgery, and Psychiatry, 42*, 151–153.

Wilson, S. A. K. (1912). Progressive lenticular degeneration: A familial nervous disease associated with cirrhosis of the liver. *Brain, 34*, 295–509.

Woods, C. G., & Taylor, A. M. (1992). Ataxia telangiectasia in the British Isles: The clinical and laboratory features of 70 affected individuals. *Quarterly Journal of Medicine, 82*, 169–179.

Woods, S. E., & Colon, V. F. (1989). Wilson's disease. *American Family Physician, 40*(1), 171–178.

Yorkston, K. M., Miller, R. M., & Strand, E. A. (1995). *Management of speech and swallowing disorders in degenerative disease.* Tucson, AZ: Communication Skill Builders.

Yorkston, K. M., Strand, E., Miller, R., Hillel, A., & Smith, K. (1993). Speech deterioration in amyotrophic lateral sclerosis: Implications for the timing of intervention. *Journal of Medical Speech/
Language Pathology, 1*(1), 35–46.

Yorkston, K. M., Strand, E. A., & Hume, J. (1998). The relationship between motor function and
speech function in amyotrophic lateral sclerosis. In M. Cannito, K. M. Yorkston, & D. R. Beukelman (Eds.), *Neuromotor speech disorders: Nature, assessment, and management* (pp. 85–98). Baltimore: Brookes.

Yorkston, K. M., Strand, E. A., & Miller, R. M. (1996). Progression of respiratory symptoms in amyotrophic lateral sclerosis: Implications for speech function. In D. A. Robin, K. M. Yorkston, &
D. R. Beukelman (Eds.), *Disorders of motor speech: Assessment, treatment and clinical characterization* (pp. 193–204). Baltimore: Brookes.

Young, R. R., & Delwaide, P. J. (1981a). Drug therapy: Spasticity, Part I. *New England Journal of
Medicine, 304,* 28–33.

Young, R. R., & Delwaide, P. J. (1981b). Drug therapy: Spasticity, Part II. *New England Journal of
Medicine, 304,* 96–99.

CHAPTER

CLINICAL EXAMINATION
OF MOTOR SPEECH DISORDERS

Clinical Issues: We regularly provide clinical training opportunities for student interns in speech pathology, medical students, and resident physicians in neurology and rehabilitation medicine. The impetus for this book has come at least in part from our attempts to help our students make the transition from students to practicing clinicians, from readers of research literature to individuals responsible for making decisions about management of communication problems. Typically, our speech pathology interns come to us well versed in the normal aspects of speech production. Students in speech–language pathology have read research literature related to motor speech disorders. If we were to ask them to list all the aspects of speech production in individuals with dysarthria or apraxia that can be measured, their lists would be long. Students, if asked, would typically have much more difficulty selecting those aspects of speech that they would measure given only a 1-hour evaluation time. The goal of this chapter is to provide a framework for deciding what aspects of speech are important to measure within typical clinical time limitations. In Chapter 1, we introduced a model of chronic disease as a way of desribing dysarthria and apraxia of speech. This model will serve as the framework for assessment. In this chapter, we will address the following questions:

- What is the nature and severity of underlying motor impairment?
- What are the consequences of those impairments for speech?
- What types of disability are imposed by the dysarthria or apraxia of speech?

PURPOSES OF THE CLINICAL EXAMINATION

While the clinical examination of speech is a process of observation and fact finding, it must go beyond description to include synthesis of information, dynamic analysis, and initial intervention planning. Adequate treatment plans can only be developed out of assessments that probe the nature of the deficits and the speaker's response to the deficits. Because clinical hypotheses are formed and tested, the examination will proceed in different directions based on initial findings. In other words, the clinician changes the assessment strategies based on what he or she has already seen. The specific goals and outcomes of the examination may vary from situation to situation. Although each examination does not address every issue, the following list contains potential reasons for assessing speakers with motor speech disorders (McNeil & Kennedy, 1984, p. 337):

- to detect or confirm a suspected problem
- to establish a differential diagnosis
- to classify with a specified disorder group
- to determine site of lesion or disease process
- to specify the degree or severity of involvement
- to establish a prognosis
- to specify more precisely the treatment focus
- to establish criteria for treatment termination
- to measure any change in the patient that accompanies treatment, lack of treatment, or exacerbation of the original etiological factor

The purposes of the clinical examination may vary depending on such factors as site of practice and phase of intervention. For example, the site of practice may be an outpatient diagnostic clinic within a department of neurology, an inpatient rehabilitation service, or a community-based rehabilitation program. In each of these sites, the clinical examination may have different goals. In the neurology clinic, contribution to a differential diagnosis and documentation of current severity may be the tasks at hand. For example, the speech–language pathologist may be asked to give an opinion about which cranial nerves are impaired. In an inpatient rehabilitation service, establishing the prognosis for improvement and developing a plan of intervention may be the goal. In a community-based rehabilitation program, the examination may have a number of goals, including understanding the pattern and severity of the impairment as well as the functional limitation and disability. A primary care team in community-based settings may be responsible for multiple aspects of the condition. Health care is increasingly being delivered in a variety of venues, and clinical examination must be tailored to the specific needs of each.

The phase of intervention may also influence the range of possible assessment questions and thus the conclusions of the clinical examination. For example, a number of critical points in the management of individuals with amyotrophic lateral sclerosis (ALS) may dictate the focus of the clinical examination. Assessment may occur at four critical points. The first occurs when the diagnosis is made. At that time, the speech–language pathologist determines the presence or absence of dysarthria and verifies that the pattern of dysarthria is consistent with the proposed medical diagnosis. The clinician assesses so that he or she will be able to discuss with the dysarthric speaker and the family the nature of the problem, and to verify that the dysarthria is currently not a functional limitation in communicative situations. The second critical point occurs after the individual has achieved some psychological acceptance of the presence of the disease. Here the general goal of assessment is to stage treatment, that is, to prepare speakers and their families for the next steps if the symptoms become more severe. Based on this assessment, the clinician also makes some initial judgments about the rate of progression of the disease. At this point, the individual with ALS is involved in an information-gathering phase regarding services available, including augmentative communication options. Guidelines are provided for a reevaluation schedule. These guidelines are general and suggest the need for reassessment when speech problems begin to interfere with any aspect of daily activities. In most cases, this occurs when intelligibility is compromised in some situations. Thus, the third critical assessment point occurs when the dysarthria becomes severe enough to become a functional limitation to the individual. At this time, assessment is carried out to establish candidacy for treatment and to specify the treatment focus. For example, the outcome of the evaluation may be identification of strategies to supplement the speaker's highly distorted speech with semantic or other types of cues. This assessment may be followed by a brief period of training in an effort to maximize intelligibility and comprehensibility. The fourth critical point occurs when speech is so severely involved that it must be replaced by other communication approaches. As an outcome of this assessment process, an augmentative communication system may be selected. The case of an individual with a degenerative dysarthria serves to illustrate the varying purposes of assessment. Purposes of assessment also vary over time in children with developmental motor speech disorders. Parents' and children's needs, roles, and expectations differ when the child is an infant or toddler compared with when he or she enters school. Assessment is done at times to confirm the presence of this disorder, and at other times to measure its severity. Still other times, clinicians assess to direct the treatment, or to identify the intervention approaches that may be effective, or to make recommendations about alternatives to verbal communication.

PRINCIPLES OF THE CLINICAL EXAMINATION

Establishing a Knowledge Base

"What one knows, one sees" (DeGown, 1987, cited in Miller & Groher, 1990). In other words, the clinical examination is extensively influenced by the knowledge of the observer. That is, each clinician brings his or her own skills and knowledge base to the task of assessment. The maxim, "what one knows, one sees," has at least two meanings. First, the broader the knowledge base brought to the task, the more effective the examination will be. Therefore, it is critical for the speech–language pathologist to have an understanding of the diseases and conditions that may be associated with motor speech disorders, and their underlying neuropathologies, etiologies, natural courses, and associated symptoms. The results of the clinical examination of speech must be viewed in the broad context of other motor and cognitive signs and symptoms. For those clinicians evaluating a potential motor component to a speech or language delay in children, this broader context includes knowledge of speech and language development. Clinicians need to pay particular attention to how cognitive, language, and motor processes interact and influence each other during development (Strand, 1992). For example, children with severe motor planning problems would not be expected to perform normally on articulation tests or tests of phonologic processing. The clinician must ask, however, whether the child's poor performance on these tests is actually due to phonologic processing deficits or to the impact of the motor planning deficit on normal acquistion of phonology.

On the other hand, the maxim, "what one knows, one sees," should also be interpreted as a caution. If clinicians see only what they expect to see, they may miss important findings. Care should be taken not to attribute all symptoms to a particular known diagnosis. For example, the diagnosis of Parkinson's disease does not preclude the occurrence of other disorders with consequences for communication. An individual with Parkinson's disease and dysarthria may also experience any number of problems unrelated to the primary diagnosis. For example, the person may experience hearing loss, which compromises his or her ability to speak at the appropriate loudness levels. If clinicians see only what they expect to see, they may fail to identify complicating and potentially treatable problems.

Speech as Part of the Neurologic Examination

Assessment of speech is an important part of the neurologic examination. A neurology colleague of Duffy's (1995) suggested that "nearly all clinical neurologic diagnosis is based on speech, either its content or its manner of expression" (pp. 64–65). Consider how much information about the neurologic status a skilled clinician can obtain by appraising the way a person communicates. For example, opinions can be formed by considering questions about a patient's cognitive status:

- What is the patient's level of consciousness—alert, drowsy, lethargic, and so on?
- What is the patient's level of cooperation?
- What is the patient's affect—depressed, anxious, labile, and so on?
- Can the patient respond to questions?
- How oriented is the patient?

Skilled clinicians also form impressions about the speaker's language skills:

- Does the patient appear to have word finding and sentence formulation problems?
- Does the patient appear to understand what is being said?

Question: What is involved in a neurologic examination?

The neurologic examination attempts to answer the following six Wh–questions (Mumenthaler, 1983):

- When was the onset and what were the symptoms at onset (case history)?

(continues)

- What can be found (physical examination)?

- Where is the lesion situated, producing this clinical picture (topical diagnosis)?

- Why is the patient ill (etiologic diagnosis)?

- What is the course of the illness (prognosis)?

- What is the management (treatment)?

Expressive communication, specifically speech, requires not only cognitive and linguistic processing, but also precise, rapid, and coordinated movements. Therefore, an impression of problems in movement and the control of movement can also be formed. The clinical examination outlined in this chapter focuses to a large extent on motor speech abilities. However, motor speech is affected by other factors including, among others, cognition, language abilities, somatosensory function, and level of hearing. Readers are encouraged to refer to other sources (e.g., Miller & Groher, 1990) for a comprehensive evaluation of a broad range of factors that have the potential of influencing motor speech performance. Throughout the process of the clinical examination, observations about cognitive, language, and hearing function need to be made.

Use of Perceptual and Instrumental Measures

Generally, the tools for measuring the function of each of the speech components are categorized as either perceptual or instrumental. Perceptual measures are those that rely on the trained eyes and ears of the clinician. Instrumental approaches to assessment, on the other hand, employ a series of devices that provide information about the acoustic, aerodynamic, movement, or myoelectric aspects of speech production. A more detailed description of the assessment of the various speech components is contained in later chapters. For this general discussion, the reader should be aware that each of the speech components can be assessed with a number of different perceptual and instrumental approaches. For example, when assessing the respiratory system in the clinical setting, perceptual measures of performance might include ratings of breath group length and loudness of samples of connected speech, as well as visual observations of the presence of clavicular breathing. Among the instrumental approaches to the measurement of respiratory function are the acoustic measures of intensity and utterance duration. Aerodynamically, respiratory performance may be assessed by estimating the subglottal air pressure generated by the speaker. Respiratory inductive plethysmography (commercially available as the Respitrace from Ambulatory Monitoring, Inc., Ardaley, NY 10502) is an instrumental means of obtaining information about the rib cage and abdominal components of the respiratory system and lung volume exchange (see Chapter 7). This instrumentation can be used to study the timing of breathing for speech, the relative contributions of rib cage and abdominal components during speech, and the lung volume level at which utterances are produced. When so many approaches to the measurement of a given phenomenon are available, the final decision about which measures to use depends upon the questions being asked. Some clinical advantages and disadvantages of each of the measurement approaches are outlined in the following discussion.

PERCEPTUAL MEASURES

The "ears of a trained clinician" are wonderful integrators that seek to categorize the phenomena they hear. At times, this ability is a real asset; at other times, it is problematic. When measures of overall speech disability are needed, clinicians usually turn to perceptually derived measures. This is quite logical when the phenomenon being measured is considered. Measures of disability reflect overall aspects of speech—intelligibility, naturalness, rate, and general articulatory adequacy. Thus, an integrative function of perceptual measures is needed. Measurement of impairment may be slightly different. Here, the integrative nature of perceptual measures may be a disadvantage. Speech scientists caution against making inferences about physiologic phenomena from perceptual measures alone. The principle of motor equivalence suggests that a single perceptual end-product may be the result of one of a number of physiologic events. For example, what the listener hears as imprecise articulatory movements may be the consequence of lack of movement as in rigidity, slow movement, or incoordinated movement. Perceptual measures are of limited use in determining the contributors to the problems. Rosenbek and LaPointe (1985) summarized some disadvantages of perceptual approaches to the assessment of dysarthria:

- Trained judges are required.

- It is difficult to separate premorbid characteristics (age, medical, and social history) from those that are related to the neurologic problem.

- Symptoms may be present under some conditions and not others.

- Certain symptoms influence others (e.g., severe articulation problems may influence judgments of hypernasality).

- The same symptoms may be the result of very different underlying conditions.

INSTRUMENTAL OBSERVATIONS

The instrumental approach to speech impairment measurement also presents problems for the clinician. Unlike the perceptual measures just discussed, some instrumental measures do not lend themselves to measurement of integrative activities. Simultaneous measures of multiple aspects of speech production are technically difficult to obtain and interpret. On the other hand, instrumental measures "bring us closer to events in the peripheral speech mechanism . . . [and] leave us guessing less about the neuromuscular deficits underlying the perceptual symptoms" (Rosenbek & LaPointe, 1985, p. 112).

Clinicians must select instrumental approaches carefully. Given sufficient equipment and time, the clinician could instrumentally measure an almost endless number of aspects of dysarthria. However, the usefulness of a given measure of dysarthric performance may depend on the answers to the following questions:

- Can this measure be obtained accurately and reliably in the clinical setting?
- How important is the information obtained from this measure?
- Will the information obtained from this measure contribute to treatment planning?

For purposes of illustration, these questions will be applied to the clinical measurement of vital capacity in dysarthria. Vital capacity can be reliably and relatively easily measured in the dysarthric population, and in most cases, these measures would reveal a problem in speakers with dysarthria in the form of reduced function relative to the normal population. However, consider the clinical importance of vital capacity—it is an important decision-making variable in relatively few speakers with dysarthria. Thus, the clinician must distinguish the important from the easy, straightforward, and perhaps trivial.

A CLINICAL COMPROMISE

Earlier in this chapter, assessment was defined as a process of placing importance on information as the clinician decides what is important and what is not. Admittedly, the assessment process is heavily dependent on subjective opinions, judgments, and hunches. Many of the opinions that we provide in this discussion await research verification. Clinicians use both perceptual and instrumental observations. Perceptual means are used to identify the problems and generate clinical hypotheses about the underlying causes. Instrumental means are used to confirm or reject these hypotheses. A more thorough discussion of instrumental observations can be found in Chapters 7 through 11.

Armed with a thorough understanding of normal aspects of speech and vocal tract impairment assessment, some possible explanations can be posed.

Use of Consistent Procedures

Use of consistent procedures for the assessment of neurologic language disorders is a common practice in the field of speech–language pathology. In fact, many clinicians would be uncomfortable assessing an individual with aphasia without consistent tasks and stimuli. Clinicians believe, and rightfully so, that many advantages come from use of such procedures. For example, documentation of performance would certainly be less consistent if different tasks were used at each testing.

There can be no substitute for an expanding experience base in the development of diagnostic sophistication (Miller & Groher, 1990). Most experienced clinicians realize that this development process is gradual and has gone on throughout their professional life. We suggest that one way of "expanding the experience base" or at least making optimal use of one's existing experience base is to use consistent assessment procedures. Experienced clinicians will suggest that use of the same procedures and tasks with hundreds of patients is an excellent way to learn about the range and variability of performance of individuals with and without neurologic deficits. Listening to a thousand speakers talk about a specific picture or line drawing provides the clinician with a fund of knowledge about aphasia that is a valuable part of the examination process. Making observations from the physical examinations of dozens of speakers with differing underlying neuropathologies will also provide a rich fund of information.

Question: By the term consistent procedures, *do you mean standardized tests?*

No, these terms have quite different meanings. In standardized tests, the examiner's procedures, the speaker's tasks, and the scoring methods are strictly prescribed. Typically, the entire testing protocol is completed during every administration. The field of aphasia has standardized tests. Use of standardized tests is especially important if the performance of the speaker is to be compared with that of a group of individuals with a similar disorder. These types of comparisons are made when scores are reported in percentiles, suggesting how the performance of the individual being tested compares with that of others and allows the clinician to make statements such as, "This person's performance is better than 60% of the comparison group." The clinical examination of speech, described later in this chapter, needs to be flexible. As suggested earlier in this chapter,

(continues)

the neurologic examination process is dynamic. That is, the examination will proceed in different directions based on initial findings, and it is unlikely that all possible procedures will be included in all examinations. Therefore, instead of standardization, we are advocating consistent procedures that can be repeated and documented in a consistent fashion.

COMPONENTS OF THE CLINICAL EXAMINATION

Several important components to the clinical examination for motor speech disorders are depicted in Figure 5.1. Note that the clinical examination of motor speech is composed of three major assessment processes: history of the speech problems, physical examination, and motor speech examination. The sources of information for each of these processes vary. Chart review and interview of the speaker are the basis for acquiring information about the history of speech problems. A comprehensive history will elicit the clients' impression about their impairments, functional limitations, and disabilities. The description of the impairment can be obtained with questions such as these: What kind of problems are you experiencing with your speech? When did the problem start? Has it gotten worse? Questions will also be asked about the functional limitation and disability imposed by the disorder: Do you ever have difficulty making yourself understood? If so, what are the circumstances? What effect has the motor speech disorder had on your daily routine? Are there activities in which you no longer participate as a consequence of the disorder?

The physical examination is a series of observations made by the speech–language pathologist about the structure and function of the speech mechanism. The goal of this examination is to understand the pattern and severity of the impairment of the components of the speech production mechanism. The physical examination typically employs nonspeech tasks and assesses the relative contribution of each subsystem, including respiratory, laryngeal, velopharyngeal, and oral articulatory structures.

Whereas the physical examination focuses on evaluating movement during nonspeech tasks, the motor speech examination focuses on how motor performance varies across speech tasks. Speech is sampled in a hierarchy of utterances. The specific utterances sampled for any speaker differ based on assumption or predictions about the underlying speech disorder (dysarthria or apraxia of speech). For the speaker with dysarthria, the clinician may ask, "How is speech production affected by the weakness, alterations in muscle tone, and

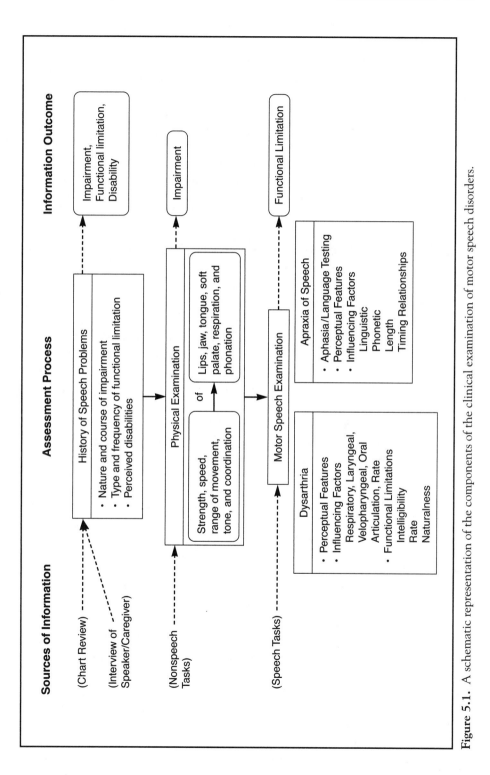

Figure 5.1. A schematic representation of the components of the clinical examination of motor speech disorders.

coordination of movements?" For a speaker with apraxia, a question may be, "How does speech performance vary when linguistic complexity is increased?" In other words, the motor speech examination assesses the disorder at the level of functional limitation. What dimensions of speech deviate from normal? What are the rate and intelligibility of speech? How is speech prosody affected?

In Chapter 1, the model of chronic disease was introduced as a means of understanding the various aspects of motor speech disorders. Both dysarthria and apraxia of speech can be viewed as an impairment, a functional limitation, and a disability. The clinical examination performed by the speech–language pathologist must address each of these levels of motor speech disorders. A review of the model of the clinical examination (Figure 5.1) suggests that different information is obtained as a result of each assessment process. For example, obtaining a history of speech problems involves interviewing the speakers for their perspectives on the impairment, functional limitation, and disability. Whereas the physical examination focuses primarily on the impairment, the motor speech examination results in information about the functional limitation. In other words, the physical examination assesses the changes in motor function of the subsystems of speech (the impairment) and the motor speech examination focuses on how those motor changes impact speech (the functional limitation).

Many of the aspects of this examination can and should be administered in a consistent fashion. With goals of increasing efficiency, we have found that checklists and forms are an effective means of both making procedures consistent and minimizing documentation time. Throughout this chapter, checklists and forms are provided as we describe the assessment of each speech subsystem.

The History of the Speech Problem

A history of the speech problem is obtained from two sources of information: (1) a review of records such as the medical chart and (2) an interview with the speaker and knowledgeable informants, such as family members, spouses, or guardians. Often referral information contains little more than the speaker's name, age, gender, and possibly medical diagnosis. This information can be supplemented by a review of the medical records. The medical records contain a chronology of medical care, including the course of the disorder, the patient's complaints, the treatment plans, and the patient's response to treatment. Because many individuals receive their health care from a number of different providers, medical records from any single source may be incomplete. An effort should be made to obtain summaries of all health care management pertinent to the current diagnosis and specifically to the motor speech disorder. A useful way to get history information about children is to send a preassessment questionnaire for parents to complete and return. Appendix 5.A provides some supplemental case history items for children with motor speech problems (Hodge & Hancock, 1994).

After the medical records are reviewed, the examination usually begins by obtaining a history from an interview with the patient and family in which they are asked to describe the communication disorder. Although the interview with the patient may vary considerably, depending on how much information is available in the medical records, history taking usually includes the topics described in the following sections (Duffy, 1995).

INTRODUCTION AND GOAL SETTING

After the appropriate introductions, the speech–language pathologist may describe his or her role and the purpose and procedures of the clinical motor speech examination. The clinical examination will often begin with the most obvious question. The clinician might ask the client, "What brought you here?" or "Why are you here?" Answers to this question will allow the clinician to begin to form an impression of the client's awareness of the deficit, and levels of alertness, orientation, and cognition. In addition, these introductory questions will help the clinician understand the client's chief complaint and determine what aspects of the problem are most troubling to the client and family.

BASIC DATA

If not already available, basic demographic data should be solicited, including age, education, occupation, family status, and perceived communication needs. Current neurologic deficits can be understood only within the framework of the patient's communication history. When interviewing an adult with an acquired neurologic communication problem, it may be beneficial to ask, "Have you ever had any other problems with communication?" Preexisting conditions, such as foreign accents, preexisting phonologic deficits, articulation changes associated with dental abnormalities, vocal nodules or polyps, chronic obstructive pulmonary disease, and childhood stuttering, may confuse the current clinical picture. When evaluating a child with delayed speech and language, it is important to get a good history of gross and fine motor skill development, early vocal behavior, chronology of language and speech development, and a history of any early feeding or swallowing problems.

ONSET AND COURSE

With acquired neurologic communication disorders, it is important to know how and when the speech problems started. What were the initial symptoms? Did they occur suddenly or did they come on gradually? How have they changed since onset? Have they improved, been stable, or gotten worse? How rapidly have changes occurred? Especially in the case of gradual onset of progressive disorders, patients may not be able to pinpoint the exact time of onset. If a diagnosis has been made, it is useful to know the length of time between the onset of symptoms and the time of diagnosis. When was the diagnosis made and by whom? When the neurologic communication disorder is developmental, it is important to know the developmental characteristics of the child's speech. Parents should be asked about periods of babbling, when first words appeared, and other developmental milestones. What is the rate of acquisition of speech and language, the resistance of the problem to treatment, and the degree to which it interfered with other aspects of development? Clinicians may also ask about early history of feeding and swallowing problems.

Hodge, Wellman, Goulden, and Heaton (1996) surveyed speech–language pathologists about the prevalence of children with motor speech disorders in their caseloads. They found that clinicians reported a large number of "suspected" cases of motor speech disorders. These were defined as unconfirmed cases where motor speech problems were observed and these signs were not explained by immature motor development alone. The signs were judged to have an adverse effect on speech intelligibility, speaking rate, and/or speech quality. If the speech–language pathologist is the first to suspect a problem, then he or she should refer the individual for an appropriate neurologic workup.

ASSOCIATED DEFICITS

During the history taking, the speech–language pathologist also obtains information about other deficits. Is the patient experiencing physical problems in addition to a speech disorder? Have any changes in walking or hand–arm function occurred? If so, when did they occur in relation to changes in speech? Have any cognitive changes occurred? Has the client or family noted any changes in memory, reasoning, or judgment? Have any changes in the ability to read or write occurred? Have any hearing problems occurred? Has the client experienced any changes in sensation? Has the client or family noted any changes in affect or emotions? Does the client laugh or cry more easily than he or she used to? Because swallowing problems frequently co-occur with motor speech disorders, it is also important to identify any changes that may have occurred in eating or swallowing. Does the patient choke or cough when eating or drinking? Has the patient changed his or her diet? Has the patient's weight been stable? Does the patient continue to enjoy eating? Is the process of eating fatiguing or excessively time-consuming?

Questions regarding associated deficits in children focus on developmental history, the current status of the child, and any changes that have recently been noticed in motor skills, language, or speech. For example, did the child babble?

What is the frequency and type of prespeech vocalization? Is canonical bab-bling present? At what age were words and phrases first spoken? When did the child walk? Has the child's speech, fine motor skill, or gait recently changed in any way? Does the child have difficulty chewing or swallowing any particular type of food or liquid?

THE PATIENT'S PERCEPTION OF DEFICIT

During the history taking, the client is asked to describe the speech problem: What aspects of your speech have changed? For example, does your voice sound different than it used to sound? Is it more difficult to move your tongue? Do you get tired when you talk? How do you feel when you speak? It is also useful to explore the compensations that the speaker is attempting to make: What do you do to improve the way you sound? How effective are these strategies? How often do you use them?

Question: Do you find that speakers with motor speech disorders vary in terms of recognition of changes in their speech?

Speakers with motor speech disorders vary greatly in the appreciation of the severity of their symptoms. For example, individuals with traumatic brain injury, Parkinson's disease, or Huntington's disease and reduced cognition may not realize the severity of their disorder. At the other end of the spectrum, individuals with amyotrophic lateral sclerosis or apraxia of speech who exhibit intact cognition and sensation may be intensely aware of changes in speech. Understanding a speaker's perception of the disorder is critical in the development of appropriate treatment plans. Children, especially those with congenital or early acquired motor speech disorders, may have little awareness of the nature or severity of their speech disorder. I had the experience of playing some tape-recorded sen-tences back to a 9-year-old girl with Moebius syndrome. After listening for three or four sentences, she said, "What is wrong with the tape? I can't understand what I am saying" (Megan Hodge, personal communication, May 1997).

CONSEQUENCES OF THE DISORDER

Less than normal speech may have a number of consequences. It is important to know what the repercussion of the motor speech disorder has been for the speaker. Does the speaker feel that he or she is difficult to understand? How does this make the speaker feel about himself or herself? Where and with whom do these difficulties occur most often? Has the speaker changed his or her activities in any way because of the speech disorder? Changes in educational, vocational, and societal activities and participation patterns should be explored.

Children with motor speech disorders, especially those who have good cognitive and receptive language skills, may be very frustrated at their inability to communicate verbally. As their language acquisition proceeds, the children may exhibit increasing challenging behaviors, such as acting out or tantrums. Other children withdraw, making few attempts to initiate communication, shrugging shoulders in response to questions, and generally avoiding additional communication failure. The clinician should ask how the child initiates requests? How does he or she attempt to repair interactions when the listener does not understand? Does he or she vary in the type and number of communication attempts in different situations?

HEALTH CARE MANAGEMENT

While gathering basic information from the speaker, we are also interested in the speaker's current health care management. What services are being provided and by whom? What medications is the client currently taking and why? What community resources is the patient aware of, interested in exploring, or currently utilizing? What adaptive equipment does the patient currently use? When was it obtained? From whom was it obtained? Does the patient have a living will or instructions regarding the level of medical care he or she wishes to receive in case he or she is no longer able to make wishes known to the health care management team? Although descriptions of current health management will vary considerably from client to client, it is especially important to identify the primary health care professionals who have responsibility for coordinating or integrating services. With children, we also ask how the health services are integrated or coordinated with educational planning and placement.

AWARENESS OF DIAGNOSIS AND PROGNOSIS

Speakers with motor speech disorders vary tremendously in terms of their awareness and understanding of the diagnosis of their disorder. Some have read extensively and know the latest developments of medical management for their disorders. Others have little or no information about their disorder or its consequences. If a diagnosis has been made, does the patient have a good understanding of the nature of his or her disease? Has the patient sought information about the disease? What are the patient's and the family's expectations? This line of questioning may help to develop the "educational" portion of the management plan. Clinical experience has taught us to appreciate the importance of clearly written educational materials for clients and families. When taken home, these materials can be read and reread. Clients and families cannot be expected to understand and retain all of the verbal information that is presented in a brief clinic visit.

In this section, we have gone into great detail about the history information that could be helpful to the speech–language pathologist. However, we must also appreciate time limitations. Clinicians must focus on the parts of the case history interview that will provide them with the most pertinent information. The extent to which the clinician gathers information can be related to the nature of the decision faced. Thus, asking every client the same list of questions may not be time-effective and may not be of assistance in focusing the clinical examination.

Physical Examination

During the physical examination, the impairment or physiologic abnormality of the speech production mechanism is evaluated. The physical examination is organized into general sections according to the subsystems of the speech mechanism: jaw, lips, tongue, velopharyngeal mechanism, and respiratory and phonatory systems. In each subsystem, the clinician evaluates the normalcy of the structure and, using largely nonspeech activities, the adequacy of the function of each speech component. Examples of forms for recording the results of the physical examination are provided throughout this chapter. For each component of the speech mechanism, the form contains a checklist of symptoms and a grid on which performance of a variety of speech functions can be rated. Both the symptoms and the performance or function are rated on a scale from 0 (*normal*) to 3 (*severe impairment*). Use of the forms and rating scale facilitates consistent record keeping and thus allows comparison of performance across time.

Question: Should I always assess and rate everything on the physical examination form?

It is good to use forms like the ones displayed in this chapter so that your assessment is consistent and you think about all of the different aspects of speech production. However, we are not advocating that you rigidly adhere to this protocol. Obviously the issues will differ depending on your site of practice and client population.

EXAMINATION OF STRUCTURE

The evaluation of the structures of the speech mechanisms involves a series of observations about the size and relative position of the jaw, lips, teeth, tongue, and hard and soft palates. The speech–language pathologist looks for the symmetry of the structures at rest. Tissue characteristics, including presence of lesions and normalcy of mucosa, are evaluated. Table 5.1 lists some abnormal tissue characteristics and provides some examples of structural abnormalities (Hodge, 1988). Although some of the characteristics listed are not necessarily

Table 5.1
Characteristics of Tissue Indicating Structural Abnormalities

Characteristic	Example
Unusual color	Red (inflammation); bluish tint (absence of underlying tissue, as with submucous cleft; cyanosis)
Rough, fissured, or furrowed texture	Ulceration; atrophy of muscular structure
Unexpected discontinuities in surface or underlying structure (especially at sites of midline union of structures)	Pits or notches in lips; clefts; fistulas; bifid uvula
Absence of structure	Velar musculature inserts anteriorly into hard palate, i.e., no palatal aponeurosis; missing teeth
Disproportionate size in relation to surrounding structures	Short velum in relation to depth of oropharynx; enlarged palatine tonsils occlude oropharynx
Asymmetry in shape or size of bilateral structures	Unilaterally reduced muscle bulk or wasting of tongue; depressed nasal ala
Misalignment of adjacent or functionally related structures	Mandibular retrusion; dental malocclusion
Unusual contour (elevations or depressions in tissue where not expected)	Peaked hard palate; torus on hard palate
Constrained range of muscular structures	Lingual or labial frenum attached over extended area of structure

Note. From "Speech Mechanism Assessment," by M. Hodge, 1988, in Decision Making in Speech–Language Pathology (p. 106), by D. Yoder and R. Kent (Eds.), Toronto: Decker. Copyright 1988 by B. C. Decker, Inc. Reprinted with permission.

within the realm of speech–language pathology, observation of such abnormalities may warrant referral for appropriate evaluation and management.

Adventitious movements are unintentional or involuntary movements that may provide information about the neuropathology of the disease. A number of these involuntary movements may be associated with structures of the speech production mechanism:

- *Chorea*—This term refers to rapid, involuntary, purposeless movements of the extremeties, head, neck, or trunk. These movements are irregular and asymmetrical. They are associated with Sydenham's chorea, a disorder of childhood, and Huntington's chorea, a hereditary disorder in adults.

- *Dystonia*—This is a group of disorders characterized by slow hyperkinesis in which individual muscles or muscle groups exhibit involuntary tonic contractions of variable duration. If they are isolated in the mouth or tongue, the term orofacial or buccolingual dyskinesia is applied. Spasmodic torticollis is a dystonia in which the patient's head and neck are twisted to one side. Athetosis is a type of dystonia commonly seen in children with cerebral palsy. It is caused by contraction of already hypertonic muscles, and is characterized by continuous, writhing movements.

- *Fasciculations*—Fasciculations are involuntary synchronous contractions of single muscle fiber groups that are visible through the skin. They may give the appearance of fine crawling twitches just under the skin. Although they may be benign, fasciculations are also associated with neuropathology of lower motor neuron disease.

- *Hemiballismus*—This term refers to sudden, centrifugally spreading, throwing movements of the extremities on one side. It is caused by lesions to the contralateral subthalamic nuclei.

- *Myoclonus*—This is characterized by involuntary, irregular, frequent, brief jerks of muscles or groups of muscles.

- *Spasms*—This is a general term for an involuntary contraction of a muscle of muscle group. They may be tonic (prolonged or continuous) or clonic (brief, repetitive, and sudden).

- *Tics*—This is a term referring to compulsive movements of small muscle groups of the face.

- *Tremors*—This term refers to rhythmic movements of parts of the body, usually at 3 to 7 Hz. Different types of tremor may occur. Resting tremor (tremor occurring when limbs are at rest) often accompanies

Parkinson's disease. Postural tremor occurs when a body part is maintained against gravity. Intention tremor (tremor occurring only during volitional movement) is common with cerebellar disorders. In children, it is much more common to see intention tremor than resting tremor, whereas resting tremor is common in adults.

EXAMINATION OF FUNCTION

In this section, the general procedures for a physical examination of the speech mechanism are outlined. Chapters 7 through 11 contain more detailed information about the in-depth assessment of each speech subsystem. It is important to examine each subsystem of speech in isolation from others in order to estimate the relative contribution of impairment in various components. During connected speech, the relative severity of the impairment is difficult to appreciate because of the complex interaction among speech subsystems. Some individuals with dysarthria have a remarkable ability to compensate for aspects of their motor impairment. For example, individuals with profound tongue weakness may attempt to compensate with jaw posturing and movement. The full extent of tongue impairment will not be appreciated unless the jaw is stabilized so that its contribution is diminished. Therefore, clinicians must examine several features of movement in speech subsystems in isolation.

Range of Movement

The speech–language pathologist observes the range of movement of the speech subsystem and judges whether the structure moves through the full range. For example, does the tongue move fully from side to side on tongue lateralization tasks? Although this movement is not critical for speech, it is very useful in diagnosing the integrity of cranial nerves. For example, asymmetries are indications of neuropathology. The extent of movement excursion may be reduced when the upper motor neurons or the extrapyramidal systems are involved. With cerebellar involvement, the range of single movements may be greater than normal.

Question: Why would you be interested in movements such as tongue lateralization, when that movement plays such a minor role in speech?

We realize that testing nonspeech movements is a somewhat controversial topic. However, there are at least two important reasons to include them in the physical examination. We observe movements such as tongue

(continues)

and jaw lateralization not because they are important contributors to speech but because they give information about cranial nerve damage, thus helping to construct a picture of the underlying neuropathology. Another reason is that lateral movements of the jaw and tongue are important in the process of chewing and swallowing. Although the physical examination we are describing here is a part of the clinical speech examination, it also provides important information about the related activity of swallowing. The issue of usefulness of nonspeech activities will be revisited in a number of the treatment chapters. In treatment activities we tend to use nonspeech activities much more sparingly than in assessment.

Strength

Muscular weakness is a common symptom of motor dysfunction. Weakness may result from a variety of underlying neuropathologies. For example, the damage to the peripheral portion of Cranial Nerve VII may cause unilateral lip weakness. In another example, upper motor neuron damage in the corticobulbar system may cause spasticity and also weakness of movement. Strength is assessed by observation of flexion and extension of muscle groups with and without resistance by the examiner. For example, upper and lower lip strength is assessed by observing the speaker's ability to resist the examiner's attempt to pull apart the lips, which are pursed together as tightly as possible. The examiner's instruction should clearly indicate that maximum effort is to be used and the patient should be encouraged to "push as hard as you can." Clinicians should also compare strength differences on left versus right sides, as well as lower versus upper lips.

Rate and Coordination of Movement

Movement rates can be observed in rapid alternating movement tasks, such as lateral tongue movements or syllable repetition. Examination of coordination of the speech mechanism involves observation of function of the components as they relate to one another during movement. Rate and coordination of various speech and nonspeech movements can be observed on these diadochokinetic tasks. Instructions for rapid alternating movement tasks should include the notions of both speed and accuracy (e.g., "Make the sounds as rapidly but also as precisely as you can"). Although individuals vary tremendously in performance of these tasks, classic descriptions of diadochokinetic performance in various clinical populations has been summarized elsewhere (Darley, Aronson,

& Brown, 1975; Kent, Kent, & Rosenbek, 1987). In lower motor neuron disease, unless weakness is severe, alternate motion rates are normal. With upper motor neuron lesions, these rates are slow but regular, whereas with cerebellar disorders, the rates are often slow and irregular. In Parkinson's disease, movement rates may be either slow or rapid with reduced range of movement excursion.

Evaluating whether rate and coordination of movement are within normal limits in children is more problematic than in adults. There is a wide range of developmental variability, and it can sometimes be a mistake to attribute a developmental speech delay to "slow movement" or "incoordination." The results of this part of the examinination should be interpreted only in conjunction with all other observations, such as estimates of language abilities.

Muscle Tone and Ability To Vary Muscular Tension

In the resting state, there is a steady background state of muscle contraction or muscle tone. Tone is reflexive in origin and is influenced by a constant stream of afferent information. Muscle tone provides the framework upon which rapid voluntary movements are superimposed (Duffy, 1995). In speakers with dysarthria, muscle tone may be excessive or reduced. It may fluctuate gradually or suddenly, unpredictably or in a regular fashion. For example, damage to the corticospinal tracts in spasticity is characterized by a clasp–knife response in which the limb resists passive motion and then suddenly gives way like the blade of a pocket knife. Again a classic picture emerges in which flaccid dysarthria is associated with reduced tone, spastic dysarthria with consistently increased tone, and hyperkinetic dysarthria with variable tone. Muscle tone and the ability to vary muscular tension are important for normal speech production. For example, some sounds are produced with the tongue in a relatively relaxed state, whereas other sounds require considerable contraction of the speech musculature. Changes in muscle tension must be made very rapidly during speech. Clinicians observe the speaker's ability to vary muscular tension, in other words to alternate between relaxed and tense muscle tone. Instructions may be to "make the muscle tight, now make it as loose and relaxed as you can." Because some adults or children may have difficulty following directions of this type, informal observations of whether changes in the lips or tongue vary in tension during other tasks should be made.

Response to Instructions

Finally, when evaluating function of the speech mechanism, the clinician is interested in the speaker's response to instructions. Can the speaker improve his or her performance on a task when asked to perform that task faster, slower, or more forcefully? Can the speaker reduce excessive muscle tone when asked to do so? Information about the speaker's ability to change performance is critical in treatment planning and in establishing the prognosis for improvement. Speakers who can modify their performance easily are better treatment candidates than those who have little voluntary control over movement abnormalities.

COMPONENTS OF THE SPEECH MECHANISM

Jaw

The physical examination of the jaw, summarized in Table 5.2, involves observation of atrophy of the temporalis or masseter muscles. These muscles are palpated during jaw opening and closing as a means of assessing the forcefulness of contraction and looking for asymmetries. Structural restrictions of the jaw opening and closing are also identified, along with presence of adventitious movements. Clients with weakness in the jaw musculature will often complain

Table 5.2
Summary of the Physical Examination of the Jaw

Symptom Checklist

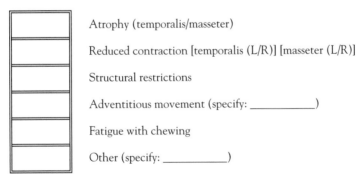

Atrophy (temporalis/masseter)

Reduced contraction [temporalis (L/R)] [masseter (L/R)]

Structural restrictions

Adventitious movement (specify: _____)

Fatigue with chewing

Other (specify: _____)

Function

	Range of Movement	Strength	Response to Instruction
Opening			
Closing			
L–lateralization			
R–lateralization			

of fatigue when chewing. Other physical findings related to the jaw include malocclusions or temporal mandibular joint dysfunction. Examination of jaw function includes observation of jaw opening, closing, and lateralization. Clinicians rate range of movement and strength, along with response to instruction if abnormalities are seen.

Lips

The physical examination of the lips, summarized in Table 5.3, includes inspection of the structural aspects, including muscle atrophy and any adventitious

Table 5.3
Summary of the Physical Examination of the Lips

Symptom Checklist

☐	Atrophy
☐	Adventitious movement: _____
☐	Resting asymmetry

Function

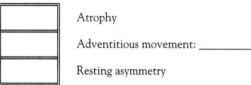

	Range of Movement	Strength	Response to Instruction
Pucker			
Retraction			
Upper Left			
Upper Right			
Lower Left			
Lower Right			

☐	Coordination of movements
☐	Ability to plose
☐	Ability to vary tension
☐	Precise labial consonants

movements. Resting asymmetry is also noted, although some degree of facial asymmetry is normal. Range of movement and strength of the lips are assessed using pucker and retraction tasks. A note should be made if voluntary lip retraction is reduced compared with a spontaneous smile. Voluntary control of facial expression may be difficult for some patients with upper motor neuron involvement. Strength of each quadrant of the lips should be tested separately using a tongue blade and asking the patient to resist the examiner's attempt to move the lips. Lip strength frequently varies as a function of left or right side, and strength of the upper lip may differ from that of the lower lip. Coordination of lip movement is also observed. Production of the pressure consonants requires rapid tensing of the lips to create a lip seal. The ability to plose the lips involves creating an adequate lip seal so that pressure can be built up in the mouth. In an effort to isolate lip function from velopharyngeal function, we occlude the nose and observe the patient's ability to produce lip closure for the /p/. Observations can also be made about the patient's ability to relax and tighten the lips. Finally, we rate the precision of plosing in labial consonants produced in CV or VC syllables.

Tongue

The physical examination of the tongue, summarized in Table 5.4, involves inspection of structural aspects, including atrophy, adventitious movements, and resting asymmetry. Function is examined by assessing range of movement and strength on tasks such as elevation, protrusion, and lateralization. During this examination, it is particularly important to isolate tongue movement from jaw movement. This can be accomplished by stabilizing the jaw with a bit block or tongue blade. Holding the jaw open approximately 2 cm in a fixed position allows observation of tongue movement alone without the contribution of jaw position. The ability to vary muscular tension of the tongue is critical for the production of many speech sounds and should be assessed by asking the speaker to relax and then tense the tongue. The ability to create an adequate lingual seal for production of plosive consonants should also be assessed. Lingual consonant precision in CV and VC syllables can be rated along with vowel differentiation. Speakers with severe lingual weakness or atrophy tend to be unable to differentiate vowels. Instead, they may neutralize vowel productions.

Velopharyngeal Function

The symptom checklist for examination of velopharyngeal function (see Table 5.5) includes perceptual features such as occurrence of nasal emission during production of pressure consonants, hypernasality during speech, and

Table 5.4
Summary of the Physical Examination of the Tongue

Symptom Checklist

Atrophy

Adventitious movements: _____

Resting asymmetry

Function

	Range of Movement	Strength	Response to Instruction
Elevation			
Protrusion			
L-lateralization			
R-lateralization			

	Ability to vary muscular tension
	Ability to plose
	Consonant precision
	Vowel differentiation
	Other: _____

changes in resonance during sustained vowels with nares occluded. Inability to drink through a straw and occurrence of nasal reflux when eating or drinking are common complaints when velopharyngeal dysfunction is severe. Palatal asymmetry at rest is noted. Adventitious movements of the soft palate, especially myoclonus, and other structural abnormalities are also noted. Function of the soft palate is evaluated during a strong, sustained phonation. It is critical to elicit a strong phonation because a less than maximum effort may not elicit sustained palatal movement. If velar elevation is not noted on simple sustained phonation, movement may be elicited in other contexts, such as asking the speaker to produce the syllable /pop/. The adequacy of initial elevation, symmetry, and the ability to sustain the elevation are observed. Each of these fea-

Table 5.5
Summary of the Physical Examination of Velopharyngeal Function

Symptom Checklist

☐	Nasal emission
☐	Hypernasality
☐	Perceptual changes with occlusion
☐	Nasal reflux
☐	Inability to use a straw
☐	Resting asymmetry
☐	Adventitious movements: _____
☐	Other (specify: _____)

Function

☐	Initial elevation
☐	Asymmetry (_____ weaker than _____)
☐	Ability to sustain (fatigue)

tures is rated separately. To identify fatigue, the clinician can not only have the speaker sustain the elevation but also look at the effects of repeated elevation in syllable chains such as /pop, pop, pop/.

Respiration and Phonation

Because respiratory and phonatory functions are difficult to isolate during the physical examination, they are examined together (see Table 5.6). Complaints of fatigue during speech, shortness of breath, and short breath groups are common with speakers with poor respiratory support. The symptom checklist for respiration and phonation includes a number of perceptual features of the voice, including abnormalities in loudness and loudness variation. Clinicians also rate sustained phonation for the features of abnormal vocal quality and stability. Vocal quality relates to the perception of type of voice, which we usually

Table 5.6
Summary of the Physical Examination of Respiration and Phonation

Symptom Checklist

☐	Abnormal loudness (reduced/excessive)
☐	Loudness variation
☐	Complaints of fatigue
☐	Shortness of breath
☐	Abnormal quality (breathy/hoarse/harsh/strained–strangled)
☐	Phonatory breaks
☐	Instability (mild/moderate/severe)
☐	Stridor (inspiratory/expiratory)
☐	Wet phonation
☐	Abnormal voluntary cough (weak/absent)
☐	Other (specify: _____)

Vital capacity (Seated): _____

Vital capacity (Supine): _____

Sustained phonation time: _____ seconds

rate on a scale of severity (0–3), and note where the quality lies on a continuum (breathy, hoarse, harsh, strained–strangled). Stability refers to variability in frequency and/or intensity. We also rate stability on a severity scale (0–3), and note whether the fluctuations are slow (about 2 Hz or less), which is called wow; medium (about 3–10 Hz), which is called vocal tremor; or fast (greater than 10 Hz), which is called flutter. Rate of occurrence of phonatory breaks is noted for sustained phonation as well as connected speech. Occurrence of inspiratory or expiratory stridor is also noted during a task in which the patient is asked to inhale and exhale rapidly but as quietly as possible. Presence of stridor indicates that the vocal folds are not abducting adequately. Presence of wet phonation is also noted. We ask the speaker to produce a strong, voluntary cough. This maneuver requires both considerable respiratory support and vocal fold adduction. We also ask the patient and family to compare the strength of the voluntary cough with a reflexive one. It is not uncommon for the voluntary cough to be much weaker than a reflexive one. Vital capacity (VC) is measured in both seated and supine positions using a hand-held respirometer. These measures may be converted to a proportion of the predicted normal vital capacity (NVC) using the following formulas (Kent, 1994):

$$\text{Men: NVC} = (-38 \times \text{age}) + (121 \times \text{height in inches}) - 2100$$
$$= \text{VC} \pm 970 \text{ cc}$$

$$\text{Women: NVC} = (-22 \times \text{age}) + (110 \times \text{height in inches}) - 2980$$
$$= \text{VC} \pm 790 \text{ cc}$$

Sustained phonation time is measured in seconds. Because patient performance can vary tremendously for this task, we give consistent instructions to "take a big breath and give me a long /ah/. Make it loud and clear and as steady as you can."

> *Question: How can I complete this examination on a child, especially if he or she is uncooperative?*
>
> Because most of the physical examination is making observations of range of motion, strength, speed, coordination of movement, and ability to vary muscular tension in nonspeech movement, it is not necessary to have a child sitting in the chair. These observations can be made while the child is engaged in play, eating, drinking, and so on. Clinicians might ask a series of questions during these observations. Does the child get good lip seal for plosive sounds, or can the child keep liquid in the mouth (even if he or she habitually has an open mouth posture)? Does the child have full range of tongue movement as noted in reflexive movement or during chewing? Is there any asymmetry of the lips or facial muscles at rest? Does the child get good volume and periodic vocal fold vibration during yelling or crying? Observations such as these will allow the clinician to make predictions about the integrity of the cranial nerves and whether other neural subsystems may be involved.

Other Functions To Note

Although production of *diadochokinetic tasks* is not associated with a single component of the speech production mechanism, we include these tasks as part of our physical examination as one means of assessing coordination. We obtain diadochokinetic rates for the syllables /pa/, /ta/, and /ka/, and for the vowel /i/. Thus we are evaluating rapid alternating movement for labial, tongue tip, and tongue back productions. Vowel diadochokinesis is a good indication of respiratory–phonatory coordination. For the syllables /pa/, /ta/, and /ka/, we note voicing errors. Speakers with poor laryngeal control have difficulty inhibiting voicing and will produce the voiced syllables /ba/, /da/, and /ga/ instead of their unvoiced cognates. We also note if respiratory symptoms, such as lack of respiratory support, contribute to poor performance. Speakers with severe respiratory weakness may need to breathe so frequently that they are unable to produce five syllables on one breath.

The contribution of *sensation* to motor speech production is important although poorly understood. There is considerable current research in speech motor control that points to the importance of afferent sensory input in motor control (Barlow & Netsell, 1989). Precise testing of sensation is difficult in a clinical setting, but guidelines are available for examination of light statis touch, kinetic touch, temperature, and double stimulation (Kent, 1997). We ask the patient about changes in sensation, and we test superficial tactile sensation by having the patient close his or her eyes and locate the light touch of a cotton swab at various facial locations. We test forehead, right and left cheeks, inside the cheek, lips, and tongue. Sensory testing is particularly important for patients with strokes or multiple lacunar infarcts who frequently have sensory changes, if the therapist is considering using a tactile stimulation approach to therapy. For example, if a speaker with apraxia of speech has no tactile sensation, treatment approaches that depend on tactile cues may be inappropriate.

Testing sensation is especially difficult with children. First, the clinician needs to rely on feedback from the child as to whether he or she felt the tactile stimulation. If this is not possible, the clinician can watch for signs of the child's unawareness of food or saliva on the lips or chin and watch for the child's reaction to having the face touched while his or her eyes and attention are diverted. Even more difficult than tactile sensation is testing proprioception. It is important to know how much proprioceptive information the child is using. For example, does the child know if his or her mouth is open wide or almost closed? Does the child know the location of the tongue in his or her mouth? Can the child "feel" particular articulatory configurations? This can be very difficult to determine conclusively, yet we know proprioceptive processing is important for motor control. Although the clinician will usually not be sure, observations can be made that suggest that the child is not using proprioceptive information well. Techniques can then be implemented in treatment to compensate for this, such as reducing speaking rate so that the child has more time to process the proprioceptive information.

Finally, because dysarthria and dysphagia co-occur frequently, the physical examination includes a brief *screening of swallowing* abilities. Reduced ability to swallow affects one's ability to speak in some fundamental ways. Swallowing problems have an impact on many of the subsystems of speech. The voice may be of different quality, and the oral articulatory subsystem may be compromised by symptoms of swallowing problems, such as presence of excess saliva. We ask the patient to swallow sips of water and note signs of aspiration such as coughing or choking. We observe strength and extent of laryngeal elevation, and signs of incoordination such as an audible swallow. Airway congestion after the swallow and the need for multiple swallows are also noted. Complete discussions of the physical examination for swallowing can be found elsewhere (Groher, 1984; Logemann, 1998).

CRANIAL NERVE FUNCTION

Thus far in this chapter, we have presented a discussion of the consistent procedures for examining the structures and function of the speech mechanism. We have viewed the physical examination as a process of observation and acquisition of information. This information may be applied in a variety of ways. For example, application of this information in differential diagnosis and treatment planning will be described in the next chapter. Information obtained in the physical examination can also be viewed as providing information about the function of the cranial nerves that are most critical to speech production. This perspective takes the viewpoint of the neurologist. Muscle function is interpreted in light of what it indicates about the integrity of the cranial nerve systems. As speech–language pathologists, we typically take a somewhat different viewpoint. Muscle function is interpreted in light of how it affects speech production. Table 5.7 is a summary of physical examination results and patient complaints for selected cranial nerves. This information is adapted from the work of Duffy (1995), who presents an excellent and in-depth discussion of the topic.

Question: Does your physical examination include testing of reflexes?

Identification of pathologic reflexes is an important part of the neurologist's physical examination because they give insight into the underlying neuropathology. It is also clear that abnormal reflexes sometimes interfere with speech production. Therefore, the speech–language pathologist needs to be aware of them. In some speakers with cerebral palsy, they may be such a significant obstacle that understandable speech is not possible. When this is the case, the speech–language pathologist will need to seek the advice of other members of the interdisciplinary team in order to develop an appropriate management plan. A more complete description of the testing of pathologic reflexes to speech can be found elsewhere (Duffy, 1995; Miller & Groher, 1990).

Table 5.7
Summary of Physical Examination Results and Patient Complaints for Cranial Nerves V, VII, X, and XII

Cranial Nerve	Function	Technique of Examination	Patient Complaints	Changes in Structure	Changes in Function		Changes in Speech	
					Unilateral	Bilateral	Unilateral	Bilateral
V—Trigeminal	Motor—masticatory muscles; Sensory—face and mucosal surfaces of the eyes, tongue, and parts of the nasopharyngeal space	Opening the mouth, clenching the teeth for palpation of the masseter and temporalis muscles	Motor—chewing difficulty, drooling, jaw difficult to close; Sensory—decreased sensation in face, cheek, tongue, teeth, or palate	Jaw may hang open at rest	Jaw deviates to weak side, partly opened jaw may be pushed easily to the weak side by the examiner; decreased contraction on palpation on weak side	Pt. may be unable to open or close jaw	None	Imprecise consonants, distorted vowels, slow rate
VII—Facial	Muscles of expression	Furrowing the brow, screwing up the eyes, sniffing, whistling, pursing the lips	Drooling, biting the cheek or lip when chewing or speaking, difficulty keeping food in the mouth	Affected side sags at rest; nasolabial fold is often flattened	During lip retraction, face will retract toward the intact side; facial asymmetry during movement	Decreased ability to retract, purse, or puff the cheeks	Mild distortion of bilabial and labiodental sounds	Distortion of bilabial and labiodental sounds, slow rate

(continues)

Table 5.7 (*continued*)

Cranial Nerve	Function	Technique of Examination	Patient Complaints	Changes in Structure	Changes in Function		Changes in Speech	
					Unilateral	Bilateral	Unilateral	Bilateral
X—Vagus (above the pharyngeal branch)	Motor and sensory—Innervation of the muscles of the soft palate, pharynx and larynx	Gag reflex symmetry; vocal characteristics; laryngoscopic examination	Changes in voice and resonance; nasal regurgitation during swallowing	Soft palate hangs lower on the side of the lesion	Soft palate pulls to the paralyzed side on phonation; gag reflex diminished on weak side	Minimal palatal movement on phonation; nasal regurgitation	Breathiness; decreased loudness and pitch; short phrases; hoarseness; diplophonia; mild hypernasality; nasal emission; mildly weak plosing	Breathiness; aphonia; short phrases; inhalatory stridor; moderate hypernasality; nasal emission; weak plosing
X—Vagus (superior branch only)		Vocal characteristics; laryngoscopic examination	Voice changes		Affected vocal fold appears shorter than normal; epiglottis and anterior larynx shifted toward the intact side	Both cords appear short and are bowed; epiglottis will overhang and obscure the anterior portion of the vocal folds	Breathy hoarseness; short phrases	Breathy, hoarse voice; decreased loudness and pitch range

(continues)

Table 5.7 (continued)

Cranial Nerve	Function	Technique of Examination	Patient Complaints	Changes in Structure	Changes in Function		Changes in Speech	
					Unilateral	Bilateral	Unilateral	Bilateral
X—Vagus (recurrent branch only)	Innervation of tongue muscles	Vocal characteristics; laryngoscopic examination			Affected vocal fold fixed in paramedian position; dysphagia may be present; cough weak; may be airway compromise	Both folds in the paramedian position; airway compromise; inhalatory stridor	Reduced loudness; diplophonia	Reduced loudness
XII—Hypoglossal	Innervation of tongue muscles	Tongue protrusion	Problem with oral articulation and chewing; difficulty handling saliva; tongue feels "thick"	Atrophy on the weak side	Tongue deviates to weak side; decreased lateral strength may be fasciculations	Atrophy and fasciculations on both sides; protrusion limited but symmetrical	Mild consonant imprecision	Mild to severe consonant imprecision; vowel distortion

Note. From Motor Speech Disorders: Substrates, Differential Diagnosis, and Management (pp. 99–128), by J. R. Duffy, 1995, St. Louis: Mosby. Copyright 1995 by Mosby. Reprinted with permission.

Motor Speech Examination

Normal speech is accomplished through a complex interaction of the movements of the components of the speech production mechanism. The goal of the physical examination previously described is to assess the function of each component in isolation, primarily in nonspeech tasks. It should be noted that the physical examination must be accompanied by an examination of connected speech. To evaluate only the components of speech production in isolation would seriously oversimplify the complex process of speech production. In dysarthria the impairment is almost never restricted to a single component. Rather, impairments of varying levels of severity may occur in various components. Further, vocal tract components do not function independently of one another (Hardy, 1967). Numerous examples of this interdependence are cited throughout this text. Consider the function of the muscles and structures of respiration as a pump to provide breath support for speech. The adequacy of respiratory support may be affected by the efficiency of all valves of the airway. Thus, inadequate laryngeal, velopharyngeal, or oral articulatory valving interact with poor respiratory support to create a cumulative negative effect.

The motor speech examination is also important in order to examine the effects of linguistic formulation on motor speech performance. A speaker with apraxia, for example, may have a normal examination of structure and function, but as linguistic demands are added, the inability to plan sequential movements for speech becomes evident.

PATTERNS OF PERCEPTUAL CHARACTERISTICS

The perceptual characteristics of motor speech disorders perhaps have received more systematic attention than any other aspect of the disorder. The procedures developed at the Mayo Clinic in the late 1960s remain today the classic method for describing the perceptual features of dysarthria (Darley, Aronson, & Brown, 1969a, 1969b, 1975). Early perceptual studies provide a detailed description of what a particular motor speech disorder sounds like and document the fact that one type of motor speech disorder sounds different from another. The 38 dimensions from the Mayo Clinic studies that appear in Table 5.8 are helpful in identifying patterns of deviant dimensions in dysarthria. Perceptual analysis is an important tool in differential diagnosis. It will be discussed in more detail in Chapter 6. In the Mayo studies, the dimensions were rated from audio recordings of a consistent passage, the Grandfather Passage, and were grouped under the following categories: pitch characteristics, loudness, vocal quality, respiration, prosody, articulation, and general impression dimensions.

Perceptual characteristics of apraxia of speech are generally articulatory and dysprodic in nature (Duffy, 1995; Itoh & Sasanuma, 1984; Johns & Darley,

Table 5.8
Speech Dimensions Used in the Mayo Clinic Studies

Pitch Characteristics

Pitch level—Pitch of voice sounds consistently too low or too high for individual's age and sex.

Pitch breaks—Pitch of voice shows sudden and uncontrolled variation (falsetto breaks).

Monopitch—Voice is characterized by a monopitch or monotone. Voice lacks normal pitch and inflectional changes. It tends to stay at one pitch level.

Voice tremor—Voice shows shakiness or tremulousness.

Loudness

Monoloudness—Voice shows monotony of loudness, lacking normal variations in loudness.

Excess loudness variation—Voice shows sudden, uncontrolled alternations in loudness, sometimes becoming too loud, sometimes too weak.

Loudness decay—There is progressive diminution or decay of loudness.

Alternating loudness—There are alternating changes in loudness.

Loudness (overall)—Voice is insufficiently or excessively loud.

Voice Quality

Harsh voice—Voice is harsh, rough, and raspy.

Hoarse (wet) voice—There is "liquid sounding" hoarseness.

Breathy voice (continuous)—Continuously breathy, weak, and thin.

Breathy voice (transient)—Breathiness is transient, periodic, intermittent.

Strained–strangled voice—Voice (phonation) sounds strained or strangled (an apparently effortful squeezing of voice through glottis).

Voice stoppages—There are sudden stoppages of voiced airstream (as if some obstacle along vocal tract momentarily impedes flow of air).

Hypernasality—Voice sounds excessively nasal. Excessive amount of air is resonated by nasal cavities.

Hyponasality—Voice is denasal.

Nasal emission—There is nasal emission of airstream.

Respiration

Forced inspiration–expiration—Speech is interrupted by sudden, forced inspiration and expiration sighs.

Audible inspiration—Audible, breathy inspiration.

Grunt at end of expiration—Grunt occurs at end of expiration.

Prosody

Rate—Rate of actual speech is abnormally slow or rapid.

Phrases short—Phrases are short (possibly due to fact that inspirations occur more often than normal). Speaker may sound as if he has run out of air. He may produce a gasp at the end of a phrase.

(continues)

Table 5.8 (*continued*)

Prosody (*continued*)

Increase of rate in segments—Rate increases progressively within given segments of connected speech.

Increase of rate overall—Rate increases progressively from beginning to end of sample.

Reduced stress—Speech shows reduction of proper stress or emphasis patterns.

Variable rate—Rate alternately changes from slow to fast.

Intervals prolonged—Prolongation of interword or intersyllable intervals.

Inappropriate silences—There are inappropriate silent intervals.

Short rushes of speech—There are short rushes of speech separated by pauses.

Excess and equal stress—Excess stress on usually unstressed parts of speech, e.g., (1) monosyllabic words, and (2) unstressed syllables of polysyllabic words.

Articulation

Imprecise consonants—Consonant sounds lack precision. They show slurring, inadequate sharpness, distortions, and lack of crispness. There is clumsiness in going from one consonant sound to another.

Phonemes prolonged—There are prolongations of phonemes.

Phonemes repeated—There are repetitions of phonemes.

Irregular articulatory breakdown—Intermittent nonsystematic breakdown in accuracy of articulation.

Vowels distorted—Vowel sounds are distorted throughout their total duration.

Overall

Intelligibility (overall)—Rating of overall intelligibility or understandability of speech.

Bizarreness (overall)—Rating of degree to which overall speech calls attention to itself because of unusual, peculiar, or bizarre characteristics.

Note. From *Motor Speech Disorders* (pp. 99–128), by F. L. Darley, A. E. Aronson, and J. R. Brown, 1975, Philadelphia: Saunders. Copyright 1975 by W. B. Saunders. Reprinted with permission.

1970; Kent & Rosenbek, 1983; Odell, McNeil, Hunter, & Rosenbek, 1990). Unlike dysarthria, respiratory and phonatory characteristics are usually not affected. As noted in Chapter 3, salient characteristics include articulation errors of substitution, omission, and distortion. Speech may sound slow, with effortful trial and error and groping for articulatory targets. The wide continuum of severity, however, makes particular perceptual characteristics for speakers with apraxia hard to define. Speakers with very severe apraxia will have few words, may make many effortful attempts at beginning a word, and may distort vowels. Speakers with mild apraxia might be able to speak in sentences, with little observable groping but with many articulatory errors. Voicing errors may also be frequent. The perceptual characteristics of speakers with apraxia and concomitant aphasia will also be complicated by the influence of language errors.

In the previous description of the physical examination, we suggested that there is no substitute for a knowledge base developed during years of clinical observation. The same notion applies to the perceptual analysis of motor speech disorders. Experienced clinicians will begin to form an impression of the perceptual patterns of speech during the initial interview when a history is being obtained from the speaker. Certain constellations of perceptual characteristics will signal the possibility of specific types of dysarthria. For example, a slow speaking rate with imprecise articulation accompanied by excess and equal stress patterning and a loud but uncontrolled voice may signal the possibility of ataxic dysarthria. The pattern of reduced loudness levels, little articulatory movement, and rapid rushes of speech will signal the possibility of hypokinetic dysarthria. Slow, labored speech with articulatory errors and groping for articulatory postures may indicate the presence of apraxia of speech.

How does the beginning clinician develop the knowledge base related to the perceptual features of motor speech disorders? As with the physical examination, we advocate consistent procedures for identifying perceptual characteristics of motor speech disorders. For speakers with dysarthria, audio recordings of a standard reading passage and use of the 38 perceptual dimensions from the Mayo Clinic studies as a checklist reminder of particular salient features may be a good place to begin. Audiotapes illustrating a series of speakers with a variety of types of dysarthria are available (Aronson, 1993). For speakers with apraxia, language may be a complicating influence. Techniques for sampling connected speech of these individuals are discussed in the next section.

A knowledge base related to perceptual characteristics of dysarthria will be just as useful for children with dysarthria as for adults. Children with acquired dysarthrias or cerebral palsy will exhibit some of the same characteristics as adults, although articulatory and language characteristics will be influenced by the child's stage of development. Perceptual characteristics of developmental apraxia of speech may be more difficult to differentiate from those of delayed articulation development or phonologic disorders. Some children with motor planning problems display articulatory groping and attempts at self-correction, but for many children, the perceptual characteristics of the pervasive articulatory disorder will overlap those of other communicative disorders.

In addition to providing evidence for making a differential diagnosis, information about the perceptual patterns of speech is also used in guiding the focus of the physical examination. If a speaker has severe hypernasality, an impairment of the velopharyngeal mechanism is probable. Therefore, particular attention to soft palate function is warranted in the physical examination. The findings of the physical examination must also be interpreted in relation to the perceptual features of connected speech. For example, what is the influence of poor velopharyngeal function on speech production? Or, how is poor respiratory support affecting the rate and intelligibility of speech? Clinicians should watch for mismatches where the functional limitation is worse (or better) than one would predict based on the level of the impairment. In other words, are the perceptual features consistent with the level of impairment that was identified in the physical examination? If the speaker is functioning better than one would predict, then questions related to compensations are appropriate. What compensatory strategies is the speaker employing to offset the level of motor impairment? If function is worse than would be predicted, then clinicians may identify potential contributors to the poor performance. Treatment plans may focus on these aspects of the speech production mechanism. For example, some speakers with dysarthria take breaths at grammatically unusual locations during connected speech. Speech intelligibility and naturalness may be compromised by inappropriate respiratory patterning even in the presence of relatively intact respiratory support. In the case of this mismatch between the level of impairment and functional limitation, treatment might focus on better use of the respiratory subsystem. Use of perceptual analysis combined with an understanding of the impairment to plan treatment is discussed in detail in Chapter 6.

INTERACTION BETWEEN LANGUAGE AND SPEECH FUNCTION

Apraxia of speech frequently co-occurs with aphasia. Consequently, it is important to understand the relative severity of aphasia in relation to the motor speech disorder. Is the major limitation related to deficits in word retrieval, syntactic construction, and auditory comprehension, or is function limited more by the inability to sequence the articulatory movements in order to produce consistent, precise, and accurate speech? Answering these questions is important because the answers will dictate the most appropriate type of treatment for the speaker. Unfortunately, answers are not always easy to obtain. Deficits in language and motor speech frequently interact. Therefore, determining the exact contribution of each is not a trivial matter. Although it is beyond the scope of this text to describe tools and techniques for assessment of aphasia, the following discussion assumes that administration of this type of testing has been completed and that information about the severity of aphasia will be considered as treatment plans are formulated.

Similarly, many children with developmental or acquired motor speech disorders exhibit concomitant delays or deficits in language. Knowledge about the child's general cognitive level, receptive language skills, and amount and type of nonverbal communication will help the clinician predict to what degree the motor speech disorder is the primary contributor to the child's communicative disorder.

Earlier in this text, apraxia of speech was defined as the reduced ability to program movements in order to produce speech. These deficits are particularly salient in connected speech. They are influenced by a number of factors, including linguistic load, length and phonetic complexity of the utterance, and temporal relationship between the stimulus and response. When performing a motor speech examination for apraxia of speech, the speech–language pathologist must consider these factors in developing hierarchies of speech tasks. As the clinician plans treatment, he or she will observe the impact of each factor of speech performance and develop a sequence of activities based on task difficulty.

Linguistic Load

For most apraxic speakers, the linguistic complexity of the task will influence the level of performance. As the linguistic demands of the task are increased, the motor performance will worsen in apraxia of speech. This is typically not the case in dysarthria. One simple hierarchy of linguistic load includes conversation, picture description, and production of narratives. Conversation is typically the easiest in terms of linguistic complexity. Speakers have control over the length of their utterances, what words they will choose, and so on. During conversation, features such as overall efficiency, syntactic complexity, word retrieval, and prosody can be observed. Keep in mind, however, that both children and adults will typically keep the linguistic context simple enough to enhance motor speech performance. In a picture description task, the speaker still has considerable structure in that particular sequences of events are depicted for them. Individuals with severe apraxia may be more understandable when describing a picture because the clinician has considerable knowledge about the content of the message and, thus, articulatory targets. The most difficult task in the hierarchy is the production of narratives. Usually, speakers are asked to tell the story of a favorite book or movie. Summary of plots of a current popular movie or perhaps a classic, such as *Gone with the Wind*, provide a shared knowledge base between the clinician and the speaker with apraxia. Clinicians might ask, "Have you ever seen *Gone with the Wind?* Tell me what it's about." This task involves a considerable linguistic load, because speakers must frame a sequence of events, use extensive syntactic construction, retrieve the words, and map the phonology of those words. At the same time, speakers are evaluating or monitoring their own narrative to make sure that they are not leaving anything out. Thus, narrative puts the considerable load on cognitive and linguistic processes and in turn on speech motor control.

Length and Phonetic Complexity of the Utterance

Long, complex utterances will be more difficult than shorter ones for individuals with apraxia of speech (Strand & McNeil, 1996). A general hierarchy of tasks in this area might begin with simple VC or CV syllables and proceed through lengthy sentences. Difficulty can be increased in a number of ways. For example, suffixes can be added. The words, *zip, zipper, zippering,* form a hierarchy of difficulty for speakers with apraxia. Difficulty can also be increased by phoneme selection. CVC words that have the same, highly visible first and last consonants (*mom, peep, bib*) tend to be easier than those with different first and last consonants (*mop, peek, big*). Finally, difficulty can be added by simply increasing the length of the utterance ("I," "I eat," "I eat lunch," "I eat lunch here," "I eat lunch here every day"). Speakers with either acquired or developmental apraxia may easily be able to say a short series of sounds (e.g., "I eat"), but if it is lengthened to "I eat lunch here," they may not be able to produce the sequence of movements for "I" that they previously did without any difficulty.

Tasks included in this portion of the motor speech examination are typically presented in an imitative format. The time between the stimulus and the response is varied depending on the performance of the speaker. In this way, demands for word finding and syntactic construction are eliminated. In the interest of clinical efficiency and in order to minimize the speaker's frustration, the entire hierarchy from VC syllables to complex sentences is typically not sampled. Rather, an appropriate starting point is selected based on the performance during conversation, picture description, and narrative. Thus, if a speaker with apraxia produces short, somewhat telegraphic sentences during conversation and displays a mild to moderate Broca's aphasia, testing would probably not start with isolated syllables, but rather with more complex utterances. Likewise, for individuals with severe apraxia, who fail to imitate single syllables even with many cues, testing would probably not proceed to multisyllabic words, phrases, and long sentences.

Question: Do you ever start your hierarchy of length and phonetic complexity with vowels in isolation?

Because apraxia of speech is considered a disorder of the programming of *sequences of movements,* testing relatively static positions such as vowels in isolation is usually not necessary except when the apraxia is extremely severe. There are some exceptions to the rule of avoiding vowels in isolation. We would start with vowels if the speaker is nonverbal or using only one or two vowels. Many speakers with severe apraxia will have four to six stereotypic utterances; if they are using only one vowel in these utterances, that might be a case where we would start with vowels. Another case might be a speaker who displays an extensive amount of vowel distortion even though he or she may be speaking at the sentence level. If the vowels are so distorted that intelligibility is greatly reduced, then we would also begin with vowels.

Temporal Relationship Between the Stimulus and the Response

Speakers with apraxia of speech often benefit from cues from the examiner. They do best when they are able to hear and see the utterance being produced by someone else and are immediately given the opportunity to reproduce that utterance. Because identification of potential cueing strategies is critical for treatment planning, considerable attention is focused on these factors during the motor speech examination. Identification of cueing strategies not only provides a starting point for treatment, but also provides a prognostic indication of how much improvement will occur and how quickly that improvement might happen. For example, speakers who can easily repeat have a better prognosis than those who cannot, and those speakers who can repeat after a long delay have a better prognosis than those who cannot repeat when a delay is imposed. More details of the use of this information in developing a treatment plan is provided in Chapter 13.

Varying the temporal relationship between the presentation of the stimulus and the response is an important aspect of the motor speech examination for apraxia of speech. The hierarchy that appears in Table 5.9 is organized from the most powerful cueing strategies to less powerful ones (Rosenbek, Lemme, Ahern, Harris, & Wertz, 1973). As in other aspects of this examination, a starting point is selected based on performance during conversation. An utterance

Table 5.9

A Potential Cueing Hierarchy Which Varies the Temporal Relationship Between the Stimulus and the Response for Speakers with Apraxia of Speech

Simultaneous production with cueing: Speakers say the utterance with the clinician, but only after tactile and visual cues are provided. The speaker is allowed to stay in the initial articulatory configuration for a second or two before production in order to take full advantage of proprioceptive feedback.

Simultaneous production: Speakers say the utterance with the clinician. Rate is slowed as needed to improve accuracy.

Immediate repetition: Speakers imitate the production of the clinician immediately after they see and hear it.

Repetition with delay: The clinician imposes a 2- to 4-second delay between modeling the utterance and requesting a response from the speaker.

Spontaneous production: The utterance is produced in response to a question.

of appropriate length and phonetic complexity is selected; for example, the word "bye" might be selected for a speaker with severe apraxia. Testing typically begins with an immediate repetition task with the clinician's statement, "I'll say a word and then you say it after me." If the speaker is unsuccessful, then more cues are provided: "Let's say the word together." If still unsuccessful, then tactile cues are provided, in this case to bring the speaker's lips together. The initial position is held for a second or two, followed by a simultaneous production of the utterance. If the speaker had initially been successful when attempting to repeat the utterance, the clinician would have made the task more difficult by imposing a delay. Many speakers with apraxia of speech will lose the motor plan if they are required to delay their response even a couple of seconds. If the speaker was successful with a delay, the utterance would be elicited spontaneously. For example, the clinician might say, "If I told you 'so long,' you might say . . ." ("bye").

In summary, during this phase of the motor speech examination, a hierarchy of syllables, words, and phrases is developed based on a sample of the connected speech. These utterances are then elicited in an imitative format. If attempts are unsuccessful, more cues are provided; if they are successful, cues are removed by imposing a delay between the stimulus and the response. Figure 5.2 illustrates a typical score sheet documenting the performance of an adult with moderate to severe acquired apraxia. Note that some words or phrases were elicited during conversation and picture description. Generally, the speech was marked by effortful production of grammatically incomplete utterances. The speaker was unable to perform the narrative task. Based on this performance, a hierarchy of words and phrases was developed. Note that the word "boy" could be produced in the immediate repetition and repetition with delay formats; however, it was not produced spontaneously. Longer phrases such as "I eat lunch" were not accurately repeated, but were accurate when produced simultaneously with the clinician. At the end of this examination, the clinician has a starting point for planning treatment both in terms of length and complexity of potential target utterances and in the level and type of cueing that may be required for accurate productions.

Figure 5.3 illustrates a typical score sheet for a child with a severe delay in speech development, although receptive language is within the normal range. This child attempts conversation, but uses mostly differentiated vowels with a few consonants. Prosody is appropriate. Imitation of vowels is excellent with little cueing. Imitation of monosyllabic words is good for easy phonetic contexts, but the child needs more cueing, especially tactile cues and simultaneous production with the clinician to produce some CVC's, bisyllabic words, and short phrases.

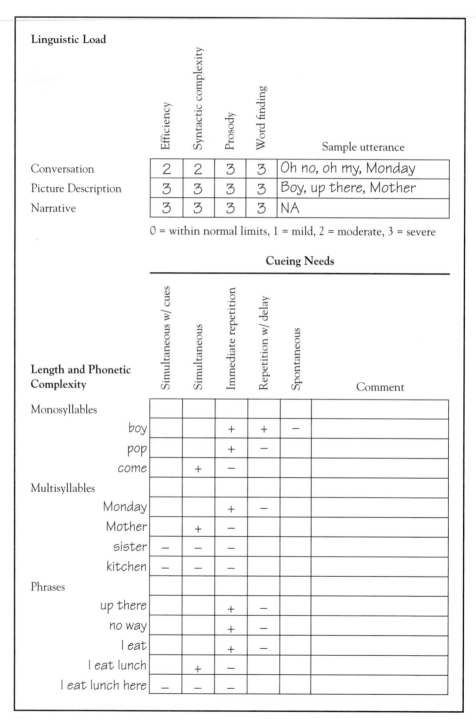

Linguistic Load

	Efficiency	Syntactic complexity	Prosody	Word finding	Sample utterance
Conversation	2	2	3	3	Oh no, oh my, Monday
Picture Description	3	3	3	3	Boy, up there, Mother
Narrative	3	3	3	3	NA

0 = within normal limits, 1 = mild, 2 = moderate, 3 = severe

Cueing Needs

Length and Phonetic Complexity	Simultaneous w/ cues	Simultaneous	Immediate repetition	Repetition w/ delay	Spontaneous	Comment
Monosyllables						
boy			+	+	−	
pop			+	−		
come		+	−			
Multisyllables						
Monday			+	−		
Mother		+	−			
sister	−	−	−			
kitchen	−	−	−			
Phrases						
up there			+	−		
no way			+	−		
I eat			+	−		
I eat lunch		+	−			
I eat lunch here	−	−	−			

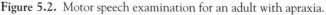

Figure 5.2. Motor speech examination for an adult with apraxia.

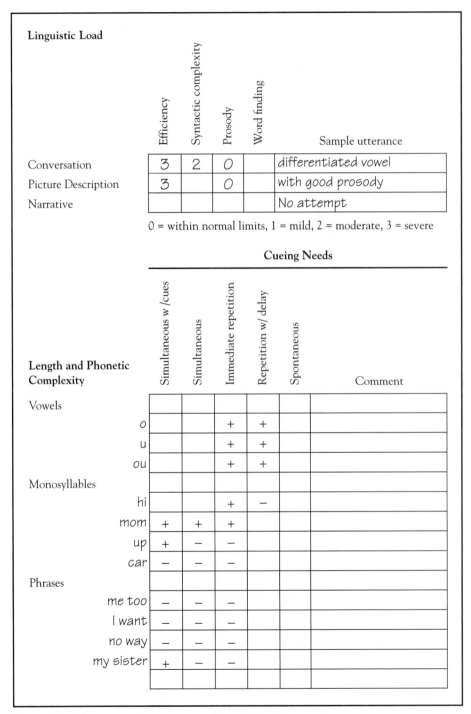

Linguistic Load

	Efficiency	Syntactic complexity	Prosody	Word finding	Sample utterance
Conversation	3	2	0		differentiated vowel
Picture Description	3		0		with good prosody
Narrative					No attempt

0 = within normal limits, 1 = mild, 2 = moderate, 3 = severe

Cueing Needs

Length and Phonetic Complexity	Simultaneous w /cues	Simultaneous	Immediate repetition	Repetition w/ delay	Spontaneous	Comment
Vowels						
o			+	+		
u			+	+		
ou			+	+		
Monosyllables						
hi			+	−		
mom	+	+	+			
up	+	−	−			
car	−	−	−			
Phrases						
me too	−	−	−			
I want	−	−	−			
no way	−	−	−			
my sister	+	−	−			

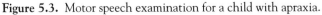

Figure 5.3. Motor speech examination for a child with apraxia.

Question: Tests of apraxia of speech are commercially available. Do you ever use them?

Yes, standard test batteries for apraxia of speech are available and we use them. Standard instruments such as the *Apraxia Battery for Adults* (Dabul, 1979) and the *Screening Test for Developmental Apraxia of Speech* (Blakeley, 1980) for children are useful tools. Standard testing is important for valid and reliable measurement, and it is essential if the clinician is going to compare one speaker with another or monitor the progress of a speaker over time. However, these tests are also constraining in that they may not allow the clinician to sample the specific utterances most appropriate for a given speaker or to vary the way speakers are asked to produce utterances. The information is often essential in treatment planning. First, the stimuli listed may not be appropriate across all speakers. For example, Dabul's battery starts with the word "dab," a word that may be phonetically too complex for speakers with severe apraxia. Second, standard batteries, when administered according to instructions in the manual, provide little information about how many cues are needed before the speaker can say the word correctly. If a speaker cannot imitate a word or phrase, can he or she produce it correctly in unison with the clinician? If a speaker can repeat a phrase correctly, can he or she also produce it correctly after a lengthy delay? In summary, although standard batteries have an important role, especially in documenting change, they must be supplemented by other tasks so that information about treatment planning can be obtained.

MEASURES OF SPEECH INTELLIGIBILITY

Rationale for Measurement of Intelligibility

Intelligibility can be defined as the extent a listener understands the speech produced by individuals with motor speech disorders. It is an overall measure reflecting not only the cumulative impact of the impairment but also the compensatory strategies used by the speaker. A more complete description of factors that may influence speech intelligibility can be found in Chapter 12. The concept of intelligibility has long been viewed as a critical one in gauging the severity of communication disorders. Kent, Miolo, and Bloedel (1994) described the central role of intelligibility: "Because the functional purpose of speech communication is to be understood, intelligibility is the functional common denominator of verbal behavior" (p. 81).

Intelligible speech is often viewed as a primary goal of speakers with dysarthria. Achieving this goal is a prerequisite for other aspects of speech performance, including naturalness. Although only intelligibility and rate are discussed in this chapter, approaches to the assessment of naturalness are reviewed in Chapter 11. A variety of reasons have been suggested for the clinical measurement of speech intelligibility and speaking rate (Yorkston, Beukelman, & Traynor, 1984). First, measures of speech intelligibility, when accompanied by measures of speaking rate, provide a useful index of the severity of the overall functional limitation. They provide a comprehensive indicator of all components of speech production, including not only oral articulatory performance, but also respiratory, phonatory, and velopharyngeal performance, which are frequently impaired in individuals with dysarthria. Second, reduced intelligibility and speaking rate are nearly universal consequences of dysarthria, regardless of the underlying neuromotor impairment. Even speakers with mild dysarthria can be distinguished from nonimpaired individuals on the basis of speaking rate (Yorkston & Beukelman, 1981). Third, intelligibility appears to be closely related to other aspects of the impairment, functional limitation, and disability. For example, work of Platt, Andrews, Young, and Neilson (1978) indicated that measures of single-word intelligibility and ratings of prose intelligibility correlated well with diadochokinetic rates, phonemes correctly identified, and judgments of speech handicap. A close relationship between transcription intelligibility scores and information transfer was also reported (Beukelman & Yorkston, 1979). Finally, speech intelligibility is used as a primary measure of functional limitation because the results of this type of assessment are easily communicated to speakers and their families. Intelligibility measures can be understood without a detailed knowledge of the physiology of the speech process. Intelligibility is usually the first area of assessment that we consider because individuals with dysarthria nearly always view the dysarthria from this functional point of view.

Clinical Measurement of Intelligibility

Although speech intelligibility and rate provide information essential for clinical management of speakers with dysarthria, their measurement is not straightforward. Despite consensus about the pivotal role of intelligibility, "consensus withers when it comes to deciding how intelligibility should be measured and assessed" (Kent et al., 1994, p. 81). A number of approaches to the measurement of intelligibility in children has been reviewed elsewhere (Kent et al., 1994). Many of these approaches emphasize phonetic contrast or phonologic analysis and were developed for use with children with hearing impairment or with phonologic disorders.

Because intelligibility can be so easily influenced, care must be taken to control for factors such as the composition of the sample, the transmission system, and listener characteristics. One attempt to control some factors that impact clinical measurement is the *Sentence Intelligibility Test* (Yorkston, Beukelman, & Tice, 1996), formerly the *Computerized Assessment of Intelligibility of Dysarthric Speech* (Yorkston et al., 1984). This instrument was designed to provide a clinician-judged technique for measuring intelligibility in the clinical setting. It provides an objective measure of sentence intelligibility and speaking rate. In developing this clinical tool, task selection involved a number of decisions. Some tasks were chosen based on research evidence, others on the basis of ease of clinical administration. Sentences varying in length from 5 to 15 words were chosen, because it was felt that they more closely approximated the demands of ordinary speaking situations than did single words. See Table 5.10 for a sentence sample. Note that the sample contains sentences that are unrelated to each other in content and that a variety of syntactic constructions are represented. The sample begins with relatively short sentences (5 words) because some

Table 5.10

Sentence Sample from the *Sentence Intelligibility Test* (SIT)

File: Smith
Date: 7/25/96
Speaker: Mary Smith
Examiner: KMY
Agency: UWMC
Comment: First clinic visit

5A. The effort is still worthwhile.

5B. He wrapped the package hastily.

6A. How many hours have you worked?

6B. Just don't fill them too full.

7A. The misguided souls have lost their way.

7B. Did dues money pay for that trip?

8A. Dreaming it, I moaned suddenly in my sleep.

8B. This year brings a change in the routine.

9A. They really don't do the job on my drains.

9B. I can easily learn to write in correct English.

10A. It is a safe and effective drug, when properly used.

(continues)

Table 5.10 (continued)

10B. You have walked all this distance just to see me.

11A. It is a safe and effective drug, when properly used.

11B. The ideal city is a place of crowds, not of highways.

12A. There was solid evidence that our quarry was right under our noses.

12B. They're asking more questions and doctors, for the most part, are answering.

13A. A clerk reads the zip code and punches three numbers on his keyboard.

13B. The vain person wants praise too much and is always angling for it.

14A. Too often, we engage in empty conversations, or sit staring vacantly at television programs.

14B. Enlightened coaches encourage players to bring their mates along with them on athletic trips.

15A. If you have a new television, you won't feel sorry for yourself because you're alone.

15B. Above all, when she receives a compliment from friends or family, she jots it down.

Note. From *Sentence Intelligibility Test* (pp. 294–295), by K. M. Yorkston, D. R. Beukelman, and R. Tice, 1996, Lincoln, NE: Tice Technology Services. Copyright 1996 by Tice Technology Services, Inc. Reprinted with permission.

severely dysarthric individuals are unable to produce long sentences. Samples may be shortened for these individuals. The speaker with dysarthria is recorded as he or she reads the sentences. Listeners who are naive to both the speaker and the sentences orthographically transcribe the sample. A sentence intelligibility score is usually reported as the percentage of the words in the sample that the listener has correctly identified.

Use of sentence stimuli also allows the measurement of speaking rate along with intelligibility. Speaking rate, a critically important variable for some speakers with dysarthria, should be considered in a number of clinical decisions. For example, reduction of speaking rate may be an important intervention technique. A measure of intelligibility combined with speaking rate (intelligible words per minute) is a useful means of distinguishing mildly dysarthric from normal speakers. Speaking rate may also be a useful indicator of progression of dysarthria. Table 5.11 illustrates data from the *Sentence Intelligibility Test* for a speaker with progressive dysarthria. Note that in the month between the first and second testing, intelligibility remained stable (93% for the first testing, and 90% for the second). However, during that interval, speaking rate declined from 88 words per minute (wpm) to 60 wpm. Because of this reduction in speaking rate, both the rate of intelligible speech and the communication efficiency ratio (Intelligible words per minute/Normal rate of intelligible speech) declined.

Table 5.11
Data from the *Sentence Intelligibility Test* for a Speaker with Dysarthria at First and Second Clinic Visit

File:	Smith	Smith–2
Date:	7/29/96	8/26/96
Sample size:	22 items	22 items
Speaker:	Mary Smith	Mary Smith
Examiner:	KMY	KMY
Agency:	UWMC	UWMC
Comment:	First clinic visit	Second visit
Judge:	JBT	JBT
Date:	7/30/96	8/27/96
Intelligible words:	205 of 220	198 of 220
Intelligibility (%):	93	90
Total duration:	2:29	3:40
Speaking rate:	88 words/min	60 words/min
Rate of intelligible speech:	82 intell wds/min	56 intell wds/min
Communication efficiency ratio:	.44	.30

Note. From *Sentence Intelligibility Test* (pp. 294–295), by K. M. Yorkston, D. R. Beukelman, and R. Tice, 1996, Lincoln, NE: Tice Technology Services. Copyright 1996 by Tice Technology Services, Inc. Reprinted with permission.

Question: Measuring intelligibility the way you suggest—that is, recording a sample and having an unfamiliar judge transcribe it—is time-consuming. Why not simply estimate intelligibility?

Although measuring intelligibility by recording a sample and having that sample transcribed is more time-consuming than a simple estimate of intelligibility, there are a number of important reasons to use this procedure. The primary reason is to ensure valid and reliable results. Kent and colleagues (1994) stated, "impressionistic statements offer rapid evaluation but sometimes fail in reliability or precision, or both" (p. 82). When listeners familiar with the sample judge intelligibility, they tend to overestimate scores (Beukelman & Yorkston, 1980). This problem is exaggerated in the mid-range of severity. That is, estimates of very mild or very severe dysarthria may be relatively accurate but estimates of moderate dysarthria may seriously inflate the intelligibility scores. Second, actual recording of speech samples allows for the measurement of speaking rate.

(continues)

The interaction of rate and intelligibility is important in making judgments about the appropriateness of speaking rate. Finally, by routinely reviewing the errors made by the judges as they transcribe the samples, you form ideas about the underlying causes of the misunderstanding. For example, consider a case where the actual sentence is, "Before I go, will you type it?" and the listener transcribes, "Before going you time it." Two types of errors occur here. The first involves a misperceived boundary, the words, "go will" become "going." If these types of errors are common, attention in treatment might focus on establishing clear word and phrase boundary signals. The second type of error appears to be phonetic; that is, the word "type" becomes "time." The listener's perception of dysarthric speech is an important topic that is only recently receiving attention in the research literature (Tjaden & Liss, 1995a, 1995b).

Because repeated administration and judging of similar speaking tasks are among the primary requirements of a clinical measurement tool, an attempt should be made to control judge familiarity with the sample. This can be done in two ways: First, a randomized sample selection procedure ensures that, although the judges have a general familiarity with the sample being produced, they do not know the specific words or sentences being spoken. Second, all samples are selected, recorded, and scored by an examiner who does not participate in judging the intelligibility samples. Because research reported earlier suggested that objective measures are less subject to interjudge differences than are estimates of intelligibility, all tasks require a response from the judge that can be scored as correct or incorrect.

Question: Does your assessment of adults with dysarthria ever include measurement of single-word intelligibility?

Because we are interested in a single measure of functional performance and because most speakers communicate in phrases rather than single words, our general rule is to use measures of sentence intelligibility. However, there are exceptions to this rule. For individuals with severe or profound dysarthria, single words may be a better reflection of their functional abilities. A technique in which words are selected from a semantic category and judged with and without semantic cues will be described in Chapter 7. There are other situations in which we are interested in the intelligibility of phonemes. For example, when considering the possibility

(continues)

of palatal lift fitting, we compare the speaker's ability to produce understandable nasal sounds with his or her ability to produce pressure sounds. This technique will be described in Chapter 10.

Question: When is single-word intelligibility measurement useful in children?

Single-word tests may be appropriate for children with short mean length of utterance. When using test items of greater length than a word, you need to make sure that the linguistic content is at or below the child's level of expressive language development. Otherwise, the test becomes a measure of language and not of speech. Also, with children who have motor coordination problems, word intelligibility scores often are greater than "sentence" scores. One useful measure of progress is the convergence of single-word and sentence scores. With children, orthographic transcription of a connected speech sample can be used to estimate speech intelligibility (Shriberg & Kwiatkowski, 1985). Complementary phonetic transcriptions can provide useful insights into the nature of subsystem impairment (Megan Hodge, personal communication, May 1997).

CONCLUSION

The clinical examination of speech is a structured series of observations where information about an individual's impairment, functional limitation, and disability is obtained. A history of the problem is obtained from chart review and an interview with the speaker. A physical examination involves assessing respiration, phonation, velopharyngeal function, and oral articulation during primarily nonspeech tasks. These tasks allow identification changes in motor function including strength, movement rate, range of movement, muscle tone, and coordination. Finally, perceptual features of samples of connected speech are identified. Observations made during the clinical examination frequently lead to other questions. Answering these questions may necessitate more in-depth testing. Details of in-depth testing can be found in other chapters. For example, assessment of the contribution of the respiratory system to speech production can be found in Chapter 7, and in-depth testing of velopharyngeal function is described in Chapter 9. The following chapter contains information about the application of the findings of the clinical examination to important clinical tasks such as differential diagnosis and treatment planning.

APPENDIX 5.A
SUPPLEMENTAL CASE HISTORY ITEMS FOR CHILDREN WITH DEVELOPMENTAL APRAXIA OF SPEECH

1. Check problems and conditions that apply to the child:

   ☐ hearing problems   ☐ vision problems

   ☐ mouth breather   ☐ drooling

   ☐ difficulty with solid foods   ☐ messy eater

   ☐ slow eater   ☐ clumsy

2. Check characteristics you have observed during the child's feeding or speech or in imitative play with sounds or facial expressions:

	Feeding	Speech	Imitative Play
spontaneous, involuntary movements			
slow, labored movements			
poor quality or incomplete, fragmented movements			
hesitation before initiating movements			
awkward or jerky movements (lack of fluidity or rhythm)			
limited diversity of movements			
"posturing" before starting movements			

3. Which of the following ways does the child use to communicate with others:

   a. Without sounds (gestures, facial expression, body movement, mime)

   b. With sounds (crying, noncry vocalizing without recognizable speech sounds, single sounds or syllables like "ma," "ba," "da," chains of sounds or syllables)

   c. Single words (Please write down 20 words that your child says. If less than 20, please note this and write these down.)

   d. Sentences (Please write five sentences that your child says during the day that you complete this form. Please write down the longest sentence that he/she said today.)

4. For which of the following reasons does the child attempt to communicate with others:

   a. To express personal needs or wants

   b. To request information or action

   c. To greet or acknowledge others (e.g., "Hi")

   d. To relate experience to others

   e. To express humor

5. Who does the child attempt to communicate with?

   a. Familiar adults (caregivers, friends, relatives)

   b. Familiar agemates (siblings, friends)

   c. Unfamiliar adults (e.g., teachers, health care professionals)

   d. Unfamiliar agemates (e.g., children in daycare, preschool, school)

6. How successful is the child in communicating with

	100%	75%	50%	25%
a. Familiar adults				
b. Familiar agemates				
c. Unfamiliar people				

7. When the child is not successful in communicating with others, how does he or she react?

   a. Abandons the communication attempt

   b. Repeats the message

   c. Tries to communicate in another way (e.g., facial expression, gesture, sounds)

   d. Appeals to other for help

8. When the child is not successful in communicating with others, how do you react?

   a. Withdraw from interaction

   b. Attempt to repair communication breakdown

   c. Offer encouragement to the child

9. Does the child appear to be aware of his or her communication problems? If yes, how is that apparent?

10. Has the child's communication problem affected the family in any way? If yes, please describe how.

11. Are there times when the child's speech is better or worse than usual? If yes, please indicate what these situations are.

12. Does anyone else in the family have a similar problem or any speech, language, or learning problems? If yes, please indicate their relationship and describe the nature of the problem.

13. Please describe the child's personality.

14. Please describe the child's ability to interact with other children.

15. Is the child enrolled in playschool, daycare, or school? If yes, please indicate:

   Those that apply:

   The child's general performance:

   If in school, describe the child's performance in:

      Math

      Spelling

      Reading

      Writing

REFERENCES

Aronson, A. E. (1993). *Dysarthria: Differential diagnosis* [Audio tape]. Rochester, MN: Mentor Seminars.

Barlow, S. M., & Netsell, R. (1989). Clinical neurophysiology in individuals with dysarthria. In K. M. Yorkston & D. R. Beukelman (Eds.), *Recent advances in clinical dysarthria* (pp. 53–82). San Diego: College-Hill.

Beukelman, D. R., & Yorkston, K. M. (1979). The relationship between information transfer and speech intelligibility of dysarthric speakers. *Journal of Communication Disorders, 12,* 188.

Beukelman, D. R., & Yorkston, K. M. (1980). Influence of passage familiarity on intelligibility estimates of dysarthric speech. *Journal of Communication Disorders, 13,* 33–41.

Blakeley, R. W. (1980). *Screening Test for Developmental Apraxia of Speech.* Tigard, OR: CC Publications.

Dabul, B. (1979). *Apraxia Battery for Adults.* Tigard, OR: CC Publications.

Darley, F., Aronson, A., & Brown, J. (1969a). Clusters of deviant speech dimensions in the dysarthrias. *Journal of Speech and Hearing Research, 12,* 462–496.

Darley, F., Aronson, A., & Brown, J. (1969b). Differential diagnostic patterns of dysarthria. *Journal of Speech and Hearing Research, 12,* 224.

Darley, F. L., Aronson, A. E., & Brown, J. R. (1975). *Motor speech disorders.* Philadelphia: Saunders.

DeGown, R. L. (1987). Methods in the physical examination. In E. L. DeGowin & R. L. DeGowin (Eds.), *Bedside Diagnostic Examination.* New York: Macmillan.

Duffy, J. R. (1995). *Motor speech disorders: Substrates, differential diagnosis, and management.* St. Louis: Mosby.

Groher, M. E. (1984). *Dysphagia: Diagnosis and management.* Boston: Butterworth.

Hardy, J. (1967). Suggestions for physiologic research in dysarthria. *Cortex, 3,* 128.

Hodge, M. (1988). Speech mechanism assessment. In D. Yoder & R. Kent (Eds.), *Decision making in speech–language pathology* (pp. 104–109). Toronto: Decker.

Hodge, M. M., & Hancock, H. R. (1994). Assessment of children with developmental apraxia of speech: A procedure. *Clinics in Communication Disorders, 4,* 102–118.

Hodge, M., Wellman, L., Goulden, K., & Heaton, E. (1996, November). *Children with motor speech disorders: Prevalence and service delivery issues.* Paper presented at the Annual Convention of the American Speech–Language–Hearing Association, Seattle.

Itoh, M., & Sasanuma, S. (1984). Articulatory movements in apraxia of speech. In J. Rosenbek, M. McNeil, & A. Aronson (Eds.), *Apraxia of speech: Physiologic, acoustics, linguistics, management* (pp. 137–162). San Diego: College-Hill.

Johns, D. F., & Darley, F. L. (1970). Phonemic variability in apraxia of speech. *Journal of Speech and Hearing Research, 13,* 556.

Kent, R. D. (1994). *Reference manual for communicative sciences and disorders.* Austin, TX: PRO-ED.

Kent, R. D. (1997). The perceptual sensorimotor examination of motor speech disorders. In M. R. McNeil (Ed.), *Clinical management of sensorimotor speech disorders* (pp. 27–48). New York: Thieme Medical.

Kent, R. D., Kent, J. F., & Rosenbek, J. C. (1987). Maximum performance tests of speech production. *Journal of Speech and Hearing Disorders, 52,* 367–387.

Kent, R. D., Miolo, G., & Bloedel, S. (1994). The intelligibility of children's speech: A review of evaluation procedures. *American Journal of Speech–Language Pathology, 3*(2), 81–95.

Kent, R. D., & Rosenbek, J. C. (1983). Acoustic patterns of apraxia of speech. *Journal of Speech and Hearing Research, 26,* 231.

Logemann, J. (1998). *Evaluation and treatment of swallowing disorders* (2nd ed.). Austin, TX: PRO-ED.

McNeil, M. R., & Kennedy, J. G. (1984). Measuring the effects of treatment for dysarthia: Knowing when to change or terminate. *Seminars in Speech and Language, 4,* 337–358.

Miller, R. M., & Groher, M. E. (1990). *Medical speech pathology.* Rockville, MD: Aspen.

Mumenthaler, M. (1983). *Neurology: A textbook for physicians and students with 185 self-testing questions.* New York: Thieme-Stratton.

Odell, K., McNeil, M. R., Hunter, L., & Rosenbek, J. C. (1990). Perceptual characteristics of consonant production by apraxic speakers. *Journal of Speech and Hearing Disorders, 55,* 345–359.

Platt, L. J., Andrews, G., Young, M., & Neilson, P. D. (1978). The measurement of speech impairment of adults with cerebral palsy. *Folia Phoniatrica, 30,* 59–64.

Rosenbek, J. C., & LaPointe, L. L. (1985). The dysarthrias: Description, diagnosis, and treatment. In D. Johns (Ed.), *Clinical management of neurogenic communication disorders* (pp. 97–152). Boston: Little Brown.

Rosenbek, J. C., Lemme, M. L., Ahern, M. B., Harris, E. H., & Wertz, R. T. (1973). A treatment for apraxia of speech in adults. *Journal of Speech and Hearing Disorders, 38,* 462–472.

Shriberg, L. D., & Kwiatkowski, J. (1985). Continuous speech sampling for phonologic analyses of speech-delayed children. *Journal of Speech and Hearing Disorders, 50,* 323–334.

Strand, E. A. (1992). The integration of speech motor control and language formulation in process models of acquisition. In R. Chapman (Ed.), *Processes in language acquisition and disorders* (pp. 86–107). St. Louis: Mosby-Yearbook.

Strand, E. A., & McNeil, M. R. (1996). Effects of length and linguistic complexity on temporal acoustic measures in apraxia. *Journal of Speech and Hearing Research, 39*(5), 1018–1033.

Tjaden, K., & Liss, J. M. (1995a). The influence of familiarity on judgments of treated speech. *American Journal of Speech–Language Pathology, 4,* 39–38.

Tjaden, K. K., & Liss, J. M. (1995b). The role of listener familiarity in the perception of dysarthric speech. *Clinical Linguistics and Phonetics, 9,* 139–154.

Yorkston, K. M., & Beukelman, D. R. (1981). Communication efficiency of dysarthric speakers as measured by sentence intelligibility and speaking rate. *Journal of Speech and Hearing Disorders, 46,* 296–301.

Yorkston, K. M., Beukelman, D. R., & Tice, R. (1996). *Sentence Intelligibility Test.* Lincoln, NE: Tice Technology Services.

Yorkston, K. M., Beukelman, D. R., & Traynor, C. (1984). *Computerized Assessment of Intelligibility of Dysarthric Speech.* Austin, TX: PRO-ED.

INTERPRETING THE CLINICAL EXAMINATION: DIFFERENTIAL DIAGNOSIS AND TREATMENT PLANNING IN DYSARTHRIA

In Chapter 5, we presented a rather detailed outline of the components of the clinical examination of motor speech disorders, including a history of the speech problem, a physical examination of the speech mechanism, and a motor speech examination. The goal of this examination is to describe the impairment, functional limitation, and disability associated with motor speech disorders. The clinical examination yields a large amount of descriptive information. However, speech–language pathologists need to go beyond description. Rather, they must interpret this information and determine the significance, importance, and value of that information to provide management directions. In this chapter, we discuss how the descriptive information obtained during the clinical examination can be used to make clinical decisions regarding differential diagnosis and treatment planning.

DIFFERENTIAL DIAGNOSIS

Differential diagnosis is particularly important because of the implications such diagnoses carry for the identification of underlying neuropathologies and for treatment planning. Speech–language pathologists are frequently called upon to provide differential diagnoses among communication disorders. At times, the differentiation involves distinguishing motor speech from language or cognitive neurologic communication problems. At other times, the differentiation involves distinguishing between the two motor speech disorders, dysarthria and apraxia of speech. Still other times, it involves distinguishing among the various dysarthrias. Neurologic communication disorders that vary in etiology, symptomatology, and management have been described elsewhere (Johns, 1985). This chapter focuses on the differential diagnosis of dysarthria; that is, dysarthria is distinguished from other neurologic communication disorders and the various types of dysarthria are distinguished from one another. A more detailed discussion of differential diagnosis of apraxia of speech can be found in Chapter 13.

Differentiating the Neurologic Communication Disorders

DYSARTHRIA VERSUS ACQUIRED APHASIA

Aphasia is a specific language disorder involving deficits that cross all language modalities, including listening, speaking, reading, and writing. Unlike speakers with dysarthria, individuals with aphasia have difficulty handling symbolic information. Critical to the distinction between acquired aphasia and dysarthria is the fact that aphasia is characterized by deficits in understanding of both verbal and written language. In dysarthria, auditory comprehension and reading skills are preserved. The word-finding difficulties, or the inability to retrieve a desired word, that characterize aphasia are typically not present in dysarthria. Some types of aphasia are characterized by articulatory errors. These errors are particularly frequent in fluent aphasia and are thought to be a problem of phoneme selection rather than production. Sound production errors are usually produced effortlessly and are often not recognized by the speaker.

Site of lesion and etiology also distinguish acquired aphasia from dysarthria. Lesions that produce aphasia are restricted to the cortical language areas and related subcortical connections, which for most speakers are located in the left hemisphere. Lesions that produce dysarthria may occur at a variety of sites in either or both the peripheral and central nervous systems. Most typical etiologies for acquired aphasia are left cerebrovascular accident (CVA), tumors, or trauma.

DYSARTHRIA VERSUS DEMENTIA

Dementia has been associated with what has been called the language of generalized intellectual impairment (Wertz, 1985). Individuals suffering from dementia exhibit language problems, but, unlike the pattern of deficits seen in aphasia, the language problems are roughly equivalent to deficits seen in other areas of intellectual functioning, including memory, reasoning, judgment, orientation, and so on. Language impairments can be observed in all stages of dementia, even though these deficits may be subtle in the early stages (Bayles, 1984). Whereas language deficits are seen in all dementias, dysarthria is observed only in a subgroup of dementias associated with movement disorders. These include parkinsonism, Huntington's chorea, and progressive supranuclear palsy, among others.

Dysarthria Versus Language of Confusion

Language of confusion is often traumatically induced. Frequent characteristics include unclear thinking, faulty memory, and irrelevant responses. Confused language may frequently coexist with dysarthria, especially in cases of traumatic brain injury. Here, locus of damage may occur in areas important to the control and regulation of movement, for example, upper motoneuron involvement or brain stem contusions. It is clear that dysarthria may co-occur with traumatic brain injury when motor control problems are among the consequences of the injury. However, others suggest that dysarthria after closed head injury may also be associated with "failure to monitor articulation" and at times may be difficult to distinguish from the consequences of cognitive deficits (Hagen, Malkmus, & Durham, 1979). Although the literature is not conclusive (see Chapter 3 for a more complete review), dysarthria associated with traumatic brain injury may frequently resolve in the first year postonset or after individuals reach a certain level of cognitive function (Dongilli, Hakel, & Beukelman, 1992; Groher, 1977).

Dysarthria Versus Apraxia of Speech

Both dysarthria and apraxia of speech are considered motor speech disorders. Apraxia of speech is a deficit of motor programming involving speech production tasks but not automatic or involuntary tasks such as chewing or smiling. Dysarthria, on the other hand, is a disorder of motor production involving abnormalities in movement rates, precision, coordination, and strength in both speech and nonspeech movements. In dysarthria, the motor control problems are present regardless of tasks or context. Perceptually, apraxia of speech has been described as a combination of features, including slow rate, variable phonemic errors, and disturbed prosody (Johns & Darley, 1970). At first glance, these characteristics appear to be quite similiar to those of dysarthria. However, the experienced observer is able to rely on a few salient differences to make a differential diagnosis in the clinical setting. Included among these are site of lesion, description of speech characteristics, pattern and type of articulatory errors, nature of error change with context, and movement deficits. The characteristics of apraxia of speech are described more completely in Chapters 2, 3, and 13.

DYSARTHRIA CONCOMITANT WITH OTHER DISORDERS

In most clinical situations, distinguishing a pure or uncomplicated dysarthria from other neurologic communication disorders is relatively straightforward. For example, clinicians typically have no difficulty distinguishing fluent aphasia from dysarthria. Differential diagnosis is much more challenging when several communication diagnoses co-occur. Further, co-occurrence of neurologic communication disorders is relatively common, especially early postonset of acquired disorders and in developmental disorders. Mild dysarthria may accompany aphasia, especially in the period immediately following a stroke. Apraxia and dysarthria may also coexist. Retrospective studies suggest that apraxia occurred with dysarthria in 8% of the sample and that apraxia of speech occurred with both dysarthria and aphasia in 14% of the sample (Wertz, 1985). Mixed dysarthrias or coexistence of two or more types of dysarthria is also common in the clinical setting.

Question: Why is it important to identify the co-occurrence of dysarthria and other communication disorders?

Perhaps the most important reason is that a correct diagnosis of a constellation of communication problems has an impact on the type of treatment plan. Let us give two case examples. The first was a 30-year-old laborer with a history of severe gastric reflux who presented to the neurology clinic with swallowing and voice problems. The neurology resident also identified "slurred speech." The patient was referred for a speech pathology evaluation with concerns about the possibility of a progressive motoneuron disorder. On examination we found, in addition to swallowing difficulty and a harsh voice, a man with evidence of craniofacial abnormalities, including micrognathia which limited the range of motion in his jaw. He also exhibited a variety of articulatory errors. When questioned more closely about his childhood, he and his family indicated that he had attended special education classes with speech therapy throughout his schooling. They indicated that speech "hadn't really changed." After medical and surgical management of the reflux, voice and swallowing problems resolved. In this case, it was critical to know about the co-occurrence of developmental articulatory problems so that his abnormal speech was not attributed to a new and possibly progressive neurologic

(continues)

condition. The second case is a 22-year-old man recently emerging from coma after a severe traumatic brain injury. In addition to confusion and disorientation, the nurses noted "slurred speech." The speech pathology evaluation report indicated "severe confusion with mild to moderate dysarthria." Because the clinician judged that the dysarthria was not a functional limitation, especially in light of confusion, treatment focused on attempts to orient the patient and to minimize his confusion. Here it was important not only to identify coexisting problems but also to estimate the relative contribution of each to the functional limitation before an appropriate treatment plan could be developed.

Differential Diagnosis Among the Dysarthrias

PERCEPTUAL DESCRIPTIONS

The Mayo Clinic Studies

Differential diagnosis among the dysarthrias is an area that has received considerable attention. Diagnosis from the Mayo Clinic perspective is based on the simple notion that one type of dysarthria sounds different from others. Darley, Aronson, and Brown (1975) provided the following perceptually based descriptions of the dysarthrias.

Spastic dysarthria (as in pseudobulbar palsy) is typically associated with speech that is slow and labored, the articulation being rather consistently imprecise, especially on more complicated groups of consonant sounds. Pitch is low and monotonous. Voice quality is harsh and often strained or strangled sounding. There may be considerable hypernasality, but usually no nasal emission is audible. Associated nonspeech signs are increase of deep tendon reflexes, appearance of the sucking reflex, increased jaw jerk, sluggish tongue movements, and activity of accessory respiratory musculature.

Flaccid dysarthria (as in bulbar palsy) is characterized by hypernasality, with associated nasal emission of air during speech as its most prominent speech symptom. Inhalation is often audible and exhalation is often breathy; air wastage is manifested also in shortness of phrases. Articulation is often imprecise on either or both of two bases: (1) consonants may be imprecise through failure to impound sufficient intraoral breath pressure because of velopharyngeal incompetence, and/or (2) consonants and vowels may be distorted because of immobility of tongue and lips resulting from impairment of the hypoglossal and facial nerves. Associated nonspeech signs include fasciculation and atrophy of the tongue, reduced rate of alternating motion of tongue and lips, poor elevation of the soft palate, and nasal alar contraction and grimacing as the patient tries to compensate for velopharyngeal incompetence.

Mixed spastic and flaccid dysarthria (as in amyotrophic lateral sclerosis) is characterized by slow rate, low pitch, and hoarse and strained–strangled quality. Oral articulation may be severely impaired. Marked hypernasality and nasal emission combine to make the speaker struggle to produce short, high-distorted phrases. There is the impression of enormous effort to overcome profound weakness.

Ataxic dysarthria (as in cerebellar disorders) usually produces one of two patterns of speech deviation, the two seldom appearing concurrently: (1) intermittent disintegration of articulation, together with dysrhythmia and irregularities of pitch and loudness in performing tests of oral diadochokinetic rate, or (2) altered prosody, involving prolongation of sounds, equalization of syllabic stress (by undue stress on usually unstressed words and syllables), and prolongation of intervals between syllables and words. Speech proceeds at an artificially even, measured pace.

Hypokinetic dysarthria (as in Parkinson's disease) is characterized by reduced vocal emphasis, peaks and valleys of pitch, and variations of loudness being flattened out monotonously. Short rushes of speech are separated by illogically placed pauses, the rate being variable, often accelerated. Consonant articulation in contextual speech and syllable repetition is blurred as muscles fail to go through their complete excursion. Difficulty in initiating articulation is shown by repetition of initial sounds and inappropriate silences. The voice is often breathy, and the loudness is reduced sometimes almost to inaudibility.

Hyperkinetic dysarthria (as in dystonia) is characterized by involuntary bodily and facial movements. These movements unpredictably cause voice stoppages, disintegration of articulation, excessive variations of loudness, and distortion of vowels. Perhaps in anticipation of these interruptions, normal prosody is altered by slowing of rate, reduction in variations of pitch and loudness, prolongation of interword intervals, and interposition of inappropriate silences.

Hyperkinetic dysarthria (as in choreoathetosis) is associated with involuntary movements that alter the normal breathing cycle and result in sudden exhalatory gusts of breath, bursts of loudness, elevations of pitch, and disintegration of articulation. The overall loudness level may be increased. Anticipated breakdowns are managed by varying the rate, introducing and prolonging pauses, and equalizing stress on all syllables and words.

For additional information, readers are referred to Chapters 2 through 4, which outline medical management, the natural course, and speech characteristics of a number of disorders that frequently result in dysarthria.

Clusters of Speech Dimensions

When making a differential diagnosis, one would wish to identify the deviant dimensions that occur in only one or two of the dysarthria groups. These features would then signal the presence of a specific type of dysarthria. According to the results of the Mayo Clinic studies, such single deviant dimensions occur only rarely. Only the following single dimensions appear to be helpful in making a differential diagnosis. Three dimensions—pitch breaks in pseudobulbar palsy, voice stoppages in dystonia, and short rushes of speech in parkinsonism—predominate in a single neurologic group. Further, four dimensions—excessive loudness variations in choreoathetosis and dystonia, nasal emission and audible inspiration in bulbar palsy and amyotrophic lateral sclerosis, and variable rate in choreathetosis and parkinsonism—predominate in only two neurologic groups. Because the remainder of dimensions are present in numerous groups, single speech dimensions are only of limited value when making differential diagnoses.

Spurred by the finding that single speech dimensions are of limited value in differential diagnosis, the Mayo Clinic group further examined the data to identify clusters rather than single deviant speech dimensions (Darley, Aronson, & Brown, 1969). These clusters are made up of groups of deviant dimensions that tend to co-occur. It was suggested that the co-occurrence or clustering of deviant dimensions reflects an underlying pathophysiology. For example, in flaccid dysarthria both the speech dimensions of nasal emission and imprecise consonants correlate with short phrases. Thus, the cluster containing hypernasality, nasal emission, imprecise consonants, and short phrases is assumed to be the result of air wastage through the velopharyngeal port. Applying this correlational method to each of the neurologic groups, eight unique clusters of three or more deviant speech dimensions were found. Unique combinations of these clusters characterized each of the neurologic groups. The clusters characterized by a combination of deviant features (in italics) include:

- **Cluster 1—Articulatory Inaccuracy,** consisting of *Imprecise Consonants, Irregular Articulatory Breakdown,* and *Vowels Distorted*. This cluster is articulatory in nature and may be the result of breakdown in coordination of activity, such as seen in ataxia or as the result of adventitious involuntary movements of dystonia or chorea.

- **Cluster 2—Prosodic Excess,** consisting of *Slow Rate* (of speech), *Excess and Equal Stress, Phonemes Prolonged, Intervals Prolonged,* and *Inappropriate Silences*. Slowness of repetitive movements is thought to be the chief neuromuscular defect responsible for this cluster.

- **Cluster 3—Prosodic Insufficiency,** consisting of *Monopitch, Monoloudness, Reduced Stress,* and *Phrases Short.* Restricted range of movement is the probable underlying neuromuscular defect responsible for this cluster.

- **Cluster 4—Articulatory–Resonatory Incompetence,** consisting of *Imprecise Consonants, Vowels Distorted,* and *Hypernasality.* This cluster is thought to result from a combination of impaired force of contraction and reduced range of movement.

- **Cluster 5—Phonatory Stenosis,** consisting of *Low Pitch, Harsh Voice, Strained–Strangled Voice, Pitch Breaks,* and *Voice Stoppages,* as well as *Excess Loudness Variation, Slow Rate,* and *Phrases Short* (which may be compensatory features). This cluster may represent the physiologic narrowing of the laryngeal outlet.

- **Cluster 6—Phonatory Incompetence,** consisting of *Breathy Voice, Audible Inspiration,* and *Phrases Short.* This cluster is thought to be the result of a reduction in the force of contraction.

- **Cluster 7—Resonatory Incompetence,** consisting of *Hypernasality, Nasal Emission, Imprecise Consonants,* and *Phrases Short.* Like Cluster 6, this cluster may result from reduction in force of muscular contraction and failure to close the velopharyngeal port.

- **Cluster 8—Phonatory–Prosodic Insufficiency,** consisting of *Monopitch, Monoloudness,* and *Harsh Voice.* Hypotonia is thought to be responsible for this cluster.

In summary, results of the Mayo Clinic study found that each of seven neurologic disorders could be characterized by a unique set of clusters of deviant speech dimensions and that no two disorders had the same set of clusters. Thus, differential diagnosis can be based on clusters of related dimensions rather than on single features. These clusters, along with the neuromuscular characteristics and a list of deviation speech dimensions for the dysarthrias studied by the Mayo group, can be found in Table 6.1. For a more complete description of the speech characteristics of various disorders, see Chapters 2 through 4.

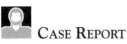

CASE REPORT

We have found that using a broader information base than perceptual judgments alone is the most effective way to assess speakers. The following case illustrates how information from the clinical examination—the history, the physical examination,

(text continues on page 260)

Table 6.1
Features Associated with the Various Dysarthrias

Dysarthria	Neuromuscular Characteristics	Characteristic Clusters	Deviation Speech Dimensions
Pseudobulbar palsy	Spasticity Weakness Exaggerated reflexes	Prosodic excess Prosodic insufficiency Articulatory–resonatory incompetence Phonatory stenosis	Imprecise consonants Monopitch Reduced stress Harsh voice Monoloudness Low pitch Slow rate Hypernasality Strained–strangled voice Short phrases
Bulbar palsy	Weakness Hypotonia Atrophy Hypoactive reflexes	Phonatory incompetence Resonatory incompetence Phonatory–prosodic insufficiency	Hypernasality Imprecise consonants Breathy voice (continuous) Monopitch
Amyotrophic lateral sclerosis	Weakness Spasticity Atrophy	Prosodic excess Prosodic insufficiency Articulatory–resonatory incompetence Phonatory stenosis Phonatory incompetence Resonatory incompetence	Imprecise consonants Hypernasality Harsh voice Slow rate Monopitch Short phrases Distorted vowels Low pitch

(continues)

Table 6.1 (*continued*)

Dysarthria	Neuromuscular Characteristics	Characteristic Clusters	Deviation Speech Dimensions
			Monoloudness Excess and equal stress Intervals prolonged
Cerebellar lesions	Incoordination Dysmetria Hypotonia Intention tremor	Articulatory inaccuracy Prosodic excess Phonatory–prosodic insufficiency	Imprecise consonants Excess and equal stress Irregular articulatory breakdowns Vowels distorted Harsh voice
Parkinsonism	Tremor Rigidity Bradykinesia	Prosodic excess Prosodic insufficiency Phonatory stenosis	Monopitch Reduced stress Monoloudness Imprecise consonants Inappropriate silences Short rushes Harsh voice Breathy voice (continuous)
Dystonia	Dyskinesis Athetosis	Articulatory inaccuracy Prosodic excess Prosodic insufficiency Phonatory stenosis	Imprecise consonants Distorted vowels Harsh voice Irregular articulatory breakdown Strained–strangled voice

(*continues*)

Table 6.1 (*continued*)

Dysarthria	Neuromuscular Characteristics	Characteristic Clusters	Deviation Speech Dimensions
			Monopitch
			Monoloudness
Chorea	Hyperkinesia	Articulatory inaccuracy	Imprecise consonants
	Variable tone	Prosodic excess	Prolonged intervals
		Prosodic insufficiency	Variable rates
		Articulatory–resonatory incompetence	Monopitch
		Phonatory stenosis	Harsh voice
		Resonatory incompetence	Inappropriate silences
			Distorted vowels
			Excess loudness variables

Note. Adapted from *Motor Speech Disorders*, by F. L. Darley, A. E. Aronson, and J. R. Brown, 1975, Philadelphia: Saunders.

and the motor speech examination—can help form an impression of the type of dysarthria. We describe this case using the chronology that unfolded in the clinical setting. Thus, the ultimate diagnosis will be presented only at the end. Jane was a 55-year-old woman who was referred for a speech examination as part of a comprehensive neurologic evaluation.

History of the Speech Problem

Jane indicated that she began to have difficulty "pronouncing words" approximately 10 months earlier. These problems had gradually worsened to the point where she indicated that she needed to "be very careful" when talking to people as part of her work as a case manager for a medical insurance company. She denied any problems with memory, reading, writing, or word finding, instead indicating that it feels like it is "something in my muscles." She also noted that in the morning, her voice felt "stiff" and took "a little while before it gets going." She reported that within the last 2 months she had choked more when eating, especially on liquids. Although she initially denied any changes in lower and upper extremity function, she commented that she had fallen several times in the last month. When questioned about her general medical history, she reported a 15-year history of asthma and long-standing depression. Other than an inhaler on an as-needed basis and antidepressants, she was on no other medications.

Physical Examination

Results of the physical examination are summarized in Figure 6.1. See Chapter 5 for details about the examination protocol. The results of the physical examination indicated that Jane's jaw function was within normal limits except for mild reduction in the range of lateral movement. Although this finding had few implications for speech, it suggested motor impairment. Lip function (both range of motion and strength) was mildly reduced in all four quadrants. This affected her ability to produce precise labial consonants, especially plosives, which require a buildup of intraoral air pressure. Tongue fasciculations were noted at rest, although there was no atrophy or asymmetry. Again, fasciculations alone would not affect speech but are suggestive of underlying neuropathology. Moderate tongue weakness was noted for elevation, protrusion, and lateralization. Some improvement in range of motion was noted with maximum effort. Reduced tongue movement resulted in imprecision in both consonant and vowel production. Velopharyngeal function was characterized by lack of complete elevation with effortful sustained phonation. Further, Jane was unable to maintain velar elevation during sustained phonation. Voice quality was rated to be severely strained–strangled, although length of sustained phonation was adequate, at 16 seconds.

Motor Speech Examination

Connected speech was characterized by a slow speaking rate, 70 words per minute (Beukelman, Yorkston, & Tice, 1997), with imprecise articulation, hypernasality, and a strained–strangled voice quality. Speech intelligibility was 85% on a sentence

Jaw

Symptom Checklist

O	Atrophy (temporalis/masseter)
O	Reduced contraction [temporalis (L/R)] [masseter (L/R)]
O	Structural restrictions
O	Adventitious movement (specify: _____)
O	Fatigue with chewing
	Other (specify: _____)

Function

	Range of Movement	Strength	Response to Instruction
Opening	O	O	
Closing	O	O	
L–lateralization	1	O	
R–lateralization	1	O	

Lips

Symptom Checklist

O	Atrophy
O	Adventitious movement: _____
O	Resting asymmetry

Function

	Range of Movement	Strength	Response to Instruction
Pucker	1	1	
Retraction	1	1	
Upper Left		1	
Upper Right		1	
Lower Left		1	
Lower Right		1	

O	Coordination of movements
1	Ability to plose
1	Ability to vary tension
1	Precise labial consonants

Codes: 0 = within normal limits, 1 = mild, 2 = moderate, 3 = severe

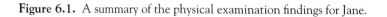

Figure 6.1. A summary of the physical examination findings for Jane.

Tongue

Symptom Checklist

0	Atrophy
1	Adventitious movements: fasciculations
1	Resting asymmetry

Function

	Range of Movement	Strength	Response to Instruction
Elevation	2	2	Some improvement
Protrusion	2	2	w/ maximum effort
L-lateralization	2	2	
R-lateralization	2	2	

1	Ability to vary muscular tension
1	Ability to plose
1	Consonant precision
1	Vowel differentiation
	Other: _____

Velopharyngeal Function

Symptom Checklist

1	Nasal emission
2	Hypernasality
2	Perceptual changes with occlusion
0	Nasal reflux
0	Inability to use a straw
0	Resting asymmetry
0	Adventitious movements: _____
	Other (specify: _____)

Function

2	Initial elevation
0	Asymmetry (_____ weaker than _____)
2	Ability to sustain (fatigue)

Codes:　0 = within normal limits, 1 = mild, 2 = moderate, 3 = severe

Figure 6.1. *(continued)*

Respiration and Phonation

Symptom Checklist

0	Abnormal loudness (reduced/excessive)
0	Loudness variation
1	Complaints of fatigue
0	Shortness of breath
3	Abnormal quality (breathy/hoarse/harsh/strained–strangled)
0	Phonatory breaks
2	Instability (mild/moderate/severe)
0	Stridor (inspiratory/expiratory)
0	Wet phonation
1	Abnormal voluntary cough (weak/absent)
	Other (specify: _____)

Vital capacity (Seated): _____2.9_____

Vital capacity (Supine): _____

Sustained phonation time: _____16_____ seconds

Codes: 0 = within normal limits, 1 = mild, 2 = moderate, 3 = severe

Figure 6.1. (*continued*)

production task (Yorkston, Beukelman, & Tice, 1996). Generally, Jane's speech pattern was consistent with the results of the physical examination. Articulatory imprecision was felt to be related to moderate tongue and velopharyngeal weakness. Respiratory support was adequate, although vocal quality suggested laryngeal spasticity. Given the level of her motor impairment, the slowed speaking rate was considered appropriate.

Impressions

As the result of this clinical examination, our impression was that Jane exhibited a mixed dysarthria with flaccid and spastic components. The pattern of the gradual onset of weakness and spasticity that affect multiple speech production subsystems was consistent with the medical diagnosis of motor neuron disease. Jane returned to our clinic 4 months later, with a confirmed diagnosis of amyotrophic lateral sclerosis. Impairment of all speech subsystems had worsened. Figure 6.2 contains a summary of the physical examination findings at the initial visit and 4 months later. Note that, although all aspects of speech had worsened, tongue and velar function were the most severely impaired. Since the initial visit, her speech intelligibility had declined to 48% and she was supplementing her highly distorted speech with handwriting for topic introduction and breakdown resolution.

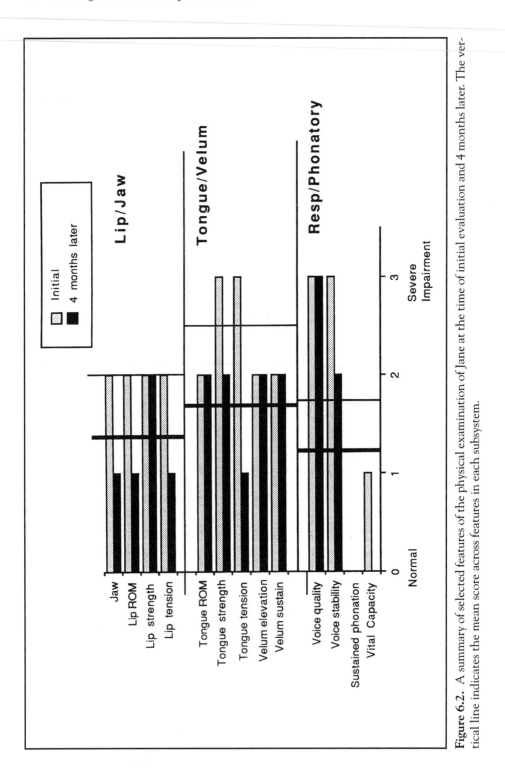

Figure 6.2. A summary of selected features of the physical examination of Jane at the time of initial evaluation and 4 months later. The vertical line indicates the mean score across features in each subsystem.

This case illustrates how differential diagnosis is typically made in the clinical setting, that is, by integrating information from the history of the speech problem, the physical examination, and the pattern and characteristics of speech to form an impression regarding type of dysarthria. This case is quite uncomplicated, with various types of information all suggesting a particular diagnosis. Although diagnoses are not always this straightforward, the principles remain the same. The process of clinically differentiating the various dysarthrias is one of integrating information from any and all sources that are available. More case descriptions that offer the opportunity to integrate the findings of the clinical examination into a communication diagnosis can be found elsewhere (Dworkin & Hartman, 1988).

Question: Can differential diagnosis be made on the basis of perceptual judgments alone?

Making a confident diagnosis of type of dysarthria based on perceptual analysis alone is difficult and may not be a prudent and reliable clinical practice. Research studies have called into question both the rating of deviant speech dimensions on a 7-point equal-appearing interval scale used in the Mayo Clinic studies (Zeplin & Kent, 1996; Zyski & Weisiger, 1987) and narrow phonetic transcription of error patterns (Miller, 1995). Results of these studies should be viewed with some caution because of the rather restricted information upon which judgments are being made. Most of these studies rely on audiotaped recordings so that no visual information is available to the rater. Further, they may rely on a rather narrow set of tasks. For example, a 30-second excerpt from a paragraph reading task was the sample judged in the Mayo Clinic studies. Fortunately, in the clinical setting, speech–language pathologists can call upon several sources of information, integrating them to make a differential diagnosis of type of dysarthria.

TREATMENT PLANNING

Assessment has been described as the process of gathering pertinent data about the impairment (the underlying neuromotor problem), the functional limitation (the decreased function resulting from the impairment), and the disability (the inability of the individual to perform expected roles). Decisions about the clinical course of action are made on the basis of that information. Thus, treatment planning in many respects can be viewed as the outcome of the assessment process. At various times in the field of dysarthria management, there has been the tendency to view approaches to intervention as unidimensional for all dysarthric individuals. For example, all speakers with dysarthria should be treated with strengthening exercises, or all speakers with dysarthria should be taught to speak more slowly. We advocate an approach to treatment planning that is individualized, based on results of the clinical examination.

Decisions about the management of speakers with dysarthria are made at a number of levels. The first level involves the most general decisions about goals of treatment. These decisions are based primarily on two types of information: the severity of the functional limitation and the disability experienced. The second level of decisions, discussed later in this chapter, involves the selection of specific treatment approaches. These approaches are selected so that the general goals of intervention can be reached. Selection of intervention techniques is heavily dependent upon an understanding of the pattern of impairment. In this section, we describe a framework for making decisions about the general goals of treatment and about specific intervention approaches to achieve those goals. Treatment planning for apraxia of speech is discussed in Chapter 13.

Goals of Treatment

Because of the chronic nature of the underlying neuromotor impairment, "normal" speech is rarely a realistic goal for individuals with dysarthria. Therefore, the clinician must find another framework for setting realistic treatment goals. In the following sections, we discuss intervention goal setting for severely, mildly, and moderately involved speakers with dysarthria.

SEVERELY INVOLVED SPEAKERS

The general goals of treatment for speakers with dysarthria vary with the severity of the disability. For severely involved speakers whose intelligibility is so reduced that they are unable to communicate verbally in ordinary situations, the general goals of treatment involve establishing a functional means of communication, using augmentative communication approaches, and educating the family and others about ways to increase communicative efficiency. Techniques to supplement severely distorted speech will be discussed in Chapter 12. Readers are referred to other texts for a description of augmentative communication approaches for children and adults with motor speech disorders (Beukelman & Mirenda, 1998; Yorkston, 1992). For the speaker with a degenerative disorder, an augmentative communication approach must be selected with an increasing level of impairment in mind. For the recovering or stable speaker with dysarthria, a second goal is to establish the motor control prerequisites for future speech development so that a transition to independent use of speech can be made.

Intervention with children who have severe dysarthria is also focused on family education, augmentative communication, and comprehensibility treatment. Similar to intervention with adult speakers, intervention techniques will vary with the type of dysarthria, the prognosis for improvement in motor speech control, and the concomitant cognitive and linguistic processing deficits that the child may have. Augmentative systems for children, for example, take into account the degree of cognitive deficit that may be present, as well as the fact that children with dysarthria are still involved in the acquisition of linguistic and motor control processes. The development of literacy in children with severe communication problems is also a critical part of intervention planning (Foley, 1993).

MODERATELY INVOLVED SPEAKERS

For those moderately involved speakers, who are able to use speech as their sole means of communication but who are not completely intelligible, the general goal of treatment is maximizing intelligibility. The term compensated intelligibility aptly describes the goal of this type of intervention (Rosenbek & LaPointe, 1985). Achieving compensated intelligibility may take a variety of forms, depending on the speaker and the nature of the underlying impairment. For example, it may include an effort to control speaking rate for some individuals with coordination problems (see Chapter 10) or may involve prosthetically managing an impaired component of the speech mechanism as it does with palatal lift fitting for individuals with little or no velopharyngeal movement (see Chapter 9).

MILDLY INVOLVED SPEAKERS

For the speaker with mild dysarthria, general treatment goals are based on both the severity of the functional limitation and the disability resulting from it. Speech of mildly involved individuals is characterized as intelligible but less efficient and natural than normal. For some speakers, this mild reduction in speech efficiency poses no problem. Such speakers are able to function adequately in all necessary communication situations; however, for those individuals who experience a disability, intervention may be warranted. The general treatment goals for individuals with mild dysarthria include maximizing communication efficiency and speech naturalness while maintaining intelligibility.

From Assessment to Treatment Planning

NATURE OF THE IMPAIRMENT

One of the chief objections to perceptually derived assessment approaches is that they generally provide little information about the nature of the problem.

Once an impairment has been identified, it must be examined in detail in order to formulate a treatment plan. For example, many individuals with dysarthria speak with short phrases, producing only a few syllables or words per breath group. This speech characteristic is easily identified perceptually. However, an understanding of the underlying problems that may be responsible for the speech disorder is best obtained as part of the physical examination. A number of different problems may result in short breath groups. In some speakers, the problem may be primarily one of respiratory insufficiency. If this is the case, the speaker may be unable to generate adequate subglottal air pressure for more than a second or two. Simple instrumental techniques for measuring a speaker's ability to sustain an adequate level of subglottal air pressure are described in Chapter 7. In other cases, respiratory function may not be the primary problem; rather, the respiratory signs may be secondary to impairments in other speech components. Short breath groups may occur in individuals with dysarthria who are attempting to compensate for spasticity in the laryngeal musculature. These individuals must "overdrive" their respiratory component in order to produce phonation. The function of the respiratory system in these individuals can be documented by aerodynamically estimating subglottal air pressure during the production of voiceless stop consonants (see Chapter 7). Often these individuals generate much greater than normal subglottal air pressure.

In still other cases, short phrase length may be the result of impairment in multiple rather than single speech components. Frequently, individuals exhibit with dysarthric impairment in all of the components. The perceptual feature of short phrases may be the result of mild to moderate respiratory support problems coupled with velopharyngeal incompetence. Thus, moderate difficulty in generating adequate breath pressure may be exaggerated by air wastage from an incompetent velopharyngeal port. This type of problem may be documented by obtaining simultaneous aerodynamic measures of intraoral air pressure and nasal airflow (see Chapter 9). These measures can be used to make inferences about the timing of velopharyngeal closure and, coupled with information about respiratory support, may provide an explanation for the perceptual measures. A gross estimate of the relative contribution of the respiratory versus the velopharyngeal components can be obtained by asking the individual to perform speech and nonspeech maneuvers with the nares occluded and then documenting changes in performance.

Finally, other individuals with dysarthria speak with short phrases for reasons not related to their current level of physiologic support. Examples of such cases frequently occur in speakers recovering from traumatic brain injury. Despite the fact that short phrases are a characteristic of their habitual speech, these individuals may demonstrate the motor control to perform in a much more normal fashion. When assessed instrumentally, they may exhibit respiratory support adequate for extended utterances. No other speech component may markedly contribute to the tendency to produce short phrases. When instructed, these individuals can produce nearly normal breath group lengths. In such cases, we speculate that these individuals with traumatic brain injury are continuing to use a respiratory pattern that they learned when their impairment was much more severe, even though their respiratory control has increased and they no longer need to use a "one-word-at-a-time" approach. What once was a useful compensatory behavior may now be maladaptive.

In summary, by reviewing the list of perceptual features related to each of the components, the reader will realize that, as with short phrases, many of the features may have multiple underlying causes. Perceptual means are used to identify the problems and generate clinical hypotheses about the underlying causes. A detailed physical examination can be used to confirm or reject these hypotheses. Armed with a thorough understanding of normal aspects of speech and vocal tract impairment assessment, some possible explanations can be posed.

An understanding of why a perceptual feature is occurring is obviously important for treatment planning. Consider the different treatment approaches for each of the speakers just described, all of whom share the common characteristic of speaking with short phrases. For the speaker with insufficient respiratory support, treatment might focus on increasing the ability to sustain adequate breath pressure either prosthetically or by training. For the speaker who uses short phrases to compensate for increased laryngeal tone, training to improve respiratory support is not needed. Rather, the laryngeal problem must be managed, perhaps through the prescription of antispasticity medications. For the speaker whose moderate respiratory support problems are exaggerated by inadequate velopharyngeal function, fitting a palatal lift may be appropriate to compensate for the velopharyngeal problem. For the speaker who has recovered physiologic support but has maintained an abnormal respiratory pattern, behavioral training may be appropriate to change the maladaptive pattern. Thus, different speakers with a common perceptual feature would each be managed differently, depending on the underlying nature of the problem.

IDENTIFYING FEATURES THAT CAN BE MODIFIED

After deviant speech features have been identified and hypotheses developed to explain them, the next phase of treatment planning involves identifying those aspects of speech where change is possible and where change will result in improved speech adequacy. This phase is necessary because it is possible to know what has gone wrong and why, and yet have no apparent means of changing that feature. Comparison between habitual performance with instructed or modified performance gives an indication of the potential value of various intervention techniques.

This discussion will not involve listing tasks or techniques that can be used with all speakers, as no such list exists. Rather, the process is illustrated with an example of two speakers who both exhibited perceptually identified characteristics related to velopharyngeal port dysfunction, including nasal emission, hypernasality, imprecise production of "pressure" consonants, and short breath group units. Although these speakers exhibited similiar perceptual features, results of the instrumental assessment suggested that different underlying problems may have caused the velopharyngeal dysfunction in each of these speakers. Results of aerodynamic studies in the first speaker suggested that this individual never achieved closure at habitual speaking rates and loudness levels. Behavioral intervention techniques appeared to have no effect. Instructions to slow the speaking rate did not result in improved performance, and instructions to speak louder or softer (to increase or decrease subglottal air pressure) resulted only in proportional increases or decreases in nasal emission as measured by increases in the volume velocity of nasal airflow and intraoral air pressure. When asked to produce contrastive phoneme pairs in single words (/mat/ vs. /bat/ vs. /pat/) and to "make them as different as possible," the speaker was unable to successfully differentiate nasals from plosives or voiced from voiceless plosives. Despite the apparent ineffectiveness of behavioral techniques, aerodynamic closure of the velopharyngeal port by occluding the nares had beneficial effects. The precision with which the speaker produced pressure consonants was judged to be improved with the nares occluded. With the nares occluded, the speaker was able to generate pressure of 5 cm H_2O during the stop phase of voiceless plosives. In summary, this speaker with consistent velopharyngeal incompetence in the presence of adequate respiratory support for speech appeared not to be able to modify the problem behaviorally. However, performance was improved by occluding the velopharyngeal port. The outcome of the assessment was a recommendation that the patient be fitted with a palatal lift.

The speech of the second individual also suggested a velopharyngeal dysfunction. However, unlike the first speaker who was consistently incompetent no matter what he was instructed to do, the second speaker's performance varied considerably, depending on the task. For example, he was able to achieve closure more consistently when speaking at a slowed rate rather than at his habitual speaking rate. Listeners were able to distinguish nasal from nonnasal productions when the speaker was producing single words, although these distinctions were not present during extended samples of connected speech. In summary, this patient appeared to be able to behaviorally modify the adequacy of velopharyngeal function along with other articulatory behaviors. Therefore, the outcome of this assessment was the recommendation for a period of therapy, focusing on slowing speech rate in an effort to increase velopharyngeal function and articulatory precision.

IDENTIFICATION OF EXISTING COMPENSATORY STRATEGIES

The speech of individuals with dysarthria is affected not only by the pattern and severity of the impairment but also by compensations made by the speaker. For example, an individual with flaccid dysarthria may use extra effort in order to compensate for weakness. An individual with poor respiratory support may make other laryngeal and articulatory adjustments in order to efficiently valve the outgoing airflow. The literature contains many examples documenting such compensations. Hixon, Putnam, and Sharpe (1983) reported a case of a speaker with flaccid paralysis of the rib cage, diaphragm, and abdomen who spoke with a mild to moderately strained–strangled voice quality, used occasional glottal stops for fricatives, and shortened the duration of fricatives. All of these modifications had the effect of conserving the airstream. Garcia, Dagenais, and Cannito (1998) reported the case of a man with severe dysarthria (sentence intelligibility = 6%) who makes subtle durational adjustments in speech when the sentences that he is producing are relatively unpredictable.

Treatment planning in dysarthria frequently involves identifying and encouraging compensatory adjustments. Clinical examination findings should be interpreted with this treatment planning goal in mind. In other words, clinicians should not only focus on areas of deficit but place equal importance on areas of preserved function. Relatively preserved areas of function may be viewed as potential means of compensation for more severely impaired subsystems.

The following case illustrated for us the remarkable ability of some speakers with dysarthria to "make the most of" residual areas of function. Larry was a 42-year-old man who was diagnosed with amyotrophic lateral sclerosis nearly 7 years before he was evaluated in our clinic. His speech was 76% intelligible when unfamiliar listeners transcribed audio recordings of Larry reading a series of unrelated sentences (Yorkston, Beukelman, & Traynor, 1984). In conversational exchanges where the topic is known and the environment is quiet, we considered him understandable with careful listening. Given this level of functioning, we were somewhat surprised by the findings of the physical examination, which are summarized in Figure 6.3. Note that tongue function is severely impaired. In fact, no lingual movement could be observed on a variety of non-speech tasks. Despite this profound impairment, Larry's speech is functional. We hypothesize that his ability to compensate was the result of jaw positioning inasmuch as jaw function was intact and that relatively preserved respiratory phonatory function allowed him to maintain prosody and provide the listener with an envelope of intonation. Although Larry had developed these compensations independently, his case illustrates how important a role preserved subsystem functions can play in maintaining speech intelligibility. The findings of the clinical examination often provide some insights that suggest what compensations may be beneficial.

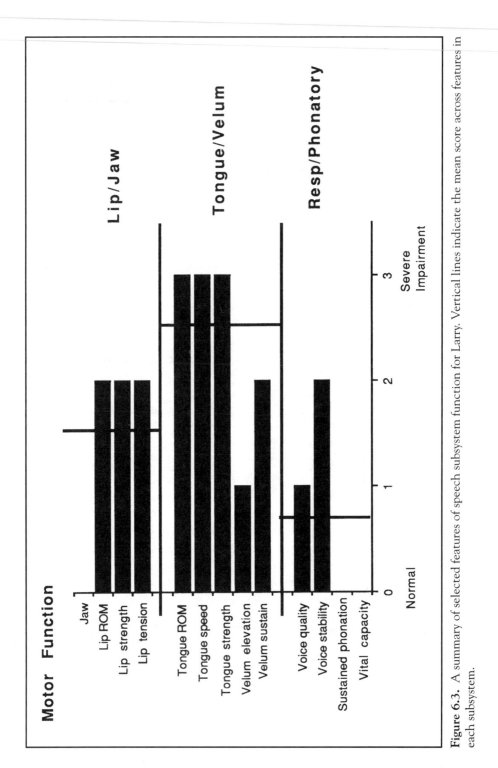

Figure 6.3. A summary of selected features of speech subsystem function for Larry. Vertical lines indicate the mean score across features in each subsystem.

Approaches to Treatment

Once the general goals of treatment have been established, the selection of specific treatment approaches is based on the severity of the disability and the pattern of speech impairment. Approaches to intervention with individuals who have dysarthria can be grouped into a few options. Development of a treatment plan involves the selection of options appropriate for the particular individual with dysarthria.

SUPPLEMENTING SPEECH WITH AUGMENTATIVE COMMUNICATION APPROACHES

Individuals with anarthria or severe dysarthria may experience such extensive impairment that natural speech alone does not serve as a functional means of communication. Augmentative communication strategies are required to meet some or all communication needs. Recently, the number of alternative communication options has increased. These options range from the "light" technology of alphabet/word boards to sophisticated computer-based systems with multiple output options. A detailed discussion of these systems of communication is beyond the scope of this book; however, this material is presented in detail elsewhere (Beukelman & Mirenda, 1998).

For some speakers with dysarthria, natural speech can meet some, but not all, communication needs. In such cases, speech is supplemented with one or more augmentative communication approaches. For example, some individuals with severe dysarthria use speech for greetings. In this type of communication, the timing of message delivery may be more critical than message intelligibility. These individuals may also speak with those partners who are very familiar with their speech and lifestyle. However, with partners who have difficulty understanding them, they may point to the first letter of each word as the word is spoken. They may use systems such as portable typewriters to communicate with strangers and to resolve communication breakdowns with everyone (see Chapter 11).

REDUCING THE IMPAIRMENT

At times, dysarthria treatment involves direct attempts to reduce the degree of impairment or to increase the physiologic support for speech in selected subsystems. These activities may involve normalizing muscle tone and/or increasing strength and movement precision. A thorough understanding of normal and disordered aspects of speech production is needed when taking this approach to treatment. Not only must the impairment be understood, but impairments noted in various components must be placed in a hierarchy so that initial treatment can focus on the most fundamental of the impairments. Discussion of such hierarchies can be found elsewhere (Netsell, 1984; Rosenbek & LaPointe,

1985). Generally, these techniques have as their goal the normalization of function. Their rationale is that reducing the impairment will produce a corresponding improvement in functional ability or a decrease in disability. Excellent case reports using this approach are available (Netsell & Daniel, 1979; Workinger & Netsell, 1992). Numerous examples of treatment tasks whose goals are reduction of impairment will be found in later chapters.

BEHAVIORAL COMPENSATION

Compensatory approaches to treatment, unlike those aimed at a reduction of impairment, do not have normalization of function as their primary goal. Rather, many of the behavioral compensatory techniques encourage the individual with dysarthria to move away from the normal range of functioning in selected parameters in order to minimize the overall functional limitation. Rate control is an example of such a compensatory technique. Despite the fact that the majority of individuals with dysarthria speak at rates slower than normal, clinicians frequently attempt to slow rates still further in an effort to increase intelligibility. Rate control techniques will be reviewed in Chapter 10. Examples of other behavioral compensations are found in certain aspects of respiratory training. Some speakers with reduced respiratory support are trained to shorten breath groups beyond their already relatively short habitual length. Behavioral compensation is also seen in prosody training. Normal speakers signal stress by subtle adjustments of the parameters of fundamental frequency, intensity, and duration adjustments. Speakers with dysarthria may be trained to select only certain parameters to signal stress patterning. They may be asked to limit use of fundamental frequency and intensity and to use only increased segment duration to signal stress. Thus, many of the treatment techniques that will be described in later chapters fall into the category of behavioral compensation. These techniques, rather than seeking normalcy in speech production, involve strategies to offset selected aspects of the impairment.

PROSTHETIC COMPENSATION

Prosthetic compensation is frequently employed to supplement or replace component function. In contrast to behavioral compensation where the speaker is trained to produce speech in a modified manner, prosthetic compensation employs a mechanical or electronic device to offset certain aspects of the impairment. Palatal lifts have been used extensively to compensate for velopharyngeal incompetence in speakers with dysarthria. Another prosthetic compensation is the use of a delayed auditory feedback device to control the excessively rapid speaking rate of certain speakers with parkinsonian dysarthria. A third example of prosthetic compensation is the use of respiratory paddles or abdominal binders. An amplification system to compensate for reduced loudness levels is yet another example of a prosthetic compensatory device. One advantage of prosthetic over behavioral compensation is the immediacy of the effect. With prosthetic compensatory techniques, little training is usually required; therefore, these techniques are particularly useful for individuals with degenerative disorders.

ELIMINATION OF MALADAPTIVE BEHAVIORS

Earlier, dysarthria was defined as a motor speech impairment resulting from abnormalities in movement rates, strength, precision, and coordination. In the clinical setting, it is useful to attempt to separate the problem into at least two aspects. The first reflects the direct result of the underlying impairment. The second reflects an attempt to compensate for that impairment. As mentioned earlier, compensatory adjustments can be beneficial. For example, consider the case of an adult with a sudden onset of ataxia. A wide-based gait may be seen to compensate for reduced balance, just as a reduced speaking rate may be a compensatory response to discoordination of the speech mechanism. However, compensatory efforts are not always beneficial. Consider the speaker with dysarthria who overdrives a poorly controlled respiratory system in an effort to compensate for reduced velopharyngeal function or increased laryngeal tone. The effort to compensate for the defective component may have the effect of increasing vocal harshness and reducing breath group length. Thus, the compensatory effort does nothing to increase the overall adequacy of speech.

Maladaptive compensatory behaviors may be a response to current physiologic problems. However, they may also be overlearned behaviors that once were adaptive but are no longer needed. We have seen a number of individuals with brain injury who exhibit respiratory compensatory patterns that are maladaptive. For example, some began to speak following their injury by producing a single word or syllable per breath. Years later, we find ourselves attempting to train them to use an extended breath group for which they now have the physiologic capability. Another example of maladaptive compensation can be found in an individual who pauses for a breath to meet her physiologic respiratory requirements without regard to the linguistic aspects of the utterance.

INTERACTION ENHANCEMENT STRATEGIES

Communication effectiveness involves both the speaker and the listener. Traditionally, dysarthria treatment has focused primarily on the speaker, with the listener being ignored or receiving a few minutes of counseling. Increasingly, we are involving the frequent listeners in interaction training activities with our clients with dysarthria. Appropriate interaction strategies cannot be assumed, and both the speaker and the listener often need guidance in developing these strategies. A more detailed discussion of interaction training can be found in Chapter 12.

COMMUNICATION SKILL MAINTENANCE

As in many areas of motor activity, skill maintenance is often required if an individual is to perform maximally. The goal of this phase of treatment must be carefully explained to the speaker and his or her important listeners. Previous treatment may have been oriented toward improving performance. When speakers fail to detect continued improvement, they will mistakenly believe that the "practice" is not working or is unimportant. We usually limit maintenance training activities to a brief time period, perhaps 10 minutes once or twice a day. Often activities include a short passage to be read aloud with notations regarding the practice objectives, such as phrase, respiratory, or articulatory patterns.

REDUCING SOCIAL LIMITATIONS

In Chapter 1, the social limitations imposed by dysarthria were introduced. A speaker with dysarthria may be prevented from participating in a desired role because of the biases and attitudes of those of the society. The reduction of these societal limitations may be brought out by changing attitudes or reformulating policies. For example, a child with dysarthria may be placed at a disadvantage by the attitudes of his or her peers, or the adult with dysarthria may find it difficult to "get past the interview" when seeking employment.

Evaluating the Treatment Plan

Treatment planning is a process in which general goals are established and specific methods selected to achieve those goals. Treatment plans for speakers with dysarthria are individualized based on communication needs, level of disability, and nature of the underlying motor impairment. Because of this individualization, treatment plans vary considerably. However, a number of general principles are used to evaluate the adequacy of treatment plans. Appropriate treatment plans must consider both present and future communication needs and must be firmly grounded in the principles of motor learning. One example of this is the move toward mainstreaming children with disabilities into the regular classrooms. For some time, children with cerebral palsy or traumatic brain injury were segregated into classrooms for the physically disabled and not allowed to participate in the regular school curriculum and activities. With the move toward mainstreaming, these children with dysarthria are facing new and challenging social and educational environments.

ATTENTION TO PRESENT COMMUNICATION NEEDS

The principle of attention to present communication needs suggests that one of the primary concerns of treatment should be to maximize the speaker's current ability to communicate. At least a portion of each training session should be devoted to developing those skills. For the speaker with severe dysarthria, this may involve training in the use of an augmentative communication approach. With the recovering speaker, this approach may initially serve temporarily as a replacement to speech when motor control problems are so severe that no functional speech is possible. Later, as recovery occurs, the augmentative system may be used to supplement speech when the speaker cannot be understood. For the speaker with moderate dysarthria, attention to present communication needs may take the form of attempts to maximize speech intelligibility through prosthetic compensation. Another general approach designed to maximize present communication is interaction training. This general category of tasks includes training both speakers with dysarthria and their listeners in such skills as topic identification and repair of communication breakdowns.

PREPARATION FOR THE FUTURE

The principle of preparation for the future suggests that, in addition to maximizing current communication skills, treatment plans should include steps appropriate for the predicted changes that may occur in the impairment, functional limitation, and disability. Preparation for the future can take a number of forms. First, it may involve establishing a hierarchy of treatment. When multiple speech components are involved, it may not be prudent to intervene at all levels at one time. Rather, the speech–language pathologist must decide where to begin. If, for example, the speech–language pathologist believes that poor respiratory control is limiting all other aspects of speech, then work in this area would have high priority. Second, preparation for the future may involve selecting specific treatment approaches based on the predicted natural course of the disorder. For example, we rarely use techniques with the intent to reduce the impairment when developing a plan for an individual with a degenerative disorder. Instead, many of the techniques we select involve prosthetic compensation. These techniques usually have immediate impact and require little training for the user. Third, planning for the future may involve an effort to prevent future problems. There are a number of patterns that are appropriate to compensate for severe motor control or coordination problems that may be counterproductive if continued as impairment severity decreases. For example, individuals with severe dysarthria are often taught to produce one word at a time or to use an alphabet board to indicate the first letter of each word as it is produced. Although this compensatory pattern may be needed early in recovery, if the pattern persists as neuromotor recovery occurs, it becomes maladaptive, interfering with natural prosodic patterns. Although it would be ideal to simply avoid training patterns that may in the future be maladaptive, in clinical practice, this is not always possible. Therefore, the experienced speech–language pathologist, aware of potential maladaptive patterns, can train the speaker to move away from them as soon as they are no longer appropriate. Finally, planning for the future may involve the selection and learning of augmentative systems for speakers with degenerative dysarthrias.

MINIMAL INTERVENTION

The principle of minimal intervention suggests that treatment should attempt to change the motor activity only so far as is needed to achieve treatment goals. This principle, when applied to training the complex motor act of speaking, suggests that the clinician does not need to "start from the ground up" in all cases. Consider, for example, the speaker with mild dysarthria who is intelligible but is not normal in terms of the naturalness of speech. In this case, naturalness may be enhanced by training the speaker to make slight modifications in breath patterning or to make slight durational adjustments. The clinician does not typically begin with the basics; that is, the clinician does not typically attempt to increase the speaker's capabilities in all components of speech. For example, respiratory–phonatory control may not improve by training the speaker to extend phonation time, and articulatory precision is not increased by asking the speaker to produce more rapid diadochokinetic movements.

The principle of minimal intervention has implications for rate control as well. Generally, the more rigid the rate control technique, the more it disrupts speech naturalness. Minimal intervention implies that if rigid techniques are not needed, they should not be employed. Rather, the speech–language pathologist should employ the least restrictive rate control techniques that produce the desired result.

Another example of the application of the minimal intervention principle can be found in the work of Ramig and her colleagues (Ramig, Countryman, Thompson, & Horii, 1995; Ramig, Pawlas, & Countryman, 1995). The overall goal of this therapy is to improve the adequacy of speech in individuals with Parkinson's disease. It is typical to see a number of deviant perceptual features in the speech of these individuals, including reduced loudness and prosody, along with reduced oral articulatory movement and, in some, rapid speaking rates. Instead of attempting to change production in all of the affected subsystems, the treatment focuses only on increasing respiratory–phonatory effort. When the speaker is successful in changing respiratory–phonatory effort (making speech louder and stronger), then other changes also occur (articulatory gestures become exaggerated and rate slows). The success of this type of treatment is attributed, at least in part, to simplicity of the training. Speakers are taught to "think loud." These minimal instructions are easy to learn. Although articulatory changes are not a focus of training, they occur as a by-product of the training.

ATTENTION TO PRINCIPLES OF MOTOR LEARNING

Speakers with acquired dysarthria have experienced important changes in their speech production mechanism. Therefore, intervention not only focuses on increasing motor performance (e.g., increasing strength or range of motion), but also must focus on establishing new motor schema. The distinction between cognitive learning and motor learning has important implications for training speakers with dysarthria. This distinction can be illustrated with examples from the sport of tennis. Learning the basic rules and strategies of tennis is an example of cognitive learning and can occur, at least on a basic level, in a brief period of time. The learner, having been told only once or twice, will have learned enough to play the game—at least from a cognitive viewpoint. Learning to produce a good backhand stroke involves an entirely different type of learning. Learning complex motor activities may require thousands of repetitions before a player is first able to adequately perform them, then be able to "hit the groove" and repeat the adequate performance time after time at will.

Modifying speech is an example of an extremely complex motor learning task. Movements have been classified as discrete movements if they have a recognizable beginning and end (e.g., throwing a ball). They are classified as continuous if they have no such recognizable points (e.g., swimming). Because it shares characteristics with both of these types of movement, speech is considered a serial movement composed of a series of discrete movements in a particular order that form a complete response (Schmidt, 1988). Studies of people as they learn novel movements give clinicians insights that can be applied to assisting individuals in learning or relearning the movements of speech. The following three experiments illustrate some aspects of motor learning that are pertinent as clinicians develop treatment plans (Schmidt & Bjork, 1992). As you read them, try to formulate an opinion about why the results occurred.

Experiment 1 (Shea & Morgan, 1979): Subjects were taught three different motor tasks under one of two conditions. In one condition, the learning trials were *blocked*; that is, all trials of Task 1 were completed, then all trials of Task 2, and finally all trials of Task 3. This is similar to what is usually considered "drills." In the other condition, although the number of total trials was the same, the trials were *randomized*.

Question: Which learning condition showed the greatest advantage during the acquisition phase?

Answer: Subjects in the blocked condition had the clear advantage during the initial phases of learning.

Question: Which learning condition showed the greatest advantage during the retention phase (10 days later)?

Answer: Subjects who learned the motor task in the randomized condition.

Experiment 2 (Schmidt, Young, Swinnen, & Shapiro, 1989): Subjects were taught a complex arm movement under three schedules of feedback of results: feedback after every trial, after every 5th trial, or after every 15th trial.

Question: Which learning condition showed the greatest advantage during the acquisition phase?

Answer: Subjects receiving feedback after every trial learned the task most rapidly.

Question: Which learning condition showed the greatest advantage during the retention phase (2 days later)?

Answer: Subjects who were given summary feedback only after every 15th trial performed best during the retention phase.

Experiment 3 (Catalano & Kleiner, 1984): Subjects were taught a motor timing task in which stimuli were presented either at one target rate (either 5, 7, 9, or 11 mph) or at variable rates (all four rates interspersed during training). All subjects received the same number of trials. Retention was tested using novel rates, outside the range of subjects' experience during the learning conditions.

Question: Which learning condition showed the greatest advantage during the retention phase?

Answer: Subjects who learned under the condition of variable practice.

The results are somewhat contradictory to what would be expected. What do all of the experiments have in common? Results of these experiments suggest that performance during learning does not necessarily predict performance later, during the retention phase. Further, they suggest that conditions that result in the greatest ease of acquisition are not always associated with greatest retention. These studies have important implications for treatment, because the primary goal in therapy is retention of learning rather than merely acquisition. One common thread that runs through all of these experiments is that the learners who had the most difficulty during learning ultimately did the best.

Some possible explanations have been offered for why introducing difficulty enhances learners' retention. In the blocked versus randomized learning experiments, it is hypothesized that randomized trials prevent learners from generating a stable "set" for the task; rather they must retrieve and organize slightly different movements for every trial. This practice of retrieving patterns during acquisition is apparently beneficial for long-term retention. In the feedback experiment, it was suggested that one of the disadvantages of frequent feedback is that it comes as part of the task. Therefore, performance without the feedback in the retention phase is disrupted. It is also possible that frequent feedback prevents learners from forming a stablized "representation" of the motor task. Learners who receive minimal feedback must evaluate their own response-produced feedback. In summary, training activities that foster "processing activities" and enhance the effectiveness of rules or schemata may be the most beneficial (Schmidt & Bjork, 1992).

The nature of motor learning dictates a number of approaches to training. Adequate performance of a specific task one time or 10 times or even 100 times may not be enough to establish a consistently successful pattern. Therefore, extensive practice often is required. This is not always easily accomplished within the time limitations of treatment sessions. When possible, it is highly desirable to structure ordinary communication situations so that they too offer the possibility of practice. For example, an individual with severe dysarthria who is not sufficiently understandable to communicate independently via speech may be afforded valuable practice by supplementing speaking efforts with an alphabet board. Thus, in using a system in which the speaker indicates the first letter of each word as it is spoken, many individuals are able to speak functionally earlier in the course of their recovery than would have been possible if a supplementary system had not been used. Still another example of the need for extensive practice of motor learning tasks is in the area of rate control. An individual with ataxic dysarthria may learn cognitively in a very brief period of time that a slow rate is best. The motor learning required to speak consistently at an appropriate rate may require an extensive period of training. Other principles of motor learning as they apply to specific treatment strategies can be found in Chapters 12 and 13.

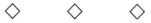

In this chapter, general approaches to interpreting results of the clinical examination and treatment planning have been described. In the following chapters, details of more in-depth assessment of each speech subsystem will be presented, along with treatment approaches that focus on the respiratory, laryngeal, and velopharyngeal aspects of speech.

REFERENCES

Bayles, K. A. (1984). Language and dementia. In A. Holland (Ed.), *Language disorders in adults* (pp. 209–244). San Diego: College-Hill.

Beukelman, D. R., & Mirenda, P. (1998). *Augmentative and alternative communication: Management of severe communication disorders in children and adults (2nd ed.)*. Baltimore: Brookes.

Beukelman, D. R., Yorkston, K. M., & Tice, R. (1997). *Pacer/tally rate measurement software*. Lincoln, NE: Tice Technology Services.

Catalano, J. F., & Kleiner, B. M. (1984). Distant transfer and practice variability. *Perceptual and Motor Skills, 58*, 851–856.

Darley, F., Aronson, A., & Brown, J. (1969). Clusters of deviant speech dimensions in the dysarthrias. *Journal of Speech and Hearing Research, 12*, 462–496.

Darley, F. L., Aronson, A. E., & Brown, J. R. (1975). *Motor speech disorders*. Philadelphia: Saunders.

Dongilli, J. P., Hakel, M., & Beukelman, D. (1992). Recovery of functional speech following traumatic brain injury. *Journal of Head Trauma Rehabilitation, 7*, 91–101.

Dworkin, J. P., & Hartman, D. E. (1988). *Cases in neurogenic communicative disorders*. Boston: Little, Brown.

Foley, B. (1993). The development of literacy in individuals with severe congenital speech and motor impairments. *Topics in Language Disorders, 12*(2), 16–32.

Garcia, J. M., Dagenais, P. A., & Cannito, M. P. (1998). Acoustic differences in dysarthric speech rated to use of natural gestures. In M. P. Cannito, K. M. Yorkston, & D. R. Beukelman (Eds.), *Motor speech disorders: Neurobases, assessment, and treatment* (pp. 213–228). Baltimore: Brookes.

Groher, M. (1977). Language and memory disorders following closed head trauma. *Journal of Speech and Hearing Research, 20*, 212.

Hagen, C., Malkmus, D., & Durham, P. (1979). Levels of cognitive functions. In *Rehabilitation of head injured adults: Comprehensive physical management*. Downey, CA: Professional Staff Association of Ranchos Los Amigos Hospital.

Hixon, T., Putnam, A., & Sharpe, J. (1983). Speech production with flaccid paralysis of the rib cage, diaphragm, and abdomen. *Journal of Speech and Hearing Disorders, 48*, 315–327.

Johns, D. F. (Ed.). (1985). *Clinical management of neurogenic communicative disorders* (2nd ed.). Boston: Little, Brown.

Johns, D. F., & Darley, F. L. (1970). Phonemic variability in apraxia of speech. *Journal of Speech and Hearing Research, 13*, 556.

Miller, N. (1995). Pronunciation errors in acquired speech disorders: The errors of our ways. *European Journal of Disorders of Communication, 30*, 346–361.

Netsell, R. (1984). Physiological studies of dysarthria and their relevance to treatment. *Seminars in Language, 5*(4), 279–292.

Netsell, R., & Daniel, B. (1979). Dysarthria in adults: Physiologic approach to rehabilitation. *Archives of Physical Medicine and Rehabilitation, 60*, 502.

Ramig, L. O., Countryman, S., Thompson, L. L., & Horii, Y. (1995). A comparison of two forms of intensive speech treatment in Parkinson disease. *Journal of Speech and Hearing Research, 38,* 1232–1251.

Ramig, L. O., Pawlas, A. A., & Countryman, S. (1995). *The Lee Silverman Voice Treatment.* Iowa City, IA: National Center for Voice and Speech.

Rosenbek, J. C., & LaPointe, L. L. (1985). The dysarthrias: Description, diagnosis, and treatment. In D. Johns (Ed.), *Clinical management of neurogenic communication disorders* (pp. 97–152). Boston: Little, Brown.

Schmidt, R. A. (1988). *Motor control and learning: A behavioral emphasis* (2nd ed.). Champaign, IL: Human Kinetics.

Schmidt, R. A., & Bjork, R. A. (1992). New conceptualizations of practice: Common principles in three paradigms suggest new concepts for training. *Psychological Science, 3*(4), 207–217.

Schmidt, R. A., Young, D. E., Swinnen, S., & Shapiro, D. C. (1989). Summary knowledge of results for skill acquisition: Support for the guidance hypothesis. *Journal of Experimental Psychology: Learning, Memory and Cognition, 15,* 352–359.

Shea, J. B., & Morgan, R. L. (1979). Contextual interference effects on the acquisition, retention, and transfer of a motor skill. *Journal of Experimental Psychology: Human Learning and Memory, 5,* 179–187.

Wertz, R. T. (1985). Neuropathologies of speech and language: An introduction to patient management. In D. F. Johns (Ed.), *Clinical management of neurogenic communicative disorders* (2nd ed., pp. 1–96). Boston: Little, Brown.

Workinger, M. S., & Netsell, R. (1992). Restoration of intelligible speech 13 years post-head injury. *Brain Injury, 6,* 183–187.

Yorkston, K. M. (Ed.). (1992). *Augmentative communication in the medical setting.* San Antonio, TX: Communication Skill Builders.

Yorkston, K. M., Beukelman, D. R., & Tice, R. (1996). *Sentence Intelligibility Test.* Lincoln, NE: Tice Technology Services.

Yorkston, K. M., Beukelman, D. R., & Traynor, C. (1984). *Computerized Assessment of Intelligibility of Dysarthric Speech.* Austin, TX: PRO-ED.

Zeplin, J., & Kent, R. D. (1996). Reliability of auditory–perceptual scaling of dysarthria. In D. A. Robin, K. M. Yorkston, & D. R. Beukelman (Eds.), *Disorders of motor speech: Assessment, treatment, and clinical characterization* (pp. 145–154). Baltimore: Brookes.

Zyski, B. J., & Weisiger, B. E. (1987). Identification of dysarthria types based on perceptual analysis. *Journal of Communication Disorders, 20,* 367–378.

CHAPTER

RESPIRATION

Clinical Issues: Two consultation requests gave evidence of respiratory impairment. In the first, we were asked to evaluate the speech of a 67-year-old woman with amyotrophic lateral sclerosis (ALS) and severely reduced vital capacity. Our evaluation confirmed a reduced vital capacity. In addition, she was able to sustain phonation for only approximately 5 seconds, was unable to increase the loudness of her speech, and complained of fatigue after relatively brief periods of speaking. Yet, despite evidence of respiratory impairment, her conversational speech was remarkably good. It was adequately loud for face-to-face conversation, the number of words she produced on one breath was nearly normal, and inhalations occurred at locations appropriate for the syntax of the message. In short, she appeared to be handling a severely compromised respiratory system as well as she could.

In the second case, we were asked to evaluate the speech of a 35-year-old man with residual ataxia from a motor vehicle accident over 10 years earlier. The physician had indicated that this man's speech sounded "explosive" and that he produced only one or two words per breath. On examination, the man presented a very different pattern of respiratory impairment from that of the woman. Our evaluation began with a perceptual evaluation of his speech. His speech pattern was typical of ataxic dysarthria and was characterized by "excess and equal" stress patterning. His voice was excessively loud and somewhat harsh, and vowels were hypernasal. Irregular articulatory breakdowns occurred frequently. Perhaps the most unique aspect of his speech was his abnormal breath patterning. In both conversational speech and oral reading, he would inhale after every word and occasionally within words. His abnormal breathing pattern, in combination with a tendency to speak too rapidly for his level of motor control, not only reduced the naturalness of his speech but also reduced his speech intelligibility. A more detailed examination of his performance indicated that he was "overdriving" his respiratory system during speech. He was initiating each word at excessively high lung volume levels and generating excessive levels of subglottal air pressure for speech. His phonatory quality was harsh. Despite the abnormal pattern of breathing during speech, he could sustain loud phonation for over 15 seconds and could count from 1 to 23 with adequate loudness on a single breath. Clearly, he was not making optimal use of his respiratory system during speech. As we reviewed the results of these two evaluations, we asked the following questions:

- Why were the respiratory impairments of these two individuals so different from one another?
- Why was the woman with ALS able to compensate so well for severe respiratory impairment?
- What intervention approaches might be useful in helping to reduce the fatigue she was experiencing?
- Why did the man with ataxia develop such an unusual respiratory pattern for conversation and oral reading?
- How did his abnormal respiratory patterning affect other aspects of speech?
- What technique would be effective in teaching him to modify his abnormal breathing pattern during speech?

The impact of respiratory impairment on speakers with dysarthria is often complex to evaluate and treat. Some individuals with severely compromised respiratory function do remarkably well during speech; others with apparently less impairment use unusual and maladaptive respiratory patterns. Some speakers are able to modify their respiratory function very well in response to training; others are remarkably rigid in their respiratory patterning. For some speakers with dysarthria, respiratory dysfunction is so severe that functional speech is impossible; for others, respiratory performance does not substantially interfere with speech. We devote this chapter to the management of respiratory aspects of dysarthric speech.

The respiratory system is the source of aerodynamic energy for speech. If respiratory performance is severely impaired, adequate speech may be impossible. When it is less severely impaired, poor respiratory performance may have an impact on other speech components, most notably the phonatory system. Optimizing respiratory performance is an important aspect of speech intervention for many speakers with dysarthria, because other speech subsystems are strongly influenced by patterns of respiratory support for speech.

Overall aspects of speech, such as naturalness, may also be compromised by respiratory impairment. Breath patterning is basic to speech naturalness because the breath group may be considered the unit upon which other aspects of prosody, such as intonation and stress patterns, are superimposed. An understanding of the respiratory component of dysarthric speech is needed in order to make appropriate intervention decisions. For selected individuals with dysarthria, focus on respiratory performance during treatment is clearly beneficial.

For some individuals with dysarthria, intervention focuses primarily on improving physiologic support for speech. The goal of such an intervention is for the speaker to develop levels of subglottal air pressure and durations of subglottal air pressure for speech that will support their communication needs. For others, intervention focuses on the development of optimal patterns of respiratory performance within the limitations of their current level of physiologic support. This includes determining the level of respiratory performance that is comfortable and nonfatiguing, so that these individuals can speak over extended periods of time and communicate effectively to support the social roles that are important to them.

Question: What aspects of respiratory function do you assess during a motor speech evaluation?

Tom Hixon discussed this issue in his 1993 teleconference presentation when he said,

> Speech breathing is complex . . . but it is possible to break it down into a set of parameters that are common to all types of speech performance. It doesn't matter whether its acting, reading, conversation, cheerleading or whatever, and it doesn't matter whether it's normal or abnormal, or even if it fluctuates between normal and abnormal as sometimes it does. In my experience four parameters capture most of what I need to know about speech breathing. This is true whether I am trying to understand a research article or the

(continues)

> problems of the next patient to come through my door. The four
> essential parameters I'm referring to are (air) pressure, lung volume,
> flow, and (respiratory) shape.
>
> We also focus on these four parameters, but pay particular attention to
> the nature of the utterance that a speaker is attempting to produce. This
> allows us to focus on the respiratory adjustments made by speakers for
> shorter versus longer breath groups, stressed versus unstressed words,
> pauses versus continuous speech, and spontaneous speech as compared to
> oral reading.

RESPIRATORY FUNCTION DURING SPEECH

Normal Speakers

SUBGLOTTAL (ALVEOLAR) AIR PRESSURE

Subglottal air pressure refers to the air pressure generated below the vocal folds
(see Figure 7.1). Generally, the respiratory goal of a speaker is to generate
steady subglottal air pressure during an utterance with slight variations to support
stress patterning. When individuals talk loudly, subglottal air pressure is
greater than when they talk at a conversational level. The relationship
between subglottal air pressure and vocal intensity is approximately 1:1 for a
given speaker. Thus, if subglottal air pressure is doubled, vocal intensity is also
doubled. Whispering involves generally lower subglottal air pressure than normal
speech (Stathopoulos, Hoit, Hixon, Watson, & Solomon, 1991).

> *Question: When I read reference material, the terms subglottal air pressure
> and alveolar air pressure are used interchangeably. Is that appropriate?*
>
> The terms subglottal air pressure and alveolar air pressure are both used
> in this text to refer to the level of air pressure in the respiratory system
> below the vocal folds. For many years, the speech–language pathology
> field has used the term subglottal air pressure, while medical fields have
> referred to the air pressure below the vocal folds as alveolar air pressure.

Normal speakers accomplish the goal of stable subglottal air pressure levels
during conversational speech quite efficiently. Functioning well within their
physiologic capabilities, they do not experience fatigue during ordinary speech

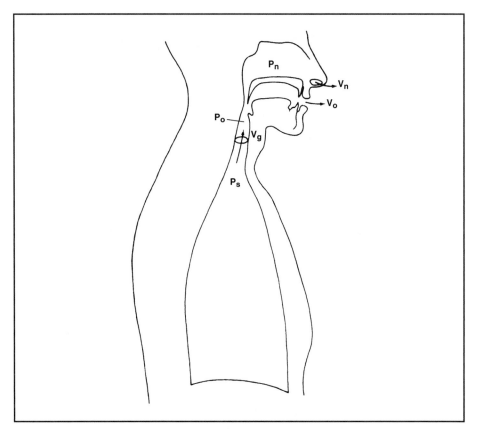

Figure 7.1. A midsagittal line drawing of the vocal tract showing pressures in nasal cavity (P_n), oral cavity (P_o), and subglottal region (P_s) and volume velocities in the glottis (V_g) and leaving the nasal (V_n) and oral tracts (V_o). From "Speech Physiology," by R. Netsell, 1973, in *Normal Aspects of Speech, Hearing and Language* (p. 215), by F. Minifie, T. Hixon, and F. Williams, Englewood Cliffs, NJ: Prentice-Hall. Copyright 1973 by Prentice-Hall. Reprinted with permission.

tasks. Although respiration for speech appears to be quite simple, adequate respiratory support and patterning requires a high level of motor control. A detailed review of the literature describing normal respiratory function for speech is well beyond the scope of this chapter. However, an understanding of the basic respiratory goals for speech and how these goals are achieved is needed if one is to understand the respiratory impairments experienced by individuals with dysarthria. Readers can find summary discussions of normal respiration for speech in a variety of sources (Folkins & Kuehn, 1982; Hixon, 1973, 1987; Hixon, Mead, & Goldman, 1976; Warren, 1996; Weismer, 1985). Commonly used respiratory volume and capacity terms are illustrated in Figure 7.2.

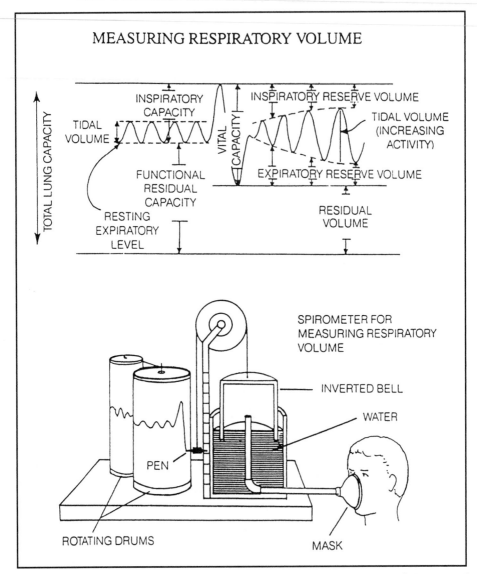

Figure 7.2. Spirogram showing lung volumes and capacities. From *Functional Anatomy of Speech, Language, and Hearing: A Primer* (p. 106), by W. Perkins and R. Kent, 1986, Austin, TX: PRO-ED. Copyright 1986 by PRO-ED, Inc. Reprinted with permission.

Respiratory Activities: The following classroom exercises assist students in understanding terminology related to speech breathing.

Exercise 1. Sit or stand quietly and do not talk.

You are *rest breathing*, that is, exchanging *tidal volume*.

Exercise 2. Continue to breathe quietly. Notice the "bottom" of the rest breathing cycle—at the end of exhalation just before you inhale. After three or four respiratory cycles, hold your breath at the bottom of the rest breathing cycle.

You are now at *resting expiratory level* (REL). Some call it *resting respiratory level* (RRL).

Exercise 3. Repeat Exercise 2 to establish your resting expiratory level. Hold your breath briefly. Now count aloud as long as you can until you need to inhale.

You are now speaking into *expiratory reserve volume*. In expiratory reserve, subglottal air pressure is generated primarily by your expiratory musculature.

Exercise 4. Continue to breathe quietly. Notice the "top" of the rest breathing cycle—at the end of inhalation just before you exhale. After three or four respiratory cycles, hold your breath at the top of the rest breathing cycle for a second and then continue to inhale before beginning to count aloud.

If you did the exercise correctly, you inhaled into the *inspiratory reserve volume* and for a time were speaking on that volume.

Exercise 5. Rest breathe for a few cycles, then inhale as deeply as possible, hold your breath for a second, and exhale as much air as you can. Work hard.

You have just experienced your *vital capacity*, that is the total amount of air that can be exhaled following maximal inhalation.

Exercise 6. Give yourself a few minutes to recover from Exercise 5. If you feel dizzy or light-headed, skip Exercise 6.

Rest breathe for a few cycles, then inhale as deeply as possible, hold your breath for a second, then speaking quietly, count aloud from 1 to 10.

(continues)

Notice how active your inspiratory muscles are at maintaining your subglottal air pressure at a low level in order to speak quietly.

You are experiencing inspiratory checking, *the action of your respiratory musculature to produce low subglottal air pressure levels at high lung volume levels.*

Exercise 7. Place the fingers of one hand on your thorax, just below your clavicle (collar bone). Place the fingers of your other hand on your abdomen. Rest breathe for a few cycles.

What was your *respiratory shape* during this activity? You should feel both your thorax and your abdomen participating in rest breathing.

Exercise 8. Using the same hand positions as in Exercise 7, rest breathe for a few cycles and then count aloud from 1 to 25.

Before beginning to count, did you feel yourself inhale to a higher lung volume level than you experienced during rest breathing? What was your respiratory shape during this activity? Did you feel both thoracic and abdominal movement? Did one movement predominate?

Exercise 9. Using the same hand positions as in Exercise 7, rest breathe for a few cycles. Hold your breath for a second when you are at REL and then count aloud from 1 to 25.

As you spoke far into expiratory reserve, what was your respiratory shape? Most people make extensive use of their abdominal muscle to generate the expiratory forces needed for this activity.

Exercise 10. Before singing a familiar song, rest breathe for a few cycles, then inhale quickly and deeply (to a high lung volume level). Sing.

During the inhalation phase of this activity, what was your respiratory shape? Did you inhale primarily using thoracic or abdominal movement? Did you expand both your thorax and your abdomen? Did you expand your thorax and collapse your abdomen? If you did, you experienced a form of *paradoxing*—the thorax and the abdomen moving in opposite directions.

ACHIEVING RESPIRATORY GOALS

The subglottal air pressure level during speech is a reflection of the driving forces of the respiratory system and the resistance to airflow imposed by the glottal and supraglottal structures.

Question: *What is the range of alveolar pressures generated during speech?*

Alveolar (subglottal) pressure can be changed by compressing and decompressing the lungs. The respiratory system movements that cause pressure changes during speech production are quite small. In fact, sometimes they are hard to see. When you talk conversationally, alveolar pressure ranges between 4 and 8 cm H_2O (Hixon, 1993).

Subglottal air pressure is generated by the compression of the volume of air in the lungs. This compression results from a combination of two forces generated by the respiratory system. One of these forces is generated by muscular activity and the other by elastic recoil of the respiratory structures. The respiratory system has many of the characteristics of a spring. The forces of elastic recoil vary depending on the lung volume level; the larger the volume of air in the lungs (lung volume level), the larger the elastic recoil force and the alveolar pressure produced by recoil forces alone. For example, at 70% lung volume level in the upright position, approximately 15 cm H_2O is generated by relaxation forces only. At 36% of lung volume level, the relaxation forces generate 0 cm H_2O.

Question: *Exactly what is meant by the term* lung volume level?

The volume of greatest importance to speech breathing is lung volume. One way to think of lung volume is that it specifies the size of the respiratory system. Lung volume is important because it represents the sum of all of the displacements of respiratory structures and because it is a manifestation of the overall "stroke" of the respiratory system for speech production. One of its strongest perceptual correlates is breath group duration. These (lung volume) excursions for speech usually cover about 10% to 20% of vital capacity and average about 5 seconds in duration. The average excursion will have about 15 syllables produced on it. Further, each syllable will involve an average lung volume expenditure of about 50 cc, which is about a third of a mouthful of air (Hixon, 1993).

Question: *What is the relation between lung volume level and vital capacity?*

Vital capacity is the volume of air that can be expelled from the lungs from a position of full inspiration. Lung volume level is the volume of air that is present in the lungs at a given point in time. Percentage of vital capacity is used as a measure of lung volume level. Lung volume level is 100% at full inspiration and 0% at full expiration.

For a given lung volume level, greater air pressures are generated in the supine as compared to the upright position. This occurs because, in the supine position, gravitational forces contribute to the net expiratory force of both the rib cage and the abdomen. In the upright position, gravitational forces contribute to the expiratory forces of the rib cage and the inspiratory forces of the abdomen. This difference in elastic recoil force, as a function of posture, is important in management of the respiratory–phonatory components of speakers with severe dysarthria. A more detailed discussion of the influence of position on respiratory function in severe dysarthria is presented later in this chapter. Readers are referred to Hixon (1973) for a complete discussion of the effects of position on the resting expiratory level in normal speakers.

In addition to the elastic recoil forces, there are forces generated by the contraction of the respiratory muscles. Subglottal air pressure is generated by the interaction of the elastic recoil and muscle contraction forces. Speech requires a constant level of subglottal air pressure throughout an utterance in the presence of a declining lung volume level. Thus, a steadily changing relationship between muscular effort and elastic recoil forces is necessary. Assume that a subglottal air pressure level of 7 cm H_2O is needed for a particular conversation. At 70% of lung volume level, elastic recoil forces generate 15 cm H_2O. Thus, at high lung volume levels, if left unchecked, forces would generate greater than necessary subglottal air pressures. Therefore, muscular activity must be in the inhalatory direction (inspiratory checking) to counterbalance the excessive contribution of the exhalatory elastic recoil forces. As lung volume levels decrease, less and less inspiratory checking is necessary. At slightly less than 60% of lung volume level, elastic recoil alone is no longer sufficient to generate adequate subglottal air pressure for speech. At this point and below, the active respiratory forces begin to act in the exhalatory direction in order to generate the appropriate level of air pressure. Thus, maximum sustained phonation, an apparently simple speech task, requires complex adjustments of the respiratory system through the course of the activity.

Maximum sustained phonation in some respects is very unlike ordinary speech utterances. Speech typically is produced by normal speakers within a relatively narrow range of lung volumes (60% to 35% of vital capacity in the seated position), which allows adequate generation of subglottal air pressure for speech with a minimal expenditure of energy (Hixon, 1987). When speech is initiated at 60% of vital capacity, the passive relaxation forces, resulting from the elastic recoil of the respiratory structures, generate subglottal air pressure nearly equal to that required for conversational speech. There is little need for contraction of the inspiratory musculature to oppose these recoil forces, as there would be if speech were initiated at 80% or 90% of vital capacity. At high lung volume levels, the associated recoil forces would generate subglottal air pressures in excess of that needed for conversational speech. During speech, as compared to rest breathing, abdominal muscles are contracted to some extent throughout the production of an utterance. The active role of the abdomen throughout speech appears to "tune" the respiratory musculature for increased efficiency during the inspiratory and expiratory phases of respiration for speech. During loud speech associated with increased subglottal air pressure, normal speakers typically inhale to lung volume levels greater than 60% of vital capacity in order to efficiently initiate speech at a subglottal air pressure level similar to that which is generated by the elastic recoil forces of the respiratory structures.

Normal speakers can achieve elastic recoil forces in a number of ways. Throughout the lung volume level range used for speech, the elastic recoil forces and muscular forces interact somewhat differently to compress the air within the respiratory system in order to generate a steady level of subglottal air pressure. The normal speaker is able to vary the relative contributions of the chest wall structures and the abdomen to the respiratory patterns for speech. For example, one speaker might increase lung volume level primarily through expansion of the thorax with minimal expansion of the abdomen, whereas another speaker might increase lung volume level primarily through expansion of the abdomen.

Question: The notion of "respiratory shape" is a new concept for me. What is the respiratory shape of a "normal" (nonimpaired) individual?

According to Hixon (1993),

> Respiratory shape . . . means the configuration of the respiratory system. . . . It is specified by the relative positions of the rib cage and abdomen. These two can be moved in and out in different combinations. When we are relaxed, the rib cage is pulled downward by gravity and the abdomen is distended outward by the weight of the abdominal mass. We take on the shape of a pear under this circumstance, but when we talk, the abdominal wall is moved inward about a fourth of the way along its range of motion. . . . When we talk we tuck our bellies in slightly and push our rib cages to expanded positions. . . . A "belly in" strategy allows me to inspire very quickly during my running speech. The reason is that my diaphragm is mechanically tuned when my abdomen is inward, so that it can contract quickly and forcefully. Quick inspirations are a hallmark of running speech.

Gender and age influence respiratory patterns during speech. In their study of speech breathing patterns of men of three age ranges (25, 50, and 75 years),

Hoit and Hixon (1987) reported that older men, when compared with younger men, used larger lung volume excursions, larger lung volume expenditures per syllable, initiations at higher lung volume levels, and fewer syllables per breath. The authors suggested that these age-related changes may be associated with changes in laryngeal function. Perhaps as men age, their laryngeal valving becomes less efficient, allowing greater expenditure of air during speech. The respiratory changes with increasing age are required to compensate for this air wastage. This hypothesis has been supported in a subsequent study. Laryngeal airway resistance is lower for men 75 years of age than for men 10 years younger (Melcon, Hoit, & Hixon, 1989). In a later study, Hoit and colleagues investigated the speech breathing patterns of women in three age ranges (25, 50, and 75 years). They concluded that the patterns of age-related differences are quite similar for the two sexes when the measures obtained are normalized for body size (Hoit, Hixon, Altman, & Morgan, 1989).

Different speaking tasks also influence respiratory performance during speech. Normal adult male speakers (ages 52 to 74 years) produced more syllables, used more time for speech per breath group, and spoke at a more rapid rate during monologue than for reading (Solomon & Hixon, 1993). Average airflow during speech was greater for monologue, possibly because speakers may use less efficient valving by the larynx and the articulators when they need to formulate thoughts and do not need to rush. Similar results have been observed for young women speakers with no known impairment (Hodge & Putnam-Rochet, 1989).

In summary, normal speakers not only are able to generate a steady level of subglottal air pressure throughout an utterance, but also are able to do so in a highly efficient manner that is well within the mid-range of their physiologic capabilities. Their speech breathing is influenced to some extent by gender, age, body type, and speaking task.

Typical Breath Group Length

In addition to the perceptual estimates of loudness, clinicians need to make judgments about breath patterning characteristics. Normal speech breathing is characterized by rapid inhalation and a prolonged period of exhalation. Typically, the ratio of inhalation to exhalation duration is approximately 1:6 for normal speakers. Figure 7.3 illustrates lung volume levels obtained as a normal speaker reads a passage. Note that this speaker inhales to slightly more than 60% of lung volume level and, depending on the utterance, speaks until she reaches approximately 35% of lung volume level. At that time, she inhales again. Note also that this speaker inhales to higher lung volume levels before beginning long utterances, and inhales to only 55% of lung volume level before initiating the final four-word utterance. Figure 7.4 shows the frequency of

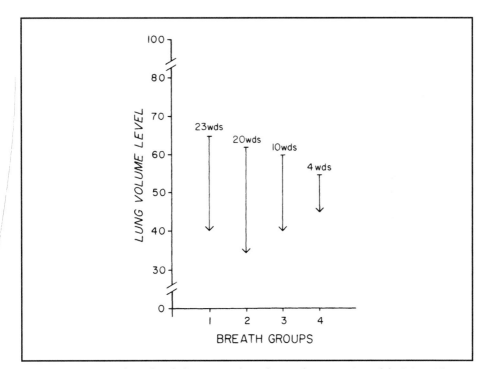

Figure 7.3. Lung volume levels for a normal speaker reading a portion of the Mount Ranier Paragraph. The following utterances correspond to breath groups 1 through 4: (1) I pointed to the mountain covered with snow, but someone said, "Don't try to show him all that snow. Show Sam some snow." (2) I picked up a handful of snow and began to show everyone but they interrupted and said, "Show Sam some snow." (3) Pretending to be angry, I questioned "Show Sam some snow?" (4) What a ridiculous idea.

occurrence of breath group lengths for groups of dysarthric and normal speakers (Hammen & Yorkston, 1994). During connected speech, normal speakers took most of their breaths (74%) at primary syntactic junctures (sentence boundaries) and only a few of their breaths (3%) within a phrase or a clause. Speakers with dysarthria, by contrast, took less than half of their breaths (39%) at primary syntactic junctures and approximately one quarter (23%) within a phrase or a clause (Hammen & Yorkston, 1994).

Patterns of Respiratory Impairment for Speakers with Dysarthria

As was apparent in Chapters 2, 3, and 4, speakers with dysarthria experience a wide range of speech symptoms depending on the type and severity of their

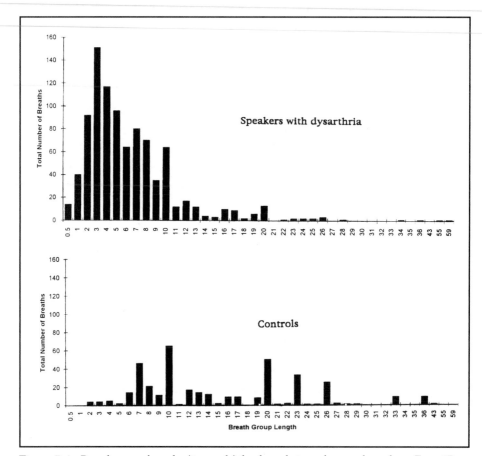

Figure 7.4. Breath group lengths (in words) for dysarthric and normal speakers. From "Respiratory Patterning and Variability in Dysarthric Speech," by V. L. Hammen and K. M. Yorkston, 1994, *Journal of Medical Speech–Language Pathology*, 2(4), p. 257. Copyright 1994 by Singular. Reprinted with permission.

dysarthria. Impairment of the respiratory system in specific speakers is often complex to understand because it is influenced by many different factors. For some, respiratory impairment is a primary symptom of the neurologic conditions that cause the dysarthria. However, for others, respiratory performance is an appropriate compensation for inadequacy of other aspects of the speech mechanism that allows excessive air wastage during speech. Finally, respiratory impairment may occur because of speakers' maladaptive attempts to compensate for current or previous speech problems.

The goals of dysarthria assessment and intervention are to identify the nature of respiratory support for speech, identify those aspects of respiratory performance that need to be modified, determine which of these factors can be modified, and engage the speaker in appropriate intervention procedures. We have found that knowledge of the type of dysarthria only (flaccid, spastic, ataxic, etc.) is an inadequate base on which to treat a speaker with dysarthria and respiratory impairment. Rather, it is necessary to assess the individual's speech performance and identify the pattern of impairment.

In our clinical practice, we have observed a number of patterns of respiratory impairment in speakers with dysarthria. Some of these patterns reflect primary neuromotor impairment, some are compensatory, and others are maladaptive.

PRIMARY RESPIRATORY IMPAIRMENTS

The respiratory symptoms associated with dysarthria may be the result of the underlying or primary neurologic impairment. Weak, unpredictable, or uncoordinated respiratory movements affect speech. For example, speakers who experience weak respiratory musculature have difficulty generating the levels and durations of subglottal air pressure needed for speech. When the impairment is severe, they are unable to produce phonation for speech. When it is moderate, they demonstrate overall reduced loudness or decreasing loudness toward the end of utterances. Fatigue during speech is common. Weak respiratory support for speech is observed in adults with flaccid and hypokinetic dysarthria. Children with spastic cerebral palsy also experience difficulty generating adequate respiratory support for speech.

Normal speakers are able to produce stable patterns of subglottal air pressure dependent upon the task. When they wish to talk loudly, they increase subglottal air pressure, and when they wish to speak softly, they decrease subglottal air pressure. Throughout an utterance the level of subglottal air pressure is relatively consistent. Speakers with dysarthria who produce inconsistent loudness or bursts of excessive loudness demonstrate unpredictable respiratory support for speech. Speakers with hyperkinetic dysarthria are the most common group to demonstrate these symptoms because of unpredictable bursts of muscle contraction resulting from the chorea or dystonia.

Speech is a highly coordinated activity. Individuals with neuromotor impairment may not have the coordination necessary for the proper timing of speech movements. Such mistiming may lead to air wastage, which involves release of a portion of air supply prior to initiation of an utterance. Children with cerebral palsy often demonstrate this pattern; that is, they inhale to relatively high lung volume levels and allow air to be expired (and wasted) before activation of the vocal tract to speak.

COMPENSATORY RESPIRATORY STRATEGIES

Changes in respiratory performance may also be the result of the speaker's attempt to make up for impairment in other aspects of speech production. When the function of vocal tract valves (laryngeal, velopharyngeal, or oral articulatory subsystems) are inefficient and excessive air is allowed to escape during speech, the function of the respiratory system is affected. If they are capable, speakers with dysarthria will attempt to compensate for vocal tract inefficiency by making increased demands on the respiratory system. In an effort to compensate, speakers may reduce the length of breath groups, speak softly, inhale to higher lung volume levels, or overdrive their respiratory systems. Speakers with flaccid dysarthria and hypokinetic dysarthria frequently face problems related to inefficient vocal tract valving.

Speakers with hyperadduction of the vocal folds due to spastic or hyperkinetic dysarthria engage in a different type of respiratory compensation. Hyperadduction of vocal folds results in increased laryngeal resistance to airflow through the glottis. Therefore, the speaker with dysarthria usually talks with increased subglottal air pressure to compensate for vocal fold hyperadduction. Typically, the speaker has no choice but to engage in this compensation, unless the level of vocal fold hyperadduction can be reduced (see Chapter 8 for a discussion of intervention at the level of the larynx).

When speakers experience neuromotor incoordination of the type associated with ataxic dysarthria, they frequently employ a simplification strategy to compensate for respiratory impairment. Typically, these individuals speak with excess and equal stress patterning during which each syllable (or word) is produced with a "pulse" of subglottal air pressure. Apparently, these speakers attempt to coordinate their upper vocal tract activity by using this one-word-at-a-time strategy.

MALADAPTIVE RESPIRATORY STRATEGIES

As was suggested in the previous section, abnormal respiratory function may reflect speakers' efforts to adjust for respiratory inadequacy or vocal tract inefficiency. At times these compensations or adjustments are maladaptive in that they cause more harm than good. Maladaptive breath patterning may be present because of either current or prior vocal tract dysfunction. The following example illustrates how a compensation that once may have been effective may later become maladaptive. One of our clients experienced extensive weakness following traumatic brain injury. Initially, her respiratory support was inadequate for connected speech because of respiratory weakness, hypoadduction of the vocal folds, and consistently inadequate velopharyngeal closure during speech. Therefore, early in her recovery, she produced one syllable per breath group. In time, she was fitted with a palatal lift, laryngeal hypoadduction was reduced, and respiratory strength returned. However, she continued to speak using a single-word-per-breath-group pattern, even though she demonstrated considerable respiratory capacity by sustaining phonation for many seconds and counting aloud from 1 to 20.

Speakers with dysarthria engage in a variety of maladaptive respiratory strategies that result in speech at inappropriate lung volume levels. Normal speakers assess the respiratory demands of an upcoming speech act and prepare their respiratory systems accordingly. For example, if the utterance will be very short, they may not inhale before speaking. However, if the utterance is to be long or loud, they inhale to a much higher lung volume level before beginning to talk. Some speakers with severe dysarthria do not engage in preparatory inhalation before beginning an utterance regardless of its length or loudness. Rather, they begin to speak at the prevailing lung volume level available at the moment. If they happen to initiate an utterance at a low lung volume level, they must either speak far into expiratory reserve or inhale after only a few words or syllables. A variation of this pattern involves the use of brief "catch" breaths during connected speech. Because these speakers do not inhale to 60% or 65% of lung volume level before initiating speech, they may try to compensate by taking repeated small inhalations (5% to 10% of lung volume level) every few syllables or words. Finally, some individuals with dysarthria engage in the maladaptive respiratory strategy of failing to inhale in a timely manner during connected speech and talking deep into expiratory reserve. Many find this pattern very fatiguing. Some experience increased vocal roughness when speaking deep in expiratory reserve. If laryngeal spasticity is present, the vocal roughness may be even more prominent.

Assessment

Perceptual Indicators of Respiratory Inadequacy

Clinical assessment of respiratory function begins with the question, "Is respiratory function adequate for speech?" Because respiratory demands for conversational speech are minimal compared with the physiologic capability of normal speakers, respiratory function that is not normal in all respects may be adequate to support conversational speech. At a preliminary level, we judge adequacy of respiration for speech with perceptual judgments of connected speech. We are fully aware of the potential for failing to identify the presence of abnormal respiratory patterns in some speakers who may sound normal in terms of the respiratory aspects of speech. However, we need more basic research before the seriousness of this risk can be evaluated. For the present, if the respiratory component of speech appears adequate to the trained eyes and ears of the clinician, the respiratory function evaluation stops. A number of visual–auditory characteristics may alert the clinician to potential respiratory impairment. If any of these characteristics appears, respiratory function is examined in depth.

> *Question: When assessing a person with a motor speech disorder, how do the self-perceptions of the speaker fit into intervention decisions?*
>
> Adequacy of speech performance must be assessed in terms of the *disability* experienced by the speaker. The performance of speakers should be judged according to their preferred roles and social contexts. Thus, communicative performance that may be adequate for the optimized clinical setting (quiet room, face-to-face, small group) may be inadequate for the contexts in which speakers routinely function or prefer to function.

LOUDNESS

As described earlier, the primary respiratory goal for speech is to generate an adequate, sustained energy source. An adequate loudness level for connected speech is a good indicator of the adequacy of respiratory support. However, reduced loudness may be the result of a variety of physiologic, psychological, and social factors. Loudness is closely related to the level of subglottal air pressure being generated. While listening to a sample of connected speech, the speech–language pathologist asks the following questions:

- Is the overall loudness level too high or too low?

- Is the loudness level consistent?

- Are sudden uncontrolled alternations in loudness present?

- Does loudness diminish over the course of a single breath group unit or over the course of extended speech?

- Can the speaker increase speech loudness (shout)?

- Can the speaker produce quiet phonation?

- Does the speaker complain of fatigue when speaking for extended periods of time at conversational loudness levels?

- Can the speaker emphasize (stress) words in a sentence by increasing loudness?

- Do some words have more prominence than others?

If the clinician identifies a loudness problem, then an in-depth examination of respiratory–laryngeal components during speech must be carried out. Particular attention should be given to the speaker's ability to produce adequate levels of subglottal air pressure.

BREATH PATTERNING

Clinicians, during the initial perceptual evaluation, should listen for evidence suggesting an abnormal pattern or timing of inhalation and exhalation for speech. The following questions pertain to this aspect of speech:

- Does the speech respiratory pattern differ from the normal pattern of quick inhalation followed by a prolonged exhalation?

- Does the speaker inhale to an appropriate lung volume level?

- At what point in the respiratory cycle does the speaker initiate an utterance?

- Is there a quick preparatory inhalation before the initiation of an utterance?

- Does the speaker use pauses for emphasis, or do all of the pauses contain an inhalation?

- Is speech interrupted by sudden, forced inspiration or expiration sighs?

- Are exaggerated respiratory maneuvers, such as excessive elevation of the shoulders during inhalation, apparent during speech?

- Does the speaker appear to run out of air before inhaling?

In addition to movement patterns during inhalation and exhalation, the clinician may find evidence of respiratory impairment by examining the phrasing or breath group units produced during connected speech. The following questions relate to breath group units:

- How many words or syllables does the speaker produce on one breath?

- What is the duration (in seconds) of each breath group?

- Do breaths occur at syntactically appropriate locations in the utterance?

The performance of some speakers with dysarthria is extremely different from the physiologically flexible, rule-governed performance of normal individuals. Figure 7.5 contains respiratory data during paragraph reading by a speaker with

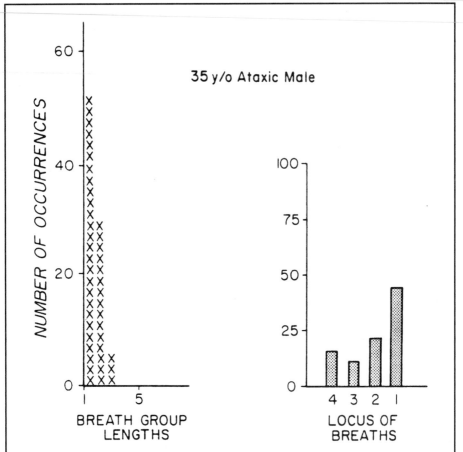

Figure 7.5. Breath group lengths (in words) and locus of breath codes for a speaker with predominantly ataxic dysarthria.

brain injury and predominantly ataxic dysarthria. Examination of the figure suggests that most of the time this speaker inhaled after only one or two words. Because short breath groups are frequently associated with reduced respiratory support in speakers with dysarthria, it is tempting to speculate that this speaker simply did not have the respiratory support for more extended breath groups. Although this may be the case for some speakers, this individual was able to sustain phonation for more than 15 seconds and to count to over 20 on a single breath when instructed to do so. Clearly, he had the physiologic capability to avoid grammatically impermissible locations for inhalation. Although this case may be extreme, many speakers with dysarthria disrupt the naturalness of their speech needlessly by taking breaths at grammatically impermissible locations.

Instrumental Examination of Respiratory Impairment

Once the presence of inadequate respiratory support has been confirmed through perceptual evaluation, an attempt is made to examine respiratory function in depth. This is typically accomplished with instrumental measurement techniques. The perceptual analysis of respiratory function during connected speech alerts the clinician to a potential problem. A more detailed series of questions is addressed in the in-depth examination. These questions may include the following:

- Is the speaker achieving the primary respiratory goals of a steady energy source during speech?

- How are pressures being generated?

- Does impairment of other speech components contribute to the perception of inadequate respiratory function during speech?

- Is the respiratory impairment physiologically based, or does the pattern appear to be related to learned maladaptive patterns?

ADEQUACY OF RESPIRATORY SUPPORT

We begin the in-depth evaluation of respiratory function by examining the energy source for speech. Measurement of subglottal air pressure is the most direct approach to assessing respiratory adequacy for speech. In speakers with tracheostomies, subglottal air pressure can be sensed through the tracheostomy tube or tracheostomy button. However, in speakers without tracheostomies, it is difficult to directly measure subglottal air pressure. Rather, subglottal air pressure levels are estimated by measuring intraoral air pressure during the stop phase of a voiceless stop consonant and estimating the corresponding level of subglottal air pressure. Consider the posturing of the speech mechanism structures during the stop phase of /p/ in "apa." The respiratory system provides the driving force for speech. The glottis is open for the voiceless phoneme /p/. The oral cavity is a sealed system, because the velopharyngeal port is closed and the lips are closed. Because the glottis is open and the remaining system is sealed, the oral and subglottal cavities can be considered to function as a single cavity from an aerodynamic point of view (Netsell, 1969; Smitheran & Hixon, 1981). During conversational speech, the normal adult's subglottal air pressure level averages between 4 and 8 cm H_2O.

Although measurement of intraoral air pressure during the stop phase of the voiceless plosive /t/ or /p/ is a good estimate of subglottal air pressure for normal speakers, care must be taken in obtaining and interpreting these measures for speakers with dysarthria. One cannot assume that reduced air pressure values for speakers with dysarthria are always indicative of respiratory weakness or incoordination. Because subglottal air pressures generated by the compression of the respiratory mechanism may be acted upon by several of the speech valves, it is possible that impairment of the larynx, velopharyngeal mechanism, or oral articulators may also contribute to reduced air pressure values (Hardy & Arkebauer, 1966).

If intraoral air pressure is to be used as an estimate of subglottal air pressure, both the velopharyngeal port and the anterior oral cavity must be completely sealed. Simultaneous sensing of nasal airflow through a full face mask is one way of verifying these seals. If nasal airflow is observed, a nose clip should be used to obstruct the nasal airflow. If, on subsequent recordings, no airflow was recorded during the stop phase of the consonant, one would assume that the velopharyngeal port had been responsible for the air leak from the oral cavity under the previous condition. With the occlusion of the nasal airflow, one could estimate subglottal air pressure from the intraoral air pressure measure. A comparison of the level of intraoral air pressure measures with and without the nares occluded would provide some indication of the effect of velopharyngeal impairment on the speaker's ability to generate adequate air pressures for speech.

If, during the measurement of intraoral air pressure with the nares occluded, airflow was still present, one would assume that the oral seal was inadequate to prevent the escape of air from the oral cavity during the production of the voiceless stop consonant. An attempt would be made to sense intraoral air pressure during the production of a different voiceless consonant in an effort to find a consonant that could be produced without escape of air during the stop phase of the consonant. If this was not possible, intraoral air pressure could not be used as an accurate estimate of subglottal air pressure.

Although aerodynamic estimates of subglottal air pressure are good indicators of the adequacy of respiratory support for speech, this technique requires instrumentation that is not always available clinically. When such instrumentation is unavailable, clinicians may estimate respiratory adequacy with simple devices such as those shown in Figures 7.6 and 7.7. Netsell and Hixon (1978) suggested the use of a manometer with a "leak" tube as an inexpensive means of estimating subglottal air pressure (Figure 7.6). Just as with the aerodynamic transduction equipment described earlier, a velopharyngeal and lip seal is assumed when using a mouthpiece. A full face mask that captures both nasal and oral airflow may be used when either the velopharyngeal or lip seal is inadequate. Using this technique, the client is asked to blow and to maintain a target level of water pressure. Netsell and Hixon gave the following clinical rule of thumb: "An individual who can generate and sustain 5 cm H_2O for 5 sec with the 'leak' tube has sufficient pressure capability to meet most speech requirements" (p. 329).

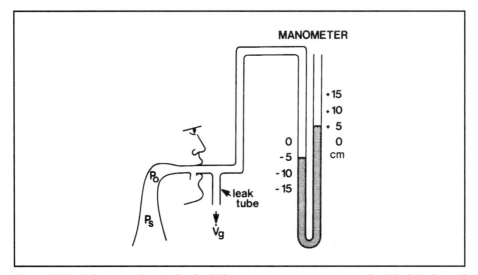

Figure 7.6. A drawing of an individual blowing into a manometer with a "leak" tube and generating 10 cm H_2O. From "A Noninvasive Method for Clinically Estimating Subglottal Air Pressure," by R. Netsell and T. Hixon, 1978, *Journal of Speech and Hearing Disorders, 43,* p. 328. Copyright 1978 by American Speech and Hearing Association. Reprinted with permission.

Hixon, Hawley, and Wilson (1982) suggested an even simpler "homemade" device for determining respiratory driving pressures using a drinking glass with a straw. After filling the glass with water, the straw is inserted into the water to the depth of the air pressure desired. For example, in Figure 7.7, an individual blowing into the straw would need to generate 5 cm H_2O in order to initiate the flow of bubbles at the end of the straw. In order to sustain 5 cm H_2O for seconds, this individual would have to blow a continuous stream of bubbles for 5 seconds. If a client is very weak, the clinician might want to insert the tube only 3 cm into the water. In order for bubbles to emerge from the tube, the client would need to produce 3 cm H_2O.

Many clinicians ask individuals with dysarthria to sustain a neutral vowel in order to obtain an indication of respiratory support on a speechlike task. A number of cautions are warranted when using this technique. As noted earlier, maximum sustained phonation is not a simple task from the standpoint of respiratory control. It reflects phonatory as well as respiratory performance. For example, a speaker with a breathy voice quality due to inefficient laryngeal control will "waste" air, with resultant reduction in sustained phonation time. On the other hand, a speaker with dysarthria and strained–strangled voice quality may be generating excessive subglottal air pressure in order to initiate

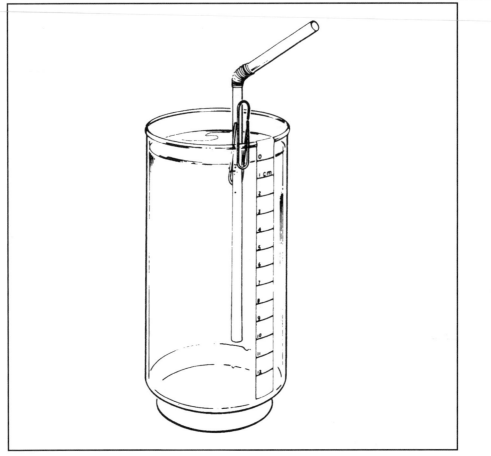

Figure 7.7. A drinking glass with a straw inserted to a depth of 10 cm. This device can be used as an indicator of respiratory driving pressure. From "An Around-the-House Device for the Clinical Determination of Respiratory Driving Pressure," by T. Hixon, J. Hawley, and J. Wilson, 1982, *Journal of Speech and Hearing Disorders, 47,* p. 414. Copyright 1982 by American Speech-Language-Hearing Association. Reprinted with permission.

and sustain phonation. It should also be noted that sustained phonation tasks more accurately reflect maximum respiratory capacity rather than breath support required for a series of breath groups during connected speech. Although most normal individuals can sustain phonation for a longer period of time, a minimum sustained time of approximately 15.0 seconds for adult males and females is acceptable (Hirano, Koike, & von Leden, 1968). Remember that the respiratory capabilities of normal individuals are far greater than the respiratory demands for conversational speech. When speakers are instructed to sustain phonation for as long as possible, they usually inhale to lung volume levels much higher than are appropriate for conversational speech. Thus, the speaker with dysarthria cannot be expected to produce consecutive breath groups in contextual speech that match in duration the maximal effort seen in sustained phonation. Our approach clinically is not to require maximum phonation, but rather to request that the speaker produce phonation for a relatively brief period of time, 4 or 5 seconds, and conversational loudness and quality. In this way, the task more closely reflects the respiratory demands of connected speech.

Respiratory Movement

APPROACHES TO MEASUREMENT

Observation of the respiratory movements of speakers with dysarthria suggests that a variety of impairments may occur. Some speakers exhibit excessive respiratory movements during speech. In some cases, excessive elevation of the shoulders and expansion of the thorax may be indicative of an effort to compensate for poor abdominal control. In other cases, observations of changes in respiratory shape may reveal paradoxical movements of the thorax and the abdomen. Paradoxing is a maneuver in which the circumference of the thorax is increased during inhalation while the circumference of the abdomen is decreased, or vice versa. Because the two movements are, in effect, working at cross-purposes, inadequate respiratory support for speech may be the result. In still other cases, speakers with dysarthria appear to be attempting to speak at lung volume levels well below those observed for tidal breathing.

Changes in chest wall shape and estimates of lung volume levels can be observed perceptually by placing one hand over the diaphragm and the other on the rib cage. Of course, these perceptual observations are extremely informal and cannot yield precise or objective measures of shape, timing, and respiratory volume. Currently, the most popular devices for objective measurement of respiratory shape are the magnetometer system used by Hixon et al. (1976), and the Respitrace unit (Hunker, Bless, & Weismer, 1981). Respiratory Inductive Plethysmography (RIP), or Respitrace, is a transduction system designed to monitor circumferential size changes in the rib cage and abdomen. The system consists of two coils of insulated wire glued to cotton mesh bands that fit snugly around the speaker's torso (see Figure 7.8). The Respitrace unit electronically sums the individual rib cage and abdominal contributions to obtain a calibrated index of total lung volume change. Results of either the magnatometer system or the Respitrace unit can be displayed in movement-by-time or movement-by-movement (rib cage-by-abdomen) displays (Abbs, Hunker, & Barlow, 1983; Putnam & Hixon, 1984).

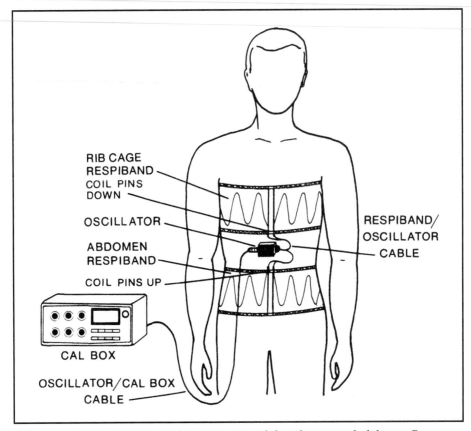

Figure 7.8. A line drawing of the positioning of the rib cage and abdomen Respitrace bands. Reprinted with permission of Ambulatory Monitoring, Inc., Ardsley, New York, NY 10502.

DESCRIPTION OF THE MOVEMENT IMPAIRMENT

Although some individuals with dysarthria initiate utterances at lung volume levels similar to those of normal speakers, many with respiratory impairment employ several different patterns.

Reduced Vital Capacity—Due to reduced vital capacity as compared to normal speakers, some speakers with dysarthria are unable to generate adequate subglottal air pressure amplitudes and durations for functional speech when utterances are initiated at 60% of this reduced vital capacity. These individuals may need to routinely initiate utterances at levels greater than 60% of vital capacity.

Inconsistent Lung Volume Level—Some speakers with dysarthria initiate utterances at the prevailing lung volume level without taking a preparatory breath prior to speech. Other individuals initiate utterances at varying lung volume levels. Figure 7.9 illustrates the lung volume levels at which utterances were initiated and terminated by a 28-year-old woman with Friedreich's ataxia as she read a paragraph. This speaker is intelligible, but is producing this passage at a slow rate (81 wpm). A comparison of this performance with that of the normal speakers in Figure 7.3 suggests many differences. Perhaps the most obvious is the increased number of inhalations produced by the speaker with dysarthria. The lung volume level at which she appears to be initiating utterances is generally reduced as compared both to the normal speakers and to her own resting breathing lung volume levels. During speech, this woman does not achieve lung volume levels as high as those she achieves during quiet breathing. The levels at which she initiates utterances are also highly variable. At times she continues to speak at low lung volume levels and fails to return to appropriate levels after inhalation. This is particularly the case with breath group units 11 through 13, where inhalations are insufficient to return the speaker to an appropriate lung volume level. When she fails to return to an appropriate lung volume level, she produces only two or three words before inhaling again.

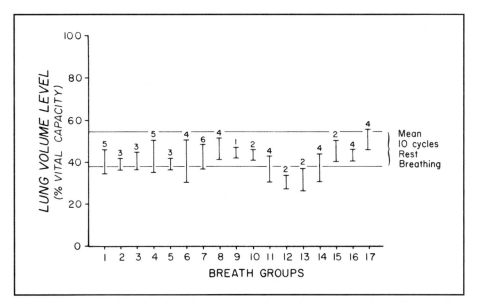

Figure 7.9. Lung volume level produced by a speaker with ataxic dysarthria who is reading a portion of the Mount Ranier Paragraph. The range indicates the lung volume levels at which the following breath groups were initiated and terminated: (1) I pointed to the mountain (2) covered with snow, (3) but someone said, (4) "Don't try to show him (5) all that snow. (6) Show Sam some snow." (7) I picked a handful of snow (8) and began (9) to show (10) everyone, (11) but they (12) interrupted and said, (13) "Show Sam (14) some snow." (15) Pretending to be angry, (16) I questioned, (17) "Show Sam some snow? What a ridiculous idea." Also noted as a referent is the range of lung volume level for rest breathing.

Inappropriate Lung Volume Level—This pattern of lung volume level use has several forms. Many individuals with severe dysarthria are unable to voluntarily modify their rest breathing patterns. Therefore, they are unable to modify volume level and initiate inhalation at approximately 60% (upper levels of tidal volume). For those with efficient phonatory and laryngeal systems, this lung volume level range may be adequate for speech. However, many individuals with dysarthria need to initiate speech at a lung volume level higher than 60%. Other individuals with dysarthria will consistently exhale partially before initiating speech. Thus, they inhale to an adequate lung volume level to support speech, but then exhale or allow air wastage before speech is initiated. This pattern may occur because of impairment of laryngeal function or a maladaptive attempt to compensate for such an impairment of laryngeal control. Finally, some individuals with severe dysarthria are unable to initiate phonation unless they are very low in lung volume level. Then, once phonation is initiated, they have a minimal respiratory reserve for the production of the remainder of the utterance. This is particularly true of persons who have difficulty adducting their vocal folds and compensate with extensive muscular effort, which results in considerable air wastage from the respiratory system.

Excessive Lung Volume Levels—In an effort to compensate for inefficient phonatory, velopharyngeal, and articulatory functions, some speakers with dysarthria inhale to excessive lung volume levels prior to the initiation of speech. The resulting high level of subglottal air pressure is associated with excessively loud speech for those who are able to initiate phonation at such high lung volume levels. For those who are unable to initiate phonation efficiently at that lung volume level, there may be excessive air wastage.

TREATMENT

The overall treatment goal for respiratory impairments in dysarthria is to achieve a consistent subglottal air pressure level, thus allowing nonfatiguing production of speech with adequate loudness and breath group length. The selection of intervention procedures is based on assessment information from each specific client. Using information about the client's respiratory pattern, the clinician selects preliminary respiratory intervention strategies.

Earlier in this chapter, three general patterns of respiratory impairment were introduced. An analysis of assessment results reveals whether the particular respiratory patterns are primary respiratory impairments, compensatory strategies, maladaptive strategies, or some combination. Primary impairments occur because of the neuromotor disorder associated with the client's disease, syndrome, or condition and include (a) weak respiratory support, (b) unpredictable respiratory support, or (c) mistiming among speech subsystems. Intervention usually focuses directly on primary respiratory impairments and, perhaps, concurrently on other speech subsystem impairments as well. Compensatory respiratory strategies occur as the speaker attempts to respond respiratorily to impairments elsewhere in the speech mechanism, such as in the laryngeal, velopharyngeal, and oral articulatory subsystems. Compensatory strategies are appropriate adjustments made by the speaker to optimize his or her speech performance. Intervention usually focuses on those aspects of the speech mechanism that are impaired rather than directly on the respiratory subsystem. Maladaptive respiratory strategies are inappropriate and/or nonproductive strategies that speakers have developed in response to impairments that are currently present or were present in the past. Occasionally, maladaptive strategies were appropriate compensatory strategies at an earlier point in recovery, but have become maladaptive as they are no longer needed. Intervention may focus only on the maladaptive strategies or on residual primary impairments as well.

Establishing Respiratory Support

As in any intervention activity, the clinician is faced with the task of choosing speakers who are candidates for a particular type of treatment program. In an effort to describe speakers for whom basic respiratory patterns for speech must be developed, we have included the following characteristics:

- The speaker has estimated levels of subglottal air pressure of 5 cm H_2O or less on speech or speechlike tasks.

- The speaker is unable to sustain consistent air pressure (at or above a given level) for 5 seconds.

- The speaker is unable to generate adequate subglottal air pressure to support phonation.

- The speaker has such limited respiratory support or control for speech that a one-word-at-a-time speech pattern is used during connected speech.

If a speaker exhibits one of more of these characteristics, respiratory intervention should be considered.

Production of Consistent Subglottal Air Pressure

The production of a consistent level of subglottal air pressure is a primary goal of the respiratory function during speech. Reports are available of a biofeedback approach to train a client with flaccid dysarthria to sustain air pressures within the range used for speech (5 to 10 cm H_2O) (Netsell & Daniel, 1979). At the beginning of treatment, their client generated only 2 to 3 cm H_2O for no more than 3 seconds. They instructed their client to blow into the pressure sensor (a water manometer) with a "leak tube" that allowed air to escape at a rate associated with normal phonation (75 to 125 cc/sec). This client was able to generate 10 cm H_2O for 10 seconds by the end of the eight 20-minute training sessions.

In our clinical practice, we have modified the simple "blow-bottle" device described by Hixon et al. (1982) by using slightly different materials. We use a plastic bottle with a hole in the cover. A tube is then inserted through the hole and into the water. We have found this approach useful as a training tool, as the plastic materials do not break when dropped, and the cover with a small vent hole allows air to escape but does not allow water to be expelled when excessive air pressures are generated by some speakers with dysarthria.

Question: *Some speakers with dysarthria are unable to seal their lips around a small tube. What adaptations can be used such that these individuals can participate in the blow-bottle task described in the previous paragraph?*

Some individuals are unable to generate oral air pressure during the tasks described above either because they are unable to seal their lips around the tubing or because they are unable to achieve velopharyngeal closure during the blowing tasks. Clinically, we have addressed these difficulties in two ways. First, for those with inadequate lip closure, we have modified the approach by inserting the tubing through a rubber or plastic stopper or by having a prosthodontist fabricate a custom mouth piece. When these approaches fail, we have sealed the tubing into a full face mask, thereby eliminating the need for a lip seal. When lip weakness is mild, the clinician may assist clients to achieve lip seal, by manually positioning their lips around the tubing. For persons who are unable to achieve velopharyngeal closure during the blowing task, we have used nose clips (clamps) during the blowing task or have used the full face mask and instructed the individual to complete the task by blowing gently into the face mask.

Another approach to training sustained air pressure generation employs an air pressure transducer similar to that described in the assessment section. The output from the pressure sensing system is displayed on an oscilloscope for feedback information to the speaker. The target air pressure levels can be set on the oscilloscopic screen using a second cursor. We have used this air pressure feedback approach with individuals following traumatic brain injury who demonstrate difficulty in maintaining consistent air pressure levels or who produce excessively large air pressure values during speech. Rather than attempt to train them during speech, we have simplified their task by initially training them during nonspeech activities. Generally, training is continued until they are able to sustain intraoral air pressures at approximately 5 cm H_2O for 5 seconds or until their performance plateaus. Although it is clear that sustaining 5 cm H_2O for 5 seconds is not normal performance, we typically stop training on this task when this "5 for 5" target has been achieved (Netsell & Hixon, 1978). We do this at least in part because our goal is "easy" production rather than maximal production. At times, maximal performances encourage the speaker to exhale to excessively low lung volume levels. We do not wish to encourage a habit that may be maladaptive for speech.

In addition to the blowing techniques, another approach to training consistent air pressure generation is to have the client produce sustained phonation. The intensity level of the sound can be monitored on a VU meter or with an intensity measurement device such as a Visipitch (available at 2 Bridgewater Lane, Lincoln Park, NJ 07035-1488). This task can be used successfully only if laryngeal control is reasonably good. It is a more difficult task than the nonspeech tasks described previously. Once respiratory support for sustained phonation can be controlled, we usually attempt to involve the client in tasks that are more speechlike, such as the repetition of syllables. Air pressure can then be monitored with a pressure sensing tube inserted through the corner of the mouth. Vocal intensity can also be monitored instrumentally.

Finally, clients can be instructed to produce consistent phonation while producing utterances. Utterance lengths are selected so that the speaker is physiologically able to produce the entire utterance in one breath. The air pressure is monitored by constructing the utterances containing many tokens of the phoneme /p/ and sensing the air pressure during those productions as described before. Measurement of vocal intensity during utterances of this type is less effective than aerodynamic measurement, because of the various levels of sound energy associated with different vowel and consonant sounds.

For an individual who speaks with excessive effort and generates subglottal air pressures in excess of that needed for the speaking task, air pressure monitoring can be used to train him or her to reduce air pressure and, thus, effort. This individual may habitually generate air pressures between 10 and 20 cm H_2O during conversational speech. By displaying air pressure levels on an oscilloscope, the client can often be trained to speak with levels below 10 cm H_2O. This air pressure reduction is often accompanied by a normalization of other parameters of respiration, such as breath group length, lung volume level, and respiratory shape. In addition, normalization of air pressure levels may be associated with a normalization of phonatory symptoms, since the phonatory subsystem is not being "overdriven" by excessive respiratory pressures.

POSTURAL ADJUSTMENTS

Posture frequently affects the respiratory support patterns for individuals with severe dysarthria. Such speakers are unable to develop and maintain adequate air pressure values in the seated position. In these situations, postural adjustments and/or prosthetic assistance may be necessary. Postural adjustment strategies vary depending on the neuromotor impairment of the speaker.

Posture for Speakers with Flaccid Dysarthria

In our clinical work, we frequently treat speakers with weak respiratory support, in the supine position.

> When the body is upright, gravity pulls the abdominal contents down and thus flattens the diaphragm. In a supine position, those contents will tend to push the diaphragm into the thoracic cavity and thus assist in expiration. There is again, a trade-off, in that inspiratory ability will not be as good since the diaphragm must push against the abdominal contents for inflation of the lungs. (Hardy, 1983, p. 153)

Although Hardy (1964) suggested that there is little difference in the respiratory function of individuals with severe cerebral palsy as a result of static differences in posture, we have observed many individuals with dysarthria, including individuals with traumatic brain injury, spinal cord injury, and multiple sclerosis, who were able to generate the respiratory support to speak with phonation in the supine and not the seated position. It appears that individuals with greater impairment of the expiratory rather than the inspiratory musculature benefit from posture adjustments. Thus, the "stronger" inspiratory musculature is able to inhale against the added pressure generated by the forces of the abdominal contents, and the "weaker" expiratory muscles are benefited by the expiratory forces created by the abdominal contents in the supine position. For the speaker with inspiratory inadequacy, such as ALS or obstructive lung disease, the supine position makes breathing and respiration for speech more difficult. Readers are referred to Putnam and Hixon (1984) for an excellent description of the effect of position on respiratory function in individuals with motoneuron disease.

For speakers who benefit from postural adjustments, appropriate position can be accomplished by placing the individual in a wheelchair or lawn chair with an adjustable back (Collins, Rosenbek, & Donahue, 1982). Some clients benefit from an adjustment in their posture to provide increased respiratory support for speech during the aspects of the treatment program that focus on phonatory or articulatory proficiency, while minimizing the demands placed on the respiratory system. However, it is often appropriate at some point in treatment that such speakers might be seated while focusing on the improvement of respiratory function. In an effort to optimize for speech performance for communication interaction, we encourage speakers (and their families) to select a position that facilitates speech intelligibility and efficiency during social situations.

Posture for Individuals with Spastic Dysarthria

The speech performance of many individuals with spastic dysarthria is facilitated when they are positioned to reduce excessive muscle tone. Physical and occupational therapists are most helpful in identifying appropriate positions and providing supports that make these positions comfortable. Positioning to reduce abnormal muscle tone often is used to reduce excessive resistance to airflow through the larynx. For speakers who must compensate for hyperadducted vocal folds, by generating elevated subglottal air pressures, treatment of the phonatory–respiratory subsystems in a facilitating posture is quite common.

Posture for Individuals with Hypokinetic Dysarthria

Persons with hypokinetic dysarthria due to Parkinson's disease may experience weak respiratory support. Their posture may contribute, in part, to this respiratory pattern. With these individuals sitting in a "hunched forward" position, the expansion of their respiratory systems may be limited. During treatment for their voice impairments (Chapter 8), these individuals are encouraged to sit upright, allowing for optimized respiratory performance.

RESPIRATORY PROSTHESES

Two types of respiratory prostheses are used to supplement expiratory forces during speech. The abdominal binder (corset) has been used routinely with individuals with spinal cord injury who have intact diaphragmatic innervation but minimal or no innervation of the expiratory musculature. As with postural adjustment, the binder is ineffective and potentially dangerous for speakers with inspiratory weakness. Because the abdominal binder potentially interferes with inspiration, its use in treatment must involve medical approval and supervision.

A second type of abdominal prosthesis is the expiratory "board" or "paddle" described by Rosenbek and LaPointe (1985). A board is attached to a speaker's wheelchair such that it can be swung into position just anterior to the abdomen. As individuals prepare to speak, they lean forward into the board, thus increasing the expiratory forces. Because individuals can lean back away from the board, this approach does not interfere with inhalation. The efficient use of the board requires some truncal strength and balance to lean forward and back at the appropriate times. We have found that occasionally the expiratory board is useful; however, usually the speakers who need it most do not have the trunk balance and strength to use it effectively. Some speakers with dysarthria can simulate this type of abdominal support with their arms by placing arms lightly over the abdomen during inspiration and squeezing during exhalation.

INSPIRATORY CHECKING

Inspiratory checking is a compensatory respiratory strategy useful for speakers with dysarthria who release excessive airflow through the larynx when they speak (Netsell, 1995). The natural tendency for persons with inefficient airway valves is to overdrive the respiratory system, thereby forcing excessive air from the lungs through the vocal tract. The larynx and other vocal tract valves do not provide sufficient resistance to airflow, so air wastage is common as the elastic recoil forces of the respiratory system push air from the lungs. These individuals are instructed to control flow of air through the larynx by using a technique called inspiratory checking, in which the inspiratory muscles are used to counter the elastic recoil forces of the respiratory system. The inspiratory checking strategy results in a gradual release of the air supply to support speech. Netsell reported the successful use of this strategy with a speaker with dysarthria due to traumatic brain injury.

Stabilizing the Respiratory Pattern

Even after speakers with dysarthria are able to produce the levels of air pressure necessary for speech, some continue to manage their respiratory systems very inconsistently. For example, speakers with severe dysarthria due to traumatic brain injury may initiate utterances at any point in the rest breathing cycle. Some individuals with cerebral palsy may initiate utterances at a variety of lung volume levels. At times, these levels are appropriate and, at times, they are not. Speakers with several different respiratory patterns associated with dysarthria are candidates for a respiratory pattern stabilization program if:

- The speaker initiates phonation at inappropriate lung volume levels that are either too high or too low.
- The speaker initiates speech without taking a preparatory inhalation.
- The speaker initiates breath groups at inconsistent lung volume levels.
- The speaker consistently produces utterances that are too loud or too quiet.
- The speaker does not terminate a breath group at an appropriate lung volume level, but rather continues to speak until reaching an excessively low level.

LUNG VOLUME LEVEL

The first step in stabilizing the respiratory pattern of speakers with moderate or severe dysarthria is to identify a functional lung volume level range. The range that is selected is an individual judgment; however, normal speakers generally inhale to approximately 60% of lung volume level. Prior to the production of an utterance, speakers with cerebral palsy inhale to "a relatively high lung-volume level where the relaxation recoil of the respiratory system will assist in generating the needed air pressure in the vocal tract" (Hardy, 1983, p. 154). Hardy recommended this pattern because few individuals with cerebral palsy are able to produce adequate support for speech below the resting respiratory level. Before an optimal inspiratory lung volume level for speech can be determined, the ability of the speaker to check the recoil air pressure generated at high lung volume levels must be assessed. Obviously, there is no reason to have an individual inhale to such high lung volume levels that air pressure cannot be controlled.

For some speakers with dysarthria and good control of expiratory musculature, the target inspiratory level for speech may be set at or above 60% of lung volume level. For individuals who do not have the ability to inhale to a lung volume level greater than peak tidal volume, the goal is to begin each utterance precisely at that referent level. The lower end of the lung volume level range for speech is also established informally. Usually, speakers are discouraged from exhaling to lung volume levels that elicit abnormal reflexes, result in a change in phonatory quality, or are excessively fatiguing.

The approach for identifying and training a speaker to achieve appropriate lung volume levels for speech depends on the equipment that is available. Water spirometry will assist the clinician in establishing lung volume levels. However, individuals with dysarthria often have difficulty speaking into the closed system of a water spirometer during the training activities. The objective approaches to assessing respiratory shape have been very useful in lung volume level training. As mentioned previously, the Respitrace and magnetometers are useful for this type of training, with results displayed on an oscilloscope for feedback purposes.

Question: I am having difficulty visualizing the use of respiration measurement technology for clinical interventions. Would you provide an example?

I met Carmen during a speech evaluation. She arrived in her wheelchair, but left it at the door and entered the room while stabilizing herself on the door jamb, the wall, and the table. She greeted me with a big smile and began to explain to me how frustrated she was about her speech

(continues)

difficulties. She was the mother of a young daughter and was concerned that her speech was not a very good example for her child. In fact, she had gotten into difficulty during the delivery process as she was allergic to the anesthesia that was used. Her severe anoxia had left her with a number of neurologic deficits. As she explained her concerns to me, she exhibited mixed ataxic and flaccid dysarthria. Her articulatory patterns were quite ataxic, her phonation was breathy and rough, and her breath groups were very short.

As the assessment and trial therapy progressed, it became clear to me that her articulatory patterns were quite resistant to change. However, her respiratory phonatory patterns were very intriguing. Using a Respitrace to estimate her respiratory shape and lung volume levels, it was clear that Carmen initiated utterances at whatever lung volume level she happened to be at the moment. If she was at the resting expiratory level when she decided to speak, she began at that point of lung volume level and spoke well into expiratory reserve. Rarely did she inhale before initiating an utterance.

Using the Respitrace system and an oscilloscope as a feedback strategy, I taught her about the rising and falling pattern of tidal volume (rest breathing). She understood quite easily. Next, I had her initiate vowel phonation at the top of a rest breathing cycle as it was shown on the oscilloscope. That was quite easy for her. We used to laugh, because she would initiate an intentional vowel production at the top of her tidal volume breathing and then drop down to resting expiratory level to initiate a comment like "That wasn't so difficult." Her habits were obviously strong.

In time, she learned to initiate single words, strings of numbers, and rote phrases at a lung volume level that was slightly higher than the upper levels of rest breathing. When she did this, her phonatory quality was normalized considerably, as it was much less rough than it was when she spoke at low lung volume levels.

In time, Carmen was able to communicate all of her intentional utterances at appropriate lung volume levels. However, when she tried to say something that she considered funny, she would tend to move to a low lung volume level, as most of us do when we laugh, and then attempt to speak without inhaling first.

As suggested earlier, the respiratory system can be considered an aerodynamic cavity within the chest wall. There is no best respiratory shape pattern for a speaker with dysarthria (Hardy, 1983). Generally, we agree, however, that there are speakers who have adopted patterns of respiratory shape that are extremely fatiguing or maladaptive. In these cases, an attempt is made to teach them a more effective respiratory pattern. For example, a woman with ALS came to our clinic complaining of reduced vocal loudness and fatigue after talking for a period of time. Our evaluation revealed that she was using a paradoxical respiratory pattern. To increase the volume of the thorax, she elevated her shoulders excessively as she attempted to increase rib cage circumference. Simultaneous with the increase in rib cage circumference, abdominal circumference decreased. Using a Respitrace system, we trained her to enlarge the circumference of the abdomen or at least to stabilize the circumference of the abdomen as the rib cage expanded during inhalation. Following two sessions, she learned the new pattern and found that she no longer needed to elevate her shoulders excessively during inhalation. The result was a speech pattern with greater vocal loudness and less fatigue.

ELIMINATING ABNORMAL (MALADAPTIVE) RESPIRATORY BEHAVIORS

The task of eliminating abnormal or maladaptive respiratory behaviors occurs throughout respiratory training. We have included a specific section because some speakers with dysarthria have compensated for their motor impairments with behaviors that are now maladaptive. This situation occurs quite frequently with individuals with cognitive impairments. A case report will illustrate this point. Betty demonstrated a maladaptive respiratory pattern after being injured during a helicopter crash. Early in her recovery, her speech mechanism was so inefficient that she spoke in single-syllable utterances and inhaled at the beginning of every syllable. When Betty came to our center, she demonstrated the unusual respiratory pattern of inhaling during or after the first syllable of each utterance, even though she had just inhaled prior to the beginning of the utterance, and her breath groups averaged about four words in length. Evidently, she retained the abnormal respiratory pattern she had adopted earlier in recovery.

Increasing Respiratory Flexibility

The speaker with mild dysarthria usually has accomplished the respiratory goals presented in the previous sections. Thus, the remaining focus of treatment is to increase the flexibility with which the respiratory system is controlled during speech, so that the naturalness of the overall speech pattern can be improved. During this phase of treatment, the stabilized respiratory patterns taught earlier to the individual with severe dysarthria may need to be modified. Candidates for this phase of respiratory intervention usually include

- Speakers who produce utterances with stereotypic breath group lengths

- Speakers who never pause without inhaling
- Speakers who are unable to manage the quick inhalation needed to support the short breath group utterance

---

Question: Can you recommend any additional references about the relationships among the respiratory and linguistic patterns during speech?

Winkworth and colleagues described breathing patterns of nondisabled individuals during reading aloud and during spontaneous speech (Winkworth, Davis, Adams, & Ellis, 1995; Winkworth, Davis, Ellis, & Adams, 1994). Their work provides insights into the associations between linguistic and physiologic factors on the control of respiratory support for speech. During spontaneous speech, 63% of breaths occur at structural boundaries; however, during reading aloud, 88% of breaths occur at structural boundaries. This pattern appears to be of benefit to the listener, such that disruptions in the flow of speech are minimized and confined to appropriate breaks corresponding to the syntactic structure of the utterance. The duration of the forthcoming breath group is anticipated by the speaker, and the depth of inspiration is coordinated with that expectation.

ADJUSTING LUNG VOLUME LEVELS

Normal speakers support their overall speech patterns with subtle adjustments of the respiratory system. For example, in anticipation of loud speech, the normal speaker will inhale to a high lung volume level to take advantage of the greater recoil pressures that will be generated. A similar respiratory maneuver occurs where the speaker anticipates an unusually long breath group. During the production of an extremely long utterance, the normal speaker may pause to inhale and replenish the air supply in the lungs. If the speaker is near the end of the utterance, however, a small inhalation will be taken. If an extensive amount of the utterance remains to be spoken, a larger inhalation will occur. The stabilized breath patterning described earlier for individuals with severe dysarthria is simply not subtle enough to support this type of flexible speech performance.

Training in respiratory flexibility occurs at three levels. The first level of training is conceptual. The client is taught the general rules that govern respiratory performance during speech. For initial practice, the speaker with dysarthria reads paragraphs in which the respiratory patterns have been marked. Next, conversational scripts for two speakers are prepared. The respiratory patterns have been marked in the speaker's lines. Finally, the speaker reads aloud or speaks conversationally without the aid of the respiratory pattern markings.

Performance is audio- or video-recorded and discussed. An attempt is made to relate the content of the passage to the interests of the client. The following paragraph was developed for a retired man with parkinsonism. The slashes signal breath group boundaries.

/ For twenty-five years / I have been a member / of the Upland Gamebird Club. / For about five years / I was the president. / We work to preserve habitat / for the birds. / We also lobby the Game Department / for fair hunting seasons. / As you can guess, / that is a matter of opinion. / I have enjoyed the Club / a great deal. / My wife and I travel a lot. / I used to do a lot of speaking, / until the Parkinson's disease / started to affect my voice. / My wife used to complain / that I worked for the Club / and sold insurance on the side.

The following is an example of a dialogue with a woman named Pat who has dysarthria as the result of a traumatic brain injury.

DAVID: Hi.

PAT: / Hello.

DAVID: How are you today?

PAT: / Okay / How are you?

DAVID: Fine. Tell me about your weekend pass.

PAT: / It was great. / We went / to the game / on Saturday. / It was / a beautiful day. / My brother / played a good game. / It was good / to be outside / again.

DAVID: Who went with you?

PAT: I went / with Mom and Dad. / Jim's girlfriend / came too.

MAXIMIZING SPEECH NATURALNESS

A second goal in increasing the flexibility of respiratory support for the speaker with mild dysarthria is to teach natural stress patterning. A detailed discussion of stress pattern training can be found in Chapter 11. Because the breath group may be the unit of prosody, adequate respiratory control and appropriate phrasing are necessary for natural speech.

Flexibility may also be added to the speech of individuals with dysarthria by teaching them to pause without inhalation. Because of the respiratory patterns developed by some speakers early in recovery, inhalation occurs during every pause. Thus, they do not produce the momentary pause without inhalations that are commonly used in speech of nonimpaired individuals to add emphasis. A report on this topic is available in which a young man was taught to increase his speech naturalness by increasing his average breath group length and including momentary pauses in his speech pattern (Rowland, 1980). The training sequences used are very similar to those described in Chapter 11.

REFERENCES

Abbs, J., Hunker, C., & Barlow, S. (1983). Differential speech motor subsystem impairments with suprabulbar lesions: Neurophysiological framework and supporting data. In W. Berry (Ed.), *Clinical dysarthria* (pp. 21–56). San Diego: College-Hill.

Collins, M., Rosenbek, J., & Donahue, E. (1982). The effects of posture on speech in ataxic dysarthria. *ASHA, 24*, 767.

Folkins, J., & Kuehn, D. P. (1982). Speech production. In N. J. Lass, L. V. McReynold, J. Northern, & D. Yoder (Eds.), *Speech, language and hearing: Vol. 1. Normal processes* (pp. 246–285). Philadelphia: Saunders.

Hammen, V. L., & Yorkston, K. M. (1994). Respiratory patterning and variability in dysarthric speech. *Journal of Medical Speech–Language Pathology, 2*(4), 253–262.

Hardy, J. C. (1964). Lung function of athetoid and spastic quadriplegic children. *Developmental and Child Neurology, 6*, 378–388.

Hardy, J. C. (1983). *Cerebral palsy.* Englewood Cliffs, NJ: Prentice-Hall.

Hardy, J. C., & Arkebauer, H. J. (1966). Development of a test for velopharyngeal competence during speech. *Cleft Palate Journal, 3*, 6–19.

Hirano, M., Koike, Y., & von Leden, H. (1968). Maximum phonation time and air usage during phonation. *Folia Phoniatrica, 20*, 185–201.

Hixon, R. (1973). Respiratory function in speech. In F. Minifie, T. Hixon, & F. Williams (Eds.), *Normal aspects of speech, hearing, and language* (pp. 73–126). Englewood Cliffs, NJ: Prentice-Hall.

Hixon, T. (1987). *Respiratory function in speech and song.* Boston: College-Hill.

Hixon, T. (1993). *Clinical evaluation of speech breathing disorders: Principles and methods—Telerounds.* Tucson, AZ: National Center for Neurogenic Communication Disorders.

Hixon, T., Hawley, J., & Wilson, J. (1982). An around-the-house device for the clinical determination of respiratory driving pressure. *Journal of Speech and Hearing Disorders, 47*, 413–415.

Hixon, T., Mead, J., & Goldman, M. (1976). Dynamics of the chest wall during speech production: Function of the thorax, rib cage, diaphragm, and abdomen. *Journal of Speech and Hearing Research, 19*, 297–356.

Hodge, M., & Putnam-Rochet, A. (1989). Characteristics of speech breathing in young women. *Journal of Speech and Hearing Research, 32*, 466–480.

Hoit, J., & Hixon, T. (1987). Age and speech breathing. *Journal of Speech and Hearing Research, 30*, 351–366.

Hoit, J. D., Hixon, T., Altman, M., & Morgan, W. (1989). Speech breathing in women. *Journal of Speech and Hearing Research, 32*, 353–365.

Hunker, C., Bless, D., & Weismer, G. (1981, November). *Respiratory inductive plethysmography: A clinical technique for assessing respiratory function for speech.* Paper presented at the annual convention of the American Speech–Language–Hearing Association, Los Angeles.

Kent, R. D. (1994). *Reference manual for communicative sciences and disorders*. Austin, TX: PRO-ED.

Melcon, M., Hoit, J., & Hixon, T. (1989). Age and laryngeal airway resistance during vowel production. *Journal of Speech and Hearing Disorders, 54*, 282–286.

Netsell, R. (1969). Subglottal and intraoral air pressures during the intervocalic contrast of /t/ and /d/. *Phonetica, 20*, 68–73.

Netsell, R. (1973). Speech physiology. In F. Minifie, T. Hixon, & F. Williams (Eds.), *Normal aspects of speech, hearing and language* (pp. 211–234). Englewood Cliffs, NJ: Prentice-Hall.

Netsell, R. W. (1995). Speech rehabilitation for individuals with unintelligible speech and dysarthria: The respiratory and velopharyngeal systems. *Special Interest Divisions: Neurophysiology and Neurogenic Speech Language Disorders, 5*(4), 6–9.

Netsell, R., & Daniel, B. (1979). Dysarthria in adults: Physiologic approach to rehabilitation. *Archives of Physical Medicine and Rehabilitation, 60*, 502.

Netsell, R., & Hixon, T. (1978). A noninvasive method for clinically estimating subglottal air pressure. *Journal of Speech and Hearing Disorders, 43*, 326–330.

Perkins, W., & Kent, R. (1986). *Functional anatomy of speech, language, and hearing: A primer*. Austin, TX: PRO-ED.

Putnam, A. H. B., & Hixon, T. (1984). Respiratory kinematics in speakers with motor neuron disease. In M. R. McNeil, J. C. Rosenbek, & A. E. Aronson (Eds.), *The dysarthrias: Physiology, acoustics, perception, management* (pp. 37–68). San Diego: College-Hill.

Rosenbek, J. C., & LaPointe, L. L. (1985). The dysarthrias: Description, diagnosis, and treatment. In D. Johns (Ed.), *Clinical management of neurogenic communication disorders* (pp. 97–152). Boston: Little, Brown.

Rowland, L. P. (1980). Motor neuron diseases: The clinical syndromes. In D. W. Mulder (Ed.), *The diagnosis and treatment of amyotrophic lateral sclerosis* (pp. 7–33). Boston: Houghton Mifflin.

Smitheran, J., & Hixon, T. (1981). A clinical method for estimating laryngeal airway resistance during vowel production. *Journal of Speech and Hearing Disorders, 46*, 138–146.

Solomon, N. P., & Hixon, T. J. (1993). Speech breathing in Parkinson's disease. *Journal of Speech and Hearing Research, 36*, 294–310.

Stathopoulos, E., Hoit, J., Hixon, T., Watson, P., & Solomon, N. (1991). Respiratory and laryngeal function during whispering. *Journal of Speech and Hearing Research, 34*, 761–767.

Warren, D. (1996). Regulation of speech aerodynamics. In N. Lass (Ed.), *Principles of experimental phonetics* (pp. 46–92). St. Louis: Mosby.

Weismer, G. (1985). Speech breathing: Contemporary views and findings. In R. Daniloff (Ed.), *Speech science* (pp. 47–71). Austin, TX: PRO-ED.

Winkworth, A. L., Davis, P. J., Adams, R. D., & Ellis, E. (1995). Breathing patterns during spontaneous speech. *Journal of Speech and Hearing Research, 38*(1), 124–144.

Winkworth, A., Davis, P., Ellis, E., & Adams, R. (1994). Variability and consistency in speech breathing during reading: Lung volumes, speech intensity, and linguistic factors. *Journal of Speech and Hearing Research, 37*, 535–556.

CHAPTER

8

LARYNGEAL FUNCTION

Clinical Issues: We were asked to evaluate the "voice" problems of a 23-year-old young man with severe dysarthria. Prior to evaluation, we reviewed his medical records and discovered that he had suffered a closed head injury with brain stem contusion 1 year earlier. Upon admission to the rehabilitation unit 3 months postonset, the list of medical problems included spastic quadriplegia, swallowing difficulty, anarthria, reduced memory, and cognitive impairment. During the course of inpatient rehabilitation, his physical recovery proceeded gradually. At the time of discharge, he was wheelchair dependent and communicated using a portable typing-based communication augmentation device. Six months after discharge, the speech–language pathologist associated with a home health agency referred the patient for a voice evaluation, because she felt that lack of voluntary phonation was limiting the return of his speech. He was beginning to mouth words and to achieve some voicing, according to his parents, "when he wanted to." These episodes of phonation usually occurred when he was lying in bed. When preparing for this evaluation with our student intern, we asked that she be prepared to answer the following questions after completing the evaluation:

- How do you assess voice production when episodes of voicing occur only once or twice per week?

- What factors appear to be contributing to the occasional episodes of voicing?

- What is this speaker's level of respiratory function, and how do you decide if respiratory function is adequate to support phonation?

- What factors other than respiratory or phonatory control need to be considered when evaluating the voice of speakers with severe dysarthria?

- What approaches may be appropriate for improving the voice of this individual?

Phonatory aspects of dysarthria are clinically important for a number of reasons. Phonatory disorders not only are very common among speakers with dysarthria but also play an important role in differential diagnosis of the dysarthrias. Identification of laryngeal signs and symptoms plays a key role in the early differential diagnosis of some progressive disorders, such as parkinsonism (Logemann, Fisher, Boshes, & Blonsky, 1978), myasthenia gravis (Aronson, 1971), and amyotrophic lateral sclerosis (ALS) (Roth, Glaze, Goding, & David, 1996). With the speaker with more severe dysarthria, examination of phonatory characteristics may yield important information about the underlying neuropathology. A thorough understanding of the phonatory aspects of dysarthria also is important when planning intervention for speakers at all levels of severity. For individuals with severe dysarthria, inability to produce voice is, at times, the feature that prevents functional speech. Without voluntary phonation, some individuals with brain injury cannot take advantage of their residual articulatory movements. For those with somewhat less severe involvement, impaired phonatory aspects of speech production warrant attention because of their potential impact on speech intelligibility (Ramig, 1992).

Increases in speech loudness or intensity are frequently reported when speakers attempt to maintain intelligible speech in the presence of background noise. Speakers with dysarthria and phonatory impairments who are unable to adjust their phonatory performance in the presence of ambient noise will experience reductions in speech intelligibility as compared to quiet, optimal conditions. Care should be taken to interview speakers and their listeners to determine if the speakers have difficulty being understood in noisy situations. Speech intelligibility testing with and without background noise allows the clinician to more completely understand the interaction between background noise and speech intelligibility.

Listeners use suprasegmental information to assign syntactic structure to an utterance before decoding the rest of the information. Therefore, if prosodic information is deviant, a listener may experience increased difficulty in decoding a message (Weismer, 1990). For speakers with dysarthria, inadequate laryngeal control, resulting in unpredictable changes in phonation, such as sudden breaks in voicing, or fundamental frequency (pitch) and intensity (loudness) variations, may reduce intelligibility. Also, equal and excess stress or monotone patterns provide listeners with little information about the syntactic structure of an utterance, thereby potentially reducing speech intelligibility.

Impairment of laryngeal timing interferes with the articulatory function of the larynx. For example, the reduced ability to achieve voiced and voiceless contrasts interferes with the differentiation of voiced cognates, such as /t/ and /d/ or /k/ and /g/. In addition, laryngeal timing interferes with the distinction of sounds and words that begin with an aspirated sound, such as "hat," as compared to words that do not, such as "at" (Kent, Weismer, Kent, & Rosenbek, 1989).

NORMAL LARYNGEAL FUNCTION

Neuromotor Function

Production of voice depends on the interaction of the respiratory, phonatory, and resonance components of speech. Although all of these components play a role in the production of the perceptual features of the voice, this chapter contains only a description of neuromotor aspects of the laryngeal system. A more detailed description of the respiratory requirements for speech is found in Chapter 7, and the resonance system is discussed in Chapter 9.

The primary vegetative function of the larynx is to protect the airway from entry of foreign material during swallowing. Superimposed on this important vegetative function is voicing. The muscles of the larynx may be divided into two groups: (1) the extrinsic muscles, innervated by Cranial Nerves V, VII, and XI, which are responsible for fixation, elevation, and lowering the position of the larynx, and (2) the intrinsic muscles, innervated by the vagus nerve (Cranial Nerve X), which are responsible for the adducting, abducting, and elongation of the vocal folds. The nerves that innervate the intrinsic laryngeal muscles, the superior laryngeal nerves, and the recurrent laryngeal nerves, have two characteristics that ensure the ability of the laryngeal muscles to move quickly and with fine motor control. The laryngeal nerves have very high conduction velocity (second only to the eye), which allows for rapid contractions. The innervation ratio per motor unit of these muscles is low, allowing for fine control (Garrett & Larson, 1991).

Readers are referred to other sources for a more comprehensive discussion of normal voice production and neurologic phonatory disorders (Aronson,

1990; Barlow, Netsell, & Hunker, 1986; Blitzer, Sasaki, Fahn, Brin, & Harris, 1992; Boone, 1977; Prator & Swift, 1984; Ramig & Scherer, 1992).

Measurement of Laryngeal Function

Generally, six parameters are useful in describing laryngeal function during speech (Smitheran & Hixon, 1981):

1. *Vocal intensity*—This is a measure of the level of sound energy produced and is perceptually interpreted as loudness.

2. *Fundamental frequency*—This reflects the number of vibratory cycles of the vocal folds per second and is perceived as pitch.

3. *Vocal quality*—This refers to the regularity of the vibratory cycle of the vocal folds and is perceptually described by a variety of terms, including breathiness, roughness, harshness, hoarseness, and strained–strangled.

4. *Timing of the initiation and cessation of glottal closure for voicing*—This aspect of phonation is particularly important in the production of distinctions between voiced and voiceless consonants.

5. *Position of the vocal folds on a moment-by-moment basis*—This involves identification of adduction (movement of the vocal folds toward the midline of the laryngeal airway) and abduction of the vocal folds.

6. *Aerodynamic resistance of the vocal folds to subglottal air pressure*—Laryngeal resistance is the extent to which the larynx offers opposition to the flow of air through it.

Normal phonation requires precise motor control. When weakness, slowness, or incoordination exists in the laryngeal musculature, deviations from normal are heard in the voice. Aronson (1985) described both normal function and deviation from normal in the following passage:

The vocal folds must be adducted to the midline and kept there with balanced and bilaterally symmetrical adductor–abductor muscle tonus. Thyroarytenoid and cricothyroid muscle tension must be optimum. Glottal opening and closing has to be precisely timed, the folds adducted at the exact moment for onset of voiced consonants and vowels, and abducted for voiceless. Should they adduct too soon, voiceless sounds would be voiced; too late, voiced sounds would be voiceless. Yet they must not overadduct, for then they would obstruct the exhaled airstream and produce transient changes in voice quality and loudness; should such adduction become extreme, phonation will cease. The extrinsic muscles of the larynx must be able to elevate and depress the larynx in the neck. Otherwise pitch variation will be restricted. On the other hand, if fluctuations are excessive, pitch will change unexpectedly and inappropriately. (p. 77)

CLASSIFICATION OF NEUROLOGIC VOICE DISORDERS BASED ON PHONATORY FUNCTION

Phonatory impairments often occur in the dysarthrias associated with neurologic diseases and syndromes. The vocal characteristics of various types of speakers with dysarthria are summarized in Chapters 2 through 4 and are not discussed in detail here. Clinically, the speech–language pathologist may be faced with several different tasks. In a neurology setting, the primary task of the clinician is to differentially diagnose phonatory impairments to determine the type of dysarthria present, to determine the consistency of the speech diagnosis with the proposed neurologic diagnoses of the medical team, to document severity of the disorder, and to make appropriate referrals.

The speech–language pathologist with a rehabilitation perspective focuses more on (a) the nature of the phonatory impairment as it impacts the overall speech performance and (b) the selection and implementation of intervention procedures that may improve phonatory function and overall speech performance. We have found the classification of phonatory impairments of speakers with dysarthria proposed by Ramig (1995; Ramig & Scherer, 1992) to be useful in guiding our assessment and intervention.

According to Ramig's system, a *hypoadduction impairment* of phonation occurs when there is reduced or weak closure of the vocal folds. It is associated with the perceptual characteristics of reduced loudness, breathy voice, and hoarse voice quality. This impairment results from lower motoneuron laryngeal paresis or paralysis, Parkinson's disease, progressive supranuclear palsy, Shy-Drager syndrome, and some traumatic brain injuries.

A *hyperadduction impairment* of phonation occurs when the vocal folds close too tightly. It is associated with pressed, harsh, strained–strangled voice that may be of reduced, normal, or excessive loudness. These impairments occur in pseudobulbar palsy, spastic cerebral palsy, Huntington's disease, adductor laryngeal dystonia, and some brain injuries.

Phonatory instability impairment is associated with tremorous voice, rough hoarse voice quality, pitch breaks, and glottal fry. Two types of instability are discussed in the literature (Strand, Buder, Yorkston, & Ramig, 1994). Short-term instability refers to the fluctuations in intensity and frequency on a cycle-by-cycle basis. It is perceived as a problem in voice quality and is present in most persons with neurologically based voice disorders. Long-term instability refers to fluctuations in vocal frequency and intensity occurring in intervals greater than one cycle. Three types of long-term instability have been reported (Hartelius, Buder, & Strand, 1997). Very slow fluctuations (wow) occur less than 2 times per second. Tremor refers to fluctuations that can be observed 3 to 10 times per second. Flutter refers to very fast (7 to 10 times per second) changes in frequency and intensity. All have been associated with dysarthric speech.

Mixed phonatory impairments involve aspects of the previous three groups in various proportions (hypoadduction, hyperadduction, and instability). Mixed impairment may occur in multiple sclerosis and ataxic (cerebellar) dysphonia, and at times in progressive supranuclear palsy and Shy-Drager syndrome.

Phonatory coordination impairments involve the coordination of the phonatory system with other aspects of articulation in order to achieve voiced–voiceless distinctions (e.g., "two" vs. "due") or to achieve aspiration–nonaspiration distinctions (e.g., "hat" vs. "at").

ASSESSMENT OF LARYNGEAL FUNCTION

A variety of assessment procedures are used by speech–language pathologists to assess laryngeal function in order to provide differential diagnoses and implement intervention programs. As reported earlier, some level of laryngeal impairment is present in a large percentage of speakers with dysarthria. This impairment ranges from mild with no associated disability, to so severe that it is a primary factor responsible for the communication disability. The assessment of phonatory performance is an integral part of each dysarthria evaluation. Generally, assessment proceeds along the same lines as clinical assessment of other speech components. The first phase involves the documentation of the presence of a laryngeal impairment, and a perceptual description of its characteristics and severity. This phase essentially serves as a screening process. The second phase of assessment involves an in-depth analysis of laryngeal function. Here, a series of questions are posed that are related to the mechanisms underlying the perceptual features of phonation and to various intervention approaches that may potentially benefit the speaker.

Approaches to Measurement

When discussing assessment of voice disorders, Aronson (1980) stated, "The trained ear and mind are, at present, the most useful instrument" (p. 182). However, increasingly, the specific characteristics of phonatory dysfunction are being assessed using instrumental measurement techniques. For example, acoustic analysis equipment is becoming more available in the clinical setting. Using this instrumentation, fundamental frequency and relative vocal intensity can be measured. Often, timing relationships (i.e., phonatory–respiratory coordination) may be described more precisely with acoustic analysis and respiratory measures than by perceptual means alone.

Question: When should a clinician use perceptual versus instrumental measurement in the assessment of laryngeal impairment for speech?

A series of perceptual, acoustic, and aerodynamic assessment techniques are presented in this chapter. Selection of one technique over another for clinical use obviously depends on a number of issues. Perhaps the most important issue is the nature of the questions being addressed in the evaluation. Other issues include the importance of the phonatory problems in relation to overall impairment, the knowledge and time available to the clinician, and the equipment at hand.

Researchers have compared and contrasted results of various measurement approaches. For example, Ludlow and Bassich (1983, 1984) studied the relationships between perceptual ratings and acoustic measures of the speech of nonimpaired individuals and those with Parkinson's disease and Shy-Drager syndrome. (For a more complete discussion of these syndromes, refer to Chapter 4.) Persons with Parkinson's disease and Shy-Drager syndrome have differing underlying neuropathology. Therefore, their speech symptoms can be differentiated. Ludlow and Bassich (1983) identified strengths and weaknesses of perceptual and acoustic approaches in the assessment of this population. For example, they found that either perceptual ratings or acoustic measures were adequate to distinguish the nonimpaired speakers from those with either type of dysarthria and to distinguish one type of dysarthria from another. They also stated,

> Somewhat different variables were identified as most useful for discriminating between the two types of dysarthria . . . . The acoustic system identified vowel-voicing errors as particularly important for distinguishing between the types of dysarthria, while the perceptual system identified differences in voice quality and overall rate as being particularly important. The perceptual rating system identified three aspects of vocal quality as useful for differentiating between types of dysarthria: breathiness, strain–strangle, and wet hoarseness. None of

(continues)

the acoustic measures of vocal quality, jitter ratio, or diplophonia ratio were included in the discriminant function for differentiating between the two types of dysarthria. Therefore, the acoustic measures may be more discrete for the analysis of different speech production factors in patients' speech. Further investigation is needed to determine if such is the case. If so, the acoustic system may be more suitable for assessing those aspects that are particularly impaired prior to treatment planning, while the perceptual system may better provide an overall indication of the degree of impairment. (Ludlow & Bassich, 1984, p. 140)

In the situation just described, instrumental (in this case acoustic) measurement has permitted an assessment of phonatory timing that is not available using the perceptual approaches alone. Further, the perceptual measures gave an indication of overall voice quality that could not be obtained instrumentally. Thus, it appears that, when assessing phonatory function in dysarthria, clinicians need to select measurement approaches dependent on the specific aspects of the impairment that are of interest to them.

Identification of Perceptual Signs of Laryngeal Impairment

Generally, the initial phase of the evaluation involves the determination of the presence or absence of a phonatory impairment. For example, when the evaluation is part of an overall assessment to detect the presence of a neurologic impairment, slight variation from normal, or at least from previous performance, is important. If no impairment is observed during speech, further assessment of phonatory performance is usually discontinued. If phonatory impairment is confirmed, further description is necessary. The impact of the phonatory impairment on overall functional limitation, disability, and handicap must also be assessed.

The assessment of phonatory function usually begins by using perceptual measures of loudness, pitch, quality, and overall instability. Clinically, these perceptual observations are usually quantified using a scale such as the 7-point equal-appearing interval scale used by the Mayo Clinic group (Darley, Aronson, & Brown, 1975). Research investigations have used magnitude estimation scaling techniques (Southwood, 1996).

The specific phonatory parameters are as follows (Darley, Aronson, & Brown, 1975):

Pitch level—Pitch of voiced sounds consistently too low or too high for individual's age and gender.

Pitch breaks—Pitch of voice shows sudden and uncontrolled variation (falsetto breaks).

Monopitch—Voice is characterized by a monopitch or monotone. Voice lacks normal pitch and inflectional changes. It tends to stay at one pitch level.

Voice tremor—Voice shows shakiness or tremulousness.

Monoloudness—Voice shows monotony of loudness. It lacks normal variations in loudness.

Excessive loudness variation—Voice shows sudden, uncontrolled alternations in loudness, sometimes becoming too loud, sometimes too weak.

Loudness decay—There is progressive diminution or decay of loudness.

Alternating loudness—There are alternating changes in loudness.

Harsh voice—Voice is harsh, rough, and raspy.

Hoarse (wet) voice—There is wet, "liquid sounding" hoarseness.

Breathy voice—Voice is breathy, weak, and thin.

Strained–strangled voice—Voice (phonation) sounds strained or strangled (an apparent effortful squeezing of voice through the glottis).

Long-term instability—Voice quality changes occur over periods of a few seconds.

The presence of perceptual changes in these speech dimensions may lead the clinician to ask questions about the mechanisms underlying the impairment and possible intervention approaches. Answers to these questions require the clinician to pursue a more in-depth assessment of phonatory function.

Question: I have the impression that perceptual measures of phonation are unreliable. How should the clinician approach this area of assessment?

We do not have a lot of information about the validity and reliability of the assessment of phonation in the dysarthria field; however, the voice field is focusing quite intensely on this issue at the moment. For example,

(continues)

recent work suggests that perceptual ratings for some parameters are quite complicated (Bielamowic, Kreiman, Gerratt, Dauer, & Berke, 1996). Clinicians may wish to review this material and be appropriately cautious regarding the measures that are used on a routine basis.

In our clinical work, we continue to use perceptual ratings of the many overall vocal parameters suggested (Darley et al., 1975). We have found it most effective to rate the various parameters separately rather than to listen to a speech sample one time and rate all of the parameters.

However, for measures of the timing aspects of phonatory performance in relation to other aspects of articulation (voiced–voiceless distinctions and aspiration–nonaspiration distinction), we rely on instrumental measurement (Strand et al., 1994).

In-depth Assessment of Laryngeal Function

CONTRIBUTION OF IMPAIRMENTS IN OTHER COMPONENTS

Because dysarthria typically is characterized by impairment in multiple speech components, it is necessary to examine the relationship of phonatory impairment with other aspects of speech production. It is possible that what appears to be an impairment in phonation instead may reflect impairment in respiratory or velopharyngeal performance. For example, poor respiratory support may result in deviations in voice loudness and length of phrases. Answers to the following questions are needed in order to interpret data derived from the assessment of phonatory performance:

- Is the level of subglottal air pressure adequate to support phonatory function?

- How flexible is the respiratory system?

- Can the respiratory system be controlled in a coordinated fashion?

- How efficient is the velopharyngeal valve?

- Is the speaker able to achieve complete velopharyngeal closure?

- Is that closure well timed in relation to other aspects of speech production?

A detailed discussion of assessment of the respiratory and velopharyngeal components can be found in Chapters 7 and 9, respectively. The following discussion of phonatory function assumes an understanding of respiratory and velopharyngeal function. Once the function of other speech components has been established, then assessment can focus on laryngeal function. A number of aspects of laryngeal function are important in the assessment of dysarthric speech. These include efficiency, flexibility, stability, and coordination. Each of these aspects, together with a number of perceptual and instrumental measurement techniques, is discussed in the following sections.

LARYNGEAL EFFICIENCY (HYPOADDUCTION AND HYPERADDUCTION IMPAIRMENTS)

Laryngeal efficiency is a term used to describe the adequacy with which the expiratory airstream is valved at the level of the vocal folds. Laryngeal efficiency is compromised when, due to motor impairment, the vocal folds do not adduct properly (hypoadduction) or when they adduct excessively (hyperadduction). Laryngeal efficiency may be assessed in a number of ways.

Perceptual Characteristics of the Voice

Several perceptual features of the voice may signal hypoadduction. These qualities may be observed in connected speech, in sustained phonation tasks, or in both. A breathy voice may indicate air wastage and thus signal hypoadduction of the vocal folds. On the other hand, a voice with a strained–strangled quality may reflect hyperadduction of the vocal folds.

Sustained Phonation Time

Maximum sustained phonation time has been used by some clinicians as an indicator of laryngeal efficiency. However, in our clinical practice, for several reasons, we are usually not very interested in maximal performance by speakers with dysarthria because speech is not a "maximal performance activity." Also, even speakers with rather severe dysarthria are able to adjust their laryngeal resistance to maximize their phonation time, and this is not the type of phonation that they use in conversational speech. The /s/ and /z/ ratios used as an index of vocal efficiency for persons with nonneurologic voice disorders are rarely used with speakers with dysarthria, because of the articulatory imprecision common in dysarthria.

Estimates of Laryngeal Resistance

The extent to which the larynx offers opposition to the flow of air through it is known as laryngeal resistance. Although it cannot be measured directly, Smitheran and Hixon (1981) described an approach to estimate the aerodynamic impedance of the laryngeal structures. Briefly, the level of subglottal air pressure for vowels is estimated from intraoral air pressure levels of voiceless consonants adjacent to the vowel in question. The volume velocity of airflow through the glottis during vowel production is measured. An estimate of laryngeal resistance is calculated using the following formula:

$$\text{Laryngeal airway resistance} = \frac{\text{Translaryngeal pressure}}{\text{Translaryngeal flow}}.$$

This measure provides information about the resistance to airflow through the larynx. Smitheran and Hixon reported that persons with harsh voices have resistance levels that are considerably higher than those with normal voices and persons with breathy voices have lower levels of resistance.

Question: As aerodynamic measurement systems become more common in clinical settings, measures of laryngeal airway resistance have become more routine. What are the normal values associated with nonimpaired speakers of various ages?

Laryngeal Airway Resistance

Men (Smitheran & Hixon, 1981)

Age Group (Years)	Resistance (cm H_2O/liters per second)		
	Mean	Range	Standard Deviation
(21–40)	35	30.0–43.1	3.3

Women (Hoit & Hixon, 1992)

Age Group (years)	Resistance (cm H_2O/liters per second)	
	Mean	Standard Deviation
25	54.88	15.94
35	51.32	16.03
45	38.00	13.74
55	55.60	20.74
65	58.37	18.12
75	54.20	12.92
85	56.67	26.01

Movement Measures

Movement of the vocal folds in speakers with dysarthria has been routinely observed through indirect laryngoscopy. In this procedure, the interior larynx is observed using a laryngeal mirror. This technique is useful when evaluating vocal fold paralysis. However, the rapid movement of the vocal folds does not permit cycle-by-cycle evaluation of the vocal fold closure using this technique. The use of a fiberscope, a stroboscopic light source, and video-recording equipment allows for visualization and description of vocal fold movement in speakers with dysarthria. This technology permits observation of laryngeal movement and, taken together with perceptual and aerodynamic measures, can provide important information regarding laryngeal dysfunction.

Electroglottography is another technique that shows promise in the laryngeal assessment of vocal fold movement (Orlikoff & Kahane, 1996). In this technique, the electrical conductance of the vocal folds is measured. From this information, the changes in vocal fold contact area can be estimated. As the contact area increases and decreases during phonation, so does the conductance. When vocal folds are completely closed, electrical conductance is high, and when the vocal folds are separated, conductance is very low (Stone, 1996). To date it has been used in research of normal speakers, persons with voice disorders, and speakers who stutter. It has not yet received widespread use as a clinical measurement tool in the dysarthria field.

VOCAL FLEXIBILITY

Aronson (1980) referred to vocal flexibility as "variations in pitch and loudness that aid in the expression of emphasis, meaning, or subtleties indicating the feelings of the individual" (p. 6). This aspect of voice can be assessed perceptually by judging parameters of pitch variation, loudness, and quality in speech contexts. Typically, habitual performance may be compared to maximum performance by asking the speaker to perform structured tasks designed to heighten flexibility. Examples of such tasks and their use in dysarthria intervention are included in Chapter 11 and are listed in Table 11.6 (Robin, Klouda, & Hug, 1991). Vocal flexibility can also be measured acoustically with parameters related to fundamental frequency, such as range of fundamental frequency within an utterance, range of peak fundamental frequencies of each syllable within an utterance, or slope of the fundamental frequency contour. Lack of vocal flexibility is a characteristic of certain types of dysarthria, including the hypokinetic dysarthria seen in Parkinson's disease.

Two general types of phonatory inflexibility are observed in speakers with dysarthria. For some, lack of variation in fundamental frequency and intensity is perceived as monotonicity. In others, a recurring (and similar) pattern of fundamental frequency and intensity is used in consecutive breath groups and perceived as a monopattern. Monotony is a feature that often reduces the speech naturalness of those dysarthric individuals whose speech is intelligible but not normal. Monopitch and monoloudness both rank among the 10 most deviant dimensions in all of the seven diagnostic groups in the Mayo Clinic study (Darley et al., 1975). Both of these features rank within the five most deviant speech dimensions in parkinsonism and pseudobulbar palsy.

The perception of monotony may be more complex than simply reduced ranges of fundamental frequency and relative intensity. Solomon, Ludolph, and Thomson (1984) acoustically analyzed the fundamental frequency of speech samples of individuals who were judged to exhibit monopitch using the perceptual methods of Darley and colleagues. They found that the range of fundamental frequency excursion was not reduced as compared to normal. This suggests that other factors contributed to the perception of monopitch.

In addition to being a phenomenon that occurs within a breath group, the perception of monotony also may be the result of excessive uniformity across breath group units. For normal speakers, the breath group unit is regulated to a large extent by the syntactic demands of the utterance being produced. In Chapter 7, data were presented that illustrated the variability of breath group length as normal individuals read a passage. Although the average number of words per breath group was just less than 10, these speakers frequently produced breath groups of only 4 words. At other times they spoke nearly 20 words before taking a breath. These data suggest that normal individuals vary their breath group durations depending on the material they are reading. Further, their breath group duration is not restricted by the limits of their physiologic support. Dysarthric speakers are quite different.

Bellaire, Yorkston, and Beukelman (1986) presented the case of a 20-year-old male who suffered a closed head injury in a motor vehicle accident. His speech was intelligible at a speaking rate of 90 words per minute (wpm), but was judged to be quite monotonous. He was able to signal stress within breath groups accurately and without exaggerating any of the suprasegmental features of fundamental frequency, relative intensity, or duration. However, when prosodic patterning across breath groups was analyzed, an explanation of the monotony was found. The speaker produced breath groups that were both shorter than normal and more regular, nearly every pause in the paragraph production contained an inhalation, and the sample was characterized by a restricted fundamental frequency range. Because the speaker appeared to have the physiologic support to produce more extended breath groups, a training program was undertaken in which he was asked to increase the number of words per breath and to increase the frequency of pauses without inhalation. Data obtained at the end of treatment suggested he had learned to do what was asked of him. Mean words per breath group increased from 5.1 to 9.8, and his speech was judged to be more natural. Figure 11.6 contains fundamental frequency × time tracings for a portion of a paragraph read pre- and posttreatment. Note that in the posttreatment sample, breath group lengths were extended and fundamental frequency excursions were greater than in the pretreatment tracings. This case illustrates the point that the perception of monotony may arise from a number of sources. It may be the result of monoloudness and monopitch within a breath group, or it may be the result of "monopatterning" across breath groups. Breath groups of equal length add to the perception of monopitch because of the repetitive fundamental frequency patterns that they create.

Question: What are the habitual fundamental frequency levels of normal adults?

Fundamental Frequency in Young and Old Adults (Benjamin, 1981)

Group	Modal Fundamental Frequency (in Hz)
Younger males	110.3
Older males	103.0
Young females	197.2
Older females	180.2

VOCAL STABILITY

Voice stability is a complex perceptual phenomenon relating to vocal fold periodicity. Aronson (1990) classified neurogenic voice disorders according to consistency or variability of vocal production. For example, there is a group of neurologic voice disorders in which the quality deviation is relatively constant. This group includes the phonatory properties of flaccid, spastic, and hypokinetic dysarthrias. Another group of phonatory disorders is characterized by irregular fluctuations and long-term instability. Ataxic, choreic, and dystonic dysphonias fall into this group. Rhythmically fluctuating dysphonias include those associated with tremor, including palatopharyngolaryngeal myoclonus and organic (essential) voice tremor. Paroxysmal neurologic dysphonia is evidenced where voice quality is altered relatively infrequently by sudden bursts.

Question: Is it better to measure instability acoustically or perceptually?

Short-term instability is routinely measured acoustically, because the human ear is not good enough to measure cycle-by-cycle phenomena. However, long-term instability is usually perceptually and acoustically measured.

Coordination

Laryngeal coordination refers to the timing of laryngeal activity with other aspects of speech production. Timing of respiratory and phonatory efforts is particularly important in dysarthria. This type of coordination can be assessed in several ways. For example, the speaker can be asked to produce in rapid succession the series of vowels /i-i-i-i-i/. This task may be difficult for many individuals with dysarthria, especially those with respiratory or laryngeal coordination problems. It requires not only rapid initiation and cessation of vocal fold vibration, but also a steady respiratory drive. In severe impairment, evidence of such incoordination is visually apparent during connected speech. For example, the individual may begin speaking toward the end of an expiratory cycle or take a breath in the middle of a word. At other times, observations of respiratory–laryngeal incoordination require instrumental measurement. Acoustic measurement has permitted assessment of phonatory timing that is not available using only the perceptual approach. For example, measures of the latency between the initiation of phonation following the beginning of the expiratory phase of respiration may be obtained using aerodynamic techniques. Some individuals with dysarthria waste their air supply by exhaling a portion of their lung volume before initiating phonation.

Still another example of phonatory incoordination can be seen in the production of voicing distinctions. Some individuals with dysarthria are unable to produce perceptually different voiced versus voiceless cognate pairs. Often, this is a consequence of poorly controlled and timed phonation. Although this type of voicing problem can be identified perceptually, acoustic analysis is often helpful in examining the details of this problem. Durational measures of the timing of phonation cessation and reinitiation (voice onset time) during the production of a voiceless consonant sound can be made.

TREATMENT

This discussion of treatment of laryngeal dysfunction is organized according to the classification of neurologic voice impairments described earlier.

Establishing Voluntary Phonation for Persons with Severe Hypoadduction of the Vocal Folds

Evaluating Reflexive Phonation

Some individuals with severe dysarthria are unable to produce phonation voluntarily. The speakers described in the following section generally exhibit reduced respiratory support, velopharyngeal incompetence, and laryngeal weakness that prevents them from forcefully adducting the vocal folds. Common etiologies include closed head injury with brain stem contusion and brain stem cardiovascular accident (CVA). With both of these etiologies, there is a sudden onset followed by a gradual course of recovery that may extend over years.

With these individuals, the various nonspeech reflex patterns that might be associated with phonation are inventoried, including laughing, coughing, sighing, and expressions of pain or discomfort. When phonation occurs, note is taken not only of the type of activity (i.e., laughing) but also of the speaker's position (supine, prone, or sitting). When respiratory drive is weak, the speaker's efforts may be supplemented with abdominal pressing to increase the subglottal air pressure being generated. Family members and caregivers are encouraged to keep a diary of the times when reflexive phonation occurs, thus carefully documenting situations that produce successful phonation, including stimulus, body position, assistance provided, and associated activity, such as response to pain or discomfort. An example of such a phonation diary appears in Table 8.1. A review of this table suggests a gradual change over a 4-month period. Voicing was initially present only in response to discomfort, phonation then became consistent in the supine position, and finally phonation became consistent and voluntary when the speaker was seated.

Table 8.1

An Example of a Phonation Diary Completed by the Family of a 23-Year-Old Individual with a Closed Head Injury and Severe Dysarthria

---

Name: Tom Matthews
Recorder: Ellen Matthews

Instruction: Remember to include information about date, voicing behavior, consistency, position, stimulus, and whether or not the speaker could continue to produce voicing.

Make an entry at least once a week. Pick a particular day each week, if that will help you be consistent.

1/15   no voicing today, supine or prone, with verbal instruction
1/22   no voicing this week in any position, with verbal instruction
1/29   voice in response to an uncomfortable transfer from bed to wheelchair
2/5   sound occurred when choking on saliva, no voluntary voicing supine or prone, with verbal instruction
2/12   cough and choking sound, supine when swallowing saliva; no voluntary sound in any position with verbal instruction
2/19   same

(continues)

Table 8.1 *(continued)*

2/26	same
3/5	same
3/12	same
3/19	voice during laughing, both prone and supine, but not seated, still voice when coughing and choking occasionally
3/26	same
4/2	same
4/9	same
4/16	same, maybe voluntary sound supine with verbal instruction and while pushing stomach
4/23	occasional voluntary sound when supine with verbal instructions and abdominal push, no voluntary sound in seated position
4/30	sound 50% of time in supine with abdominal push, sound occasionally without abdominal push, occasional sound in seated position with abdominal push
5/7	consistent voluntary sound in prone and supine, sound 30% of time in seated position with abdominal push
5/14	consistent sound in seated position, voice is almost a whisper
5/21	voice stronger every day, especially after a coughing spell

DEVELOPING VOLUNTARY PHONATION

The transition from reflexive to voluntary phonation varies from individual to individual. For some, the transition is almost immediate; for others, the transition takes months or years. Our first approach is usually to have individuals attempt to produce a reflexive behavior on a repetitive basis. For example, a cough or laugh may produce increased adduction. We can create opportunities for this to occur, help speakers to be aware of the movements involved, and reinforce their effort. Next, we ask them to produce the phonation voluntarily. Commonly, these speakers are simultaneously participating in a program designed to increase their ability to generate and control subglottal air pressure. During phonatory practice sessions, we position the individual for optimal generation of subglottal air pressure when attempting phonation. Many persons are positioned supine with an abdominal press to increase subglottal air pressure. Rarely is initial phonatory initiation produced in the upright or seated position.

Because the goal of this phase of intervention is more forceful vocal fold adduction, traditional pulling–pushing exercises such as those described by Prator and Swift (1984) may be used. These exercises typically involve forceful muscular activity, such as lifting, pulling, or pushing. Pushing the hand, arms, or legs against resistance may facilitate vocal fold closure for those who are unable to achieve it under other circumstances. Because individuals with severe dysarthria may have arm and leg weakness, the anatomic site used and the specific pushing activity will vary from speaker to speaker. Some individuals push against the arm rests or lap tray of the wheelchair; others pull against overhead slings mounted to hospital beds or wheelchairs (see Figure 8.1).

Once speakers with severe dysarthria are able to consistently initiate phonation voluntarily, they are asked to attempt to shape the oral cavity to produce a number of different vowel sounds and to initiate phonation when assuming various articulatory postures. Once they have demonstrated the ability to do this, they are introduced to vowel intelligibility drills such as those discussed in Chapter 11.

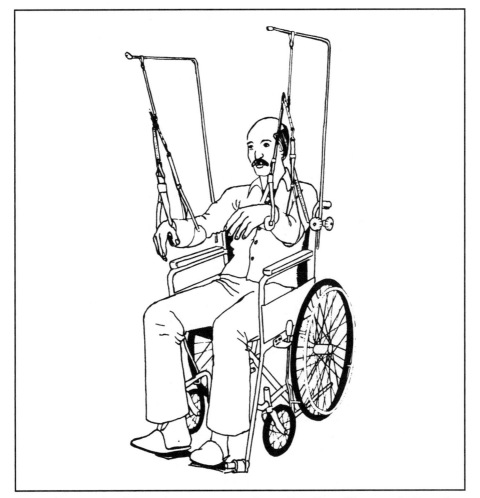

Figure 8.1. Overhead slings for increasing speaking effort. From "Treating the Dysarthric Talker," by J. Rosenbek, 1984, *Seminars in Speech and Language, 5*, p. 377. Copyright 1984 by Thieme-Stratton, Inc. Reprinted with permission.

CASE PRESENTATION

Sam was 72 years old when he suffered an extensive brain stem stroke. He was admitted to the rehabilitation unit 1 month postonset. At that time, he was anarthric and was communicating with a yes/no eye blink system. He had severely compromised respiratory support, bilateral vocal fold paralysis, no observable velopharyngeal movement, and some bilabial weakness. After an augmentative communication approach had been established using a head-mounted light pointer and an alphabet board, focus of attention turned to speech production. Goals of initial rehabilitation included increasing respiratory support for speech, increasing ability to produce spontaneous phonation in the supine position, and increasing ability to produce understandable vowels. At the time of his discharge, he was able to consistently initiate voluntary phonation in the supine position. Although he was able to produce two or three syllables per utterance when lying down, he was not able to vocalize voice when seated.

Five months after his discharge, he was readmitted for management of an unrelated medical problem. When we evaluated him, we found that he had made some small but important gains. He and his wife reported that speech had become sufficiently understandable so that the augmentative communication system was no longer needed when he was lying down. However, he was still unable to initiate phonation in the seated position. This lack of phonation was posing more and more of a problem because he wished to spend the majority of his day seated in the wheelchair. Our next goal was to develop phonation in the seated position. As is frequently the case, both respiratory and phonatory impairments were implicated in Sam's lack of phonation.

Evaluation of respiratory function revealed that, although his ability to generate adequate levels of subglottal air pressure was severely compromised in both positions, it was considerably worse in the seated than in the supine position. Observations of respiratory movements were made using the Respitrace unit. (See Chapter 7 for a more detailed discussion of this instrument.) This examination indicated that rest breathing was accomplished almost exclusively with abdominal movements. Rib cage movements appeared to contribute only minimally during rest breathing.

Several pushing techniques were explored in an effort to facilitate the initiation of voicing in the seated position. Most of these were unsuccessful. First, Sam did not have the trunk control to push a respiratory paddle. Likewise, he did not have sufficient arm strength to push against his own abdomen when attempting to initiate phonation. Only one technique appeared to be associated with consistent production of phonation. This technique involved both pushing and an attempt to initiate phonation at maximum lung volume. Sam was asked to push his legs against his footrests and his arms on his lap tray. When performing this maneuver, he displaced his rib cage and presumably initiated phonation at a higher lung volume level than when relying on his abdominal musculature alone. Further, the generalized pushing movement appeared to increase Sam's overall muscle tone. This may have been responsible for better adduction of the vocal folds. Once voluntary phonation was established, we began to consider techniques to manage the incompetent velopharyngeal mechanism. These efforts are described in Chapter 10. Sam quickly learned to use this technique during conversational speech, and began to use it consistently and successfully in day-to-day communication. Although more effort was required to speak when seated, Sam considered this part of his "exercise routine."

Increasing Loudness for Persons with Hypoadduction of the Vocal Folds Due to Flaccid Dysarthria

BEHAVIORAL TRAINING

Respiratory support and control are critical aspects in determining vocal loudness. The respiratory capabilities of individuals with dysarthria who are not sufficiently loud should be examined carefully. Behavioral training for loudness may involve training the speaker to generate greater levels of subglottal air pressure or to initiate phonation at appropriate lung volume levels or at appropriate times in the respiratory cycle. These and other techniques are discussed in detail in Chapter 7. Increases in subglottal air pressure must be coordinated with appropriate increases in the medial compression (adduction force) of the vocal folds.

> *Question: I work in an acute hospital and see patients who have previously been orally intubated and are emerging from coma. They often have a breathy voice. Would voice intervention be effective?*
>
> Prolonged periods of oral intubation may cause swelling of the vocal folds. This swelling and, therefore, the breathiness typically resolve spontaneously in a few days. Typically, we do not intervene with this laryngeal impairment; however, we monitor the patients' progress. If the laryngeal impairment does not resolve, these speakers should be referred to an otolaryngologist for a laryngeal examination and appropriate referrals.

INCREASING MEDIAL COMPRESSION IN SPEAKERS WITH FLACCID DYSARTHRIA

Increasing the medial compression (adduction force) of the vocal folds is also a component in intervention programs designed to increase vocal loudness for persons with flaccid and hypokinetic dysarthria. Exercises using "effortful closure techniques" have traditionally been used to increase medial compression of the vocal folds for speakers with adductory weakness (paresis) or paralysis in persons with flaccid dysarthria (Duffy, 1995). These techniques include pushing, lifting, pulling, grunting, and controlled coughing. While these techniques are used during intervention sessions, some speakers may use them during nearly all speaking activities. For these individuals, wheelchairs, traditional chairs, and beds must often be modified so they have something convenient to grasp, pull on, or push against. Other speakers are able to increase medial compression of the vocal folds by pressing their elbows down on the conventional armrests of a wheelchair or by pressing their hands together. Effortful closure techniques are employed temporarily by some speakers with flaccid dysarthria; however, others use these techniques during all speech efforts over an extended period of time.

Question: At times we have difficulty setting up speakers with diffuse motor impairment such that they can independently use effortful closure techniques. How have you dealt with that problem?

We mount a handlebar grip from a bicycle anterior to the armrest(s) of a speaker's wheelchair. While resting arms on the armrests, the speaker can grasp the handlebar grip and pull on it as he or she initiates phonation. The pulling activity increases the medial compression of the vocal folds, thereby reducing vocal breathiness, improving vocal quality, and increasing vocal loudness.

When such a speaker is in bed, a Striker Frame can be mounted over the bed. The speaker can then grasp a handle attached to the Striker Frame and pull gently while initiating phonation.

Some speakers with flaccid dysarthria improve the loudness of their phonation by rotating the head to the left or the right during phonation, or by manipulating the larynx (thyroid cartilage) with their fingers. These postures may increase tension in the weak vocal fold and enhance vocal fold closure (Aronson, 1990; McFarland, Holt-Romeo, Lavorato, & Warner, 1991). Speakers often resist the use of such intervention strategies for conversational speech because of their unusual appearance.

Once the medial position of the vocal folds has been optimized, speakers with dysarthria should be taught to speak in such a way that their subglottal air pressure level is appropriate for the degree of medial compression of the vocal folds. Speakers and their clinicians may need to experiment to achieve this balance. Often, speakers must learn to reduce their level of subglottal air pressure to match the level of medial compression offered by weakened vocal folds. In an effort to increase the loudness of their speech, some individuals with laryngeal weakness will attempt to increase their loudness by increasing the subglottal air pressure only. If the level of subglottal air pressure is excessive relative to the level of medial compression, phonation will increase in roughness with minimal (if any) increase in loudness. Often loudness and voice quality are maximized when subglottal air pressure and medial compression of the vocal folds are "balanced." Some individuals who have been "overdriving" their laryngeal subsystems in an effort to increase their loudness may resist initial efforts to encourage them to decrease their respiratory drive during speech.

SURGICAL PROCEDURES

Laryngoplasty is a surgical procedure that may be used to move one or both vocal folds medially and improve phonation. Laryngoplasty is the placement of an implant (cartilage or alloplastic) between the thyroid cartilage and the inner thyroid perchondrium on the weak side in order to move the vocal fold medially. This laryngoplasty procedure is reversible, as the implant(s) can be removed (Duffy, 1995).

Teflon, collagen, or autogenous fat can be injected into the weak or paralyzed vocal fold in order to increase the bulk of the fold, thereby reducing breathiness and improving loudness (Ford & Bless, 1986; Remalce, Marbaix, Hamoir, Declaye, & van den Eeckhaut, 1989). These procedures are not reversible and are not recommended until a year postonset.

Reinnervation techniques, such as nerve–muscle pedicle (surgical implantation of a strip of muscle with its blood and nerve supply intact into a weakened or paralyzed muscle) and nerve anastamosis (surgical connection between nerves), address the problem of the loss of vocal fold body and tonicity due to atrophy and weakness. Transplanted muscle blocks can provide innervation to a paralyzed muscle. Neuromuscular pedicle reinnervation usually involves the lateral cricoarytenoid or thyroarytenoid, the main vocal fold adductors.

Nerve to nerve reinnervation of two types may be considered for persons with laryngeal paralysis. Recurrent laryngeal nerve to recurrent laryngeal nerve reinnervation is not consistently successful (Stemple, Glaze, & Gerdmeman, 1994). Crumley (1991) developed a procedure connecting the ansa cervicalis to the recurrent laryngeal nerve. The procedure yields a "quiet" tonicity of the vocal fold body, which is a good vibratory source for voice production. Reinnervation techniques are used with persons with laryngeal paralysis only and not usually with persons who have a dysarthria that involves multiple speech subsystems.

Question: I have used the techniques described above to increase the loudness of speakers with flaccid dysarthria. However, how do I approach speakers who demonstrate mixed (flaccid–spastic) dysarthria?

Speakers with mixed dysarthria often experience a unique problem when attempting to increase their respiratory drive and optimize their laryngeal function. When speakers with mixed dysarthria, who have a weakness component to their impairment, increase their effort to achieve a more adequate level of respiratory drive, they may simultaneously increase the resistance at the level of the larynx due to the spastic component of their dysarthria. Such speakers require instruction to increase their respiratory drive while relaxing their laryngeal structures. Few speakers with mixed dysarthria can manage this on their own, without instruction.

Increasing Vocal Loudness and Voice Quality in Persons with Hypoadduction of the Vocal Folds Due to Hypokinetic Dysarthria

Reduced vocal loudness is commonly experienced by persons with hypokinetic dysarthria. During the past 10 years, Ramig and colleagues have focused on an intervention program, called the Lee Silverman Voice Treatment for Parkinson's Disease, to improve the vocal performance of these speakers. This program focuses on increasing vocal effort in order to enhance vocal fold closure and loudness (Ramig, Pawlas, & Countryman, 1995). While the primary goal is to increase loudness and decrease breathiness by increasing vocal fold adduction, a secondary goal is to improve intonation by increasing cricothyroid muscle activity. A third goal is to improve voice quality by increasing stability of vocal fold vibration. This intervention approach is intense (four times a week for a month) to reach the habitual use of the loud voice. To encourage loud voice with good quality, adduction exercises that may include "pushing" exercises are often used. Ramig and Dromey (1996) reported that the combination of increased vocal fold adduction and increased subglottal air pressure is key in generating increases in vocal intensity following treatment.

Once the louder voice is established, use of the respiratory and laryngeal subsystems at high effort levels is encouraged by having the speaker engage in exercises requiring maximum duration of vowel phonation with constant levels of loudness and steadiness. Fundamental frequency range exercises (habitual pitch to lowest pitch and habitual pitch to highest pitch) are practiced.

Speakers with Parkinson's disease are encouraged to talk with the same effort level in conversation as during the sustained phonation exercises. Increased effort during phonation encourages increased accuracy in articulation as well; therefore, the Lee Silverman Voice Treatment approach does not focus on articulatory interventions directly.

To habituate and generalize the "loud" voice, there is often the need to recalibrate the individual so that he or she is comfortable with the louder voice. Activities helpful in the calibration phase are feedback with a tape recorder, activities of self-monitoring, and group therapy after the initial 16 sessions (Ramig, Pawlas, & Countryman, 1995). The beneficial influence of group therapy on the recalibration process has also been reported (Sullivan, Brune, & Beukelman, 1996).

Ramig and colleagues have suggested several factors that increase the likelihood that patients will improve with the Lee Silverman Voice Treatment program. Persons with classic Parkinson's disease and the classic hypoadducted (bowed) vocal folds with anterior glottal gap respond well. Persons who are motivated to improve their speech function and who value speech are good candidates. Many persons may not be motivated initially, because they may have already been unsuccessful in improving their speech; however, they may become motivated when they observe initial progress. Persons who are stimulable to produce voices louder than their habitual voices are good candidates (Countryman & Ramig, 1993; Ramig, Countryman, Thompson, & Horii, 1995). Mead, Ramig, and Beck (1989) have reported that persons with adequate cognition respond well to treatment; however, positive posttreatment results also occur with persons who are mildly or moderately demented.

PROSTHETIC MANAGEMENT

In cases where speakers are unable to change their vocal loudness pattern, speech intensity may be enhanced by portable amplification systems. Figure 8.2 illustrates one such amplifier. The system is small enough to be carried in a pocket or purse, and a microphone small enough to be mounted on eyeglasses or behind the ear may be used. We have found that such amplifiers are successful for some speakers with parkinsonism. The amplifiers appear to be much more effective when quiet phonation is present than when the speaker produces only a whisper.

> Question: What type of technology do you use when a speaker is unable to produce phonation consistently during speech?
>
> Recently, the Voice Enhancer has been introduced with a high-quality, directional microphone that has amplified whispered speech quite effectively for some clients.

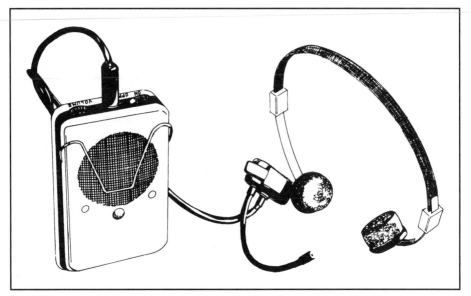

Figure 8.2. A portable, battery-operated voice amplifier (Cooper-Rand), by Luminaud, Inc., 8688 Tyler Boulevard, Mentor, OH 44060.

SURGICAL PROCEDURES

During the past few years, pallidotomy surgery has been used with increasing frequency to reduce the symptoms of Parkinson's disease. Schulz, Sapienza, and Peterson (1996) reported the impact of pallidotomy surgery on six individuals with Parkinson's disease. They reported that surgery has more consistent positive results on limb movement and tremor than on the voice and speech symptoms. Three of the six speakers showed improved acoustic evidence of phonatory improvement and three did not. Barlow, Iacono, Paseman, Biswas, and D'Antonio (1998) reported reductions in laryngeal resistance for some speakers with Parkinson's disease following pallidotomy. Once pallidotomized, speakers (with Parkinson's disease) frequently reported that speech required less effort.

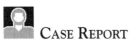 **CASE REPORT**

Ken was diagnosed with Parkinson's disease 10 years before he was referred to our clinic. He was the supervisor of a custom tool shop in a local industry. He found that he was unable to speak loudly enough to be heard in the noisy environment, so for at least a year, he had invited all of his employees into his office to communicate with them. In Ken's opinion, his method of staff communication was inadequate, because it did not allow him to discuss problems and solutions in the shop where the work was being done.

The problem that brought Ken to us was his increasing inability to communicate effectively at management team meetings. He was concerned that he was losing his ability to represent his area well. A brief conversation revealed the presence of a voice impairment. Ken's voice was characteristic of many people with Parkinson's disease. His voice was breathy and vocal intensity was low; however, phonation was consistently present. A more complete assessment revealed that Ken's estimated subglottal air pressure during speech averaged between 2 and 3 cm H_2O. His respiratory pattern was unusual in several ways. He frequently initiated speech at 40% of lung volume level or lower. To complete utterances of reasonable breath group lengths, he frequently spoke to lung volume levels of 20% or lower before inhaling. His inhalations were often minimal, raising his lung volume levels only 10% or 15%.

Ken was involved in a trial of respiratory treatment described in Chapter 7. Using the Respitrace unit, he was instructed to initiate phonation at approximately 60% of vital capacity and end the breath group at no lower lung volume level than 30%. In addition, he was instructed to inhale to approximately 60% of lung volume level before each breath group, and thus to eliminate the minimal inhalations that he had used habitually. With biofeedback, Ken achieved those objectives with remarkable ease. In the treatment room, he was speaking and achieving the objectives without constant feedback, and he reported that in group meetings, he was able to speak with acceptable loudness. However, during conversation, he frequently neglected to exercise the level of respiratory control that he achieved in group meetings or in treatment. Ken was provided with a portable voice amplifier and a boom microphone mounted on his glasses for communication in the shop. Depending on the progression of his disease, the portable amplification system may become a regularly worn prosthesis.

Reducing Hyperadduction of the Vocal Folds

Speakers with spastic dysarthria often hyperadduct their vocal folds, with a resulting harsh voice or, in severe cases, a strained–strangled voice. When treating such individuals, the clinician should make an initial determination as to whether they are overdriving their laryngeal mechanisms by speaking with excessive effort and vocal loudness. If so, one aspect of the intervention process is to attempt to instruct these speakers to talk with less effort, hopefully reducing the hyperadduction of their vocal folds and the associated harsh, rough voice quality. In some speakers, reduction in effort can be accomplished through direct instruction. However, others require feedback to change their habitual speaking patterns. Feedback can be provided with a sound level measuring device or a system to monitor oral air pressure during speech as an estimate of subglottal air pressure (see Chapter 7). Traditional relaxation procedures have been recommended with strained voices (Brookshire, 1992; Rosenbek & LaPointe, 1985). However, in our experience, the success of these approaches is inconsistent. Effortful closure techniques (pulling, pushing, and lifting) are not recommended for speakers with spastic dysarthria, because hyperadduction of the vocal folds is already a problem for many of these speakers.

IMPROVING VOICE QUALITY

Dysarthric speech is frequently characterized as rough, hoarse, harsh, or breathy. Often, these symptoms are not treated. For speakers with severe dysarthria, other aspects of speech production may be more critical to the improvement of speech intelligibility. For speakers with mild dysarthria, the presence of a slight phonatory impairment may not be an important handicap. When voice quality impairment is present and it is felt to contribute to overall disability and handicap, intervention may be warranted. When voice quality disorders are associated with hyperadduction of the vocal folds, traditional voice therapy techniques designed to reduce laryngeal hyperadduction and to increase airflow through the glottis may be appropriate (Prator & Swift, 1984).

Smitheran and Hixon (1981) reported intervention with a 57-year-old man who had had multiple bilateral CVAs. Among the characteristics of his mixed dysarthria was a markedly strained–strangled voice quality. Estimates of laryngeal airway resistance suggested excessive laryngeal obstruction of airway, with a resistance score 85% higher than that of normal individuals. It was assumed this high resistance value was associated with the probable spastic component of his laryngeal problem. Voice quality was judged to be perceptually better when the speaker was asked to perform under one of the following conditions: to raise his fundamental frequency, to rotate his head backward, or to initiate his utterance from a high lung volume level. These perceptual changes also were associated with decreases in laryngeal airway resistance. Smitheran and Hixon stated, "It was assumed that this improvement was related to passive abduction of the vocal folds brought about by the tracheal tug associated with a lower diaphragm position at a high lung volume level" (p. 145).

Question: Are pharmacological approaches ever used to treat the phonatory problems of persons with spastic dysarthria?

Antispasticity medications are occasionally used to reduce hyperadduction of the vocal folds in persons with spastic dysarthria. Dworkin (1991) reported that Dantrium may be beneficial for some patients. In our experience, the benefits of antispasticity medications, taken orally for improvement in voice quality, are often outweighed by side effects, such as increased swallowing problems. Recent improvements in the delivery of antispas-

(continues)

ticity medication with an intravenous pump have yielded encouraging results in controlling spasticity in general. No studies on the impact of such a medical regime on phonation have been reported.

As reported in Chapter 4, botox injections may result in dramatic improvement in speech for persons with spasdomic dysphonia. However, adverse effects may include decreased loudness, breathiness, and difficulty swallowing liquids.

Improving Laryngeal Coordination

RESPIRATORY–LARYNGEAL TIMING

Appropriate laryngeal timing usually involves two issues for speakers with dysarthria. One is the prompt initiation of phonation at the beginning of the exhalation phase of respiration for speech. Prompt initiation of phonation reduces air wastage and fatigue during speech. We have found respiratory biofeedback using the Respitrace unit particularly helpful in training this aspect of phonatory timing. With a respiratory signal displayed on one channel of a scope and a raw acoustic waveform or intensity contour from an intensity analysis system, such as the Visipitch, on the second channel of a storage scope, the respiratory–phonatory timing patterns can be "captured" and presented to the speaker as biofeedback.

Some speakers, who experience difficulty initiating phonation promptly upon initiation of exhalation, are able to initiate phonation by using an effortful closure technique such as pulling or pushing. As mentioned previously, one of our clients initiated phonation by pulling on a bicycle hand grip that was attached to the anterior portion of his wheelchair armrest. Once phonation was initiated, he relaxed his pulling effort for the remainder of the utterance. At the beginning of the next utterance, he pulled on the hand grip again. A second man with dysarthria due to traumatic brain injury was unable to consistently initiate phonation in a timely manner at the beginning of utterances. He learned to initiate phonation promptly by pushing his hand against the hand of his listener as though he were giving the listener a "high-five" gesture. In time, this gesture was no longer needed to initiate phonation.

ARTICULATORY DISTINCTIONS

A second aspect of phonatory timing is voice onset and cessation during the production of voiceless consonants in vowel environments. Many individuals with dysarthria have extreme difficulty producing perceptually different voiced–voiceless cognate pairs or producing the /h/ sound in the initial position of words. Because the phonatory timing requirement for this task is so demanding, we have successfully taught some individuals to exaggerate other aspects of the voiced–voiceless distinction. For example, some speakers may produce the distinction by aspirating final unvoiced plosives and producing final voiceless plosives without aspiration. Rosenbek and LaPointe (1985) have listed some other differences that may be useful training techniques. For example, voiced plosives are usually accompanied by greater intraoral breath pressure and airflow than their voiceless counterparts. Vowel duration before voiceless productions are typically longer than before unvoiced productions. We typically train individuals with dysarthria to produce voiced–voiceless or aspiration distinctions within the framework of the intelligibility drill (see Chapter 11). Briefly, when voicing contrasts such as "cap" and "cab" are present, a listener naive to the target utterance is asked to transcribe the utterance produced by the speaker. The speaker is informed of the perceived message as an indication of whether or not the target distinction was adequately produced.

REFERENCES

Aronson, A. (1971). Early motor unit disease masquerading as psychogenic breathy dysphonia: A clinical case presentation. *Journal of Speech and Hearing Disorders, 36*, 115–124.

Aronson, A. E. (1980). *Clinical voice disorders: An interdisciplinary approach.* New York: Thieme.

Aronson, A. E. (1985). *Clinical voice disorders: An interdisciplinary approach* (2nd ed.). New York: Thieme.

Aronson, A. E. (1990). *Clinical voice disorders* (3rd ed.). New York: Thieme.

Barlow, S. M., Iacono, R. P., Paseman, L. A., Biswas, A., & D'Antonio, L. (1998). The effects of posteroventral pallidotomy on force and speech aerodynamics in Parkinson's disease. In M. Cannito, K. M. Yorkston, & D. R. Beukelman (Eds.), *Neuromotor speech disorders: Nature, assessment, and management* (pp. 117–156). Baltimore: Brookes.

Barlow, S. M., Netsell, R., & Hunker, C. (1986). Phonatory disorders associated with CNS lesions. In C. Cummings, J. Fredrickson, L. Harker, C. Krause, & D. Schuller (Eds.), *Otolaryngology—Head neck surgery* (Vol. 3, pp. 2087–2093). St. Louis: Mosby.

Bellaire, K., Yorkston, K. M., & Beukelman, D. R. (1986). Modification of breath patterning to increase naturalness of a mildly dysarthric speaker. *Journal of Communication Disorders, 19*, 271–280.

Benjamin, B. (1981). Frequency variability in the aged voice. *Journal of Gerontology, 36*, 722–726.

Bielamowic, S., Kreiman, J., Gerratt, B., Dauer, M., & Berke, G. (1996). Comparison of voice analysis systems for perturbation measurement. *Journal of Speech and Hearing Research, 39*, 126–134.

Blitzer, A., Sasaki, C., Fahn, S., Brin, M., & Harris, K. (Eds.). (1992). *Neurological disorders of the larynx.* New York: Thieme Medical.

Boone, D. (1977). *The voice and voice therapy* (2nd ed.). Englewood Cliffs, NJ: Prentice-Hall.

Brookshire, R. (1992). *An introduction to neurogenic communication disorders* (4th ed.). St Louis: Mosby–Year Book.

Countryman, S., & Ramig, L. O. (1993). The effects of intensive voice therapy on voice deficits associated with bilateral thalomotomy in Parkinson's disease: A case study. *Journal of Medical Speech-Language Pathology, 1*, 233–250.

Crumley, R. L. (1991). Update: Ansa cervicalis to recurrent laryngeal nerve anastomosis for unilateral laryngeal paralysis. *Laryngoscope, 101*, 384–387.

Darley, F. L., Aronson, A. E., & Brown, J. R. (1975). *Motor speech disorders.* Philadelphia: Saunders.

Duffy, J. R. (1995). *Motor speech disorders: Substrates, differential diagnosis, and management.* St. Louis: Mosby.

Dworkin, J. P. (1991). *Motor speech disorders: A treatment guide.* St. Louis: Mosby.

Ford, C., & Bless, D. (1986). A preliminary study of injectable collagen in human vocal fold augmentation. *Otolaryngology, Head and Neck Surgery, 94,* 104.

Garrett, J., & Larson, C. (1991). Neurology of the laryngeal system. In C. N. Ford & D. Bless (Eds.), *Phonosurgery* (pp. 43–76). New York: Raven Press.

Hartelius, L., Buder, E., & Strand, E. (1997). Long-term phonatory instability in individuals with multiple sclerosis. *Journal of Speech, Language, and Hearing Research, 40,* 1056–1072.

Hoit, J. D., & Hixon, T. J. (1992). Age and laryngeal airway resistance during vowel production in women. *Journal of Speech and Hearing Research, 35,* 309–313.

Kent, R. D., Weismer, G., Kent, J. F., & Rosenbek, J. C. (1989). Toward phonetic intelligibility testing in dysarthria. *Journal of Speech and Hearing Disorders, 54,* 482–499.

Logemann, J. A., Fisher, H. B., Boshes, B., & Blonsky, E. (1978). Frequency and cooccurrence of vocal tract dysfunction in the speech of a large sample of Parkinson patients. *Journal of Speech and Hearing Disorders, 43,* 47–57.

Ludlow, C. L., & Bassich, C. J. (1983). The results of acoustic and perceptual assessment of two types of dysarthria. In W. Berry (Ed.), *Clinical dysarthria* (pp. 121–154). Austin, TX: PRO-ED.

Ludlow, C., & Bassich, C. (1984). Relationship between perceptual ratings and acoustic measures of phyokinetic speech. In J. R. M. McNeil & A. Aronson (Ed.), *The dysarthrias: Physiology, acoustics, perception, management* (pp. 163–197). Austin, TX: PRO-ED.

McFarland, S., Holt-Romeo, T., Lavorato, A., & Warner, L. (1991). Unilateral vocal fold paralysis: Perceived vocal quality following three methods of treatment. *ASHA, 1*(1), 45–62.

Mead, C., Ramig, L., & Beck, J. (1989). Parkinson's disease with severe dementia: Effectiveness of intensive voice therapy. *ASHA, 31,* 118.

Orlikoff, R., & Kahane, J. (1996). Structure and function of the larynx. In N. Lass (Ed.), *Principles of experimental phonetics* (pp. 112–118). St. Louis: Mosby.

Prator, R. J., & Swift, R. (1984). *Manual of voice therapy.* Boston: Little, Brown.

Ramig, L. (1992). The role of phonation in speech intelligibility: A review and preliminary data from patients with Parkinson's disease. In R. D. Kent (Ed.), *Intelligibility in speech disorders* (pp. 119–156). Philadelphia: John Benjamins.

Ramig, L. (1995). Voice therapy for neurologic disease. *Otolaryngology—Head and Neck Surgery, 3,* 174–182.

Ramig, L. O., Countryman, S., Thompson, L. L., & Horii, Y. (1995). A comparison of two forms of intensive speech treatment in Parkinson disease. *Journal of Speech and Hearing Research, 38,* 1232–1251.

Ramig, L. O., & Dromey, C. (1996). Aerodynamic mechanisms underlying treatment-related changes in vocal intensity in patients with Parkinson disease. *Journal of Speech and Hearing Research, 39,* 798–807.

Ramig, L. O., Pawlas, A. A., & Countryman, S. (1995). *The Lee Silverman Voice Treatment.* Iowa City, IA: National Center for Voice and Speech.

Ramig, L., & Scherer, R. (1992). Speech therapy for neurological disorders of the larynx. In A. Blitzer, C. Sasaki, S. Fahn, M. Brin, & K. Harris (Eds.), *Neurological disorders of the larynx* (pp. 248–278). New York: Thieme Medical.

Remalce, M., Marbaix, E., Hamoir, M., Declaye, X., & van den Eeckhaut, M. (1989). Initial long-term results of collagen injection for vocal and laryngeal rehabilitation. *Archives of Oto-Rhino-Laryngology, 246,* 403–406.

Robin, D. A., Klouda, G. V., & Hug, L. N. (1991). Neurogenic disorders of prosody. In M. P. Cannito & D. Vogel (Eds.), *Treating disordered speech motor control: For clinicians by clinicians* (pp. 241–271). Austin, TX: PRO-ED.

Rosenbek, J. (1984). Treating the dysarthric talker. *Seminars in Speech and Language, 5,* 359–384.

Rosenbek, J. C., & LaPointe, L. L. (1985). The dysarthrias: Description, diagnosis, and treatment. In D. Johns (Ed.), *Clinical management of neurogenic communication disorders* (pp. 97–152). Boston: Little, Brown.

Roth, C. R., Glaze, L. E., Goding, G. S., & David, W. S. (1996). Spasmodic dysphonia symptoms as initial presentation of amyotrophic lateral sclerosis. *Journal of Voice, 10,* 362–367.

Schulz, G., Sapienza, C., & Peterson, T. (1996, November). *Effects of pallidotomy surgery on parkinsonism voice production.* Paper presented at the Annual Convention of the American Speech-Language-Hearing Association, Seattle, WA.

Smitheran, J., & Hixon, T. (1981). A clinical method for estimating laryngeal airway resistance during vowel production. *Journal of Speech and Hearing Disorders, 46,* 138–146.

Solomon, J. R., Ludolph, L. B., & Thomson, F. E. (1984, February). *How "mono" is monopitch: An acoustic analysis of motor speech disorders tapes.* Paper presented at the Biennial Clinical Dysarthria Conference, Tucson, AZ.

Southwood, M. H. (1996). Direct magnitude estimation and interval scaling of naturalness and bizarreness of the dysarthria associated with amyotrophic lateral sclerosis. *Journal of Medical Speech-Language Pathology, 4*(1), 13–27.

Stemple, J., Glaze, L., & Gerdmeman, B. (1994). *Clinical voice pathology: Theory and management* (2nd ed.). San Diego: Singular.

Stone, M. (1996). Instrumentation for the study of speech physiology. In N. Lass (Ed.), *Principles of experimental phonetics* (pp. 495–524). St. Louis: Mosby.

Strand, E. A., Buder, E. H., Yorkston, K. M., & Ramig, L. O. (1994). Differential phonatory characteristics of four women with amyotrophic lateral sclerosis. *Journal of Voice, 8,* 327–339.

Sullivan, M. D., Brune, P. J., & Beukelman, D. R. (1996). Maintenance of speech changes following group treatment for hypokinetic dysarthria of Parkinson's disease. In D. A. Robin, K. M. Yorkston, & D. R. Beukelman (Eds.), *Disorders of motor speech: Assessment, treatment and clinical characterization* (pp. 287–310). Baltimore: Brookes.

Weismer, G. (1990, March). *Keynote address.* Paper presented at the Clinical Dysarthria Conference, San Antonio.

CHAPTER

9

VELOPHARYNGEAL FUNCTION

Clinical Issues: A speech–language pathology student was invited to observe a palatal lift fitting for a young adult with severe dysarthria due to traumatic brain injury. The fitting involved several modifications of the lift. Gradually, the prosthodontist and speech–language pathologist agreed that their intervention goals for this speaker had been met, the lift was given a final polish, and the speaker was sent on his way.

The student was full of questions about the fitting:

- When multiple speech components are impaired, where should intervention begin?

- Who is a candidate for a palatal lift?

- How do you know when you have a well-fitting palatal lift?

- Can speakers with dysarthria and velopharyngeal incompetence be managed successfully with behavioral methods alone?

- How do velopharyngeal management options differ for speakers with dysarthria and for speakers with cleft palate?

Velopharyngeal dysfunction is frequently, but not universally, associated with dysarthria. Although the incidence of velopharyngeal dysfunction is unavailable for most populations of speakers with dysarthria, it is reported that approximately 40% of children with cerebral palsy have velopharyngeal closure problems that are considered important to their speech problems (Hardy, Rembolt, Spriestersbach, & Jaypathy, 1961). Perceptual evidence of hypernasality and nasal emission has been reported in many types of dysarthria, including flaccid, spastic, ataxic, hyperkinetic dysarthria of chorea, and some mixed dysarthrias such as in amyotrophic lateral sclerosis (ALS) (Darley, 1984). Although some researchers have suggested that nasal resonance disorders are absent or present only in mild form in Parkinson's disease (Logemann, Fisher, Boshes, & Blonsky, 1978; Mueller, 1971), others conclude that disordered resonance occurs systematically in speakers with Parkinson's disease and may be a severe problem for some individuals (Hoodin & Gilbert, 1989; Ludlow & Bassich, 1983; Morrison, Rigrodsky, & Mysak, 1970; Netsell, Daniel, & Celesia, 1975). This research suggests that velopharyngeal dysfunction occurs not only in those individuals with lower motor neuron damage affecting innervation of the soft palate, but also in individuals with other underlying neuropathologies, including damage to the cortex, basal ganglia, and cerebellum.

Although velopharyngeal dysfunction does not occur in all speakers with dysarthria, an understanding of the velopharyngeal mechanism, its disorders, and its management is extremely important clinically. Velopharyngeal dysfunction of speakers with dysarthria is of critical interest to the clinician because it tends to exaggerate the impairment of other speech mechanism components. For example, a speaker with an impaired respiratory system may perform adequately to produce functional speech if the laryngeal, velopharyngeal, and oral articulatory valves are functioning efficiently. However, in the presence of velopharyngeal dysfunction, the speaker may not be able to maintain adequate respiratory drive for speech. Velopharyngeal dysfunction distorts the production of vowel and consonant sounds even though they may be produced with accurate oral articulatory gestures. In the presence of velopharyngeal dysfunction, vowels will be perceived as hypernasal and many consonants will be perceived as imprecise.

Case reports of interventions ranging from prosthetic management to behavioral training and surgery suggest that the velopharyngeal mechanism can be managed successfully in selected individuals and that this management positively influences other aspects of speech production. These interventions will be described in detail later in this chapter. Although it is encouraging to read reports of successful interventions, a review of the literature also suggests that there is no single best approach to velopharyngeal management. Rather, because velopharyngeal dysfunction in dysarthria may vary widely in its characteristics, interventions must also be tailored to the specifics of the dysfunction. Thus, the clinician not only must be able to verify whether there is a velopharyngeal problem, but also must be able to carefully describe the extent and consistency of the deficit before an appropriate intervention can be recommended.

VELOPHARYNGEAL FUNCTION DURING SPEECH

Normal Speakers

THE MECHANISM

The velopharyngeal mechanism consists of the soft palate and that portion of the pharynx that approximates the soft palate. The velopharyngeal mechanism functions to couple the nasal cavity with the oropharyngeal cavity during speaking and swallowing. At times, this coupling involves separately the two cavities. At other times, it involves opening for linking the two.

A number of different patterns of velopharyngeal closure occur in both normal speakers and speakers with disorders. Using multiview videofluoroscopy, Croft, Shprintzen, and Rakoff (1981) classified large groups of normal speakers into the following valving categories:

- *Coronal*—The velum or soft palate approximates to the posterior pharyngeal wall, which remains immobile. The lateral pharyngeal walls move medially to approximate the lateral edges of the velum. The major component of velopharyngeal valving occurs in the antero-posterior direction. This pattern occurred in 55% of normal speakers.

- *Sagittal*—Marked movement of the lateral pharyngeal walls occurs posterior to the velum, which moves posteriorly only slightly, approximating to the anterior edge of the abutted lateral walls. This pattern occurred in 16% of normal speakers.

- *Circular*—There are equal amounts of movement in the velum and the lateral pharyngeal walls, creating a circular closure pattern. This pattern occurred in 10% of normal speakers.

- *Circular with Passavant's Ridge*—As in the circular pattern, there is equal contribution to closure of the velum and the lateral walls, but there is also anterior movement in the posterior pharyngeal wall (Passavant's ridge), resulting in a truly sphincteric closure pattern. This pattern occurred in 19% of normal speakers.

Although differing patterns of velopharyngeal closure are observed in normal speakers, the roles, anatomy, and histology of the muscles of velopharyngeal closure are well known and are reviewed in Figure 9.1 and Table 9.1. Kuehn and Kahane (1990) presented an excellent review of the anatomy, histology, and physiology of the velopharyngeal mechanism.

The shape of velopharyngeal closure is influenced by the structural anatomy of the speaker and the coordination of velopharyngeal muscle activity. The anatomical differences of the oral and nasal cavities of normal adult speakers are extensive. Given their differing anatomies, speakers must achieve velopharyngeal closure by coordinating the movement of their muscular structures. The positioning of the velopharyngeal mechanism during speech is determined by the relative contributions of several muscles: levator, palatoglossus, palatopharyngeus, and pharyngeal constrictors. The levator is the primary muscle involved in the elevation of the soft palate during speech. The contributions made by the palatoglossus muscle depend on the vowel sound being produced.

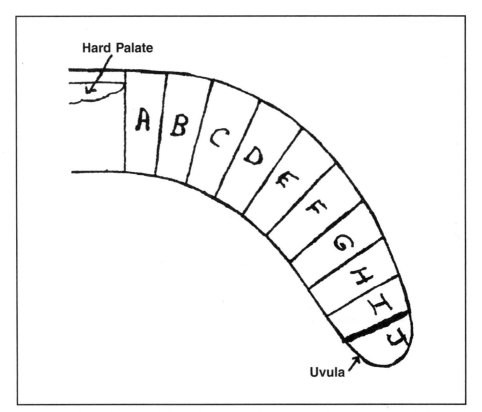

Figure 9.1. Line drawing of the soft palate with Segments A through J (see Table 9.1) identified.

Table 9.1

Presence of Muscle Tissue in 10 Segments (A–J) of the Soft Palate

	Segments of the Soft Palate									
Muscle	A	B	C	D	E	F	G	H	I	J
Tendon of tensor muscle	10	10	9	0	0	0	0	0	0	0
Levator muscles	10	10	10	10	10	10	5	0	0	0
Palatoglossus muscle	0	0	0	4		5	4	4	0	0
Palatopharyngeus muscle	0	0	0	P	10	10	10	10		0
Uvular muscle	0	0	1	10	10	10	5	10	10	4

Note. Segment A adjoins the hard palate, and Segment J is the most posterior portion of the soft palate. The number in each cell refers to the number of persons ($N = 10$) whose tissue samples contained the presence of muscle fiber in a given segment.

Data from "Histologic Study of the Normal Human Soft Palate," by D. Kuehn and J. Kahane, 1990, *Cleft Palate Journal, 27*, p. 27.

The soft palate is a richly innervated structure. The levator veli palatini, uvula, and superior pharyngeal constrictor muscles are dually innervated by the facial nerve and the branches of the pharyngeal plexus derived from the glossopharyngeal and vagus nerves (Nishio, Matsuya, Ibuki, & Miyazaki, 1976). Studies conducted on rhesus monkeys suggest that the movements observed on stimulation of the vagus or glossopharyngeal nerve were similar to those observed in swallowing in humans, whereas stimulation to the facial nerve resulted in velopharyngeal movement similar to that observed in human phonation (Nishio et al., 1976). Thus, the motor nerves innervating the velopharynx may be responsible for different types of movements.

Question: In our clinical practice, we see individuals across the age range. During nasoendoscopic examination, there is a wide variation among the velopharyngeal closure patterns for different clients. Are any of these differences in velopharyngeal performance due to age?

The impact of age on velopharyngeal function has been studied by two research groups with somewhat different results. Hoit, Watson, Hixon, McMahon, and Johnson (1994) concluded from their aerodynamic measurements that there are no age-related differences in nasal airflow during consonant production. However, Hutchinson, Robinson, and Nerbonne (1978) measured sound pressure levels using two microphones, one near the nose and one near the mouth. They reported that older speakers had higher nasalance scores than younger speakers.

The Speaking Task

The role of the velopharyngeal mechanism for normal speakers varies, depending on the speaking task. During the production of nonnasal consonant sounds, the velopharyngeal mechanism can be viewed as an aerodynamic valve that usually is completely sealed to prevent the escape of air from the oral cavity through the nasal cavity (Thompson & Hixon, 1979; Warren, 1975; Warren & DuBois, 1964). Although the pattern and duration of closure vary from speaker to speaker, the velopharyngeal seal is usually complete during some aspects of "pressure consonant" production. However, normal speakers occasionally demonstrate very small velopharyngeal openings during the production of nonnasal consonants (Hoit et al., 1994).

Question: Recently an otolaryngologist and I examined a woman who played a clarinet professionally and who experienced air escape through her velopharyngeal mechanism when she played. Why did this happen?

Playing a brass or wind instrument requires a great deal more intraoral air pressure than does speech (Fiz et al., 1993). In our clinical experience, we have evaluated a number of brass and wind musicians who experience velopharyngeal incompetence while playing, but were velopharyngeally competent during speech. Given that normal speakers produce 5 to 8 cm H_2O during speech and musicians often produce 70 or 80 cm H_2O while playing, the demands on the velopharyngeal mechanism are much greater for musicians than for speakers. One of our clients who played clarinet had an experience similar to the woman described above, in that he became velopharyngeally incompetent when he increased the stiffness of his reeds. With wind instruments, increased stiffness of the reed is associated with increased resistance to airflow through the instrument, thereby requiring greater intraoral air pressure. In the presence of heightened intraoral air pressure, this man experienced velopharyngeal incompetence after playing for only a few minutes. When he played for extended periods of time, his velopharyngeal incompetence became worse as his velopharyngeal mechanism fatigued.

During the production of nasal consonants, the velopharyngeal mechanism is opened to allow the coupling of the oropharyngeal and nasal cavities to form the primary acoustic resonator for these sounds. The oral cavity is the occluded side branch resonator (Shoup, Lass, & Kuehn, 1982). This resonance pattern yields the acoustic patterns that are associated with hypernasal speech: low first formant, high sampling of formants, and high density of formants that are associated with nasal consonants.

During vowel and semivowel production, the status of the velopharyngeal mechanism is influenced by the velopharyngeal requirements of the adjacent consonants. Some nasalization of the vowels is common. In fact, the complete closure of the velopharyngeal mechanism results in denasality, which is judged to be abnormal. However, excessive nasality during vowel production is also judged as abnormal. Normal (balanced) nasality in English varies for different regional dialects.

Speakers with Dysarthria

In Chapters 2 through 4, the speech characteristics associated with a wide variety of neurologic conditions were discussed. Symptoms of velopharyngeal dysfunction are quite common for speakers with dysarthria. In contrast to the speaker with a cleft palate, the speaker with dysarthria has adequate palatal tissue to achieve velopharyngeal closure; however, motor control impairments are responsible for several different patterns of velopharyngeal function. Clinically, we classify velopharyngeal dysfunction into five categories and plan our interventions depending on the pattern of dysfunction observed.

1. *Consistently Adequate Closure*—Speakers included in this group demonstrate essentially normal function without hypernasality, nasal emission, or abnormal movement patterns during habitual speech.

2. *Consistently Inadequate Closure with Extensive Velopharyngeal Dysfunction*—The speakers in this group exhibit consistent velopharyngeal dysfunction. Speakers with severe flaccid dysarthria may show little or no evidence of movement of the velopharyngeal structures during speech. This impairment is associated with the extreme weakness that is characteristic of such disorders as brain stem stroke and ALS. Other speakers with moderate weakness due to flaccid or spastic impairments exhibit consistently inadequate closure of the velopharyngeal mechanism, although movement of the velopharyngeal structures may be observed.

3. *Consistently Inadequate Closure with Minimal Velopharyngeal Dysfunction*—Speakers in this group exhibit consistent velopharyngeal inadequacy; however, their degree of dysfunction is minimal under optimal speaking conditions and more pronounced when they are fatigued.

4. *Delayed Closure*—Speakers in this group exhibit delayed closure of the velopharyngeal mechanism during speech. This pattern may be observed in speakers with mild to moderate slowness of movement, perhaps due to the moderate weakness or stiffness of muscles.

5. *Inconsistent Closure*—Speakers who demonstrate inconsistent velopharyngeal closure patterns due to incoordination–timing patterns or
fatigue are included in this group. Persons with hypokinetic and ataxic
dysarthria demonstrate inconsistent velopharyngeal function during
speech. Velopharyngeal (as well as articulatory) function of these two
groups is often influenced by speaking rate. When these speakers
attempt to talk at rates that are excessive for them, velopharyngeal
incompetence may occur due to articulation timing problems. However, during the production of single words or sentences spoken at a
reduced rate, velopharyngeal function is more consistently adequate.

The various patterns of velopharyngeal closure clinically observed in speakers
with dysarthria are not completely understood. Several authors have addressed
this issue. Kuehn and Moon (1993) discussed the fatigue effect as they responded
to the common anecdotal report that clients often have the capability of producing sustained phonemes or isolated words with no evidence of velopharyngeal
incompetence but that the velopharyngeal competence breaks down in connected speech. It may be that these individuals are experiencing muscular fatigue.
The authors suggested that such individuals may not necessarily be within a state
of fatigue, but rather have developed a pattern of velopharyngeal control to *avoid*
a fatigue state that might occur very rapidly in the presence of increased or sustained muscle force generation. Perhaps because of weaker velopharyngeal
muscles, these individuals may have a lower threshold of fatigue than individuals
who have normal strength, and they may have developed a pattern of neuromotor control to remain below the fatigue threshold. Warren, Dalston, and Mayo
(1993) also considered the fatigue option. They wrote that one way to alleviate
fatigue of the velopharyngeal closure muscles is to avoid excessive opposition to
gravity and other forces that naturally tend to open the velopharyngeal port.

Reports of velopharyngeal dysfunction in speakers with dysarthria are quite
common. A series of studies from the University of Iowa focused on the velopharyngeal function in speakers with cerebral palsy (Hardy, 1983). In addition
to many of the patterns described by Netsell (1969), Hardy indicated that
velopharyngeal closure may be associated with vowel height, in that there may
be velopharyngeal closure during the production of high back vowels and adjacent consonants, but not for high front vowels, neutral vowels, and the consonants adjacent to these vowels. Hardy also suggested that velopharyngeal function might be affected by speaking rate. He suggested that there may be greater
velopharyngeal competence at rapid than at slow speaking rates, or vice versa.
In addition, he observed that patterns of velopharyngeal closure may be com-
pounded by head position.

The implication is that the velopharyngeal component of speech must be
considered in relation to other aspects of speech production. Not only may

velopharyngeal incompetence exaggerate impairment in other speech components, but such incompetence may bring about maladaptive compensatory adjustments in other aspects of speech. Velopharyngeal dysfunction in dysarthric speech resulting from various etiologies is described in detail in Chapters 2 through 4. The remainder of this chapter focuses on assessment and intervention of velopharyngeal function in specific speakers with dysarthria.

Assessment of Velopharyngeal Function

During the assessment to develop the intervention plan for a speaker with dysarthria, the clinician usually attempts to address several questions:

- Is there evidence of velopharyngeal dysfunction in this speaker?

- What are the extent, pattern, and consistency of the dysfunction?

- Does the velopharyngeal dysfunction influence other aspects of speech performance?

- What is the potential for improved velopharyngeal function to enhance overall speech performance?

- What options are available to improve velopharyngeal function for this speaker?

As in the evaluation of other aspects of dysarthria, a number of approaches to measurement are available, including perceptual and instrumental techniques. The specific measurement approach depends on the nature of the clinical question. The general question, "Is there a velopharyngeal problem?" can best be answered perceptually as the clinician listens to the speech and identifies the presence or absence of those features that are typically associated with velopharyngeal dysfunction. However, after the clinician has confirmed the presence of a problem and is seeking information regarding the extent and pattern of the dysfunction, approaches other than perceptual ones are appropriate.

Perceptual Adequacy

The first phase of assessment is the confirmation of the presence of a velopharyngeal dysfunction. The adequacy of velopharyngeal function during speech is often perceptually assessed. As discussed in the following sections, ratings of hypernasality, occurrence of nasal emission, and patterns of articulatory errors can be employed as indicators of adequacy of velopharyngeal function.

HYPERNASALITY

The term *hypernasality* refers to the perception of excessive nasality. In the field of dysarthria, it has traditionally been assessed by rating samples of connected speech on the 7-point equal-appearing interval scale used by the Mayo Clinic group (Darley, Aronson, & Brown, 1975). Presence of hypernasality may also be identified clinically by alternate pinching of the nostrils while the speaker is producing a sustained vowel (Moser, 1942). A fluttering vowel quality signals the presence of hypernasality. A word of caution is warranted, however, when using such a task because sustained phonation is a speechlike task and may not reflect the degree of hypernasality in contextual speech.

The use of perceptual ratings of hypernasality is associated with a number of limitations, one of which is judge reliability. Kuehn (1982) noted that

> one of the main disadvantages of perceptual measures, specifically listener judgments, is that they are difficult to calibrate. Perceptual judgments depend on training and experience, among other factors, and different listeners may not agree as to the severity of a particular problem. (p. 505)

In addition, mild to moderate hypernasality is an aspect of some dialectic patterns of normal speakers. In this case, hypernasality is not associated with velopharyngeal dysfunction. Perceptual judgments of hypernasality may be influenced by factors unrelated to velopharyngeal function. Noll (1982) grouped these factors into the following categories for individuals with cleft lip and palate: phonetic aspects, pitch level, loudness level, and articulatory proficiency. Although unconfirmed in the research literature, the same factors may affect judgments of hypernasality in speakers with dysarthria. Hypernasality ratings are no doubt influenced to some extent by the severity of the articulatory deficit of speakers with dysarthria. Judges tend to inflate hypernasality ratings for speakers with extensive articulation errors. Hypernasality ratings may also be affected by loudness level. If respiratory drive and, therefore, loudness levels are reduced, the extent of hypernasality may be underestimated. However, if loudness is excessive, hypernasality may be exaggerated.

Question: What types of stimulus materials have been used clinically to elicit a speech sample for judging nasality?

To elicit an adequate speech sample for judging hypernasality and hyponasality, we use paragraph as well as sentence stimuli, which include the Grandfather Passage (Darley et al., 1975) and the Rainbow Passage (Fairbanks, 1960). The "Pittsburgh Sentences" were developed to assess resonance and velopharyngeal function (Phillips, 1986):

(continues)

1. Mamma made lemon jam.
2. Put the baby in the buggy.
3. Kindly give Kate the cake.
4. Go get the wagon for the girl.
5. Sissy sees the sun in the sky.
6. The ship goes in shallow water.
7. Jim and Charlie chew gum.
8. Please tie the stamps with string.

The problems associated with perceptual ratings of hypernasality have led researchers to seek objective or instrumental means of measurement. To date, however, no substitute for perceptual ratings of hypernasality has been developed. Kuehn (1982) wrote about this issue and pointed out that, while resonance is an acoustic phenomenon with underlying structural correlates, there are no explicit standards for normal resonance patterns in either the acoustic or the anatomic–physiologic domain.

Hyponasality

Hyponasality is a reduction in normal nasal resonance that usually results from complete or partial blockage of the nasal airway. Blockage may result from upper respiratory infection, a hypertrophied turbinate, or an obstructing pharyngeal flap, palatal obturator, or palatal lift. When hyponasality is present, clients and their families or attendants should be questioned to determine if the symptoms are transient or chronic. Care should be taken to clarify the cause of hyponasality before proceeding with intervention procedures for velopharyngeal dysfunction.

Nasal Emission

The term *nasal emission* refers to airflow through the nose during production of nonnasal consonants. Nasal emission may appropriately be considered an articulatory rather than a resonance problem. However, both nasal emission and hypernasality may be consequences of velopharyngeal incompetence, although the two features may exist independently (Peterson-Falzone, 1982). A speaker may exhibit moderate hypernasality without audible nasal emission, or inconsistent nasal emission with hypernasality. The presence of nasal emission is frequently associated with velopharyngeal dysfunction. Because nasal emission during production of the nasal consonants is not associated with normal speech, the perceptual identification of this feature is usually taken as an indication of dysfunction. However, inability to perceptually detect nasal emission should not be taken as an indication of adequate velopharyngeal function. If the nasal emission is minimal, it may not be audible and can be detected only by instrumentation that measures airflow. If a speaker is unable to impound air pressure in the oral cavity due to severely reduced respiratory drive or inability to achieve a constriction or obstruction of airflow in the oral cavity, only a minimal amount of air will escape through the nasal cavity, regardless of the degree of velopharyngeal dysfunction.

ARTICULATORY ERROR PATTERNS

Velopharyngeal incompetence results in the inability to generate sufficient intraoral air pressure to produce certain consonants, particularly the plosives, fricatives, and affricates. Evaluation of the pattern of consonant articulation errors, with particular emphasis on the pressure sounds, has long been used in the field of cleft palate research (Morris, Spriestersbach, & Darley, 1961; Prins & Bloomer, 1968; Van Demark et al., 1985).

Analysis of articulatory patterns may indicate the presence of velopharyngeal dysfunction. Most obvious of the articulatory patterns is the nasalization of voiced consonants such as /b/, /d/, and /g/. Because of the effect of neuromotor impairment on the overall articulation performance of the speaker with dysarthria, determining the contribution of the velopharyngeal dysfunction to the specific articulatory pattern may be somewhat more difficult in the speaker with dysarthria than in the speaker with cleft palate. In an effort to deal with this issue, Shprintzen (1995) investigated the articulatory performance of two groups of speakers with dysarthria. One group included those who were determined through aerodynamic studies not to achieve velopharyngeal closure, and the other group achieved velopharyngeal closure at least occasionally. For those speakers who achieved some velopharyngeal closure, the percentage of nasal sounds that were correctly produced was very similar to the percentage of pressure consonants that were correctly produced. However, for the group of subjects with dysarthria who did not achieve complete velopharyngeal closure, the percentage of nasal and glide sounds correctly produced was much greater than the percentage of pressure consonants correctly produced.

Figure 9.2 contains a scattergraph of actual (attempted) versus perceived consonants produced by an individual with velopharyngeal incompetence, as well as other impairments in the respiratory, phonatory, and oral articulatory components of speech. The scattergraph is typical of those obtained from speakers with velopharyngeal incompetence. Examination of the figure suggests that the judge misidentified many of the pressure consonants as nasals. Overall scores for consonant production indicate that the judge is able to identify 17% of the consonant productions correctly. Further analysis reveals a marked difference between accuracy of the nasal/glide category (45% accurate) and that of the pressure consonants (7% accurate).

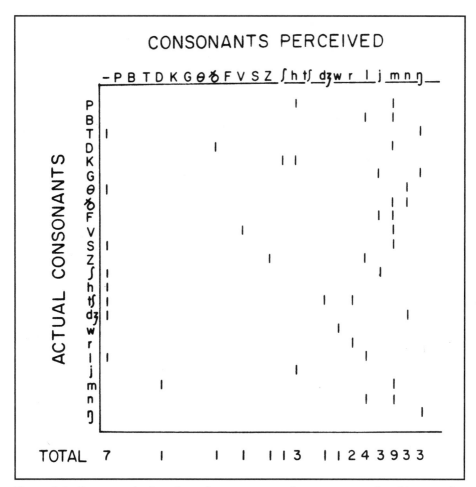

Figure 9.2. Scattergraph plot of actual versus perceived consonants produced by a speaker with severe dysarthria and velopharyngeal incompetence.

Patterns of Velopharyngeal Dysfunction

After the presence of velopharyngeal dysfunction has been identified, an attempt is often made to describe the pattern of dysfunction. The velopharyngeal port cannot be viewed directly during connected speech. Further precise inferences about the size of the velopharyngeal port and the timing of closure in relation to other aspects of speech production cannot be made solely on the basis of perceptual judgments. Therefore, a number of instrumental measurement techniques are typically used to supplement perceptual judgment and to give a more detailed description of the pattern of the dysfunction. The following discussion will be restricted to those techniques that are routinely employed clinically when evaluating speakers with dysarthria. Kuehn (1982) wrote an excellent review of approaches to assessment of resonance disorders, including acoustic analysis and those techniques that assess resonance by comparing nasal and oral sound pressure levels.

Aerodynamic Measures

Because the velopharyngeal port is one of the most important valves that interrupts the breath stream during the production of speech sounds, measurement of oral air pressure and volume velocity of airflow across the port are useful indicators of velopharyngeal function. Aerodynamic techniques do not provide a direct measure of velopharyngeal movement; rather they are used to make estimates of velopharyngeal resistance and/or area of the velopharyngeal orifice.

Equipment

The basic components for aerodynamic measurement include an airflow meter, an air pressure transducer, and a microphone. The pneumotachometer is the most frequently used type of airflow meter. Use of this device requires that the speaker wear a nose mask that traps nasally emitted air. Measurement of airflow is based on the detection of pressure difference across the wire screen of the pneumotachometer. Airflow rate measures alone are not a good index of velopharyngeal adequacy because these measures are affected by such factors as nasal or oral cavity resistance and intraoral air pressure. Therefore, intraoral air pressure measures are obtained simultaneously with those of nasal airflow. This is accomplished by placing a small, flexible polyethylene tube on the tongue, oriented perpendicularly to the flow of air in the oropharynx. Pressures are sensed within this tube and are converted to electrical voltage by a transducer. The simultaneously obtained measures of nasal airflow rates and intraoral air pressure may be used in standard equations to calculate velopharyngeal orifice area or velopharyngeal resistance (Barlow, Suing, Grossman, Bodmer, & Colbert, 1989; Warren & DuBois, 1964; Warren & Ryon, 1967).

> *Question: My graduate program had a system for measuring the aerodynamics of speech, but it was composed of many different electronic components. Are such systems currently available for clinical use for persons who are not electronics experts?*
>
> Several aerodynamic assessment systems are available:
>
> (continues)

Aerowin
Neurologic, Inc.
3420 Ashwood Dr.
Bloomington, IN 4740
812/333-3103

Aerophone II
Key Elemetrics Corp.
12 Maple Ave., P.O. Box 2025
Pine Brook, NJ 07058-2025

Computer Assisted Speech
Evaluation and Rehabilitation (CASPER)
Speech Research Laboratories
VA Medical Center
Long Beach, CA 90822
310/494-2611

Speech Sample

Netsell (1969) suggested the use of a speech sample that varied both speaking rate and the phonetic context of speech. Table 9.2 lists utterances to be produced, including voiceless and voiced plosive and nasal consonant productions accompanied by a neutral vowel. Utterances are to be produced at conversational levels of pitch and loudness.

Table 9.2
A List of Utterances Produced During Aerodynamic Measurement Procedures

Procedure	Utterance	Rate
Rate Variation	/ta/	1, 2, 4, and 5 seconds
	/da/	1, 2, 4, and 5 seconds
	/na/	1, 2, 4, and 5 seconds
Phonetic Context Variation	/atada/	Conversational
	/adata/	Conversational
	/andantan/	Conversational
	/antandan/	Conversational
	/atana/	Conversational
	/adana/	Conversational
	/anata/	Conversational
	/anada/	Conversational

Note. From "Evaluation of Velopharyngeal Function in Dysarthria," by R. Netsell, 1969, *Journal of Speech and Hearing Disorders, 34,* p. 113. Copyright 1969 by American Speech and Hearing Association. Reprinted with permission.

Interpreting the Results

Figure 9.3 contains results of simultaneous recording of nasal airflow and intra-oral air pressure for a normal speaker who is repeating the utterance /apapapa/. For ease of interpretation, an audio signal is also displayed. Examination of this figure reveals that no nasal emission is present during any of the stop phases of the voiceless plosive /p/. Further, the speaker is consistently achieving intraoral air pressures of approximately 7 cm H_2O.

In contrast to the measurements obtained from a normal speaker, the measurements shown in Figure 9.4 are from a speaker with dysarthria. This figure illustrates the audio signal, nasal airflow, and intraoral air pressure as the speaker repeated the sentence, "Buy a pie," two times. Note that consistent nasal emission occurs simultaneously with the buildup of intraoral air pressure during the stop phase of the plosive sounds. Further, increases in intraoral air pressure are associated with proportional increases in the level of nasal airflow.

Limitations of the Technique

Although aerodynamic measures allow the clinician to make precise inferences about the extent and timing of velopharyngeal closure, the technique has certain limitations. For the clinician to interpret the results, the speaker must be able to achieve either tongue tip to alveolar ridge contact for /ta/ or bilabial

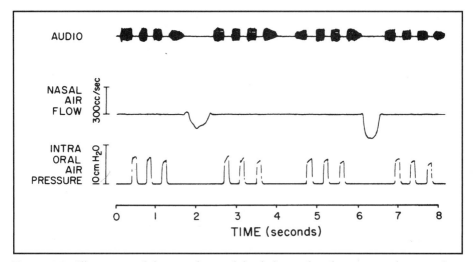

Figure 9.3. Illustration of the speech signal (audio), nasal airflow rate, and intraoral air pressure from a normal speaker repeating the utterance /apapapa/ four times.

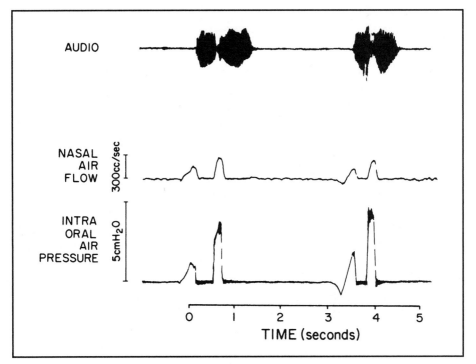

Figure 9.4. Illustration of the speech signal (audio), nasal airflow rate, and intraoral air pressure from a speaker with dysarthria repeating the sentence "Buy a pie" two times.

contact for /pa/. If the speaker is unable to achieve an airtight seal, accurate measures of intraoral air pressure cannot be obtained.

RADIOGRAPHIC TECHNIQUES

In addition to aerodynamic measures of velopharyngeal dysfunction, radiographic techniques have been used extensively with speakers with cleft palate and speakers with dysarthria. Rather than relying on inference about movement from perceptual observation, these techniques allow for the examination of movements in speech structures typically hidden from view. Cineradiographic or videofluoroscopic approaches have been used extensively to evaluate velopharyngeal function in speakers with cleft palate. These procedures are reviewed elsewhere (Kuehn, 1982; Shprintzen, 1995). In the dysarthria field, radiographic procedures have been used somewhat more sparingly. Typically, radiographic procedures are not used as a routine part of our examination of an individual with dysarthria. Radiographic procedures are employed in some centers during the fitting of palatal lifts.

DIRECT VISUALIZATION

Endoscopic (fiberoptic) equipment allows the direct visual observation of structures without radiation exposure. To assess velopharyngeal function, the flexible shaft of the endoscope is inserted through the nares and nasal cavity until the soft palate and pharyngeal wall movement can be observed (Miyazaki, Matsuya, & Yamaoka, 1975; Shprintzen, 1995). Reports of the usefulness of this technique are beginning to appear in the literature (D'Antonio, Chait, Lotz, & Netsell, 1987; Ibuki, Karnell, & Morris, 1983; Karnell, Ibuki, Morris, & Van Demark, 1983; Shprintzen, 1995). This technique also allows the movement of the structures to be viewed.

The endoscope (Figure 9.5) contains several components. The portion that is inserted into the nose (about 30 cm in length) has a viewing end and light guide. At the end of the light guide, a lens gathers the image and a light-conducting apparatus illuminates the area (soft palate and pharynx). The light guide attaches to a light source. The viewing end can be positioned before the eye of the examiner for direct viewing or it can be attached to a video camera, so that the image can be video recorded and viewed on a video screen.

Following the application of a topical anesthesia (which is usually applied with an atomizer or with cotton packing or swabs) into one nostril, the endoscope is passed through the middle meatus so that the scope does not rest on the soft palate and is not moved during speech. A superior position of the tip of the endoscope provides a more complete view of the velopharyngeal space (Figure 9.6). During speech, the soft palate can be seen to elevate toward the posterior pharyngeal wall during rest breathing, speech, and swallowing. The endoscope may need to be maneuvered or rotated to obtain a view of the entire area in order to determine the degree and type of velopharyngeal closure. While fitting a palatal lift, endoscopic evaluation can be particularly helpful in determining extent and pattern of velopharyngeal closure.

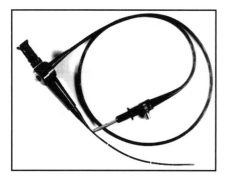

Figure 9.5. Photograph of an endoscope.

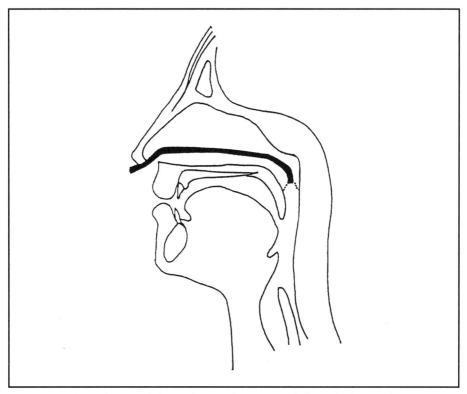

Figure 9.6. Lateral view of the endoscope being passed through the nasal cavity. From "Instrumental Assessment of Velopharyngeal Valving," by R. Shprintzen, 1995, in *Cleft Palate Speech Management: A Multidisciplinary Approach* (p. 232), by R. Shprintzen and J. Bardach (Eds.), St. Louis: Mosby–Year Book. Copyright by Mosby–Year Book. Reprinted with permission.

Question: Do you use the endoscope in your research and clinical work?

Yes, we do. We find endoscope assessment particularly useful during the fitting of palatal lift prostheses. During palatal lift fitting, the shape of the pharyngeal space can be observed at rest and during speech attempts. Because the weakness present in these individuals is often not bilaterally symmetrical, the palatal lift must be shaped to position the soft palate to maximize velopharyngeal closure during speech. Visualization of velopharyngeal space with and without the prosthesis in position is very useful during the final stages of fitting.

Estimating the Impact of Intervention

The final phase of assessment is a process of estimating the impact of improved velopharyngeal function on other aspects of speech production. A number of informal techniques are available. For example, the nares are occluded to eliminate the escape of air through the nasal cavity. Speech loudness and articulatory precision are assessed with and without the nares occluded. Although valving the speech mechanism in this way does not precisely mimic adequate velopharyngeal function, it does provide a gross estimation of improved function, if one selectively observes such features as adequacy of pressure consonant production. The speaker with flaccid dysarthria may experience improved velopharyngeal function in the supine position, with gravity assisting the soft palate to approximate the posterior pharyngeal wall. Also, for the flaccid speaker, a dental mirror can be inserted into the oral cavity and the soft palate elevated into the position approximating the pharyngeal wall. Change in vowel quality may be noted as the velopharyngeal port is occluded. Finally, we instruct the client to speak at a variety of rates, in an attempt to determine the impact of speaking rate on velopharyngeal function.

TREATMENT OF VELOPHARYNGEAL DYSFUNCTION

Earlier in this chapter, five patterns of velopharyngeal function commonly observed in dysarthria were described. One goal of the assessment of the velopharyngeal mechanism is to identify the pattern of velopharyngeal function that is exhibited by a specific speaker and then to tailor the intervention to that pattern. In the following discussion, readers will find that a number of general principles are pertinent. The first is that the severity of the velopharyngeal impairment has an important influence on the approach to intervention. Generally, behavioral interventions are reserved for those with mild or inconsistent velopharyngeal dysfunction, whereas prosthetic or surgical management is typical in cases with severe and consistent dysfunction. The selection of an intervention approach also depends to some extent on the stability of the problem. If a speaker is improving rapidly (e.g., following brain injury), the decision not to intervene directly to improve velopharyngal function is frequently made. Likewise, if a speaker is deteriorating rapidly, complex prosthetic or surgical intervention with the velopharyngeal mechanism may not be considered. Thus, the interventions described below are usually selected for speakers with relatively stable conditions.

Behavioral Intervention

A Caution

Behavioral approaches for the management of velopharyngeal dysfunction in speakers with dysarthria appear to be as controversial as they are in managing speakers with cleft palate. Similarities exist in management of speakers with dysarthria and those with cleft palate (Noll, 1982). If the speaker is unable to achieve closure, because of neuromotor deficits or lack of tissue, behavioral intervention may not be appropriate. According to Noll (1982),

> The only way to modify the problem is to improve the position of the soft palate with the pharyngeal walls, regardless of whether it is due to a structural deficiency of the palatal mechanism (as in cleft patients) or to a neuromuscular dysfunction of the soft palatal (as in some dysarthric patients). If the structural defect is of such a degree that there is insufficient anatomic tissue to accomplish velopharyngeal closure whatsoever, then no amount of speech therapy will result in significantly altering the problem of excessive nasality. By the same token, if there is severe neuromuscular involvement such that the patient cannot possibly accomplish closure, then a program of speech therapy is undoubtedly futile. (p. 566)

Exercises

With the caution that the following approaches are likely to succeed only with those speakers with mild velopharyngeal dysfunction who are able to achieve adequate closure, a number of behavioral approaches can be found in the literature. Some researchers suggest a pushing technique for speakers with velar paralysis (Froeschels, 1943; Froeschels, Kastein, & Weiss, 1955; Ruscello, 1982). Their rationale is that voluntary contraction of one group of muscles will overflow onto other groups. However, such direct exercises may be ineffective because speech and nonspeech velopharyngeal closures involve different underlying mechanisms, and no evidence exists that increasing soft palate strength improves speech performance (Shelton, Hahn, & Morris, 1968).

Kuehn and Wachtel (1994) introduced an intervention for persons who demonstrate velopharyngeal incompetence due to cleft palate or motor speech disorder. Continuous positive airway pressure, commonly called CPAP, has been used routinely to treat patients with obstructive sleep apnea. CPAP involves an air pressure–flow device to deliver air to the nasal cavities via a hose and nasal mask assembly. The person with apnea wears the mask during sleep. The positive air pressure delivered to the nasal cavities presents collapse of the upper airway, thus keeping the airway patent and allowing the person to breathe while sleeping. During CPAP intervention for velopharyngeal dysfunction in speakers with dysarthria, the positive air pressure provides a resistance against which the muscles of velopharyngeal closure must work. Theoretically, this activity is used in a resistance exercise paradigm to strengthen the muscles of velopharyngeal closure. Kuehn and Wachtel suggested that, if effective, CPAP intervention has several advantages over traditional treatment using palatal lift prostheses, including (a) increased subject comfort, (b) greater convenience, and (c) more active subject and care provider participation.

Kuehn and Wachtel (1994) reported on the outcome of CPAP intervention with a speaker with dysarthria. He was seen $1^1/_2$ years following head injury. He wore a palatal lift. A lateral cephalometric study with the lift in place revealed soft palate movement with contact against the posterior pharyngeal wall while he sustained the /s/ sound. Even with the palatal lift inserted, he demonstrated hypernasality (rated as 4 on a 5-point scale). Within the first 4 weeks of therapy, he reduced his hypernasality from 4 to 2. He maintained reduced hypernasality and his rating of 2 at 1 year post–CPAP therapy.

Speakers with severe velopharyngeal dysfunction typically experience weakness associated with flaccid or spastic dysarthria. For those with stable dysarthria, behavioral intervention is inadequate to achieve velopharyngeal closure for speech. Therefore, prosthetic or surgical methods are employed to reduce velopharyngeal dysfunction.

FOCUS ON OTHER ASPECTS OF SPEECH PRODUCTION

At times, it is appropriate to treat mild velopharyngeal dysfunction using articulatory or speaking rate intervention procedures. Many of the techniques reported in Chapter 10 may be employed to improve the production of nasal as well as nonnasal consonants. Rate control may also have an impact on velopharyngeal performance. A reduction in velopharyngeally associated symptoms (hypernasality) was reported in selected subjects with ataxic dysarthria when their speaking rate was reduced (Yorkston & Beukelman, 1981). Because these speakers spoke at an excessively rapid rate, they may have been unable to achieve articulatory targets and the velopharyngeal movements for closure were not accomplished. However, when speaking rates were reduced, with the resultant increase in speech intelligibility, articulatory targets were achieved by oral and velopharyngeal structures and hypernasality was within the normal range. As mentioned earlier, excessive loudness may exaggerate hypernasality in some speakers with dysarthria. Thus, individuals with ataxic dysarthria may benefit from intervention focusing on reducing their excessive respiratory drive. In some cases, this treatment also reduces the perception of hypernasality.

Prosthetic Methods

THE PALATAL LIFT

When speakers with dysarthria are unable to achieve velopharyngeal closure by voluntarily modifying their speech pattern, better function can be accomplished by prosthetically managing the dysfunction with a palatal lift, a rigid acrylic appliance fabricated by a prosthodontist (see Figure 9.7). The palatal lift consists of a retentive portion that covers the hard palate and fastens to the maxillary teeth by means of wires and a lift portion that extends along the oral surface of the soft palate. At times, orthodontic bands or acrylic ridges are added to selected teeth to improve the retention capability of the palatal portion of the lift. The lifting action of the device is illustrated in Figure 9.8.

The palatal lift is usually constructed in a series of steps:

1. The speaker's teeth and gums are checked, and needed restoration is completed.

2. Orthodontic bands or acrylic (composite) ridges are secured to selected teeth (optional).

3. An oral cavity desensitization program is begun for those speakers with hyperactive gag reflexes (Daniel, 1982).

4. An impression mold of the maxillary arch is taken.

5. A dental retainer (the portion covering the hard palate) of the lift is fabricated with a wire loop extending posteriorly as an anchor for the posterior portion.

6. The posterior portion of the lift is customized to meet the needs and tolerances of the individual speaker.

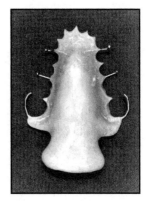

Figure 9.7. Photograph of a palatal lift.

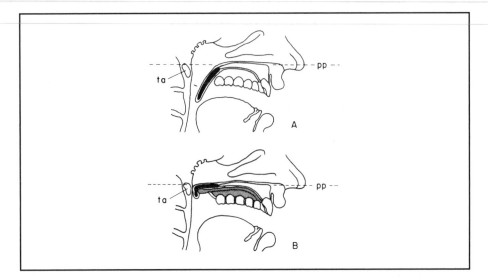

Figure 9.8. The lifting action of the palatal lift device. From "Palatal Lift Prosthesis for Treatment of Anatomic and Neurologic Palatopharyngeal Insufficiency," by J. Gonzalez and A. Aronson, 1970, *Cleft Palate Journal, 7*, p. 94. Copyright 1970 by American Cleft Palate Association. Reprinted with permission.

For individuals with minimal tolerance of objects in their mouth, the palatal lift may be fitted in several stages, with the patient wearing the partially completed lift for several days or weeks to adjust to it, before the next adjustment is made.

Question: Although I have referred a couple of speakers with dysarthria for palatal lift fittings, I have never observed the process because the prosthodontics clinic is located across the state from my practice. How are palatal lifts typically fabricated?

The anterior (retainer) portion of the lift is fabricated using traditional dental procedures. An impression is taken, and the retainer is fabricated of metal or acrylic in a dental laboratory. Because the retainer will eventually support the palatal lift, retention on the teeth may be more substantial than for a dental retainer typically worn as part of an orthodontic intervention.

Two techniques are commonly used to fabricate the posterior portion of a palatal lift. In the first technique, the posterior portion is formed using temperature-sensitive wax. The wax is shaped when warm and becomes

(continues)

firm when cool. The lift is adjusted using the wax until an optimal fit is achieved. The posterior portion of the lift is then cast in acrylic and polished.

In the second technique, the posterior portion of the lift is shaped from a Triad material (Triad Hi-Flow Resin, Dentsply, York Division) that is flexible and moldable prior to exposure to intense ultraviolet light. When the appropriate shape has been achieved, the material is hardened in a light chamber. In about 7 or 8 minutes, the lift can be polished and is ready for use.

An alternative palatal lift design was reported in a series of 16 cases with moderate or severe dysarthria (Aten, McDonald, Simpson, & Gutierrez, 1984). The purpose of this research was to evaluate the efficacy of a specially designed palatal lift in treating patients with a wide variety of neurologic conditions. The traditional lift was modified so that the lift portion was attached to the body of the maxillary retainer with wire connectors instead of traditional solid acrylic material. This design allowed the lift to be adjusted by bending the wires to achieve the desired height and anterior–posterior dimensions. The authors reported that palatal lifts were demonstrated to reduce hypernasal resonance in all of the patients but one.

HISTORICAL REVIEW

The use of the palatal lift prosthesis to manage velopharyngeal dysfunction has a relatively long history. The prosthetic approach to palatal dysfunction in dysarthria was initiated 40 years ago with the development of a lift for an individual with palatal paralysis due to bulbospinal poliomyelitis (Gibbons & Bloomer, 1958). Later, detailed descriptions of palatal lift fitting and construction were presented (Kipfmueller & Lang, 1972; Lang, 1967). In an effort to fit 11 children with cerebral palsy with palatal lifts, Hardy, Netsell, Schweiger, and Morris (1969) reported successful intervention in 10 of the 11 cases. Schweiger, Netsell, and Sommerfeld (1970) wrote a summary article describing the general methods of prosthetic management and speech improvement in individuals with dysarthria. They reviewed construction of the lift, fitting considerations, and radiographic and aerodynamic measurements of velopharyngeal function. Successful palatal lift fitting has also been reported for individuals with velopharyngeal dysfunction of unknown etiology (Lawshe, Hardy, Schweiger, & Van Allen, 1971). Gonzalez and Aronson (1970) reported on the successful fitting of 19 individuals with flaccid, spastic, and mixed dysarthria. They noted reductions in hypernasality and nasal emission symptoms in response to palatal lift fitting. However, some patients with progressive disease lost their speech gains over time following palatal lift fitting. Kerman, Singer, and Davidoff (1973) constructed palatal lifts for two young adults with neurologic impairments and severe dysarthria. Fletcher, Sooudi, and Frost (1974) included the results of four speakers with dysarthria in a report of prosthetic management of nasalance in speech. They described improvement for all four subjects, but the most severe of the degenerative subjects (familial spastic paraplegia) responded less satisfactorily to the prosthesis than did her less involved sister.

GUIDELINES FOR CANDIDACY

The candidacy requirements for palatal lifts appear to differ from center to center. Generally, the following guidelines cover the major considerations that appear in the literature (Gonzalez & Aronson, 1970; Netsell & Rosenbek, 1985; Rosenbek & LaPointe, 1985).

Severity of the Dysfunction

A palatal lift should be considered for speakers who demonstrate consistent inability to achieve velopharyngeal closure. For such individuals, behavioral intervention, in the absence of spontaneous recovery, is usually ineffective. For individuals who are able to achieve closure during some, but not all, speech attempts, palatal lift intervention is less clear-cut. If the disorder is mild, behavioral intervention may be useful. Typically, a brief period of trial intervention can indicate whether the behavioral approach is likely to succeed.

Impairment in Other Speech Components

Palatal lifts are most likely to succeed immediately with those individuals who exhibit a relatively isolated velopharyngeal impairment. Unfortunately, for most speakers with dysarthria, velopharyngeal impairment is most frequently accompanied by respiratory, phonatory, and oral articulatory impairments. Although speakers with severe articulatory or respiratory disorders may be considered for palatal lift fitting, clinicians should not expect more from the lift than the speaker's symptom complex will allow (Rosenbek & LaPointe, 1985). When multiple speech components are involved, palatal lift fitting must be followed by a traditional program of respiratory or articulatory training. For the severely involved speaker, managing the velopharyngeal mechanism may serve to improve the efficiency of the respiratory system and to allow for progress in the modification of oral articulation. At our center, we do not require good oral articulation and respiratory function before proceeding with palatal lift fitting for stable or gradually recovering speakers. However, we do not typically recommend palatal lifts for individuals who are unable to achieve voluntary phonation.

Potential Impact on Other Intervention Strategies

At times, the decision to fit a palatal lift is made in an effort to make other intervention strategies more effective. Usually, these decisions are made in conjunction with three different intervention options: vowel differentiation, positioning of the soft palate to enhance behavioral intervention, and reduction or elimination of nasal air escape to enhance articulatory, phonatory, and respiratory performance during speech.

The first strategy of differentiating vowel production (Chapter 11) occurs early in the intervention of individuals with flaccid and mixed flaccid–spastic dysarthria who have achieved consistent initiation of phonation. For some individuals with extensive weakness and flaccidity, the soft palate rests on the posterior tongue during rest breathing and efforts to speak. As the speaker attempts to produce the different vowel sounds, each production is completely nasalized and the vowel cannot be perceptually differentiated from other vowels, even though the speaker can approximate oral shapes for the appropriate vowel. In this case, the palatal lift is fitted to lift the soft palate off the posterior tongue, so that sound can be radiated through the oral cavity and vowel sounds can be approximated. Usually, at this time in treatment, the soft palate does not need to be positioned so that it approximates the posterior pharyngeal wall if it is uncomfortable for the speaker.

A second palatal lift fitting strategy is to position the soft palate so that the rather minimal palatal movements that are present can effectively close the velopharyngeal port. Some individuals with dysarthria achieve limited velopharyngeal movement that is not adequate to appropriately position the soft palate for speech. However, when the soft palate is positioned near the target position, the minimal movements of the velopharyngeal mechanism approximate velopharyngeal closure. This second strategy for palatal lift fitting is also used when the speech–language pathologist wishes to employ a behavioral intervention to complete velopharyngeal closure, but needs to facilitate movement patterns by positioning the palate near the pharyngeal walls.

Question: Would you illustrate palatal lift fitting with a clinical example?

Herman was in his 60s when he was admitted to the rehabilitation center. He had survived a brain stem stroke that left him with extensive brain

(continues)

stem damage. He was very weak, unable to sit without support, unable to produce voluntary phonation, and unable to swallow. Using the blow-bottle technique to develop his ability to produce and control air pressure, he was able to develop some level of respiratory control. At times he was able to produce short voluntary phonation in the supine position and we began to assist him to differentiate vowels.

About this time, his personalized wheelchair arrived and he was able to sit at about a 120-degree angle with considerable support. He was delighted with the opportunity to view the world from a somewhat vertical position; however, during his next speech intervention session, we realized that all of his vowel sounds were severely nasalized. In fact, we were unable to differentiate the vowels that he was practicing.

While Herman was in the supine position, gravity apparently positioned his very flaccid soft palate away from his tongue so that he was able to radiate sounds through the oral cavity and differentiate vowels. However, in the more upright position, gravity apparently positioned his soft palate on the posterior part of his tongue and he radiated all of his sound through his nasal cavity.

We had not expected to refer Herman for a palatal lift this early in his treatment, although we knew that his muscles were so flaccid that he would probably need it at some point. Under the circumstances, we referred him for a palatal lift with the goal of simply lifting his soft palate off his posterior tongue so that we could continue with his speech intervention program. Following his palatal lift fitting, Herman practiced differentiating vowels and producing words that contained vowels, nasals, glides, semivowels, and so on. In time, his palatal lift was modified in an effort to position his soft palate closer to the pharyngeal wall in order to create greater velopharyngeal closure that would allow him to produce the pressure consonants. By this time, he was speaking more extensively, was stronger, and could tolerate the modification of the palatal lift prosthesis.

A third strategy is to position the soft palatal fitting such that velopharyngeal closure can be achieved or approximated to enhance articulation and respiratory intervention. In this situation, the palatal lift is positioned to achieve as complete velopharyngeal closure as is possible during speech while maintaining the speaker's ability to produce nasal sounds, swallow comfortably, turn his or her head comfortably, and breathe through the nose if desired. With the increasing availability of endoscopic equipment, nasoendoscopic assessment is often used to evaluate the palatal lift fittings (Turner & Williams, 1991). The nasoendoscopic view allows the prosthodontist and speech–language pathologist to observe the position of the velopharyngeal structures during rest with the palatal lift removed and inserted during various speaking tasks. Of particular interest is the movement pattern of the velopharyngeal walls in relation to the velum during speech.

Cooperation

Lack of motivation and failure to cooperate are frequently cited as contraindications for palatal lift fitting (Dworkin & Johns, 1980; Gonzalez & Aronson, 1970). We do not consider palatal lifts for speakers with severe brain injuries who are still easily agitated, unable to tolerate minimal amounts of discomfort, or unable to understand the purpose of the intervention.

Palatal Spasticity

Speakers with extremely spastic palates may be difficult to fit with a palatal lift. The result of spasticity is a stiff soft palate that may not tolerate elevation and may make retention more difficult.

Course of the Disorder

When considering a palatal lift for a speaker with a degenerative disease, the clinician should consider the natural course of the disease and realize that the benefits of the lift may be of short duration. We are particularly conservative when the speaker's articulation capability is deteriorating rapidly. Unlike individuals with a stable recovery course, for speakers with rapidly degenerating disorders, we typically require good oral articulation before proceeding with palatal lift fitting.

Swallowing Difficulties

In speakers who have difficulty swallowing secretions without aspiration, the presence of a palatal lift will reduce swallowing efficiency to some extent. Typically, the flow of saliva is increased during the phase in which the speaker is accommodating to the lift. This period is typically a brief one.

Dentures

Edentulous persons are considered difficult to fit with palatal lifts by some centers, whereas other centers report considerable success with this group of speakers.

Ill-fitting dentures are particularly problematic when combined with a spastic soft palate.

Documenting the Effects of the Lift

When the goal of a palatal lift fitting is to position the soft palate away from the posterior tongue so that vowels can be differentiated, the goals of the intervention are as follows:

- Production of differentiated vowel sounds that are not excessively nasalized

- Painless, efficient, comfortable swallow of secretions (food and drink if appropriate)

When the goal of a palatal lift fitting is to maximize velopharyngeal resistance and reduce nasal escape of airflow during pressure consonant production, the goals of the palatal lift intervention are as follows:

- Velopharyngeal closure during the production of the pressure consonants of speech

- Velopharyngeal opening during the nasal sounds of speech

- Painless, efficient, comfortable swallow of secretions, food, and drink

- Ability to breathe through the nose during rest breathing (if desired)

- Ability to rotate the head to the left and right without pain from the prosthesis

- Improvement in overall speech function in terms of improved intelligibility, normalized nasality, elimination or reduction in nasal emission, improved precision of consonant production, and more efficient valving of the breath stream during speech

---

Question: Does the strategy for fitting a palatal lift differ depending on the residual movement patterns of the pharyngeal walls?

Typically, the intervention team uses two different strategies depending on the movement patterns of the posterior and lateral pharyngeal walls. When the walls are relatively active, the palatal lift is used to position the soft palate such that residual movement of the pharyngeal walls allows for

(continues)

maximal velopharyngeal closure. When the pharyngeal walls are relatively inactive, the palatal lift positions the soft palate to optimize the obturation of the velopharyngeal port. However, care is taken not to position the lift (and soft palate) such that speakers experience pain, difficulty swallowing or turning their heads, or tissue trauma.

Successful achievement of these goals can be documented in a variety of ways. Nearly all of the measures used to assess velopharyngeal function may also be used to document the effects of palatal lift fitting. Perhaps the most direct means of documenting the impact of a palatal lift is aerodynamically. Such measures provide an indication of change at the level of the impairment. The relationship between rate of nasal airflow and intraoral air pressure generation can be seen in Figure 9.9. This figure contains measures obtained from a speaker with severe dysarthria as a result of closed head injury. This speaker was 6 months postonset when first evaluated. Aerodynamic measures were again obtained at 9 months postonset. On both occasions, the speaker was unable to generate

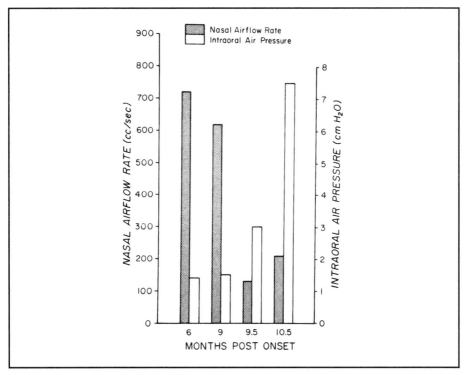

Figure 9.9. Nasal airflow and oral air pressure for a speaker with a palatal lift.

more than 1.5 cm H_2O intraorally. These low intraoral air pressures were produced in the presence of high nasal airflow rate, thus indicating velopharyngeal
incompetence. Further, these measures obtained 3 months apart indicated
essentially no change over time. The initial fitting of the palatal lift was completed at 9.5 months postonset. Measures obtained at that time indicated that,
with the lift in place, the speaker was able to generate intraoral air pressure values as high as 3 cm H_2O in the presence of airflow rates, approximately one third
of those obtained without the lift. Aerodynamic measures were obtained once
again at 10.5 months postonset. At that time, the speaker was able to generate
7.5 cm H_2O of intraoral air pressure during the stop phase of voiceless plosives.

Another useful technique for measuring palatal lift effect is the examination of articulatory error patterns for speakers with and without the lift in place.
Figure 9.10 illustrates data obtained during the first 3 months after fitting of a
palatal lift for a speaker with severe dysarthria. The palatal lift was initially
fitted at 23 months postonset of closed head injury. An inventory of perceived
articulatory adequacy was obtained using a task in which judges without knowl-

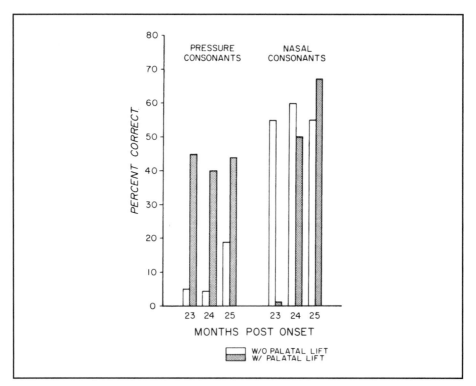

Figure 9.10. Data obtained during the first 3 months after fitting of a palatal lift for an individual with severe dysarthria.

edge of the target attempted to identify the phoneme produced (Yorkston, Beukelman, Honsinger, & Mitsuda, 1989; Yorkston, Honsinger, Beukelman, & Taylor, 1989). Immediately following fitting, results suggested a marked improvement in nonnasal consonant production. Judges identified only 5% of these sounds when the speaker was not wearing the lift compared with 45% when the lift was in place. However, accuracy of production of nasal consonants was markedly reduced when the lift was first introduced.

Over the next 2 months, performance with and without the lift was monitored. Results indicated that adequacy of nonnasal consonant production remained relatively stable; however, production of nasal consonants with the lift in place consistently improved to the point that performance on these sounds with the lift in place was better than without the lift. This case illustrates the point made by many clinicians that optimal speech results come only after a period of accommodation and, in this case, speech training (Kerman et al., 1973; LaVelle & Hardy, 1979; Shaughnessy, Netsell, & Farrage, 1983).

Improvement in the overall adequacy of speech intelligibility is perhaps the best means of assessing the functional changes brought about by the palatal lift. Figure 9.11 contains longitudinal speech intelligibility data for the speaker just described (Yorkston, Beukelman, & Traynor, 1984). The graph plots single-word intelligibility, with and without the palatal lift, from 23 to 30 months post-onset. Examination of the figure suggests that the speaker consistently demonstrated a 15% to 20% increase in single-word speech intelligibility when wearing the lift. Although some improvement is noted over the course of time without the lift, the speaker continued to benefit from the lift.

In 1989 Yorkston, Honsinger, and colleagues reported on the long-term follow-up of persons with brain injury who had been fitted with palatal lifts. The speaker whose articulatory performance is illustrated in Figure 9.12 was a 20-year-old individual with dysarthria due to traumatic brain injury. Initial lift fitting occurred 23 months after the injury. Her articulatory adequacy was plotted at 23, 25, and 85 months postinjury. Of particular interest is the improvement in pressure consonant production over this period. The presence of the palatal lift improved pressure consonant accuracy from 4% to 47% at the initial fitting. At 85 months, pressure consonant accuracy had improved to 100% with the lift in place and 32% with the lift removed.

In a second case report (Figure 9.13), the same authors described the impact of palatal lift fitting on a 28-year-old woman with traumatic brain injury who was fitted with a palatal lift at 96 months postinjury. Her articulatory performance was monitored for 3 months. At the initial lift fitting, her articulatory accuracy increased from 5% to 44% with the lift in place. In 3 months (at 99 months postinjury), her pressure consonant accuracy was 90% with the lift inserted and 30% with the lift removed.

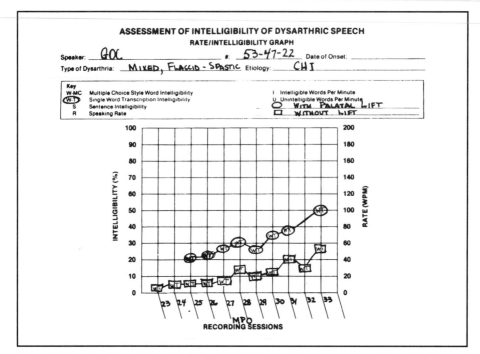

Figure 9.11. Single-word intelligibility (judged using the transcription format) obtained from a speaker with severe dysarthria with and without a palatal lift. Measures were obtained from 23 through 33 months postonset.

Question: Does the fitting of a palatal lift affect multiple speech parameters?

We have observed that palatal lift fittings in speakers who are severely dysarthric and velopharyngeally incompetent often result in changes in articulatory error patterns. Although these errors may not be eliminated, error patterns following lift fitting closely resemble those of speakers who are more velopharyngeally competent. Case reports of these speakers who are neurologically stable but traumatically brain injured suggest that increased benefits can come after a period of accommodation to the palatal lift and speech treatment. It is possible to bring about important changes in speech performance in neurologically stable patients with a combination of palatal lift fitting and behavioral intervention (Yorkston, Honsinger, et al., 1989).

Still another potential impact of palatal lift fitting is the suggestion made by some authors (Dworkin & Johns, 1980; Lang, 1967; Mazaheri & Mazaheri,

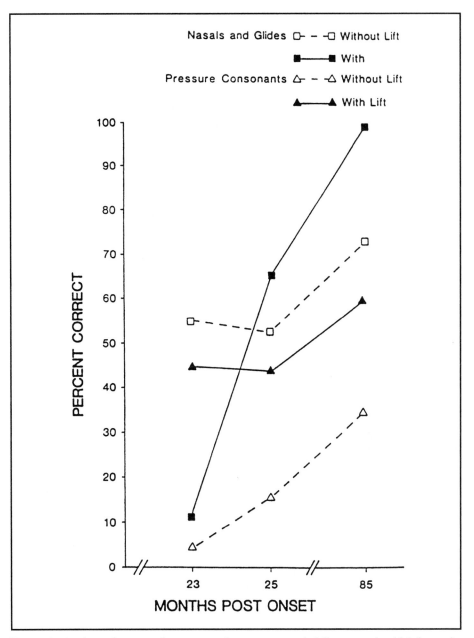

Figure 9.12. Articulatory performance at three time periods following palatal lift fitting for a 20-year-old woman with dysarthria due to traumatic brain injury. From "The Effects of Palatal Lift Fitting on the Perceived Articulatory Adequacy of Dysarthric Speakers," by K. M. Yorkston, M. J. Honsinger, D. R. Beukelman, and T. Taylor, 1989, in *Recent Advances in Clinical Dysarthria* (p. 92), by K. M. Yorkston and D. R. Beukelman (Eds.), Boston: College-Hill. Copyright 1989 by College-Hill Press. Reprinted with permission.

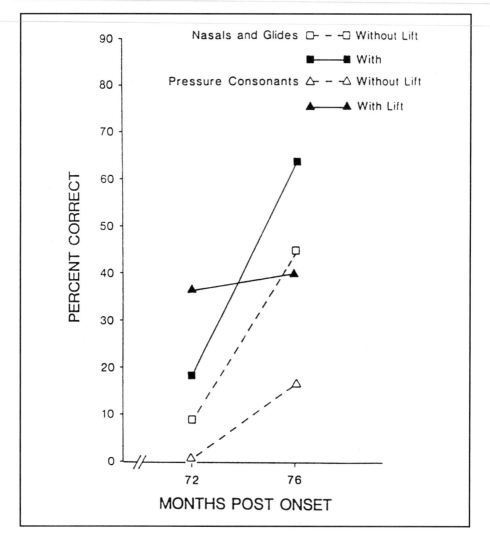

Figure 9.13. Articulatory performance for 3 months following palatal lift fitting for a 28-year-old woman with dysarthria due to traumatic brain injury. From "The Effects of Palatal Lift Fitting on the Perceived Articulatory Adequacy of Dysarthric Speakers," by K. M. Yorkston, M. J. Honsinger, D. R. Beukelman, and T. Taylor, 1989, in *Recent Advances in Clinical Dysarthria* (p. 94), by K. M. Yorkston and D. R. Beukelman (Eds.), Boston: College-Hill. Copyright 1989 by College-Hill Press. Reprinted with permission.

1976) that placement of the lift stimulates or facilitates development of lateral and posterior wall movements in some speakers. Lateral wall movement may contribute in an important way to the success of the outcome. With an optimally fitting lift, velopharyngeal contact is made in the anteroposterior dimension, but lateral airways are left in order to maintain nasal breathing and nasal sound production. Schweiger and colleagues (1970) reported that many speakers with dysarthria and well-fitted lifts are able to close off the velopharyngeal orifice completely during speech duration. Presumably, this is accomplished with lateral wall movements.

DIFFICULT POPULATIONS TO SERVE WITH PALATAL LIFTS

Edentulous Speakers

Through the years, attempts have been made to fit edentulous speakers with palatal lifts. Rosenbek and LaPointe (1985) reported that their clinical group had attempted to fit five patients who were edentulous and had flaccid dysarthria with palatal lifts, but that only one was successful. The others were unable to retain the prosthesis. Aten and colleagues (1984) reported fitting palatal lifts for 16 patients, 9 of whom wore dentures. They concluded that for 15 of the 16 speakers, the palatal lifts were effective in reducing hypernasality. One subject with ataxic dysarthria was judged to be more nasal with than without the lift. The authors reported that denture seals were maintained and retention was not a major problem.

Very Young Children

Shaughnessy and colleagues (1983) reported the successful palatal lift fitting of a 4-year-old boy with severe dysarthria. They summarized an intervention program that involved a variety of treatment approaches, including the palatal lift. Although this 4-year-old boy appears to be the youngest child with palatal lift fitting thus far reported in the literature, a 7-year-old boy with a "lifelong history of grossly nasal speech" of unknown etiology was successfully fitted with a palatal lift. This boy's hypernasality was "greatly reduced" and "speech intelligibility was improved" (Holley, Hamby, & Taylor, 1973). A case report has been published that describes the successful palatal lift fitting of a 7-year-old child with signs of developmental apraxia (Hall, Hardy, & LaVelle, 1990). This child's speech symptoms included excessive nasal resonance and nasal emission of air because of velopharyngeal port dysfunction. In addition to the palatal lift, this child was involved in an extensive speech intervention program.

Changing Neurologic Status

The need to adjust palatal lifts to meet the requirements of the changing client has been a long-standing problem. At times, clients become frustrated with the repeated visits needed to achieve a properly fitting lift. Then, as the neurologic status of the individual changes, further adjustment often is needed.

Persons with Difficulty Adjusting to the Prostheses

Patients who have difficulty adjusting to the presence of a palatal lift are managed quite differently, depending on the philosophy of the intervention team. There is no research supporting one approach over the others. Daniel (1982) suggested that individuals who have difficulty adjusting to a palatal lift include persons with spasticity of the soft palate, hypersensitivity to touch, and hyperactive gag reflexes. For those individuals, she suggested a palatal desensitization program prior to palatal lift fitting. In the program, someone other than the patient applies pressure in a rubbing motion on the alveolar ridge of the patient with a cotton swab placed on the index finger. Gradually, the hard palate is stimulated at the midline farther and farther posteriorly. When the patient feels the urge to gag, he or she is instructed to utter a sound and the posterior progression of the stimulating finger is stopped and lateral movements begun. After 30 seconds of lateral massage, a 15-second rest period is provided. The stimulation pattern then begins again. Daniel suggested that exercises should be completed for 5 minutes, 4 times per day, 7 days per week, and that desensitization, if it is going to occur, usually takes 2 or 3 weeks.

Hardy and colleagues have adopted an approach in which the completed palatal lift is inserted without a desensitization program. Although the adaptation process may be difficult, the gag reflex is gradually inhibited (Hardy, 1983). In our clinical practice, we have taken a moderate position on this issue. For individuals, especially those with head injury who have difficulty tolerating discomfort, we initiate a program of desensitization during the tooth brushing routine. This familiarizes the patients with another person stimulating their oral area. In addition, during the initial insertions of the palatal lift, we have the individual wear the lift for very brief periods of time (often 5 to 10 seconds). During each subsequent insertion, the duration is doubled. With two or three insertions per day, the duration of palatal lift wearing soon reaches several hours.

A topical gel anesthesia has been applied to the upper surface of the lift for persons having difficulty retaining their prostheses. The resulting reduction in sensation allows the individual to retain the lift for several hours. The anesthesia was reapplied each time the lift was reinserted (Brand, Matsko, & Avart, 1988).

FOLLOW-UP APPROACHES

After the palatal lift is optimally fitted, a follow-up program should be initiated to meet several needs. First, the fit of the lift should be checked, especially during the first months of use. Some speakers who are not experienced in managing the prosthesis bend the wires that attach the dental portion of the lift to the teeth, and the lift does not fit properly. Second, although lift users may be somewhat uncomfortable initially, they should no longer experience pain after they adapt to the lift. If pain or discomfort persists, the lift probably will need to be modified slightly. Third, the condition of the tissues of the soft palate should be checked to ensure that the fit of the lift is appropriate. For speakers with severe impairment in multiple speech components, follow-up to palatal lift fitting takes the form of speech treatment. Typically, this treatment focuses on attempting to achieve increased respiratory support and on increasing the precision of pressure consonant production. Finally, long-term follow-up is necessary, especially with speakers gradually recovering from closed head injury or stroke, because for many, the palatal lift is a temporary device worn until adequate velopharyngeal function returns. It is essential to follow these individuals so that return of function can be adequately monitored.

Surgical Methods

Although surgical procedures are used infrequently in the United States with speakers with dysarthria, pharyngeal flap surgeries and pharyngeal wall injections are reviewed briefly.

PHARYNGEAL FLAP

Hardy and colleagues reported their experience with pharyngeal flaps for three children with cerebral palsy in 1961. Two children, both over 10 years of age, showed good speech gains. The child under 10 years of age was able to attain intraoral air pressure following surgery. Later, however, Hardy (1983) wrote that the results of the pharyngeal flap program proved disappointing and that the palatal lift prosthesis proved to be a viable alternative.

Crikelair, Kastein, and Cosman (1970) reported successful inferiorly based pharyngeal flap surgery for an individual 2 years postonset of closed head injury. Their patient had previously undergone a period of "voice therapy" without success. A "marked" improvement was noted, although a "slight residual dysarthria" persisted. Johns (1985) reported a case study of a patient with dysarthria following a gunshot wound to the left frontal region of the brain, as well as the left shoulder and left mandible. He exhibited severe mixed dysarthria. A superiorly based pharyngeal flap surgery was performed. From perceptual and acoustic analysis, Johns concluded that improved postoperative velopharyngeal closure correlated with perceptual judgments of clarity, improved intelligibility, and decreased nasality.

Noll (1982) summarized his review of surgical management of velopharyngeal dysfunction in dysarthria by saying,

It would appear from a review of the published reports that any form of surgical treatment of the velopharyngeal system for dysarthric patients is less than totally successful. It is true that some authors report good results with their patients. However, other studies indicate that some postoperative hypernasality or impaired speech persists. At any rate, this form of management certainly does not seem to be as successful with patients who have an impaired velopharyngeal mechanism due to neuromotor problems as it is with those patients who have structural deficits. (pp. 561–562)

PHARYNGEAL WALL INJECTIONS

In an effort to reduce velopharyngeal dysfunction, a Teflon and glycerin mixture has been injected into the area of Passavant's line in patients with neurologically based dysfunction (Lewy, Cole, & Wepman, 1965). They reported improved speech as a result. Bluestone, Musgrave, McWilliams, and Crozier (1968) injected Teflon into the nasopharynges of 12 individuals with velopharyngeal incompetence. They excluded from their sample any persons with poorly defined or erratic levator action.

> *Question: I have heard that there are some problems with Teflon injections. Is this technique still used?*
>
> The injection of Teflon to enhance velopharyngeal closure is now extremely rare. Concerns about the migration of the Teflon within the tissues of the body and the human body's potential reaction to the presence of Teflon have contributed to this change of practice.

A number of approaches to management of velopharyngeal dysfunction in dysarthria have been described in this chapter. In addition to eliminating or reducing such features as nasal emission and excessive hypernasality, effective management of this component is often necessary before effective treatment of oral articulation problems can be carried out.

REFERENCES

Aten, J., McDonald, A., Simpson, M., & Gutierrez, R. (1984). Efficacy of modified palatal lifts for improved resonance. In M. McNeil, J. Rosenbek, & A. Aronson (Eds.), *The dysarthria: Physiology, acoustics, perception, management* (pp. 231–242). Boston: College-Hill.

Barlow, S. M., Suing, G., Grossman, A., Bodmer, P., & Colbert, R. (1989). A high-speed data acquisition and protocol control system for vocal tract physiology. *Journal of Voice, 3,* 283–293.

Bluestone, C., Musgrave, R., McWilliams, B., & Crozier, P. (1968). Teflon injection pharyngoplast. *Cleft Palate Journal, 5*, 19–22.

Brand, H. A., Matsko, T. A., & Avart, H. N. (1988). Speech prosthesis retention problems in dysarthria: Case report. *Archives of Physical Medicine and Rehabilitation, 69*, 213–214.

Crikelair, G. F., Kastein, S., & Cosman, B. (1970). Pharyngeal flap for post-traumatic palatal paralysis. *Plastic and Reconstructive Surgery, 45*, 182–185.

Croft, C., Shprintzen, R., & Rakoff, S. (1981). Patterns of velopharyngeal valving in normal and cleft palate subjects: A multi-view videofluoroscopic and nasendoscopic study. *Laryngoscope, 91*, 265–271.

Daniel, B. (1982). A soft palate desensitization procedure for patients requiring palatal lift prostheses. *Journal of Prosthetic Dentistry, 48*, 565–566.

D'Antonio, L., Chait, D., Lotz, W., & Netsell, R. (1987). Perceptual–physiologic approach to evaluation and treatment of dysphonia. *Annals of Otology, Rhinology and Laryngology, 2*, 182–190.

Darley, F. (1984). Perceptual analysis of the dysarthrias. *Seminars in Speech and Language, 5*, 267–278.

Darley, F. L., Aronson, A. E., & Brown, J. R. (1975). *Motor speech disorders*. Philadelphia: Saunders.

Duffy, J. R. (1995). *Motor speech disorders: Substrates, differential diagnosis, and management*. St. Louis: Mosby.

Dworkin, J. R., & Johns, D. F. (1980). Management of velopharyngeal incompetence in dysarthria: A historical review. *Clinical Otolaryngology, 5*, 61.

Fairbanks, G. (1960). *Voice and articulation drillbook*. New York: Harper & Brothers.

Fiz, J. A., Aguilar, J., Carreras, A., Teixido, A., Haro, M., Rodenstein, D. O., & Morera, J. (1993). Maximum respiratory pressures in trumpet players. *Chest, 104*, 1203–1204.

Fletcher, S., Sooudi, I., & Frost, S. (1974). Quantitative and graphic analysis of prosthetic treatment for "nasalance" in speech. *Journal of Prosthetic Dentistry, 32*, 284–291.

Froeschels, E. (1943). A contribution to the pathology and therapy of dysarthria due to certain cerebral lesions. *Journal of Speech Disorders, 8*, 301–321.

Froeschels, E., Kastein, S., & Weiss, D. A. (1955). A method of therapy for paralytic conditions of the mechanisms of phonation, respiration, and glutination. *Journal of Speech and Hearing Disorders, 20*, 365–370.

Gibbons, P., & Bloomer, H. (1958). The palatal lift: A supportive-type prosthetic speech aid. *Journal of Prosthetic Dentistry, 8*, 362–369.

Gonzalez, J., & Aronson, A. (1970). Palatal lift prosthesis for treatment of anatomic and neurologic palatopharyngeal insufficiency. *Cleft Palate Journal, 7*, 91–104.

Hall, P. K., Hardy, J. C., & LaVelle, W. E. (1990). A child with signs of developmental apraxia of speech with whom a palatal lift prosthesis was used to manage palatal dysfunction. *Journal of Speech and Hearing Disorders, 55*, 454–460.

Hardy, J. C. (1983). *Cerebral palsy*. Englewood Cliffs, NJ: Prentice-Hall.

Hardy, J., Netsell, R., Schweiger, J., & Morris, H. (1969). Management of velopharyngeal dysfunction in cerebral palsy. *Journal of Speech and Hearing Disorders, 34*, 123–137.

Hardy, J., Rembolt, R., Spriestersbach, D., & Jaypathy, B. (1961). Surgical management of palatal paresis and speech problems in cerebral palsy: A preliminary report. *Journal of Speech and Hearing Disorders, 26*, 320–325.

Hoit, J., Watson, P., Hixon, K., McMahon, P., & Johnson, C. (1994). Age and velopharyngeal function during speech production. *Journal of Speech and Hearing Research, 37*, 295–302.

Holley, L. R., Hamby, G. R., & Taylor, P. P. (1973). Palatal lift for velopharyngeal incompetence: Report of case. *Journal of Dentistry for Children*, 467–470.

Hoodin, R. B., & Gilbert, H. R. (1989). Nasal airflows in parkinsonian speakers. *Journal of Communication Disorders*, 22, 169–180.

Hutchinson, J., Robinson, K., & Nerbonne, M. (1978). Patterns of nasalance in a sample of normal gerontologic speakers. *Journal of Communication Disorders*, 11, 469–481.

Ibuki, K., Karnell, M. P., & Morris, H. L. (1983). Reliability of the nasopharyngeal fiberscope (NPF) for assessing velopharyngeal function. *Cleft Palate Journal*, 20, 97–104.

Johns, D. F. (1985). *Clinical management of neurogenic communicative disorders* (2nd ed.). Boston: Little, Brown.

Karnell, M. P., Ibuki, K., Morris, H. L., & Van Demark, D. R. (1983). Reliability of the nasopharyngeal fiberscope (NPF) for assessing velopharyngeal function: Analysis of judgment. *Cleft Palate Journal*, 20, 199–208.

Kerman, P., Singer, L., & Davidoff, A. (1973). Palatal lift and speech therapy for velopharyngeal incompetence. *Archives of Physical Medicine and Rehabilitation*, 54, 271–276.

Kipfmueller, L. J., & Lang, B. R. (1972). Treating velopharyngeal inadequacies with a palatal lift prosthesis. *Journal of Prosthetic Dentistry*, 27, 63–72.

Kuehn, D. P. (1982). Assessment of resonance disorders. In N. Lass, L. McReynolds, J. Northern, & D. Yoder (Eds.), *Speech, language and hearing: Vol. 3. Pathologies of speech and language* (pp. 499–525). Philadelphia: Saunders.

Kuehn, D., & Kahane, J. (1990). Histologic study of the normal human soft palate. *Cleft Palate Journal*, 27, 26–35.

Kuehn, D., & Moon, J. (1993, November). Levator veli palatini muscle activity in relation to intra-oral air pressure variation. NCVS *Status and Progress Report*, pp. 1–10.

Kuehn, D. P., & Wachtel, J. M. (1994). CPAP therapy for treating hypernasality following closed head injury. In J. A. Till, K. M. Yorkston, & D. R. Beukelman (Eds.), *Motor speech disorders: Advances in assessment and treatment* (pp. 207–212). Baltimore: Brookes.

Lang, B. R. (1967). Modification of the palatal lift speech aid. *Journal of Prosthetic Dentistry*, 17, 620–626.

LaVelle, W. E., & Hardy, J. C. (1979). Palatal lift prostheses for treatment of palatopharyngeal incompetence. *Journal of Prosthetic Dentistry*, 42, 308–315.

Lawshe, B., Hardy, J., Schweiger, J., & Van Allen, M. (1971). Management of a patient with velopharyngeal incompetency of undetermined origin: A clinical report. *Journal of Speech and Hearing Disorders*, 36, 547–551.

Lewy, R., Cole, R., & Wepman, J. (1965). Teflon injection in the correction of velopharyngeal incompetencey of velopharyngeal insufficiency. *Annals of Otology, Rhinology & Laryngology*, 78, 874.

Logemann, J. A., Fisher, H. B., Boshes, B., & Blonsky, E. (1978). Frequency and cooccurrence of vocal tract dysfunction in the speech of a large sample of Parkinson patients. *Journal of Speech and Hearing Disorders*, 43, 47–57.

Ludlow, C. L., & Bassich, C. J. (1983). The results of acoustic and perceptual assessment of two types of dysarthria. In W. Berry (Ed.), *Clinical dysarthria* (pp. 121–154). Austin, TX: PRO-ED.

Mazaheri, M., & Mazaheri, E. H. (1976). Prosthodontic aspects of palatal elevation and palatopharyngeal stimulation. *Journal of Prosthetic Dentistry*, 35, 319–326.

Miyazaki, T., Matsuya, T., & Yamaoka, M. (1975). Fiberscopic methods for assessment of velopharyngeal closure during various activities. *Cleft Palate Journal*, 12, 107–114.

Morris, H., Spriestersbach, D., & Darley, F. (1961). An articulation test for assessing competency of velopharyngeal closure. *Journal of Speech and Hearing Research, 4*, 48.

Morrison, E., Rigrodsky, S., & Mysak, E. (1970). Parkinson's disease: Speech disorder and released infantile oroneuromotor activity. *Journal of Speech and Hearing Research, 13*, 655–666.

Moser, H. M. (1942). Diagnostic and clinical procedures in rhinolalia. *Journal of Speech and Hearing Disorders, 7*, 1–4.

Mueller, P. (1971). Parkinson's disease: Motor-speech behavior in a selected group of patients. *Folia Phoniatrica, 23*, 333–346.

Netsell, R. (1969). Evaluation of velopharyngeal function in dysarthria. *Journal of Speech and Hearing Disorders, 34*, 113.

Netsell, R., Daniel, B., & Celesia, G. G. (1975). Acceleration and weakness in parkinsonian dysarthria. *Journal of Speech and Hearing Disorders, 40*, 170–178.

Netsell, R., & Rosenbek, J. C. (1985). Treating the dysarthrias. *Speech and language evaluation in neurology: Adult disorders* (pp. 363–392). New York: Grune & Stratton.

Nishio, J., Matsuya, T., Ibuki, K., & Miyazaki, T. (1976). Roles of the facial, glossopharyngeal and vagus nerves in velopharyngeal movement. *Cleft Palate Journal, 13*, 201–214.

Noll, J. D. (1982). Remediation of impaired resonance among patients with neuropathologies of speech. In N. Lass, L. McReynolds, J. Northern, & D. Yoder (Eds.), *Speech language and hearing: Vol. 3: Pathologies of speech and language* (pp. 556–571). Philadelphia: Saunders.

Peterson-Falzone, S. J. (1982). Resonance disorders in structural defects. In N. Lass, L. McReynolds, J. Northern, & D. Yoder (Eds.), *Speech, language and hearing: Vol. 3: Pathologies of speech and language* (pp. 520–553). Philadelphia: Saunders.

Phillips, B. (1986). Speech assessment. *Seminars in Speech and Language, 7*, 297–317.

Prins, D., & Bloomer, H. H. (1968). Consonant intelligibility: A procedure for evaluating speech in oral cleft subjects. *Journal of Speech and Hearing Research, 11*, 128–137.

Rosenbek, J. C., & LaPointe, L. L. (1985). The dysarthrias: Description, diagnosis, and treatment. In D. Johns (Ed.), *Clinical management of neurogenic communication disorders* (pp. 97–152). Boston: Little, Brown.

Ruscello, D. (1982). A selected review of palatal training procedures. *Cleft Palate Journal, 19*, 181–194.

Schweiger, J. W., Netsell, R., & Sommerfeld, R. M. (1970). Prosthetic management and speech improvement in individuals with dysarthria of the palate. *Journal of the American Dental Association, 80*, 1348–1353.

Shaughnessy, A. L., Netsell, R., & Farrage, J. (1983). Treatment of a four-year-old with a palatal lift prosthesis. In W. Berry (Ed.), *Clinical dysarthria* (pp. 217–230). San Diego: College-Hill.

Shelton, R. L., Hahn, E., & Morris, H. L. (1968). Diagnosis and therapy. In D. C. Spriestersbach & D. Sherman (Eds.), *Cleft palate and communication* (pp. 225–227). New York: Academic Press.

Shoup, J., Lass, N., & Kuehn, D. (1982). Acoustics of speech. In N. Lass, L. McReynold, J. Northern, & D. Yoder (Eds.), *Speech, language, and hearing* (pp. 193–218). Philadelphia: Saunders.

Shprintzen, R. (1995). Instrumental assessment of velopharyngeal valving. In R. Shprintzen & J. Bardach (Eds.), *Cleft palate speech management: A multidisciplinary approach* (pp. 221–256). St. Louis: Mosby–Year Book.

Thompson, A., & Hixon, T. J. (1979). Nasal air flow during normal speech production. *Cleft Palate Journal, 16*, 412–420.

Turner, G., & Williams, W. (1991). Fluoroscopy and nasoendoscopy in designing palatal lift prostheses. *Journal of Prosthetic Dentistry, 66,* 63–71.

Van Demark, D., Bzoch, K., Daly, D., Fletcher, S., McWilliams, B. J., Pannbacker, M., & Weinberg, B. (1985). Methods of assessing speech in relation to velopharyngeal function. *Cleft Palate Journal, 22,* 281–285.

Warren, D. (1975). The determination of velopharyngeal competence by aerodynamic and acoustic techniques. *Clinical Plastic Surgery, 2,* 299–304.

Warren, D. W., Dalston, R. M., & Mayo, R. (1993). Hypernasality in the presence of adequate velopharyngeal closure. *Cleft Palate–Craniofacial Journal, 30,* 150–154.

Warren, D. W., & DuBois, A. (1964). A pressure-flow technique for measuring velopharyngeal orifice area during continuous speech. *Cleft Palate Journal, 1,* 52–71.

Warren, D. W., & Ryon, W. E. (1967). Oral port constriction, nasal resistance, and respiratory aspects of cleft palate speech: An analog study. *Cleft Palate Journal, 4,* 38–49.

Yorkston, K. M., & Beukelman, D. (1981). Ataxic dysarthria: Treatment sequences based on intelligibility and prosodic considerations. *Journal of Speech and Hearing Disorders, 46,* 398–404.

Yorkston, K. M., Beukelman, D. R., Honsinger, M. J., & Mitsuda, P. A. (1989). Perceived articulatory adequacy and velopharyngeal function in dysarthric speakers. *Archives of Physical Medicine and Rehabilitation, 70,* 313–317.

Yorkston, K. M., Beukelman, D. R., & Traynor, C. (1984). *Computerized assessment of intelligibility of dysarthric speech.* Austin, TX: PRO-ED.

Yorkston, K. M., Honsinger, M. J., Beukelman, D. R., & Taylor, T. (1989). The effects of palatal lift fitting on the perceived articulatory adequacy of dysarthric speakers. In K. M. Yorkston & D. R. Beukelman (Eds.), *Recent advances in clinical dysarthria* (pp. 85–98). Boston: College-Hill.

CHAPTER

10

SPEAKING RATE CONTROL

Clinical Issues: Two individuals who differed in etiology and type of dysarthria were scheduled for outpatient evaluations one afternoon when a new student intern had the opportunity to observe. Despite the apparent differences between the two speakers, the general intervention approaches recommended were surprisingly similar. The first individual was a 70-year-old retired executive with Parkinson's disease whose speaking rate was excessively rapid (150% of normal rate). The speaking rate interfered with intelligibility, especially when speaking on the telephone. His wife, who had accompanied him to the evaluation, stated, "I tell him to slow down, but he just doesn't remember to do it." The second individual was a 25-year-old mother who had experienced an episode of anoxia during childbirth. Living in a rural area, she had not received speech treatment in the 4 years since onset. However, she had been practicing, as she put it, "talking as fast as I can," because she was aware that her speaking rate was about half that of normal. Unfortunately, this strategy had not been effective. Reading a short paragraph was an exhausting task in which she would pause only when a breath was mandatory physiologically. Speaking trials at various rates during the evaluation suggested that intelligibility increased and articulatory breakdowns decreased when she slowed her speaking rate. Recommendations for both of these individuals included rate control as part of intervention. For the speaker with Parkinson's disease, a trial with delayed auditory feedback was recommended, and for the young woman with ataxia, a behavioral rate reduction training program was recommended. The questions asked by the student observing these evaluations were the following:

- Is rate reduction appropriate for all speakers with dysarthria?
- If it is not, what factors make an individual a good candidate for rate control?
- What techniques are appropriate for those speakers who "can't seem to learn" to slow down voluntarily?
- What are the negative consequences of rate reduction and how can they be minimized?
- How is an optimum speaking rate selected for an individual with dysarthria?

The instructions to "slow down" or "speak more slowly" have been uttered by many generations of listeners as they attempt to understand dysarthric speech. Rate control is a long-standing strategy in dysarthria treatment for a simple reason—some speakers with dysarthria are much easier to understand when they slow their rate of speech. Many speech–language pathologists have treated individuals similar to the speaker whose data appear in Figure 10.1. This figure represents data from a speaker with ataxia who read a series of sentences at different rates (Yorkston & Beukelman, 1981a). All recordings were completed during a single session. At his habitual rate (A) of approximately 125 words per minute (wpm), speech intelligibility was low. As he was instructed to slow his rate more and more, intelligibility increased until, at approximately 75 wpm (C), the speaker was over 90% intelligible. Without a doubt, this sort of performance change is highly reinforcing for the clinician. Rarely in clinical treatment can such a dramatic change be brought about by manipulating one variable.

Rate control is a frequently employed strategy in treating speakers with dysarthria, yet the effects of rate control have only recently begun to receive critical research attention. Our clinical experience has taught us that, although rate control may be beneficial for some speakers, it is not a panacea for the problems faced by all speakers with dysarthria. For some speakers, slowing down does not help at all. For others, reducing the speaking rate has some advantages if speakers and their partners are willing to accept the disadvantages. The advantages may include an increase in speech intelligibility; however, the disadvantages frequently involve a reduction in speech naturalness. For still other speakers, only certain rate control techniques are effective and the clinician must carefully choose the technique that is the best compromise between benefits and drawbacks.

In some populations of speakers with dysarthria, rate control interventions may have variable results from speaker to speaker. For example, Turner, Tjaden,

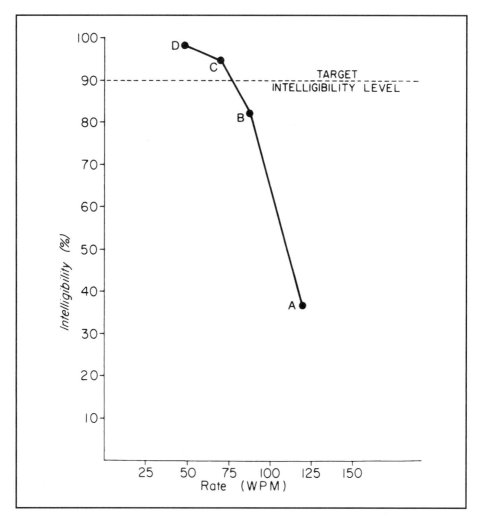

Figure 10.1. Intelligibility scores (percent correct) for sentences read at various speaking rates by a speaker with ataxic dysarthria.

and Weismer (1995) reported that for persons with amyotrophic lateral sclerosis (ALS) the relation between speaking rate and intelligibility is quite varied. Half of their speakers were more intelligible at a slower rate than at the habitual rate, while the other half were more intelligible at the habitual rate. Given the gradual deterioration of speech performance, many speakers with ALS adjust their speaking rate to maximize their speaking performance. Perhaps the results obtained by Turner and colleagues can be explained by noting that some ALS speakers independently make optimal rate adjustments for their degree of neuromotor impairment, and any further manipulation of their rate results in reduced speech intelligibility. However, others may not have made an optimal adjust-ment, and further manipulation of their speaking rate results in improvements in speech intelligibility.

Recent research involving the relationship between speaking rate and "clear speech" attempts to address in detail the interaction between rate and accuracy of speech performance. Although a discussion of clear speech research is beyond this chapter, the following references are of interest: Payton, Uchanski, and Braida (1994), Picheny, Durlach, and Braida (1985, 1986, 1989), Schum (1996), and Uchanski, Choi, Braida, Reed, and Durlach (1996).

Until research provides some clearly defined guidelines about when and with whom to use rate control techniques, clinical experience and trials with various techniques and rates must guide our management decisions. Before pre-senting information regarding rate control for speakers with dysarthria, we will review selected literature related to normal speaking rate and how speakers without neurologic impairment adjust their speaking rates. It is hoped that this information will help to provide a rationale for selection of rate reduction tech-niques in dysarthria and offer some possible explanations of the effectiveness of rate control for some speakers.

NORMAL SPEAKERS

Normal Rates

Perhaps it is best to begin to think about speaking rate and rate control by con-sidering normal speech. Normal speaking rates depend on the task: Normal paragraph reading rates range from 160 to 170 wpm (Fairbanks, 1960), and sen-tence reading rates are approximately 190 wpm (Yorkston & Beukelman, 1981b). Sentence reading rates are somewhat more rapid than paragraph rates because measures based on single sentences do not include intersentence pause times. The normal range of conversational speaking rate varies from 150 wpm to as rapid as 250 wpm (Goldman-Eisler, 1968). Undoubtedly, spontaneous speaking rate depends on the cognitive load of the task in which the speaker is engaged. Well-rehearsed passages are often spoken rapidly, whereas passages that deal with complex or novel information are usually spoken much more slowly.

Writers have long cautioned that it is misleading to consider only an over-all speaking rate when measuring speaking performance (Kelly & Steer, 1949). Overall speaking time consists of two components: speaking or articulation time and pause time. Of these two components, pause time is the most elastic. Articulatory movement rates, on the other hand, are remarkably constant within a particular individual (Goldman-Eisler, 1961). Although articulatory movement rates may vary from one speaker to another, they generally range from 4.4 to 5.9 syllables per second. Normal speakers increase articulatory movement rate only if the text material is highly practiced.

Importance of Pauses

Although movement rates are considered stable within an individual for a specific task, overall speaking rates may vary considerably, depending on the task. This variability is, to a large extent, the result of the changing proportion of pause time to total time in different tasks. Pauses may occupy 30% of prose reading and as much as 50% of the spontaneous speech in normal individuals (Klatt, 1976). Pauses are neither randomly distributed throughout normal speech nor tied closely to maximum respiratory potential. In other words, normal speakers do not pause at random locations or simply because they need to take a breath. Instead, pauses are systematically related to syntactic boundaries (Hammen & Yorkston, 1994; Hammen, Yorkston, & Minifie, 1994). For example, in spontaneous speech we pause at locations related to what have been called "cognitive strides" (Henderson, Goldman-Eisler, & Skarbeck, 1966). Thus, pauses give us time to organize and structure what we are about to say.

For the speaker, pauses may serve an organizational function. For the listener, they may serve another function. Pauses chunk utterances into meaningful units. This chunking of information is important for the intelligibility of the message. When speakers do not supply the proper pauses or give the listener durational miscues, intelligibility is reduced. Huggins (1978) referred to this as the "garden path" effect. Suddenly the listener is lost and has no points of reference to find the way out of the maze.

Pauses also are important for the naturalness of speech. When a person speaks, he or she chunks utterances into breath groups, which frequently have a falling fundamental frequency pattern. The speaker then imposes on that breath group a pattern of stress by making some words or syllables in the utterance more prominent than others.

Comparison to Speakers with Dysarthria

In comparing the speaking rates of normal individuals with speakers with dysarthria, some facts are obvious. Speakers with dysarthria tend to be slower than normal speakers. Of the 212 speakers studied by the Mayo Clinic group, 170 were said to deviate from normal speaking rates (Darley, Aronson, & Brown, 1975). With all but a subgroup of speakers with hypokinetic dysarthria, this deviation represents a trend toward slower than normal speech. Linebaugh and Wolfe (1984) studied the speech of groups of individuals who were normal speakers and individuals with spastic or ataxic dysarthria. Their results confirmed the clinical impression that individuals with dysarthria speak more slowly than normal speakers. Mean syllable durations were 198, 246, and 249 msec for the normal, spastic, and ataxic groups, respectively. Their analysis further concluded that mean syllable durations for the spastic and ataxic groups did not differ from one another. Their hypothesis that the two groups may have different pause times is an important area for future investigation.

Question: Although many speakers with dysarthria talk at rates that are slower than speakers without impairment, don't some speakers with Parkinson's disease speak at excessively rapid rates?

Yes, perceptually it seems that some persons with hypokinetic dysarthria speak at excessive rates. However, often it is clinically useful to examine perceptual judgments before making diagnostic or intervention decisions based on perceptions only. It is useful to measure overall speaking rate objectively. In some cases measurement of overall speaking rates may reveal that the individual is speaking at rates that exceed those of normal speakers. In other cases, the individual may be speaking with a rate at or somewhat below that of normal speakers. However, because of the distortions (blurring) present in hypokinetic dysarthria, listeners perceive the rate to be excessive. When a listener's categorical perception of phonemes becomes difficult, in this case because of an imprecise speech signal, the listeners often judge the speaking rate to be higher than what it really is. Although some individuals with hypokinetic dysarthria speak at overall rates within normal limits, listeners may perceive them to be speaking with excessive rate, because they are pausing more than the normal speaker, and articulating more rapidly, thus speaking at an overall normal rate. In this situation, the articulation rate of the individual may be excessive.

Finally, the clinician should think about what is meant by the notion of excessive speaker rate. So far in our response, we have implied that excessive speaking rate is more rapid than that of normal speakers. However, we often view speaking rate as excessive for an individual when it results in an attempt to speak at a rate that is excessive for that individual's neuromotor control system. For example, a speaker with dysarthria may be talking more slowly than normal speakers but still be speaking at an excessive rate, given his or her neuromotor impairment. In this case, appropriate intervention may result in a further reduction in speaking rate.

Assuming that articulatory movement rates may be physiologically "locked in" for speakers with or without dysarthria, pause time becomes critical when speakers are asked to modify their rates. When normal speakers are asked to speak as rapidly as possible, they can increase their overall rates by approximately 30% (Lane & Grosjean, 1973). They do so almost entirely by reducing pause time. It appears that certain speakers with dysarthria may adopt this same strategy in an effort to increase their slower than normal overall speaking rate. Thus, they may pause only when physiologically necessary. Unfortunately, this compensatory pattern may be maladaptive, as pauses appear to play an important role in both speech intelligibility and naturalness. When using pause reduction strategy, speakers substantially increase effort level during speech. Clearly, further investigation of the role of pauses in the perceived adequacy of dysarthric speech is critical in designing appropriate rate control intervention programs.

Although individuals with dysarthria may talk more slowly than normal speakers, their speaking rates may still be excessively rapid given their impaired motor system. Intervention for such individuals focuses on the selection and habituation of a rate that is appropriate for each speaker.

CANDIDACY FOR RATE CONTROL

Throughout this chapter a number of case studies are used to illustrate situations in which rate control has been judged to be effective. Generally, these cases exhibit either ataxic or hypokinetic dysarthria. Rate control might be effective for a number of reasons. Perhaps the most obvious explanation is that rate reduction might improve intelligibility by increasing precision of movement. Slowed rate might give speakers with dysarthria a better opportunity to move through the full articulatory range and, thus, to achieve targets more adequately (Hardy, 1983). Slower speaking rates may prevent a phenomenon labeled "undershoot," where at fast rates, a signal for one speech gesture arrives at the periphery before a preceding gesture is complete. The result is that gestures may be aborted before their completion.

> *Question: For some of my clients with Parkinson's disease, it seems that their articulatory accuracy is nearly normal when their speaking rate is appropriately controlled. Have others made that observation?*
>
> Ackermann, Grone, Hoch, and Schonle (1993) investigated the movement patterns of a speaker with Parkinson's disease, akinetic–rigid movements, and intermittent speech freezing during a diadochokinetic speaking task. When rates of 8 to 10 Hz were attempted by the speaker, the undershooting gestures failed to establish a sufficient occlusion of the vocal
>
> *(continues)*

tract for the production of the consonant /t/. However, when speaking rates were reduced to 3 to 4 syllables per second, the labial movements were normal.

Caligiuri (1989) studied the influence of speaking rate on articulatory movements of speakers with hypokinetic dysarthria. He reported that labial movements were normal at the slower of the two speaking rates. However, labial movements became hypokinetic as speaking rate was increased to a rate consistent with conversational speech.

Slowed rate might increase the ability of speakers with dysarthria to coordinate the various speech components. Improper timing of the various speech subsystems is a characteristic deficit in speakers with ataxia (Kent, Netsell, & Bauer, 1975). Many types of intersystem coordination are necessary for adequate speech. For example, respiratory efforts must be precisely timed with phonatory efforts, voicing must be properly timed with oral articulatory gestures, and velopharyngeal closure must be timed to correspond with voicing and oral gestures.

Rate control might improve intelligibility because of its effect on respiratory patterning. Selected rate control techniques enable certain speakers to produce more appropriate breath group units and to intersperse pauses at appropriate junctures. Appropriate phrasing may chunk the dysarthric utterance into appropriate syntactic units, thus increasing the redundancy of the information provided to the listener. Another explanation of the effect of rate control may also relate to the listener. The extra processing time provided by the slowed rates may give the listener the opportunity to "fill in the gaps" when attempting to interpret a distorted signal. Finally, rate control techniques may pace certain speakers and keep speech moving forward. This may be particularly important for speakers with hypokinetic dysarthria. Clearly, the list of speculations could go on.

Question: At the beginning of the previous paragraph, you indicated that speaking rate control may impact respiratory function in some speakers with dysarthria. I am not sure that I understand. Could you give an example?

Hardy (1967) presented the case of a 24-year-old individual who, at the time of evaluation, was 2 years post–brain injury with cerebral concussion–contusion, right hemiparesis, and probable brain stem injury. His unintelligible speech was characterized by an extremely rapid rate with an initial "explosive" burst followed by rapidly diminishing loudness. Cine-

(continues)

fluorographic films revealed "gross immobility of the tongue and velum" at habitual rates. However, an increase in the extent of lingual and palatal movement was noted at reduced speaking rates. Hardy offered a possible explanation for the severely impaired movements of the oral articulators. He suggested that the patient "attempts to compensate for his physiological speech problems, during recovery from the severe neurological damage, by completing an utterance 'before he ran out of air'" (p. 154). Hardy further stated that the patient's inappropriate speaking rate worked against his compensatory efforts. This case illustrates an instance where severely restricted movements of the oral articulators may not have been the direct result of damage to the neuromotor control of these structures.

At first glance, encouraging speakers who already speak more slowly than normal to reduce their speaking rates still further may seem counterproductive. However, readers are reminded that a frequent goal with speakers with dysarthria is not "normalcy" but "compensated intelligibility" (Rosenbek & LaPointe, 1985). Their physiologic impairment may necessitate a slower than normal rate. The critical question in assessing the appropriateness of speaking rate of individuals with dysarthria is not "How does it compare to normal?" but rather "Can speaking performance be improved (be made more intelligible and/or more natural) by modifying the rate?" Candidacy for rate control must be determined empirically because we cannot consistently predict who will benefit from a reduced rate and who will not.

Question: When making an intervention decision regarding speaking rate control, is the impact on speech intelligibility always the deciding factor?

Clinical decisions about speaking rate control usually involve compromise. Often the compromise involves the optimization of speech accuracy (intelligibility) at the expense of other parameters, such as naturalness or consistency. However, occasionally a different compromise is made. For example, one of our clients with ALS reported that he sensed an improvement in his neuromotor control for speech when he made a conscious effort to reduce his speaking rate to enhance his articulatory precision. However, he reported that "people looked at me like I was nuts." So, he sacrificed speech accuracy for naturalness as he returned to his habitual rate.

ASSESSING SPEAKING RATE

Speaking rate is influenced by a number of factors. As was apparent from the previous section, the type and severity of neuromotor impairment influence the rate at which individuals with dysarthria speak. In addition, many speakers with dysarthria employ compensatory strategies to improve their speech performance. Some of these strategies involve adjustments in speaking rate. Measurement of speaking rate is accomplished in several ways.

Perceptual Judgments

The perceptual judgment of overall speaking rates is still probably the most commonly used technique for measuring rate in the clinical setting. Typically, clinicians listen to a speaker and judge whether speaking rate is excessively rapid or slow and whether it is appropriate for a given speaker. However, perceptual judgment as the only measure of speaking rate has several limitations. First, these judgments do not provide objective measures of rate and, therefore, do not provide a basis for comparison as an individual's speech deteriorates or improves. Second, judgments of rate are affected by articulatory precision, with speech samples containing imprecise articulation typically being judged more rapid than those with more precisely articulated speech even though the actual speaking rates are similar. Third, as with all perceptual measures, there is little assurance that different clinicians judge rate similarly. Given the limitations of perceptual judgments, several computerized strategies have been developed to measure speaking rate.

Computerized Measures

ASSESSING SPEAKING RATE DURING SENTENCE READING TASKS

Measurement of speaking rate during sentence reading tasks is common, because speech intelligibility has often been assessed in sentence formats, and clinicians often wish to measure rate and intelligibility from the same speech sample in order to assess the relation between these two parameters. Although a stopwatch can be used to measure speech durations, and a calculator to compute speaking rate for a known speech sample, the *Sentence Intelligibility Test* (Yorkston, Beukelman, & Tice, 1996) was developed to measure rate and intelligibility and to computerize many of the measurement and computational tasks.

ASSESSING SPEAKING RATE DURING PARAGRAPH READING TASKS

Paragraph reading has been used traditionally for the assessment of speakers with dysarthria. Although a variety of paragraphs have been used, the Mayo Clinic group made the "Grandfather Passage" quite famous (Darley et al., 1975).

As with sentence reading tasks, stopwatches and calculators can be used to measure speaking rates during paragraph reading. However, the *Pacer/Tally Rate Measurement Software* (Tally) was developed to automate many of the functions involved in this task (Beukelman, Yorkston, & Tice, 1997). For example, the program automatically computes the number of words and syllables in a passage entered into the computer. When the speaker begins to read the passage, which is displayed on the screen, the computer program is activated, and when the passage is completed, the program is deactivated. Speaking rates for words and syllables are computed automatically.

ASSESSING SPEAKING RATE DURING SPONTANEOUS SPEECH

Speaking rate during spontaneous speech can be measured by (1) recording the speech sample, (2) transcribing the sample to determine the number of words or syllables, (3) measuring the duration of the sample with a stopwatch, and (4) computing speaking rate. A computerized option is available in the Tally program (Beukelman et al., 1997). As a client speaks, the clinician activates a button on the computer keyboard, as each word is spoken. At the end of the passage, the computer determines speaking rate.

ACOUSTIC MEASURES

For research purposes, speaking rates are often measured using acoustic analysis software. The speech sample is digitized into the computer and the acoustic waveform is displayed on the screen. With a cursor, the waveform is "marked" at the beginning and the end of the utterance, and the computer automatically measures the duration of the speech sample.

SELECTING THE APPROPRIATE TECHNIQUE

The selection of the most appropriate rate control technique is highly related to the question of candidacy for rate control. Again, management decisions must be based on clinical trials. We evaluate rate control techniques by examining the following issues: effectiveness, training requirements, and consequences.

Effectiveness

The first question that must be answered is obvious: Does the technique actually elicit the desired speaking rate? In a sense, all of the other questions become meaningless if the technique does not produce the desired rate or does not maintain that rate for a period of time. On the surface, this question is relatively easy to answer. Overall speaking rates are obtained for habitual speech and for speech controlled by the selected technique. However, knowing the overall speaking rate is not sufficient. Other factors also must be considered. For example, pause time and distribution of pauses appear to be important for both the intelligibility and the naturalness of normal speech. Consider the individual with Parkinson's disease using a pacing board. In this case, the articulatory rate is very rapid but pauses are interspersed between every pair of words. This speaker's overall rate may be identical to that of a speaker with a much slower articulatory rate who pauses only at phrasal boundaries. Despite similar overall speaking rates, these two individuals manage the durational aspects of speech quite differently. Because pause time as well as the distribution of pauses may have an important impact not only on intelligibility but also on the perceived naturalness of speech, it is essential to consider these durational aspects of speech. Measures of pause time and articulation time may be obtained instrumentally. However, for clinical purposes, it is usually adequate to make perceptual judgments by listening to the sample and estimating the frequency and distribution of pauses during the sample.

In summary, to evaluate the effectiveness of a rate control technique, the clinician must document changes in the overall speaking rate. Additional considerations include the changes that occur in pause time and articulation time and the distribution of pauses throughout the utterance. Knowing as precisely as possible how the rate is being slowed may allow for a better understanding of the consequences of the technique.

Question: How can pause time and articulation time be measured efficiently in the clinical setting? My graduate training program owned some of this equipment, but it is too expensive and cumbersome for clinical use.

Acoustic analysis programs are particularly useful for efficiently analyzing the durational characteristics of speech samples (Turner et al., 1995). With the wide range of computer-based acoustic analysis programs now commercially available, these systems are becoming increasingly common in clinical settings. These applications can be hosted by the same computer used to measure speech intelligibility, control speaking rate, and take speech physiologic measurements.

Training Requirements

The second question important in selecting a particular rate control technique is, Are the training requirements of the technique reasonable, considering the speaker's communication needs and availability of training time? Some rate control techniques, particularly the rigid rate control technique described later, and techniques such as delayed auditory feedback, require very little training. In effect, they are prosthetic devices. When they are removed, speakers are expected to return to their habitual speaking rates. Effective prosthetic techniques are acceptable in certain cases, but they clearly are a compromise and often are not as desirable as an independent, client-controlled speaking rate. Prosthetic devices typically are considered when they are the only rate control technique that is effective.

Many of the rate control techniques, particularly those that attempt to preserve prosody, require commitment to an intensive and perhaps extended period of training. Training to control rate independently is not a quick process. As will be apparent in the discussion of rate control drills that follow, independent control of rate requires many hours of practice.

Question: Don't most individuals with excessive speaking rates due to Parkinson's disease experience great difficulty in voluntarily controlling their speaking rate in social situations?

Yes, many do; however, some speakers with dysarthria are able to incorporate speaking rate changes into their (adjusted) habitual speech. One of our clients was a physician with Parkinson's disease who was beginning to experience communication breakdowns with his elderly patients. He spoke habitually at about 160 wpm. When he reduced his speaking rate to 110 to 125 wpm, his intelligibility was normalized and his articulation was quite precise. With coaching, he was able to reduce his speaking rate; however, he had difficulty maintaining his adjusted rate, until we helped him prepare an audio practice tape. Three times each day, he practiced his adjusted speaking rate, upon arriving at his office, during a morning "coffee break," and over the lunch hour. Occasionally, he would practice in the evening before attending a social event.

Consequences

The third and final question to ask when evaluating a rate control technique is, What are the consequences of slowing this speaker's rate? Because research has provided few predictors of success or failure of particular rate control techniques, evaluation of any technique must rely on a trial examination of its consequences. Of primary concern are the consequences in two overall aspects of speech: intelligibility and naturalness. Each of these areas is discussed in greater detail later as individual cases are described. Briefly, however, rate control is typically considered only for those individuals who are not completely understandable or whose excessive rate makes listening and comprehending very difficult. Improvement in speech intelligibility is the primary goal. If intelligibility does not improve, rate control may not be appropriate for that individual, and other management approaches must be considered. Speech intelligibility and its measurement is discussed in detail in Chapter 5.

Rate control may also affect speech naturalness. Intelligibility is expected to improve with rate control; however, just the opposite is true with speech naturalness. Many rate control techniques interfere with the speaker's ability to produce natural speech. At times, the negative consequences of rate control are acceptable because of the associated improvement in intelligibility. A slight reduction in naturalness may be an acceptable compromise in order to achieve increases in intelligibility. Not all rate control techniques adversely affect naturalness to the same degree. Therefore, the naturalness of speech produced under a given rate control technique must be carefully considered. The clinician usually assesses the naturalness of speech under a specific rate control strategy by asking questions such as the following:

- Does the overall naturalness of speech decrease using this technique?

- Does this rate control technique negatively affect the speaker's ability to produce breath groups that are closely associated with the meaning of the utterance?

- Is the speaker able to signal stress on the most prominent words of the utterance within the breath group?

The relationships among speaking rate, speech intelligibility (accuracy), and naturalness are illustrated in Figure 10.2. At very slow rates of speech, the risk of compromising speech naturalness increases, whereas at more rapid rates of speech, the intelligibility or accuracy of the speech signal may be compromised. For an individual speaker, the intervention goal is to select a target speaking rate range that will allow an optimal level of intelligibility without degrading naturalness unnecessarily. Of course, the target speaking rate range varies from speaker to speaker depending upon the individual's neuromotor capability and ability to compensate for these neuromotor impairments.

RIGID RATE CONTROL TECHNIQUES

In this section, we review some of the rate control techniques that have been reported in the clinical and research literature. We highlight the advantages

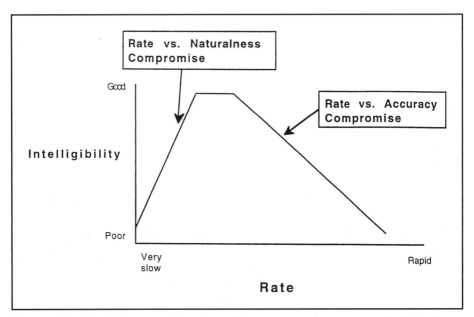

Figure 10.2. Graph illustrating the relationships among speaking rate, intelligibility (accuracy), and naturalness.

and disadvantages of each, and describe with brief case studies the types of speakers for whom these techniques have been successful. The discussion is organized according to the amount of control needed to achieve the desired rate. Few speakers with dysarthria can reduce their speaking rate and maintain a slowed rate after simply being instructed to "slow down." Training and practice are needed for nearly everyone. The technique selected depends on how rigidly the speaker's rate must be controlled to maintain the desired target speaking rate. A general word of caution is warranted: The more rigid the control technique, the more unnatural the resulting speech. Rigid rate control techniques include those that impose a one-word-at-a-time style upon the speaker. These techniques are usually reserved for the most severely involved and often involve some sort of external pacing.

Pacing Boards

Helm (1979) presented a case study of a speaker with Parkinson's disease who was thought to be demented but instead was severely palilalic, in that words or phrases were repeated several times with increasing rate. Palilalia has been compared to the festinating gait pattern in some individuals with Parkinson's disease. Helm introduced a pacing board to impose the necessary "stop/go" control over speech production, thus bringing an automatic act under voluntary control. The pacing board is a simple device consisting of a series of colored slots separated by ridges (Figure 10.3). The speaker is instructed to touch one slot per word. This technique meters speech and separates each word of the utterance.

Question: I have a client with Parkinson's disease who has not been very successful using a pacing board. Have you experienced that also?

When speakers with dysarthria use the pacing board well and have reasonably good motor control of their hands, they can achieve speaking rates up to 70 wpm. Speakers who are unsuccessful with this procedure often continue to speak at their habitual rates and then attempt to point rapidly enough to "keep up" without causing the desired reduction in speaking rate. If these individuals cannot learn to pace their speech with their pointing pattern, they usually require a more rigid form of rate control, such as alphabet board supplementation.

Alphabet Board Supplementation

Another rigid rate control technique is the alphabet board supplementation approach described by Beukelman and Yorkston (1977). The speaker is instructed to identify the first letter of each word on an alphabet board or alternative and augmentative communication (AAC) device as the word is spoken. See Chapter 12 for more details about the board and issues of partner training.

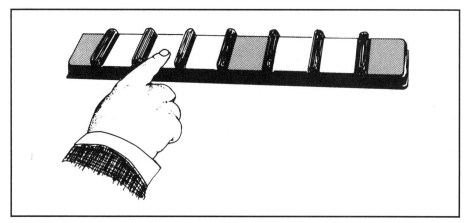

Figure 10.3. A pacing board.

The alphabet board supplementation approach not only forces speakers into a slowed rate as they locate and point to the letters of the alphabet, but also provides their listeners with extra information in the form of the first letter of each word. With some speakers, intelligibility increases depending on the listener's ability to identify the first letter of each word. In this situation, the alphabet board must be large enough for the listener to easily visualize the individual letters as the speaker points to them. For other speakers, the slowed speaking rate alone appears to be the major contributing factor to improved intelligibility. For these speakers, the alphabet board can be quite small, as it is not necessary for the listener to view the board.

Question: What speaking rate do your clients achieve with alphabet board supplementation?

In our experience speakers achieve a rate of up to 40 wpm using the alphabet board supplementation technique. Many speakers with severe flaccid or spastic dysarthria who require alphabet board supplementation do not prefer or are unable to speak very rapidly, so a rate of 40 wpm or less (on average) is acceptable to them. However, we have served numerous speakers with Parkinson's disease whose excessive speaking rate (200 to 300 wpm) was associated with intelligibility problems. During assessment, their speech was highly intelligible at rates between 110 and 125 wpm. However, they were unable to control their speaking rate without the rigid rate control of alphabet board supplementation. Unfortunately, the resulting speaking rate of approximately 40 wpm was much lower than we, or they, would have preferred. Thus, a slower than desired rate is one of the disadvantages of the board. Another disadvantage is that speakers must look at it as they use it. Some speakers dislike this feature because they lose eye contact with their listeners.

CASE REPORT

This case study illustrates the clinical application of rigid rate control techniques. Of particular interest is the compromise between perceived benefits and drawbacks. Amy was 25 years old when she participated in a job sampling program through our rehabilitation medicine department. Her duties included work as a cashier in a small shop, and thus involved extensive public contact. Understandable speech was mandatory. She came to us after many years of speech treatment during her school-age years. With the encouragement of her vocational counselor, she indicated that she was willing to give speech treatment "one last try."

Her medical history was sketchy. Her birth was normal, but early neurologic degeneration followed, which was soon stabilized. Amy's diagnosis was cerebral palsy with dystonic posturing. Her speech was characterized by rapid rate, rushes of speech, monoloudness, reduced loudness levels, monopitch, little articulatory excursion, and reduced stress patterning. Speech intelligibility measures confirmed her reports that listeners frequently asked her to repeat. Single-word intelligibility was 76%, and sentence intelligibility was 24% at her habitual rate of 145 wpm (Yorkston & Beukelman, 1981b). The large discrepancy between single-word and sentence intelligibility suggested that rate control might be an appropriate strategy. At Amy's level of severity, sentences should be more intelligible than single words because sentences provide contextual cues that a single-word production task does not provide.

The clinician who served Amy chose a rigid rate control technique as a trial for a number of reasons. Extended periods of training with other rate control techniques had not been successful, Amy could master the rigid rate control technique with little training, and time was limited to the 6-week period of job sampling. The clinician first chose a finger tapping method, which required that Amy touch her thumb to each finger in succession in a metered fashion as she produced each word of an utterance. Her clinician chose this particular technique because Amy had sufficient fine motor control in her hands to accomplish the maneuver, and this technique did not require her to carry a device such as a pacing or alphabet board. By the end of the evaluation session, Amy had learned the technique and sentence intelligibility measures were obtained once again. Figure 10.4 contains measures of speech intelligibility and speaking rate for both habitual and slowed sentence production. A review of the figure indicates that by slowing her rate from 145 to 70 wpm using finger tapping, her sentence intelligibility improved from 24% to 68%.

Encouraged by these results, the clinician scheduled Amy for a weekly training session, hoping to stabilize her performance with the finger tapping technique. By the end of the first training session following the evaluation, Amy's sentence intelligibility had increased to 95%. Unfortunately, during the second training session, intelligibility fell to 85%. When another 10% decrease in intelligibility was observed during the third training session, her clinician began to realize that finger tapping was no longer a powerful enough pacing technique for Amy. As she became increasingly practiced with the simple motor activity of finger tapping, the activity became more and more automatic. By the end of the third training session, the clinician felt that a more powerful pacing technique was needed and she introduced the small pacing board described earlier (Helm, 1979). It took only a few minutes to train Amy to use the new system. During the fourth training session, intelligibility was again measured, and this time Amy paced herself with the board. Figure 10.4 contains sentence intelligibility and speaking rate measures that had been obtained during the initial evaluation and during each of the successive training sessions. Introduction of the new pacing board improved her intelligibility from 75% to 90%. Note the reciprocal relationship between Amy's speaking rate and intelligibility. As her rate increased, her intelligibility systematically decreased. Further, with practice, those pacing systems that involved simple repetitive movements appeared to lose their effectiveness over time. Unfortunately, use of the pacing board became as automatic as the finger

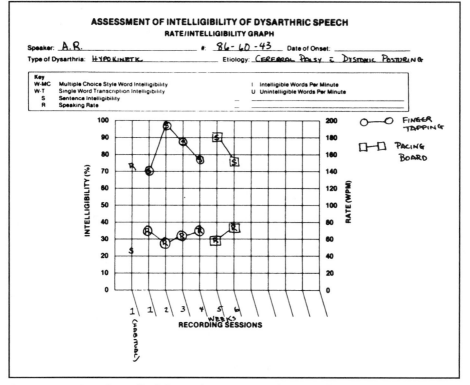

Figure 10.4. Speech intelligibility and rate measures for Amy when using various rigid rate control techniques.

tapping pacing method had become. After a relatively short time, it no longer appeared to pace her speech adequately.

The pacing board also had another important drawback, at least in Amy's opinion. She found the board cosmetically unacceptable. In fact, she called it "just another badge of disability," despite the clinician's endorsement and long discussion of the importance of understandable speech. As a final resort, the clinician introduced the alphabet board. Although the alphabet board was clearly no more cosmetically acceptable than the pacing board, the motor activity required to point to the letters on the board is not routine or repetitive, and thus cannot become automatic as the two other pacing techniques had become. With the alphabet board, Amy was nearly 100% understandable, when she would use it. It quickly became apparent to the clinician that Amy's dislike of the board would frequently result in her "forgetting" to use it when she was on the job. With some discussion, a compromise was reached. Amy would use the alphabet board at home and with friends. When she was on the job, rate control techniques were rotated, so that every third day she was able to use the preferred finger tapping technique. This compromise was one attempt to minimize the "overlearning" that reduced the effectiveness of the repetitive pacing techniques.

Advantages and Disadvantages of Rigid Techniques

As with many management decisions involving speakers with dysarthria, the selection of a rigid rate control technique represents a compromise between the advantages and disadvantages. On the positive side, a number of advantages of the rigid rate control techniques are apparent. First, these techniques often are effective in slowing a speaker's rate when other techniques fail. Second, speech intelligibility increases for certain speakers as a consequence of the slowed rates. The alphabet board supplementation system goes one step beyond other rigid rate control techniques by providing listeners with extra information in the form of the first letter of every word. This extra information often further increases intelligibility. Third, most of the rigid rate control techniques are not highly technical and therefore are inexpensive. Fourth, the rigid rate control techniques require little user training. Finally, these techniques allow for continual practice of slowed rate. Individuals are able to leave the therapy room and continue to use their system for all of their daily communication.

Despite their major advantages, rigid rate control techniques are not without their drawbacks. In fact, the drawbacks often are considered so important that these techniques may justifiably be used only as the last resort when nothing else is effective. First, rigid rate control techniques disrupt the naturalness of speech. By encouraging a one-word-at-a-time style with pauses between each word, they disrupt the breath group units that are important in normal prosody. Rigid rate control techniques also may be perceived as being unnatural because they encourage a disproportionate amount of pause time. Many speakers with severe parkinsonism who use rigid rate control techniques do not prolong articulation time; rather, they merely expand their pause time. Second, many of the rigid rate control techniques rely on a device that many users find cosmetically unacceptable. For others, the advantage of communication without frequent breakdowns is so appealing that the need for a device is accepted willingly. Finally, adaptation to the rate control technique may be a problem, especially when the technique depends on a simple movement that may easily be overlearned. Once the movement is overlearned, the technique may no longer serve as an effective pacer.

Question: Some persons are aware of their dysarthria, whereas others are unaware of their speech disorder and its impact on their listeners. What do you suggest for those individuals who are unaware of the extent of their dysarthria?

Some speakers with excessive habitual speaking rates are relatively unaware of the increase in intelligibility achieved through the use of rigid

(continues)

rate control techniques. Because they are unaware of the benefits and frustrated by the cosmetic and procedural difficulties of the techniques, at times they are unwilling to use the techniques routinely, unless their listeners insist on it.

One of our clients with Parkinson's disease often talked with his son's family over the phone. He used an alphabet supplementation strategy in order to control his speaking rate and speech intelligibility; however, he was unaware of the improvement this strategy made in his speech intelligibility. When his grandchildren would call him on the phone, they insisted that he get his board before they would talk with him. He was surprised that they knew when he was not using supplemented speech even when they could not see him.

TECHNIQUES THAT PRESERVE PROSODY

The following rate control techniques do not impose the one-word-at-a-time speaking style. Thus, these techniques are not as disruptive to speech naturalness as the rigid rate control techniques. Because, for the most part, the following techniques depend on speaker training rather than on a device that imposes the desired rate, additional demands are placed on the speaker. The speaker must demonstrate learning ability and must devote time to master the new motor skill.

Oscilloscopic Feedback

Berry and Goshorn (1983) presented the case study of an individual who had severe ataxic dysarthria secondary to several cerebrovascular episodes 6 months prior to treatment. These authors hypothesized that their patient was "overdriving" his poorly controlled speech mechanism by speaking too rapidly and too loudly. They developed a training program in which he received visual feedback from the intensity × time tracing on an oscilloscopic screen. The clinician modeled the sentence on the top half of the screen. The speaker with dysarthria was instructed to (1) "fill up the screen," that is, increase the overall duration of his utterance to the target duration, and (2) keep his loudness level below a preset line. Berry and Goshorn measured intelligibility using sentences from the SPIN list (Kalikow, Steven, & Elliot, 1977). Audio-recorded sentences produced by the speaker with dysarthria were played for a judge, who attempted to transcribe the last word of the sentence. Some of the sentence-final words were highly probable, whereas others were considered to have low probability.

Results of a 5-week training period indicated that the patient was able to slow his speaking rate. An increase in intelligibility was associated with this decrease in rate.

Of particular interest in this case was how the speaker adjusted his rate. When given no instructions other than to slow down and prolong the entire utterance (fill the screen), he developed a very interesting strategy of durational adjustments. The average duration of key words (words in the sentence-final position) did not change from pre- to posttreatment recording. Instead, he systematically prolonged the pauses prior to key words in the posttreatment condition. Further, he appeared to pause longer prior to words that were unlikely to occur in that sentence (low-probability words) than prior to high-probability words. This clinical finding illustrates the importance of strategically placed pauses to improve intelligibility and suggests that increasing word duration may not be the only goal of rate control programs. This case also illustrates another important advantage of the less rigid rate control techniques. Techniques that do not impose rigid timing on speakers allow them to develop their own compensatory strategies. Often these strategies are both effective and subtle.

Rhythmic Cueing

THE TECHNIQUE

In an effort to move away from rigid pacing techniques, we began to use a training technique called rhythmic cueing (Yorkston & Beukelman, 1981a). The technique is simple. The clinician signals the desired speaking rate by pointing to the words of a passage in a rhythmic fashion. The clinician gives more time to prominent words and intersperses pauses where appropriate. This technique must, of course, be used with printed passages. However, one disadvantage of the use of printed material is the difficulty in precisely cueing the desired speaking rate. Usually, the clinician simply estimates appropriate rates when using the technique with printed material.

COMPUTERIZATION

The rhythmic cueing technique was computerized by Beukelman et al. (1997). Passages are entered or imported into the computer. The program analyzes the passage to determine the number of syllables in each word, and then assigns duration information based on the number of syllables and type of punctuation. In addition, the clinician can type in additional pause markers to signal the speaker (via the computer) regarding the location of additional pauses. The clinician then enters a target rate and the passage appears on the computer screen with a cursor cueing (underline, highlight, or bold) that target rate. The computerization of the rhythmic cueing technique has two advantages over the printed material. First, precise rates can be selected, and second, speakers can practice independently once a set of practice materials and the appropriate rates have been established by the clinician. Typically, many hours of practice are necessary to establish a new optimum speaking rate.

> *Question: Occasionally, I have audiotaped myself demonstrating computerized rate control strategies to my clients. It is my impression that by controlling my speaking rate this way, I degrade my speech naturalness considerably. Has the relative impact of external pacing on the speech naturalness of normal individuals and speakers with dysarthria been studied?*
>
> Using a computer program, we reduced the speaking rate of normal speakers as well as those with ataxic and hypokinetic dysarthria to 60% and 80% of habitual rates. As speaking rate was reduced, sentence intelligibility improved for both groups. Reduced speaking rates were not associated with improved consonant or vowel intelligibility. Mean phoneme intelligibility scores changed little as a function of reduced speaking rates. The speech of both of the dysarthric groups was judged to be quite unnatural during the habitual condition, and slowing their speaking rate even further did not cause the judges to rate their speech as significantly more unnatural; however, the naturalness of the group of control speakers was reduced in response to computerized pacing (Yorkston, Hammen, Beukelman, & Traynor, 1990).

 CASE REPORT

This case study illustrates the use of rhythmic cueing as a training technique. Donna was a 24-year-old woman with a 10-year history of Friedreich's ataxia. At the time of our evaluation, she was wheelchair dependent and exhibited such severe ataxia in her upper extremities that the use of a typewriter or pointing to letters on an alphabet board was not possible. Although her speech was severely dysarthric, speech was her sole means of communication. During our evaluation, speech intelligibility and rate were measured (Yorkston, Beukelman, & Traynor, 1984). At her habitual rate, Donna spoke at 57 wpm with a sentence intelligibility score of 23%. A similar series of sentences was computer presented using a rhythmic cueing technique. The rate of the second sample was slowed to 45 wpm or approximately 80% of her habitual rate. When her rate was reduced in this manner, intelligibility increased to 45%.

Although we are typically cautious about embarking on an extended period of training in rate control with an individual who is suffering from a degenerative disorder such as Friedreich's ataxia, we chose to initiate treatment because Donna did not have the hand function to benefit from any of the rigid pacing techniques, all of which required manipulation of a device. She practiced for 30 minutes each day for 6 weeks, reading sentences of varying lengths presented to her by the computer in a rhythmic manner at 45 wpm. At the end of this training period, the pacing was removed and a third sentence sample was recorded and scored for intelligibility. Results of this posttreatment sample (see Table 10.1) indicated that Donna was now speaking at a habitual rate of 46 wpm with a sentence intelligibility score of 52%.

In an effort to understand more completely the changes that are brought about by rate control techniques, we further analyzed the samples produced by Donna. Acoustic analysis revealed that, although pauses represented only 23% of the total sample during the pretreatment habitual condition, this percentage increased to 40% and 41% during the pretreatment paced condition and the posttreatment habitual condition, respectively. Six months after our intervention, this young woman continued to speak at a rate that approximated the target rate during training. She resolved communication breakdowns by verbally indicating the first letter of each word that her listener did not understand.

McHenry and Wilson (1994) described an intervention program for a 34-year-old man with severe dysarthria following traumatic brain injury. At habitual speaking rates, this man was 44% intelligible; at 75% of habitual rate, he was 62% intelligible; and at 50% of habitual rate, he was 72% intelligible. He was taught to use a pacing board to control his speaking rate in conversational situations.

"Backdoor" Approaches to Rate Control

A number of rate control techniques come under the general heading of "backdoor" approaches because, although they have the effect of reducing rate, rate

Table 10.1
Sentence Intelligibility Measures Obtained for Donna

	Pretreatment		Posttreatment: Unpaced
	Unpaced	Paced	
Rate (words per minute)	73	44	46
Intelligibility (%)	23	46	52
Rate of intelligible speech (Intelligible words per minute)	16	18	23

Note. From Computerized Assessment of Intelligibility of Dysarthric Speech (p. 37), by K. M. Yorkston, D. R. Beukelman, and C. Traynor, 1984, Austin, TX: PRO-ED. Copyright 1984 by PRO-ED, Inc. Reprinted with permission.

control is not their primary focus. One illustration of such a case was a 26-year-old speaker with closed head injury and ataxic dysarthria (Simmons, 1983). Treatment focused on improving the naturalness of his speech. Initial acoustic analysis suggested that the speaker's perceived monotony was related to flat fundamental frequency contours and lack of high-frequency energy. Listeners also perceived his speech to be "excess and equal." This characteristic was attributed to his slower than normal rate and essentially equal syllable durations. Simmons outlined a four-phase treatment program that included, as a first phase, training loudness and pitch variation and, as a second phase, altered word and sentence stress patterns. Acoustic analysis was carried out after each treatment phase. Results of the analysis after the first and second phases of treatment suggested that the most striking changes were brought about in the time dimension, despite the fact that rate control was not the goal of intervention. This led Simmons to suggest that "target behaviors were not independent; working on a specific aspect of speech, such as intonation or pitch variation, caused changes in other areas, such as time and articulation" (p. 290).

> *Question: I have been using the Lee Silverman Voice Treatment Approach with some of my clients with hypokinetic dysarthria. Does this approach impact speaking rate as well as speech loudness?*
>
> Ramig, Pawlas, and Countryman (1995) suggest that for some speakers with parkinsonism, the Lee Silverman Voice Treatment Approach is a backdoor strategy to reduce speaking rate. The speaker, who is instructed to talk with increased effort and intensity by using a "Think Loud" or "Think Shout" strategy, often reduces speaking rate.

Another backdoor approach to rate control training is appropriate phrasing and breath patterning. Chunking utterances into meaningful units based on breath groups has been shown to be important for the intelligibility of normal speech. Speakers with dysarthria frequently fail to do this. The relationship between speaking rate and respiratory control is clinically important. Hardy (1983) discussed rate control in individuals with developmental dysarthria and compromised respiratory support. He suggested that, although one might predict that speakers would produce fewer units on a single breath if rates were reduced, this is not necessarily the case. Decreasing speaking rates prolonged the phonated elements of speech more than the nonphonated elements. Because the laryngeal valving of the phonated elements in some speakers tends to be more aerodynamically efficient than the valving for the nonphonated elements, rate reduction may not negatively affect respiratory support. Also, it should be noted again that some rate control techniques, particularly the ones that impose rigid rate control, may disrupt respiratory patterning for speech. Other rate control techniques, especially those that encourage appropriate phrasing, may improve speech-related respiratory function.

Delayed Auditory Feedback

RESEARCH FINDINGS

Delayed auditory feedback (DAF) is an intervention technique that has been used with a number of different communication disorders, most notably stuttering (Soderberg, 1969). Curlee and Perkins (1969) studied the effects of DAF on a group of stutterers and found that DAF reduced the stutterers' rate of speech and frequency of stuttering. Trials of DAF use have been reported with neurogenically involved populations, including subjects with aphasia (Stanton, 1958), patients with left or right hemisphere lesions (Vrtunski, Mack, Boller, & Kim, 1976), and a group of speakers with dysarthria of varying types (Singh & Schlanger, 1969). These studies generally report mixed results, with large variability in effect from speaker to speaker. Although a number of the studies of the effects of DAF included heterogeneous subject groups, other studies restricted themselves to a more homogeneous population. Downie, Low, and Lindsay (1981) tested DAF with 11 patients with parkinsonism. They reported "dramatic improvement in intelligibility" in two of the patients. These patients were described as having a "festinating" type of speech.

Hanson and Metter (1980) reported the use of a small, solid-state, battery-operated DAF unit, similar to the one that appears in Figure 10.5, with two

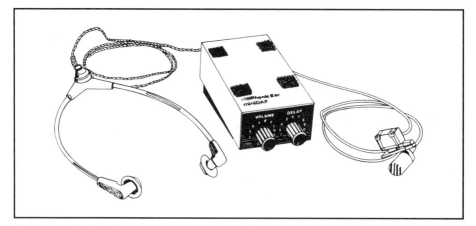

Figure 10.5. Portable delayed auditory feedback unit (MiniDAF, Phonic Ear, Mill Valley, CA).

patients with supranuclear palsy and hypokinetic dysarthria. With the delay at 100 milliseconds (msec), speech was slowed, vocal intensity increased, and speech intelligibility improved.

Hanson and Metter (1983) reported on a DAF application with two speakers with Parkinson's disease. For both of these speakers, the intervention had an impact on speech performance, including improvement in intelligibility and an increase in intensity. Measures of these changes are summarized in Table 10.2. Hansen and Metter suggested that, when using DAF, both speakers increased their physiologic effort.

A question that logically follows from the positive case reports of Hansen and Metter relates to how universally helpful DAF is for speakers with dysarthria. Both clinical experience and a review of the literature suggest that it is effective in only selected cases of hypokinetic dysarthria. Specific data related to the proportion of the population benefiting from DAF are not yet available. However, Hanson, Metter, and Riege (1984) presented an acoustic profile of a typical candidate who benefited from DAF. Acoustic features of this speech included the following:

- duration and articulation time both more than 2.5 standard deviations below normal

- pause time, number of pauses, and mean length of pauses approximately at a normal level of performance

- percent of voicing 2.0 standard deviations above normal

Table 10.2
A Summary of Changes Seen in Parkinson Subjects A and B
With and Without Delayed Auditory Feedback

	Subject A	Subject B
Reduction in speaking rate	255 to 139 wpm	184 to 122 wpm reading
		242 to 161 wpm conversation
Increased speech intelligibility	5.0 to 2.0 (7-point scale)	Increased or same
Increased speech intensity	66 to 72 dB SPL	77 to 79 dB SPL reading
		78 to 71 dB SPL conversation

Note. From "DAF Speech Rate Modification in Parkinson's Disease: A Report of Two Cases," by W. Hanson and E. Metter, 1980, in *Clinical Dysarthria* (pp. 231–251), by W. Berry (Ed.), Austin, TX: PRO-ED. Copyright 1980 by PRO-ED, Inc. Reprinted with permission.

Thus, their patient's speech was excessively rapid and voicing was consistently present throughout speech. When speaking with DAF, the following acoustic features of this individual's speech moved toward normal: duration, articulation time, fundamental frequency variability, mean intensity, and intensity variability (Hanson & Metter, 1983).

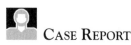

CASE REPORT

Clinical trials remain critical in assessing the benefits and drawbacks of any of the rate control techniques that attempt to preserve prosody. To illustrate this point, we present the case of a 72-year-old man with a 10-year history of Parkinson's disease. A number of different rate control strategies were tried. Habitually, his rate, as measured on a sentence production task, was excessively rapid at 262 wpm (Yorkston et al., 1984). This rate represents 138% of normal rate and is over 3.0 standard deviations above the mean of normal male speakers. At this rapid rate, speech intelligibility was 67%. The first rate control technique evaluated was rhythmic cueing. Initially, we were interested in the question, "Does reducing this speaker's rate improve intelligibility?" A computerized pacing program was used in conjunction with the intelligibility measurement task to answer this question. When sentences were presented at 127 wpm, approximately 60% of his habitual rate, he spoke at 137 wpm. At this slowed rate, he was 94% intelligible. Judges who rated speech naturalness felt that the slowed rate was more natural than the excessively rapid speech.

The initial trial with pacing had indicated that slowing his rate had beneficial consequences for both intelligibility and naturalness. Our next question was "How do we translate the result of this clinical trial, which was carried out under highly controlled conditions, into a training program that will slow his rate in real communication situations?" Three options were considered. The first was the training program described earlier for Donna. Choosing this alternative would mean an extended period of training and practice, using the computer to slow his rate. We did not choose this alternative because the patient demonstrated only limited awareness of his rapid rate and there seemed to be no carryover from the reading of computer-presented paced passages to unpaced reading or conversation. The second alternative would also require a period of training, but on a task that the speaker appeared to be able to learn more quickly. This training would involve one of the backdoor approaches to rate control and would involve the speaker learning to pause at appropriate phrasing boundaries, and thereby chunking his speech into syntactically appropriate, but short, breath groups. The third alternative for this speaker would be the use of a DAF system. We chose to begin our exploration of rate control strategies with the DAF because, if effective, it would require the least amount of training. Results of these trials will be illustrated with a variety of measures to describe as fully as possible the impact of DAF on this speaker.

As with the evaluation of any rate control technique, our first question—Does DAF control rate at the target level?—concerned the effectiveness of DAF. To answer this question, the speaker was recorded as he read passages with the sidetone of the DAF unit set at a number of different levels. Figure 10.6 illustrates the results we obtained. This figure displays the sidetone setting of the DAF versus the speaking rate (in syllables per minute) that was produced at each sidetone. Examination of the figure suggests that a reduction in speaking rate occurred when the delay was increased from a normal sidetone (no delay) to a 100-msec delay. An additional reduction occurred when the delay was increased from a 100- to a 150-msec delay. No additional reduction in rate occurred as the sidetone delay was increased from 150 to 200 msec. This information not only confirmed the effectiveness of DAF on this task, but also allowed the selection of a sidetone delay setting that produced the greatest effect in terms of rate control.

Our next question was, What are the consequences of DAF? Our hope was that the reduced rate brought about by DAF would result in an increase in intelligibility. This proved to be the case. Speech intelligibility was measured as the speaker read

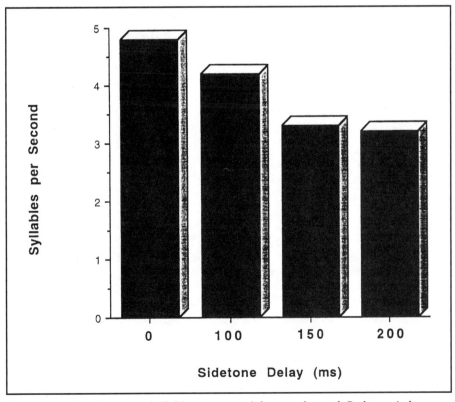

Figure 10.6. Speaking rates (syllables per minute) for a speaker with Parkinson's disease at 0-, 100-, 150-, and 200-millisecond (ms) sidetone delays.

sentences at a DAF sidetone delay of 150 msec. This DAF setting produced a speaking rate of 135 wpm and an intelligibility score of 97%. Thus, DAF produced both a higher intelligibility score and a more rapid rate than either of the other rate control strategies: computerized rhythmic cueing or insertion of pauses at the appropriate locations related to breath groups.

Although increased intelligibility is certainly important when evaluating the consequence of rate control, the effect of rate control on the naturalness of our patient's speech was also of concern. Perceptually, reducing the speaking rate with DAF appeared to improve the naturalness. The rapid rushes of speech that were present during habitual speech were gone, and the pattern of breath groups and intonation contours was preserved. To acoustically document these changes, we selected a short segment embedded in a paragraph read by the speaker for further measurement. The fundamental frequency and intensity contours were analyzed for the habitual reading and for a sidetone delayed condition (150 msec). Fundamental frequency and intensity × time plots for these segments appear in Figure 10.7. A review of this figure reveals that the speaker does not intersperse pauses in the DAF-slowed speech. Further, fundamental frequency excursion on the DAF-slowed speech was slightly greater than for habitual speech. Generally, the acoustic measures suggest that the speaker increased overall speaking time, while maintaining natural prosodic patterns.

Further acoustic analysis was performed on another short sample of habitual and DAF-slowed speech. In this analysis, consonant and vowel–nasal segment durations were obtained from an acoustic analysis for two speakers with Parkinson's disease. Table 10.3 contains the percentage change in duration of consonant and vowel–nasal segments for the habitual and three DAF-slowed conditions. For Speaker 1, the speaker we have been discussing in this case presentation, consonant and vowel–nasal segments were slowed in a roughly equivalent proportion under the 150- and 200-msec delay conditions. For Speaker 2, however, the vowel–nasal segments were increased proportionally more than the consonant segments. Thus, there appears to be individual differences among speakers and the effect of DAF on segment duration. However,

Table 10.3

Percent Changes in Consonant (C) and Vowel–Nasal (V–N) Durations for Two Speakers with Parkinson's Disease at Three DAF-Slowed Speaking Rates

Delay (in milliseconds)	Speaker 1			Speaker 2		
	C	V–N	Total	C	V–N	Total
50				9	46	28
100	−10	9	1	16	108	65
150	45	39	40	29	110	72
200	29	34	31			

Note. From *The Effects of Rate Control on Dysarthric Speech,* by D. Beukelman, K. Yorkston, and M. McClean, 1984, paper presented at the Annual Convention of the American Speech-Language-Hearing Association, San Francisco. Reprinted with permission of the authors.

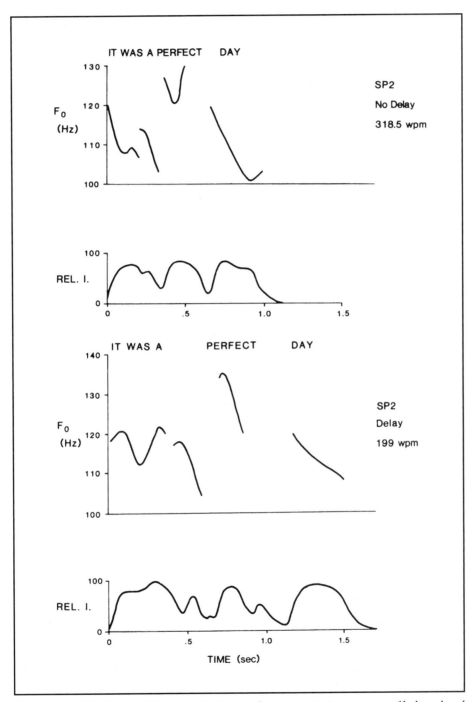

Figure 10.7. Fundamental frequency × time and intensity × time tracings of habitual and DAF-slowed speech of a speaker with Parkinson's disease.

in both speakers, DAF had the effect of increasing total articulation time rather than simply increasing pause duration. The increase in articulation time rather than pause time may be an important contributor to perceived naturalness of DAF-slowed speech.

When considering the data just presented, DAF appears to have many advantages for selected speakers over other rate control strategies. DAF effectively slows speaking rates without extensive training, it improves intelligibility while maintaining a somewhat faster speaking rate than other rate control techniques, and it preserves, and may even improve, the overall naturalness of speech. However, to clinically measure intelligibility and to compare, acoustically, speech samples produced under different conditions, structured samples must be used. In this case, our speaker was asked to read material that had been prepared for him. Unfortunately, the DAF unit did not control his rate as effectively during conversation. This reduction in effectiveness may have been due, in part, to the telegraphic nature of his spontaneous speech. Utterances were typically so short that the DAF effect did not occur. However, DAF pacing during conversation was judged to be superior to unpaced productions. To bring conversation under more control with DAF, we attempted to train this speaker in strategies that we felt would allow the DAF unit to be a more effective pacer of his speech. These strategies included producing the initial word of an utterance with relatively strong intensity, not attempting to speak rapidly in an effort to "overdrive" the DAF system, and speaking in full phrases rather than single-word utterances.

SELECTING AN OPTIMUM SPEAKING RATE

Intelligible speech at normal rates is rarely an attainable goal for speakers with dysarthria. Throughout this chapter, we have suggested that the selection of rate control techniques often reflects a compromise between the positive and the negative consequences of those techniques. Likewise, the selection of an optimum speaking rate, once the training technique has been chosen, requires a clinical compromise. In seeking the best compromise between intelligibility and naturalness, it is clear that equal weight cannot be given to each. If there is a choice between intelligibility and naturalness, intelligibility must be the deciding variable. Relatively natural but unintelligible speech is not acceptable. When speech intelligibility reaches an acceptable range (over 90%), we find ourselves compromising slightly in terms of intelligibility in order to achieve naturalness.

Data presented at the beginning of this chapter illustrated the case of a speaker with ataxic dysarthria who clearly benefited from rate control. A review of that data (Figure 10.1) reveals that the highest intelligibility score for this speaker was obtained at a rate of approximately 50 wpm. Because the speaker felt, and the clinician agreed, that this rate was too disruptive of naturalness, a slightly more rapid rate was selected as a target during training. A rate of approximately 70 wpm was selected because, at that rate, the speaker was over 90% intelligible and was able to achieve at least some degree of natural breath patterning and stressing within breath group units.

Many of the speakers with dysarthria we serve clinically are not neurologically stable. The course for some is improving, but for others it is degenerative. Because our goal is to maximize speech performance regardless of the course of the disorder, the selection of an optimum rate and rate control technique must be reevaluated periodically. Figure 10.8 contains data illustrating the recovery pattern of a speaker with head injury and dysarthria (Yorkston & Beukelman, 1981a). At 1 month postonset, when the patient was speaking at about 140 wpm, intelligibility was low, approximately 20%. At that point, a training program

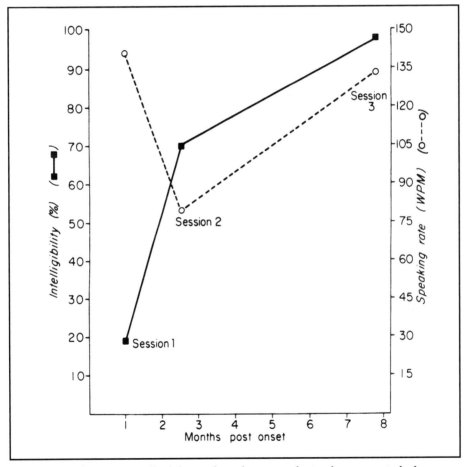

Figure 10.8. Sentence intelligibility and speaking rate obtained over a period of recovery for a speaker with ataxic dysarthria.

utilizing rhythmic cueing was initiated. By the second recording session, this patient had reduced his rate to 80 wpm with an accompanying increase in intelligibility to approximately 70%. As the speaker continued to improve, his target speaking rate was systematically increased. By 8 months postonset, he was nearly completely intelligible at a speaking rate of over 130 wpm. Thus, the target speaking rate must continue to change as long as the speaker is able to maintain an acceptable level of intelligibility. Once intelligibility has been achieved at a particular rate, treatment can appropriately focus on increasing the rate and naturalness of speech.

Although the speaker just discussed was recovering from head injury, management frequently involves individuals with degenerative disorders such as Parkinson's disease. For these individuals, optimum speaking rates and rate control strategies also need to be periodically reevaluated. More rigid rate control techniques are selected as the severity of the speech disability increases. As a consequence of the more rigid rate control techniques, target speaking rates are progressively slowed.

REFERENCES

Ackermann, H., Grone, B. F., Hoch, G., & Schonle, P. W. (1993). Speech freezing in Parkinson's disease: A kinematic analysis of orofacial movements by means of electromagnetic articulography. *Folia Phoniatrica, 45*(2), 84–89.

Berry, W., & Goshorn, E. (1983). Immediate visual feedback in the treatment of ataxic dysarthria: A case study. In W. Berry (Ed.), *Clinical dysarthria* (pp. 253–266). Boston: College-Hill.

Beukelman, D. R., & Yorkston, K. M. (1977). A communication system for the severely dysarthric speaker with an intact language system. *Journal of Speech and Hearing Disorders, 42,* 265–270.

Beukelman, D., Yorkston, K., & McClean, M. (1984). *The effects of rate control on dysarthric speech*. Paper presented at the Annual Convention of the American Speech-Language-Hearing Association, San Franciso.

Beukelman, D. R., Yorkston, K. M., & Tice, R. (1997). *Pacer/tally rate measurement software*. Lincoln, NE: Tice Technology Services.

Caliguiri, M. P. (1989). The influence of speaking rate on articulatory hypokinesia in parkinsonian dysarthria. *Brain and Language, 36,* 493–502.

Curlee, R., & Perkins, W. (1969). Conversational rate control therapy for stuttering. *Journal of Speech and Hearing Disorders, 34,* 245–250.

Darley, F. L., Aronson, A. E., & Brown, J. R. (1975). *Motor speech disorders*. Philadelphia: Saunders.

Downie, A. W., Low, J. M., & Lindsay, D. D. (1981). Speech disorders in parkinsonism: Usefulness of delayed auditory feedback in selected cases. *British Journal of Disorders of Communication, 16,* 135–139.

Fairbanks, G. (1960). *Voice and articulation drillbook*. New York: Harper & Brothers.

Goldman-Eisler, F. (1961). The significance of changes in the rate of articulation. *Language and Speech, 4,* 171–174.

Goldman-Eisler, F. (1968). *Psycholinguistics: Experiments in spontaneous speech*. New York: Academic Press.

Hammen, V. L., & Yorkston, K. M. (1994). Respiratory patterning and variability in dysarthric speech. *Journal of Medical Speech-Language Pathology, 2*(4), 253–262.

Hammen, V. L., Yorkston, K. M., & Minifie, F. D. (1994). Effects of temporal alterations on speech intelligibility of parkinsonian dysarthria. *Journal of Speech and Hearing Research, 37,* 244–253.

Hanson, W., & Metter, E. J. (1980). DAF as instrumental treatment for dysarthria in progressive supranuclear palsy: A case report. *Journal of Speech and Hearing Disorders, 45,* 268–276.

Hanson, W., & Metter, E. (1983). DAF speech rate modification in Parkinson's disease: A report of two cases. In W. Berry (Ed.), *Clinical dysarthria* (pp. 231–254). Austin, TX: PRO-ED.

Hanson, W., Metter, E., & Riege, W. (1984). *Variability in Parkinson's disease*. Paper presented at the annual convention of the American Speech-Language-Hearing Association, San Francisco.

Hardy, J. (1967). Suggestions for physiologic research in dysarthria. *Cortex, 3,* 128.

Hardy, J. C. (1983). *Cerebral palsy*. Englewood Cliffs, NJ: Prentice-Hall.

Helm, N. (1979). Management of palilalia with a pacing board. *Journal of Speech and Hearing Disorders, 44,* 350–353.

Henderson, A., Goldman-Eisler, F., & Skarbeck, A. (1966). Temporal patterns of cognitive activity and breath control in speech. *Language and Speech, 8*(4), 207–216.

Huggins, A. (1978). Speech timing and intelligibility. In J. Requin (Ed.), *Attention and performance VII*. Hillsdale, NJ: Erlbaum.

Kalikow, D., Steven, K., & Elliot, L. (1977). Development of a test of speech intelligibility in noise using sentence material with controlled predictability. *Journal of the Acoustic Society of America, 61,* 1337–1351.

Kelly, J., & Steer, M. (1949). Revised concept of rate. *Journal of Speech and Hearing Disorders, 14,* 222–226.

Kent, R., Netsell, R., & Bauer, L. (1975). Cineradiographic assessment of articulatory mobility in the dysarthrias. *Journal of Speech and Hearing Disorders, 40,* 467–480.

Klatt, D. H. (1976). Linguistic uses of segmental duration in English: Acoustic and perceptual evidence. *Journal of the Acoustic Society of America, 59,* 1208–1221.

Lane, H., & Grosjean, F. (1973). Perception of reading rate by listeners and speakers. *Journal of Experimental Psychology, 97,* 141–147.

Linebaugh, C. W., & Wolfe, V. E. (1984). Relationships between articulation rate, intelligibility, and naturalness in spastic and ataxic speakers. In M. McNeil, J. Rosenbek, & A. Aronson (Eds.), *The dysarthrias: Physiology acoustics perception management* (pp. 197–206). Austin, TX: PRO-ED.

McHenry, M., & Wilson, R. (1994). The challenge of unintelligible speech following traumatic brain injury. *Brain Injury, 8,* 363–375.

Payton, K. L., Uchanski, R. M., & Braida, L. D. (1994). Intelligibility of conversational and clear speech in noise and reverberation for listeners with normal and impaired hearing. *Journal of the Acoustical Society of America, 95*(3), 1581–1592.

Picheny, M., Durlach, N., & Braida, L. (1985). Speaking clearly for the hard of hearing: I. Intelligibility differences between clear and conversational speech. *Journal of Speech and Hearing Research, 28,* 96–103.

Picheny, M., Durlach, N., & Braida, L. (1986). Speaking clearly for the hard of hearing: II. Acoustic characteristics of clear and conversational speech. *Journal of Speech and Hearing Research, 29,* 434–446.

Picheny, M., Durlach, N., & Braida, L. (1989). Speaking clearly for the hard of hearing: III. An attempt to determine the contribution of speaking rate to differences in intelligibility between clear and conversational speech. *Journal of Speech and Hearing Research, 32,* 600–603.

Ramig, L. O., Pawlas, A. A., & Countryman, S. (1995). *The Lee Silverman Voice Treatment.* Iowa City, IA: National Center for Voice and Speech.

Rosenbek, J. C., & LaPointe, L. L. (1985). The dysarthrias: Description, diagnosis, and treatment. In D. Johns (Ed.), *Clinical management of neurogenic communication disorders* (pp. 97–152). Boston: Little, Brown.

Schum, D. J. (1996). Intelligibility of clear and conversational speech of young and elderly talkers. *Journal of the American Academy of Audiology, 7*(3), 212–218.

Simmons, N. (1983). Acoustic analysis of ataxic dysarthria: An approach to monitoring treatment. In W. Berry (Ed.), *Clinical dysarthria* (pp. 283–294). Austin, TX: PRO-ED.

Singh, S., & Schlanger, B. B. (1969). Effects of delayed sidetone on the speech of aphasic, dysarthric, and mental retarded subjects. *Language and Speech, 12,* 167.

Soderberg, G. (1969). Delayed auditory feedback and the speech of stutterers: A review of studies. *Journal of Speech and Hearing Disorders, 34,* 20–29.

Stanton, J. B. (1958). The effects of DAF on the speech of aphasic patients. *Scotish Medical Journal, 3,* 378–384.

Turner, G. S., Tjaden, K., & Weismer, G. (1995). The influence of speaking rate on vowel space and speech intelligibility for individuals with amyotrophic lateral sclerosis. *Journal of Speech and Hearing Research, 38,* 1001–1013.

Uchanski, R. M., Choi, S. S., Braida, L. D., Reed, C. M., & Durlach, N. I. (1996). Speaking clearly for the head of hearing: IV. Further studies of the role of speaking rate. *Journal of Speech and Hearing Research, 39,* 494–509.

Vrtunski, P. B., Mack, J. L., Boller, F., & Kim, Y. (1976). Response to delayed auditory feedback in patients with hemispheric lesions. *Cortex, 12,* 395–404.

Yorkston, K. M., & Beukelman, D. (1981a). Ataxic dysarthria: Treatment sequences based on intelligibility and prosodic considerations. *Journal of Speech and Hearing Disorders, 46,* 398–404.

Yorkston, K. M., & Beukelman, D. R. (1981b). Communication efficiency of dysarthric speakers as measured by sentence intelligibility and speaking rate. *Journal of Speech and Hearing Disorders, 46,* 296–301.

Yorkston, K. M., Beukelman, D. R., & Tice, R. (1996). *Sentence intelligibility test.* Lincoln, NE: Tice Technology Services.

Yorkston, K. M., Beukelman, D. R., & Traynor, C. (1984). *Computerized Assessment of Intelligibility of Dysarthric Speech.* Austin, TX: PRO-ED.

Yorkston, K. M., Hammen, V. L., Beukelman, D. R., & Traynor, C. D. (1990). The effect of rate control on the intelligibility and naturalness of dysarthric speech. *Journal of Speech and Hearing Disorders, 55,* 550–561.

ARTICULATION AND PROSODY: SEGMENTAL AND SUPRASEGMENTAL ASPECTS OF DYSARTHRIC SPEECH

Clinical Issues: In preparation for their internships with us, students are given a reading list designed to familiarize them with the nature and management of disorders frequently occurring in our clinical practice. Often this reading list is the students' first exposure to management of speakers with dysarthria. At times, students who are more familiar with management of developmental articulation disorders than adult motor speech disorders are confused by the dysarthria literature. For example, as they read the research reports of Darley, Aronson, and Brown (1975), students find that the speech dimension of imprecise consonants is consistently listed among the most deviant dimensions across all of the dysarthrias. Yet, despite the apparent frequency of occurrence of articulatory impairment, they will also read the following statement representing a philosophy of management: "Indeed, traditional articulation treatment alone is seldom salutary for the dysarthric talker even if the impairment involves only his tongue, lips, or jaw" (Rosenbek, 1984). Thus, students may ask the following questions:

- How can the apparent prevalence of articulation impairment in dysarthria be reconciled with the lack of clinical focus on oral articulation in intervention programs?

439

- How is the ability to produce speech sounds influenced by other components, such as respiration, phonation, and the velopharyngeal system?

- What is prosody and why is it important to speakers with dysarthria?

- When is treatment focused on the articulatory or segmental aspects of speech, and when is it more appropriately focused on the prosodic or suprasegmental aspects?

This chapter focuses on two important aspects of intervention: segmental features and suprasegmental aspects of speech. Intervention associated with the segmental aspect of speech focuses on enhancing the speaker's ability to produce speech sounds. Both consonant imprecision and distorted vowels are among the most common characteristics of speech of individuals with dysarthria (Darley et al., 1975). Despite the frequency with which these segmental features are disordered in dysarthria, treatment does not typically focus on segmental aspects or articulation alone. Rosenbek (1984) advocated viewing dysarthria as more than an articulatory disorder and its treatment as more than articulatory training.

Treatment of the prosodic or suprasegmental aspect of dysarthric speech is also a clinically important but poorly understood topic. Suprasegmental aspects of speech are those that go beyond the boundaries of individual segments or speech sounds and include features such as stress patterning, intonation, and rate–rhythm. Rosenbek and LaPointe (1985) suggested that it is a mistake to consider prosody the "formal wear" of speech and to attend to it only after all other aspects of treatment have been completed. Some speakers with dysarthria find that efforts to maintain normalized patterns of prosody enhance their speech intelligibility. By using prosody to signal important words and syntactic junctures, their listeners are provided important information to decode the speaker's messages.

ARTICULATION IN DYSARTHRIA: THE SEGMENTAL ASPECTS OF SPEECH

Broadly defined, articulation is considered the movement of speech structures employed in producing the sounds of speech. The oral articulatory component of speech provides an excellent illustration of the interdependencies among various speech components. For example, Hardy (1967) presented the case of a 24-year-old individual who, at the time of evaluation, was 2 years post–brain injury with cerebral concussion–contusion, right hemiparesis, and probable brain stem injury. His unintelligible speech was characterized by an extremely rapid rate with an initial "explosive" burst followed by rapidly diminishing loudness. Cinefluorographic films revealed "gross immobility of the tongue and velum" at habitual rates; however, an increase in the extent of lingual and palatal movement was noted at reduced speaking rates. Hardy offered a possible explanation for the severely impaired movements of the oral articulators. He suggested that the speaker "attempts to compensate for his speech physiological problems during recovery from the severe neurological damage by completing an utterance 'before he ran out of air'" (p. 152). Hardy further stated that the patient's inappropriate speaking rate worked against his compensatory efforts. This case illustrates an instance where severely restricted movements of the oral articulators may not have been the direct result of damage to the neuro-motor control of these structures. Rather, those severely restricted movements may have been the consequence of a poorly controlled respiratory system and the attempt to compensate for that impairment.

The interdependence of the oral articulators and other speech components can also be illustrated with an example related to phonation. The perceptual distinction between voiced and voiceless cognate pairs is based on precise laryngeal timing, as well as subtle adjustments in the duration of oral articulatory gestures. Voiced versus voiceless distinctions are often difficult for a speaker with dys-arthria to achieve, perhaps because of the complex timing and coordination required between a number of speech components. Imprecise production of speech sounds is not simply an oral articulatory phenomenon, but is the result of laryngeal, velopharyngeal, and oral articulatory impairments. Respiratory and phonatory examples have been provided to illustrate that the management of oral articulation must be considered only in the context of other aspects of speech. Often the sequence of treatment requires focus on training other compo-nents first, or on prosthetic management of other components, before training of oral articulation can be expected to result in perceptually acceptable productions.

In brief, our approach is to optimize the function of other aspects of speech performance, such as respiratory support, laryngeal timing, velopharyngeal clo-sure, and speaking rate (for the current stage of neuromotor function), before directly focusing on the articulation performance of speakers with dysarthria. This is often a cyclic process as the speaker's neuromotor status improves or deteriorates. For a speaker, several efforts may be made to optimize speech mechanism function in order to support articulatory function. This cyclic pro-cess is supported with careful assessment of speech subsystem function.

Assessment

In this section, we review measures of articulatory performance available to the speech–language pathologist and discuss interpretation of the information obtained from each of these measures. For a more general discussion of approaches to assessment, see Chapters 5 and 6. Although a variety of articulatory measurements and strategies have been used by researchers in the motor speech disorders field, perceptual measurements of articulatory performance are widely used for clinical assessment. As discussed in Chapter 5, most clinicians use consistent, although not necessarily standardized, assessment tasks across their clients with motor speech disorders. In this way, they can familiarize themselves with the types of different performance patterns that they expect from speakers with various types of neuromotor impairments.

PERCEPTUAL RATING OF SPEECH COMPONENT PERFORMANCE

The first level of clinical assessment involves obtaining an overall assessment of the adequacy of articulatory performance and comparing that to ratings of other components of speech performance. General questions that are asked by the clinician in this portion of the evaluation include the following:

- Is there an oral articulatory impairment? If so, how severe is it?

- How does the severity of the articulatory impairment compare to the respiratory, phonatory, or velopharyngeal impairment?

Thus, during assessment the first measures obtained are global ones in which the clinician confirms the presence of an articulatory impairment and ranks its severity in relation to other components of performance. This step is important for treatment planning because it allows the clinician to sequence treatment tasks and deal first with those aspects of the problem that have the most potential for changing the overall adequacy of speech. In many cases, this means beginning with treatment that focuses on aspects of speech other than articulation. Our intervention philosophy usually is to optimize the performance of the other speech subsystems, if possible, before focusing too much attention directly on oral articulation. We have found, for example, that when aerodynamic support for speech is compromised because of respiratory impairment or because of inefficiency of laryngeal and velopharyngeal performance, articulation is negatively impacted. When respiratory support is optimized, articulation is often improved with little direct attention to the articulatory subsystem.

Estimation of the relative contribution of the oral articulatory impairment to overall communication disability typically is based on informal assessment and relies heavily on subjective clinical judgment. By selecting various sounds and sound combinations, the clinician can sample movements of the lips (by asking the speaker to repeat /papapa/), the tongue tip (/tatata/), the tongue back (/kakaka/), and a combination (/pataka/). Movement rates for single structures can be compared and contrasted with one another and with combinations of sounds. These simple tasks can also be performed with and without voicing to estimate the contribution of inadequate respiratory and phonatory control to articulatory movement impairments. Typically, an individual with dysarthria and inadequate respiratory support will perform much more poorly when attempting to speak a series of syllables than when simply "mouthing" the syllables. When this is the case, the clinician may choose to work on increasing respiratory and laryngeal control before focusing on articulatory movements in treatment.

Simple alternating movement tasks also may be used to estimate the contribution of various articulatory components to overall articulatory adequacy. For example, asking a speaker to repeat the bilabial consonant–vowel combination /papapa/, with and without a bite block, may give an indication of the contribution of abnormal jaw movement to articulatory impairment. Additional interpretation of bite block use has been provided in the literature (Netsell, 1985). In addition to overall diadochokinetic movement rates, the clinician may also make judgments about the range of excursion of the movements and the variability of the movement rates.

Alternating movement tasks are particularly useful for eliciting types of abnormal movement patterns. For example, many persons with hypokinetic dysarthria due to Parkinson's disease demonstrate patterns of excessively rapid speech with minimal articulatory excursion. These abnormal movement patterns are often accentuated during alternating movement tasks; as the syllable productions become even more rapid, they become habitual, and the articulatory excursions are further reduced. Also, alternating movement tasks often reveal the coordination problems faced by many speakers with ataxic dysarthria. This is particularly obvious on a task such as /pataka pataka/ where the speaker is expected to coordinate a variety of different articulatory postures.

Clinically, tasks used for assessment of articulatory movement are, for the most part, perceptually judged. The clinician initially confirms the existence of an articulatory impairment and estimates its severity in relation to other components of speech production. As is apparent, we have not included acoustic, aerodynamic, radiographic, or movement transduction in the list of clinical approaches for assessment of articulation in dysarthria. Although these measures have been used in research, they have not found their way into routine clinical practice, probably because the necessary instrumentation to make these measurements is only now routinely becoming clinically available.

ARTICULATION INVENTORIES

Administration of traditional articulation inventories, such as *The Fisher–Logemann Test of Articulation Competence* (Fisher & Logemann, 1971), or less formal word lists that sample all of the speech sounds (Johns & Darley, 1970; Platt, Andrews, Young, & Quinn, 1980) appear not to have been accepted as a routine part of clinical assessment of speakers with dysarthria. However, measures of perceived articulatory adequacy have a place in dysarthria management because the information obtained from them may provide answers to specific questions. For selected individuals, information about articulatory performance would allow the clinician to document the impact of intervention. For example, consider the speaker with severe flaccid dysarthria. Treatment may have focused on lip strengthening exercises in order to achieve bilabial closure. An articulation inventory would allow the monitoring of changes in the perceived adequacy of bilabial sounds. Or, consider the severely involved individual for whom a palatal lift has been fitted. An articulation inventory would allow the comparison of articulatory adequacy with and without the lift. Use of an articulation inventory to make decisions regarding palatal lift management is discussed in Chapter 8. Finally, consider the individual with severe dysarthria recovering from brain injury for whom treatment has focused on inclusion of final consonants. An articulation inventory would allow for the monitoring of change in final consonant production and for comparison of that change with changes in nontreated sounds. In short, articulation inventories may provide answers to specific questions, usually involving the performance of speakers with severe dysarthria. To date, there are no reports in the literature on the performance of speakers with dysarthria on structured articulation inventories as compared to free speech sampling techniques.

In our opinion, there are a number of reasons why articulation inventories have not enjoyed widespread clinical use in dysarthria. First, traditional articulation inventories often require judges to transcribe speech samples using the International Phonetic Alphabet and a number of modifiers for such features as dentalization, lip rounding, and tongue position. This type of transcription is based on the assumption that a speaker's articulatory movements can be inferred from a judge's perception of the speech end-product. Speech physiologists have repeatedly cautioned against making such inferences. Second, distortions rather than substitutions, omissions, or other error categories predominate in dysarthria. Traditional articulation inventories, in which the target phoneme is known to the judge, often fail to adequately make the critically important distinction between a phoneme that is distorted but recognizable and one that is distorted but no longer within phoneme boundaries. Finally, in traditional articulation inventories, judges who know the target phoneme may overestimate the accuracy of productions as compared to listeners who are naive to the phoneme targets.

To circumvent some of these measurement problems, we routinely use the *Phoneme Identification Task* (Yorkston, Beukelman, & Tice, 1998) to obtain a measure of perceived articulatory adequacy. Speakers are recorded as they produce a series of single words or sentences containing 57 target phonemes (22 prevocalic consonants, 19 postvocalic consonants, and 16 vowels and diphthongs). Judges view a word frame such as "ma" and are asked to identify the missing phoneme. All frames are selected so that a variety of real-word options are possible. For example, possible words for the frame "ma__" include "mass," "mat," "mad," "mack," "map," "mash," "match," and so forth. In addition to attempting to identify the phoneme, judges score each attempt according to the following distortion scale:

3—Correct, undistorted phoneme

2—Correct but distorted (judges are confident that they have identified the correct phoneme, but the production is distorted)

1—Guess (the phoneme is so distorted that the judge's response is a guess)

0—No basis for a guess

Kent and colleagues have described a single phonetic intelligibility protocol that has been used in full or modified form in a variety of clinical research projects (J. F. Kent et al., 1992; R. D. Kent, Kent, Weismer, & Martin, 1989; R. D. Kent et al., 1990; R. D. Kent et al., 1991). This test was designed to assess 19 acoustic–phonetic contrasts that are likely to be sensitive to dysarthric impairments (R. D. Kent, Weismer, Kent, & Rosenbek, 1989; see Table 11.1). Speakers audio record a list of single words. During judging, listeners are given response forms that contain four words (a target word and three foils) for each intelligibility judgment. After hearing a specific word, the listeners select the word that most closely approximates the speaker's word production. The overall percent-correct score is taken as a measure of overall accuracy of a "speaker's word transmission." The phonetic contrast error profile reflects the error rate for the contrasts listed in Table 11.1. Although this protocol has been described in some detail in the articles cited earlier in this paragraph, it has not been released in a form for widespread clinical use including stimuli, administration instructions, and analysis instructions.

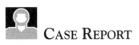 CASE REPORT

To illustrate how the results of the Phoneme Identification Task (Yorkston et al., 1998) can be used to make clinical decisions, the case of an 18-year-old individual with brain injury is presented. Table 11.2 contains a chronology of some important events in Brian's recovery. To summarize briefly, Brian began making some voluntary verbal responses 3.5 months postonset (MPO). One month later (4.5 MPO), his

Table 11.1
Listing of Phonetic Contrasts Used in the Intelligibility Test and Their Articulatory Correlates

Phonetic Contrast	Example	Articulatory Correlate
1. Front–back for vowels	feed–food	Anterior–posterior positioning of tongue
2. High–low for vowels	geese–gas	Tongue height, superior–inferior positioning of tongue
3. Vowel duration: long vs. short	feet–fit	Inherent vowel duration (also called tense–lax distinction)
4. Voicing contrast, initial consonant	bat–pat	Relative duration of vowel preceding consonant and presence or absence of vocal fold vibration during consonant
5. Voicing contrast, final consonant	feed–feet	Relative duration of vowel preceding consonant and presence or absence of vocal fold vibration during consonant
6. Alveolar consonant vs. palatal consonant	see–she	Lingua–alveolar vs. lingua–palatal constriction for consonant
7. Place of articulation for stop consonants	cake–take	Location of constriction for stops: bilabial, alveolar, or velar
8. Place of articulation for fricative consonants	sigh–thigh	Location of constriction for fricatives: labiodental, dental, alveolar, palatal, or glottal
9. Fricative–affricate articulation	mush–much	Production of fricative (noise) vs. affricate (stop + noise)
10. Stop–fricative articulation	tell–sell	Production of stop (complete closure of vocal tract) vs. fricative (narrowed constriction)
11. Stop–affricate articulation	tear–chair	Production of stop (no frication) vs. affricate (frication)
12. Stop–nasal articulation	side–sigh	Production of stop consonant (made with velopharyngeal closure) vs. nasal consonant (made with velopharyngeal opening)
13. Syllable-initial [h] vs. syllable-initial vowel	hate–ate	Laryngeal adjustment for high airflow ([h]) or voicing with low airflow (vowel)

(continues)

Table 11.1 (continued)

Phonetic Contrast	Example	Articulatory Correlate
14. Presence or absence of syllable-initial consonant	sin–in	Articulation of consonant or vowel in syllable-initial position
15. Presence or absence of syllable-final consonant	sign–sigh	Articulation of consonant or vowel in syllable-final position
16. Initial consonant vs. consonant	sit–spit	Production of a single consonant vs. a sequence of consonants in syllable-initial position
17. Final consonant vs. consonant	rock–rocks	Production of a final consonant vs. a sequence of consonants in syllable-final position
18. [r] vs. [l]	rock–lock	Differential lingual articulation: retroflex [r] vs. lateral [l]
19. [r] vs. [w]	read–weed	Differential lingual articulation: liquid [r] vs. glide [w]

Note. From "Toward Phonetic Intelligibility Testing in Dysarthria," by R. D. Kent, G. Weismer, J. F. Kent, and J. C. Rosenbek, 1989, *Journal of Speech and Hearing Disorders, 54*, p. 490. Copyright 1989 by the American Speech-Language-Hearing Association. Reprinted with permission.

speech was characterized by his primary speech clinician as unintelligible, grossly hypernasal, and produced with little oral articulatory movement. Spontaneous speech was marked by short utterances. Although initial portions of utterances were adequately loud, the patient frequently appeared to "run out of air," finishing the utterance without phonation.

At approximately 4.5 MPO, Brian's primary clinician consulted us regarding the possibility of evaluating him for palatal lift fitting. A Phoneme Identification Task was recorded and judged. Results of this and other subsequent recordings appear in Figure 11.1. This figure contains the perceived adequacy of three consonant groups: (1) labials and bilabials; (2) stops, fricatives, and affricates; and (3) nasals and others. Results of the first recording indicated severely impaired performance, with a mean score across consonants of approximately 20% correct. Both labial–bilabial and stop–fricative–affricate categories were only 10% correct. Aerodynamic measures of velopharyngeal performance could not be obtained at that time because of the patient's inability to achieve lip closure. See Chapter 9 for a detailed description of these measurement techniques. It was recommended that treatment focus on attempts to achieve bilabial closure during speech production.

Table 11.2
Chronology of Brian's Recovery

Months Postonset	Event
1.5	Began arousing from coma
3.0	Vocalized to discomfort No yes/no responses
3.5	Used an alphabet board Some verbal responses
4.5	Palatal lift first considered First recording of Phoneme Identification Task
4.6	Training focused on achieving lip closure
5.0	Second recording of Phoneme Identification Task Aerodynamic assessment of velopharyngeal function
5.5	Third recording of Phoneme Identification Task
6.0	Spasticity medications increased Increased swallowing difficulties noted Fourth recording of Phoneme Identification Task
6.5	Fifth recording of Phoneme Identification Task
7.5	Sentence intelligibility reached 97% at a speaking rate of 67 words per minute

After a 2-week interval, Brian's clinician indicated that she felt he could achieve sufficient lip closure to be tested aerodynamically. During this testing, Brian demonstrated the ability to consistently achieve lip closure and to produce air pressure in the oral cavity during the stop phase of the /p/ at 10 cm H_2O or more. This supported the observation that Brian had adequate respiratory control to support speech. However, he demonstrated nasal flow of air each time he attempted to impound intraoral air pressure during speech. This suggested that his velopharyngeal mechanism was not functioning adequately. A visual examination of the soft palate revealed some movement during sustained phonation. The Phoneme Identification Task was recorded again at the time of the aerodynamic evaluation. Results of this recording at 5.0 MPO indicated that the labial–bilabial group of consonants had improved to 60% accurate. Thus, the clinician's intervention appeared to have had the desired effect. Because of the improvement that had been observed over a 2-week period of time, the decision was made to delay palatal lift fitting and closely monitor the changing performance.

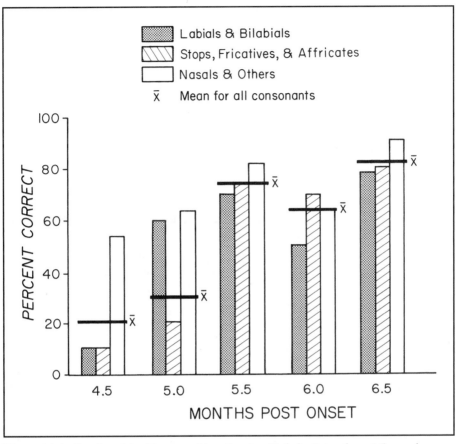

Figure 11.1. Results of the Phoneme Identification Task for Brian from 4.5 months post-onset to 6.5 months postonset.

The third recording of the Phoneme Identification Task, along with aerodynamic measures, was obtained 2 weeks later at 5.5 MPO. Results indicated that Brian was achieving adequate velopharyngeal closure, at least at times, during connected speech. Perceived accuracy of stop, affricate, and fricative consonants was now over 70%.

Close examination of Figure 11.1 suggests that performance at 6.0 MPO was lower than at testing 2 weeks earlier. This decrease in articulatory performance was coincident with an increase in Brian's antispasticity medications. Subjectively, Brian's clinician also observed increased drooling and swallowing difficulties. She reported the measures of articulatory performance as evidence of undesirable drug effects, and dosages of medications were lowered. This case illustrates the usefulness of articulation inventories for providing answers to specific questions related to intervention for individuals with severe dysarthria.

Treatment

The treatment of oral articulation disorders to improve the production of speech sounds may take on many forms. For purposes of this discussion, procedures will be reviewed under two general headings. The first set of techniques contains those that attempt to normalize function by reducing the impairment. Included in this category are those procedures that employ medical management, biofeedback training, or strengthening exercises in order to restore muscle function as nearly as possible to normal. The second set of techniques contains those that are compensatory. These techniques utilize behavioral training or prosthetic management in an effort to help speakers with dysarthria compensate for their motor impairment. The selection of specific techniques and their sequencing in relation to other training tasks are dependent on a number of factors, including the underlying neuropathology of the articulatory system deficit and the severity of articulatory impairment in relation to other components of the speech mechanism. In presenting the following techniques, we attempt to provide a framework for deciding for whom a technique is appropriate and when it should be applied.

Normalizing Function

More often than not in dysarthria treatment, intervention programs involve compensatory adjustments rather than attempts to achieve normalcy. With this caution in mind, some approaches will be reviewed that are designed to normalize the muscular function in dysarthria. These are the articulatory techniques that come to mind first when the clinician asks if anything can be done to reduce the physiologic impairment.

Normalizing function or reducing the overall impairment may occur in a number of ways. Many disorders resulting in dysarthria are characterized by a natural course of spontaneous recovery or reduction of the impairment. For example, Guillain-Barré syndrome typically involves a course of rapid recovery following the acute paralytic phase. Strokes typically involve a sudden onset, followed by a slow course of natural recovery that may last months and even years. Multiple sclerosis may be characterized by periods of exacerbations and remissions. In other disorders that cause dysarthria, the impairment may be reduced by medical management. For example, the rigidity seen in parkinsonism may be reduced by medication and the impairment seen in Wilson's disease is typically managed with diet and medication.

For some speakers with dysarthria, surgical management is used to reduce or eliminate the impairment. Neural anastamosis is occasionally employed to restore function to a damaged nerve. The most common nerve to be the target of such treatment is the facial (VIIth) cranial nerve. Usually, a branch of the normally functioning damaged hypoglossal nerve is connected to the facial nerve in order to improve appearance. Yorkston (1989) documented the experience of a woman with a facial weakness to hypoglossal anastamosis following a brain stem stroke. Immediately following surgery, the woman's speech intelligibility decreased from the 90% she had achieved before surgery. In time, intelligibility returned to baseline.

The techniques described in the following section involve attempts to reduce impairment, thus normalizing function, through training. This training is typically carried out in the presence of a natural course that is either stable or improving and typically involves some form of biofeedback. Biofeedback has been defined as "a process of transducing some physiologic variable, transforming the signal to extract useful information, and displaying that information to the subject in a format that will facilitate learning to regulate the physiological variable" (Rubow, 1984, p. 207).

Reducing Tone

At times, the goal of biofeedback is to reduce abnormally high muscle tone. For example, Netsell and Cleeland (1973) presented the case of a 64-year-old woman with a 15-year history of parkinsonism who exhibited bilateral lip retraction as the result of bilateral thalamic surgeries 6 years prior to intervention. Her speech was said to be characteristic of parkinsonism with imprecise consonants, reduced loudness, monopitch, and monoloudness.

Intervention involved placement of surface electrodes over the levator labii superioris. The speaker was presented with a tone whose frequency was analogous to the voltages recorded from the electrodes. During each intervention session, she performed both nonspeech tasks involving the lip and four speech tasks that did not involve the upper lip. The subject's task was to concentrate on lowering the audible tone, thus reducing the hypertonicity in the lip. At the end of 2.5 hours of treatment, the authors reported, "the subject was able to modify this [lip] condition in the direction of normalcy" (p. 138). She demonstrated complete control of the lip in nonspeech activities and some instances of normal lip activity while repeating structured phonetic material not requiring lip movement. Spontaneous speech was still characterized by some excessive contraction.

A case in which biofeedback training not only reduced hemifacial spasm but also had a marked effect on speech production has been reported (Rubow, Rosenbek, Collins, & Celesia, 1984). The case was described as a geriatric individual with an 18-year history of hemifacial spasm characterized by paroxysmal bursts of involuntary tonic or clonic activity. Moderately severe dysarthria was felt to be secondary to the spasm. Training involved biofeedback-assisted relaxation of the frontalis muscle. No speech treatment was undertaken. The authors suggested that, when deciding whether to treat speech per se or whether to treat the coexisting abnormal neurologic signs, at least two factors must be considered. Treatment focusing on elimination of the underlying neurologic problems is likely to be successful only if it is obvious, or at least hypothesized, that it is causing all of the speech symptoms and if the neurologic condition is amenable to treatment.

In the cases presented thus far, the biofeedback has focused on reducing tone in specific muscle groups. Finley, Niman, Standley, and Ender (1976) reported the results of a study in which a more general relaxation was sought, using a biofeedback approach in training six patients with athetoid cerebral palsy. Pre- and posttraining measures of speech and motor performance were obtained. Results indicated that the less impaired subjects showed better "acquisition curves" than subjects with more severe impairments. In all but one case, frontalis tension was significantly reduced across sessions. Only the two subjects with the most severe impairments did not improve on the speech measures.

Reduction in tone in specific muscle groups may be accomplished using botulinum toxin injections. Usually, these injections are employed to reduce the abnormal movements and tone associated with certain hyperkinetic dysarthrias. The speech performance of three speakers with dystonia of the orofacial and mandibular muscles has been studied (Schulz & Ludlow, 1991). Following botulinum toxin injections, acoustic analysis of their speech revealed improvements in words and sentence duration and a reduction of abnormal and inappropriate silences during speech.

Muscle tone reduction can also be achieved pharmacologically. A number of antispasticity medications sometimes are useful in decreasing limb spasticity, but their effects on articulation are uncertain (Duffy, 1995; Rosenfield, Viswanath, Herbrick, & Nudelman, 1991).

Optimizing Speaking Rate

As described in detail in Chapter 10, speaking rate has a marked impact on speech intelligibility and articulatory proficiency for some speakers with dysarthria. Darley and colleagues (1975) reported that approximately 13% of their patients with hypokinetic dysarthria demonstrated accelerating speech. Use of delayed auditory feedback, behavioral instruction, and computerized pacing have all been shown to be effective in controlling the speaking rate of some speakers and improving their intelligibility, as well as articulatory proficiency (Adams, 1994; Beukelman, Yorkston, & Tice, 1997; Downie, Low, & Lindsay,

1981; Hanson & Metter, 1983). Speaking rate control has also been shown to improve the intelligibility of speakers with ataxic dysarthria, although similar improvements in performance were not observed in articulatory proficiency (Yorkston, Hammen, Beukelman, & Traynor, 1990).

> *Research Note:* The interaction between the perceived speaking rate and the articulatory performance of speakers with dysarthria has some interesting clinical implications (Ziegler, Hoole, Hartmann, & Von Cramon, 1988). Ziegler and colleagues studied the acoustic dimensions of 12 speakers with dysarthria (following acquired brain injury) who were perceived to exhibit accelerated speech, although they spoke at normal or near-normal rates. The most obvious acoustic finding was that these speakers demonstrated an impaired ability to "reduce the energy of radiated speech sound" during voiceless stop plosives. Specifically, there was either (a) the presence of inappropriate voicing or (b) a continuing friction noise (spirantization) during the closures for voiceless stops, probably because of articulatory undershoot and thus failure to achieve complete lip closure.

Strengthening

In the cases presented thus far, the goal of biofeedback was relaxation or reduction of tone either generally or to specific muscle groups. Biofeedback approaches also have been reported in cases where the clinical goal is strengthening. Some of these studies have involved the facial musculature, but not specifically speech-related activities. For example, Booker, Rubow, and Coleman (1969) described a biofeedback approach to treat left facial nerve damage. They reported beneficial results both cosmetically and functionally. In other cases, improvement in speech gestures was the goal of treatment (Ziegler et al., 1988). The case of a 25-year-old male who had a surgical anastamosis involving the connection of the peripheral portion of Cranial Nerve VII to the central portion of Cranial Nerve XII has also been reported (Daniel & Guitar, 1978). The goal of this program, which took place 5 years after surgery, was symmetry in facial gestures for nonspeech and speech activities. Substantial increases in muscle action potentials over the course of treatment for both nonspeech and speech gestures were reported.

Both biofeedback to the jaw and lips and strengthening exercises have been recommended for individuals with flaccid dysarthria as the result of involvement of Cranial Nerves V, VII, and XII. A series of exercises are available, starting with assistive force as needed to achieve desired movement and advancing to movement against resistance (Linebaugh, 1983). For the jaw, depression and elevation were recommended. Bilabial closure, rounding retraction, and labiodental approximation were recommended for the lips. Interdental protrusion, retraction, apical elevation, and dorsal elevation were recommended for the tongue. These strengthening exercises may be accompanied by electromyographic biofeedback.

> The Iowa Oral Performance Instrument (IOPI) (available from Breakthrough, Inc., Oakdale, Iowa) is a pressure sensing instrument with digital and LED (light-emitting diode) displays. The IOPI measures strength and endurance. Endurance (fatigue) is assessed by measuring the speaker's ability to maintain pressure exertion on the bulb at 50% of his or her maximum strength. Percent pressure is represented by the LED or digital display. The IOPI has been used as a nonspeech strengthening instrument in a number of research projects (Robin, Goel, Somodi, & Luschei, 1992; Robin, Somodi, & Luschei, 1991; Robinovitch, Hershler, & Romilly, 1991; N. P. Solomon, Lorell, Robin, Rodnitzky, & Luschei, 1996; Stierwalt, Robin, Solomon, Weiss, & Max, 1996).

Historically, the question of when to use strengthening exercises has been controversial. This debate will no doubt continue, especially in light of the lack of clinical studies investigating the impact of strengthening exercises on the overall adequacy of articulatory performance. However, we have found a number of simple guidelines useful in making such clinical management decisions. The first question that we ask is obvious: Is weakness a problem? Weakness is by no means universally present in dysarthria. Many neuromotor disorders are characterized by increased tone and by reduced coordination rather than by weakness. If strength is reduced compared with normal levels, then the next question is, Does the weakness interfere with speech function? The presence of weakness does not necessarily imply a speech disability. Speech is a skilled motor task that is much more demanding in terms of movement precision and coordination than strength. In fact, speech requires only 10% to 20% of maximum force of lip movement (Barlow & Abbs, 1983). If weakness is present and it appears to interfere with speech production, then the clinician must ask if there are any contraindications to strengthening exercises. For example, myasthenia gravis is a disorder characterized by progressive weakness following muscular activity; strengthening exercises are obviously contraindicated. In other cases, the natural course of the disorder may make strengthening exercises futile. Such may be the case in degenerative disorders such as amyotrophic lateral sclerosis (ALS). After ruling out cases in which weakness is not a problem or does not interfere with speech and cases in which exercises are contraindicated because of the underlying neuromotor problems or course of the disorder, the clinician is left with a relatively small group of speakers with dysarthria for whom strengthening exercises may be appropriate. These individuals typically exhibit flaccid dysarthria with etiologies including such disorders as peripheral nerve damage and brain stem cerebrovascular accidents.

Rosenbek and LaPoint (1985) cautioned against other abuses of strengthening exercises, including delaying of other intervention approaches until strengthening is "finished," and increasing the strength of certain muscles so they "overwhelm" the efforts of others. Finally, strengthening exercises are an appropriate management approach only for those individuals who are willing to invest the daily time for the repetitive drills necessary for increasing strength.

> *Question: During my practicum assignment, nonspeech exercises were routinely recommended for speakers with dysarthria. The rationale provided was that the exercises improved the motor control and motor strength needed to enhance speech performance. When do you recommend nonspeech exercises for speakers with dysarthria?*
>
> The use of nonspeech activities to improve speech performance has been controversial for many years. Our discussion above has been limited to strengthening activities because, in a limited number of cases where weakness is a problem for clients with stable or improving conditions, such exercises are appropriate. Even so, an attempt should be made to include speech or at least speechlike activities as soon as possible. However, there is little evidence to support the generalization of nonspeech intervention on speech improvements for persons with spastic, hyperkinetic, hypokinetic, or ataxic dysarthria. We strongly recommend that intervention for these individuals involve speech or speechlike movements.

COMPENSATING FOR THE IMPAIRMENT

Many of the traditional approaches to the treatment of individuals with dysarthria have as their goal compensation for a neuromotor impairment that cannot be treated medically or with behavioral approaches such as strengthening exercises. At the center of the compensatory approach to articulation training lies the capability to make adjustments in movement patterns in order to achieve an acceptable speech end-product. Evidence is also accumulating to suggest that speakers with dysarthria were able to modify their articulatory productions in response to certain types of feedback. For example, it has been shown that speakers with dysarthria were able to modify acoustic features such as voice onset time after specific feedback indicated that certain sounds were not being understood (Till & Toye, 1988). Because those changes were made immediately, it is apparent that compensation, rather than a reduction in impairment, was responsible.

Kennedy, Strand, and Yorkston (1994) examined the acoustic changes produced by individuals with reduced speech intelligibility due to progressive dysarthria (ALS and progressive basal ganglia degeneration) when they made verbal repairs in response to perceived communication breakdowns. Longer interword-interval durations were most consistent across speakers when repairing breakdowns and when responding to a verbal model. However, the speakers did not increase the intensity of stress syllables even in response to a model. The most intelligible of the speakers produced the most changes during repairs; the least intelligible speakers made the fewest changes.

Contrastive Production and Intelligibility Drills

A number of training techniques attempt to take advantage of a speaker's ability to modify production depending on the adequacy of the final speech end-product. These approaches do not attempt to train the speaker to change specific movement patterns. Rather, general information about the adequacy of speech is provided. Thus, it is assumed that the speaker will make the necessary changes. A rationale for such an approach is based on the fact that speech, as a motor task, is apparently learned by adjusting the movement patterns based on the success of the perceived output, that is, knowledge of results.

Question: How do principles of motor learning influence the construction and administration training tasks, such as contrastive productions and intelligibility drills?

Chapter 13 contains an extended discussion of how the principles of motor learning can assist the clinican in making practical decisions about treatment tasks for individuals with apraxia of speech. These principles should also be applied in the area of articulatory intervention. Briefly, these include a brief period of prepractice followed by intensive practice. During the prepractice phase, the client is (1) instructed regarding the task, (2) informed of the success criterion (e.g., 80% accuracy) for the practice session, and (3) instructed on one or two important aspects of the movement to be practiced, usually with models provided by the clinician or practice partner.

(continues)

During the practice phase, tasks are distributed such that a variety of different tasks are practiced, thereby avoiding repeated practice on a single word, sound, or movement. During this phase, the client is provided with knowledge of results (e.g., intelligibility) rather than detailed information about performance (specific movement pattern). Depending on the judgment of the clinician, knowledge of results may be provided frequently or infrequently, influenced by the age and motivation requirements of the client. Generally, an effort is made to provide the client with substantial, systematic practice opportunities, as occasional or inconsistent practice is usually not sufficient to develop and refine the motor programs. See McNeil, Robin, and Schmidt (1997) for a more complete discussion of this topic.

De Feo and Shaefer (1983) provided an excellent example of the compensatory adjustments made by an individual with neurologic impairment specific to certain speech components. They presented the case of a young child with Moebius syndrome who was 3 years 8 months old at the time of initial evaluation. Moebius syndrome is characterized by congenital bilateral facial paralysis and abducens palsy. Hypotonicity was noted in the child's cheek and lip musculature; however, sensation of the lip, face, and lingual regions was not impaired. Aside from Cranial Nerve VII, no other cranial nerves appeared to be involved. An articulatory program was developed in which the child was presented with a correct model of the phoneme he misarticulated and was asked to produce a sound to match that model. Without specific instructions to do so, the child quickly adopted a lingual–dental place of articulation for /p/, /b/, /f/, and /m/. Other compensations developed more slowly. For example, contrastive production drills were used to refine the distinction between bilabial and apical stops. Two compensatory strategies were adopted. One was the insertion of a glottal stop between the target plosive and the ensuing vowel. The other was an increase in articulatory force when producing /p/ and /b/ versus /t/ and /d/. In an interesting note, the authors found that they more readily perceived the distinctions if they were not watching the child's face. This impression was confirmed when they compared perceptual judgments of production adequacy made from video–audio presentation with those made from audio presentation only. At the end of 1 year of treatment, listeners, given an audio presentation, judged as correct 89%, 65%, and 46% of the /m/, /p/, and /b/ productions, respectively. When they judged the video–audio presentation, 54%, 44%, and 33% of the productions were judged to be correct for the same phonemes. Thus, the child appeared to be making acoustically acceptable compensations despite the fact that his movement patterns, as perceived visually by the judges who viewed videotapes, remained nonstandard.

In the case just presented, a child with an impairment restricted to the muscles innervated by a single cranial nerve learned to compensate for that deficit and to produce acceptable sounds. We have found a similar approach useful with individuals who exhibit more generalized articulatory impairment. Contrastive production drills are tasks in which two sounds are produced in juxtaposition to one another. The speaker is asked to make these sounds as different as possible. For example, the voiced–voiceless distinction can be practiced with consecutive productions of /bin/ versus /pin/. See Chapter 8 for a more complete description of techniques to aid speakers with dysarthria in making voiced–voiceless consonant distinctions.

Intelligibility drills are slightly different from the contrastive production drills and involve the production of a small set of words similar except for a single phoneme. The sets may include two or more words. See Table 11.3 for examples of such word lists. Each word is printed on a card and the cards are shuffled. Unlike contrastive production tasks, the clinician is naive to the specific sound or word being produced. Thus, instead of making a judgment of "correctness" or "incorrectness," the clinician attempts to identify the utterance being produced.

Intelligibility drills provide a useful framework for treatment of articulation disorders for a number of reasons. First, they do not require specific instructions about how to produce the sound. Rather, they depend on the speaker's ability to compensate for the motor impairment and to find ways to produce a perceptually acceptable sound. In the clinical setting, the clinician rarely has detailed information about movement control and movement patterns of the various

Table 11.3
Examples of Word Lists for Intelligibility Drills

Vowels			Initial Consonants			Final Consonants		
mail	hole	feel	ban	Paul	beer	lab	map	rub
Mel	heal	file	pan	ball	tear	lack	mat	rut
mall	hail	foil	tan	tall	dear	lag	mad	Russ
mule	hall	fowl	Dan	call	gear	lap	Mack	rust
mole	hill	fuel	can	stall	fear	lad	mass	rough
mile	Hal	fill	ran	fall	mere	lass	mash	run
mill	who'll	fall	Stan	mall	near	last	match	rum
meal	hell	fail	span	shall	we're	lash	mast	rush
mull	howl	fool	man	small	cheer	latch	Madge	rug
			fan	hall	shear	laugh	ma'am	runs

articulators that can be provided to the client. Even if such information were available, it is questionable that knowledge of performance makes much difference in clinical practice. For example, the speaker simply may not be able to modify a severely impaired lip movement and, instead, may need to compensate for such impairment by making a complex series of adjustments in the movements of other structures. Tasks such as intelligibility drills allow the speaker to attempt compensation in the presence of perhaps the most important kind of feedback—knowledge of results, that is, whether or not the listener has understood the attempt.

The second feature of intelligibility drills that makes them practical and useful in the clinical setting is that the difficulty of the task can be adjusted easily to meet the needs of the speaker with dysarthria. If a target accuracy of 80% to 90% is the goal, then the clinician can select phonemes and a list length in order to achieve the target accuracy. Intelligibility drills may be used with the most severely involved speaker as the first practice in speaking.

The third clinical advantage of intelligibility drills is that they allow early training in communication breakdown resolution strategies. Because the drill is based on a "quasi-realistic" communication situation, the speaker learns to provide feedback to the listener about the correctness of the listener's perception. Thus, the speaker with dysarthria is active in the breakdown resolution process rather than merely a recipient of the clinician's feedback. When participating in an intelligibility drill, the speaker with dysarthria is required to produce the word, watch for a reaction, indicate to the listener the accuracy of the listener's guess, and repeat the word one time if the listener's guess is incorrect. If the listener erroneously guesses the second production, the speaker must resolve the breakdown in some other way. For example, the speaker with dysarthria might indicate the correct answer on the alphabet board. Thus, as soon as attempts to speak are begun in the treatment session, speakers with dysarthria are practicing the management of their listeners.

Ince and Rosenberg (1973) described a procedure in which two speakers with dysarthria were asked to spontaneously produce one sentence at a time. Following the production, the experimenters gave the speakers general feedback by indicating to the speakers whether the production was "clear" or "unclear." Over a period of 38 sessions, the proportion of intelligible sentences increased from 1.8% to 100% for one speaker and 5% to 100% for the other. It is clear that such studies need to be replicated with careful descriptions of the speakers with dysarthria and perceptual, acoustic, and physiologic documentation of changes in speech production over time.

Improvements in motor performance usually require extensive and regular practice. Although speech–language pathologists are responsible for developing the intervention program and the practice strategies, some of the practice will need to be monitored by practice partners such as parents, attendants, or volunteers. Preliminary efforts to use computer-based speech recognition systems as intelligibility drill "practice partners" for persons with dysarthria have been reported (Jones, 1997).

Prosthetic Compensation

In the previous section, techniques for behaviorally training speakers with dysarthria to compensate for their motor impairment were reviewed. At other times in dysarthria treatment, a prosthetic device can be used to compensate for speech component impairment. Use of a palatal lift to compensate for inadequate velopharyngeal function (described in Chapter 9) is perhaps the most common example of prosthetic management. In the oral articulation system, the jaw may be managed prosthetically via a bite block in those individuals in whom jaw control is disproportionally impaired relative to other structures (Netsell, 1985). A bite block is a small, custom-fitted piece of hard, rubberlike material, which is held between the upper and lower teeth. Its purpose is to maintain a constant jaw position during speech. Barlow and Abbs (1983) described the case of an individual with cerebral palsy with and without a bite block. They recorded simultaneous measures of jaw movement, intraoral air pressure, and raw acoustic signal. Their results indicated that the lip movements are much more regular when the jaw is stabilized.

The final example of prosthetic management of oral articulation is drawn from the large number of techniques designed to control speaking rate. For certain speakers, rate reduction has the effect of increasing the precision of articulatory movements. Prosthetic devices to control speaking rates and improve articulatory precision are described in Chapter 10. These techniques include pacing and alphabet boards in which the user must point to a different location for each word spoken, thus reducing overall speaking rate. Also included among the prosthetic rate control devices is the Delayed Auditory Feedback Unit, worn while speaking to reduce the excessively rapid rates of some speakers with parkinsonism.

PROSODY AND THE SUPRASEGMENTAL ASPECTS OF SPEECH

Thus far, this chapter has focused on intervention to improve the segmental aspects of dysarthric speech, that is, the production of speech sounds. Focus now turns to those aspects of speech production that extend beyond segmental boundaries to include the suprasegmental features of stress patterning, intonation, and rate–rhythm. Clinical researchers have only recently begun to focus on the prosodic aspects of dysarthria. Rosenbek and LaPointe (1985) suggested that it is a mistake to consider prosody the "formal wear" of speech and to attend to it only after all other aspects of treatment have been completed. Some speakers with dysarthria find that efforts to maintain normalized patterns of prosody enhance their speech comprehensibility. By using prosody to signal important words and syntactic junctures, their listeners are provided important information to decode the speaker's messages.

Clinical Note: Jerry is 40 years old and has been diagnosed with ALS for about 7 years. He has essentially no residual movement of his tongue, which is severely atrophied. He has sufficient strength to position his jaw, to speak with adequate intensity for conversational speech, and to speak in sentences of average length. His phonatory quality is only mildly impaired. Because of his severe tongue impairment, the segmental aspects of his speech are severely limited. Despite this limitation, his speech intelligibility is measured at 85%. When questioned about his ability to speak this intelligibly with little tongue movement, he first describes his experiment with "hyperenunciation" in which he attempted to speak such that each sound in a word would be individually enunciated. He reported that the "hyperenunciation" was not effective because it "drove his listeners crazy" and was not very intelligible. Now he focuses on maintaining the prosodic information in his speech signal. He speaks in sentences that are uncomplicated linguistically and maintains appropriate intonational contours for different sentence types. He is careful to signal syntactic junctures with intonational contours and pauses. Given the residual capability of his respiratory and phonatory subsystems, he is successful in this effort.

Numerous authors have documented prosodic aspects of speakers with specific types of dysarthria (Barnes, 1983; Caligiuri & Murry, 1983; Linebaugh & Wolfe, 1984; Murry, 1983; Odell, McNeil, Rosenbek, & Hunter, 1991; Robin, Klouda, & Hug, 1991; Simmons, 1983; Southwood, 1996; Southwood & Weismer, 1993; Yorkston et al., 1990). We believe that attention to prosody is important at all severity levels. For individuals whose speech is difficult to understand, attention to prosodic features that signal stress patterns and syntactic boundaries may improve intelligibility. For those with less severe involvement, attention to prosody may improve the naturalness of speech and thus be important in reducing the handicap.

Terminology

Individuals from such widely differing disciplines as linguistics, poetry analysis, neurology, and speech–language pathology have been interested in the study of speech prosody. Perhaps because of the varying interests of these professionals, terminology associated with prosody may be confusing. Therefore, we begin this section by providing some definitions related to prosody and dysarthria.

PROSODY

The term *prosody* is taken from the Greek and literally means "to add song." Thus, prosody refers, in part, to the melodic aspects of speech that signal linguistic and emotional features. Prosody includes a number of features that extend across a series of sound segments and are usually referred to as suprasegmentals. These include stress patterning, intonation, and rate–rhythm. Despite the rather poetic origin of the term, prosody is now considered a linguistic phenomenon. The prosodic code, although it is much less fully understood than the phonemic code, carries its own meaning. Prosodic features signal syntactic distinctions that indicate to the listener whether an utterance is a statement or a question with a descending or rising pitch at the end of the utterance. Prosody also signals which words in the utterance are the most important with an increase in loudness, increased relative duration, and perhaps a complex pitch contour. Prosodic features are also used to signal syntactic structure, no doubt contributing to a listener's ability to identify the speech sound segments and, therefore, to understand speech. In short, prosody, which is characterized by a series of suprasegmental features, carries unique information and plays an important role in the perception of segmental information.

CORRELATES OF PROSODY

The prosodic features of stress patterning, intonation, and rate–rhythm have perceptual, acoustic, and physiologic correlates. These are listed in Table 11.4.

Stress Patterning

Stress patterning, when measured perceptually, indicates the level of prominence of one syllable or word in an utterance in comparison to the rest of the utterance. Stress patterning can be measured acoustically by analyzing adjustments made in fundamental frequency, intensity, and duration throughout the course of an utterance. The roles of these variables in coding syllable prominence in normal speech are reported elsewhere (Fry, 1955; Lehiste, 1970; Lieberman, 1960, 1967; Morton & Jassem, 1965; O'Shaughnessy, 1979). Gen-

Table 11.4

Correlates of Prosodic Features

| Prosodic Features | Correlates | | |
	Perceptual	Acoustic	Physiologic
Stress patterning	Prominence	Fundamental frequency Intensity Duration	Effort
Intonation	Pitch	Fundamental frequency	Respiration Vocal fold activity
Rate–rhythm	Perceived speaking	Segement duration	Movement rates

erally, syllables that are stressed within an utterance are longer in duration and higher in fundamental frequency and voice intensity than unstressed syllables within the same utterance. However, the relationship between these features and perceived stress is not simple. For example, some prosodic features serve a number of functions in addition to signaling prominence. Fundamental frequency shifts and syllable lengthening may serve as boundary features. In many instances, an unstressed syllable in the final position of a sentence may be of greater duration than stressed syllables occurring elsewhere within the utterance. Physiologically, syllable stress reflects heightened effort compared with other syllables within an utterance. However, it is extremely difficult to measure subtle changes in physiologic effort against a background of speech movement. The physiology of the production of stressed syllables is not well understood in either normal or dysarthric speakers.

Intonation

Intonation "is the perception of changes in fundamental frequency of vocal fold vibration during speech production" (Netsell, 1973, p. 224). Thus, perceptually, intonation is an indicator of changes in pitch; acoustically, it is an indicator of changes in fundamental frequency; and physiologically, it is the result of respiratory and vocal fold action. Each speaker has an average variation in pitch or fundamental frequency. Intonational contours within a breath group signal such features as declarative or interrogative forms. In English, the simple declarative utterance has a rise–fall intonational pattern. According to the breath group theory of intonation (Lieberman, 1967), fundamental frequency is reset to the higher level after each inhalation.

Rate–Rhythm

Netsell (1973) defined rhythm as the "perception of the time program applied to the phonetic events of the speaker" (p. 228). Thus, perceptually, rhythm is a timing pattern; acoustically, it is relative segmental and pause durations; and physiologically, it is an indicator of movement rates and patterns. Netsell further suggested that phrases have the rhythm they do in English because of the "stress-timed" nature of the language. A more detailed discussion of speaking rate and the durational adjustments in normal and dysarthric speech is found in Chapter 13.

Naturalness

Naturalness, as the term is used here, is a perceptually derived, overall description of prosodic adequacy. Speech is natural if it conforms to the listener's standards of rate, rhythm, intonation, and stress patterning, and if it conforms to the syntactic structure of the utterance being produced. It is considered unnatural or bizarre if it deviates from the expected or is unconventional in terms of these prosodic features. Bizarreness is one of the two overall speech dimensions examined in the Mayo Clinic studies (Darley et al., 1975).

Several descriptors have been used to refer to the concept that we term naturalness. They include the dimensions of *bizarreness*, *acceptability*, and *normalcy*. Southwood and Weismer (1993) compared listener judgments of these dimensions in the speech of persons with ALS. They reported that there were strong correlations among the four dimensions, "suggesting that listeners may not perceive them as being different qualities of dysarthric speech" (p. 159). The listeners in their study were able to reliably judge the dimensions. Further, speech intelligibility was strongly related to these dimensions, reflecting the relationship of all of these dimensions to the severity of a speaker's speech disorder.

Clinically, it is important to consider clients' opinions regarding the terminology used to describe them and their performance. We have found that most speakers with dysarthria prefer the word naturalness. Acceptability is a judgmental term, and bizarreness is considered the most offensive of all.

Prosody in Dysarthria

PERCEPTUAL CHARACTERISTICS

Prosodic deficits are common in the speech of individuals with dysarthria. A number of the speech dimensions studied by the Mayo Clinic group relate to prosody (Darley, Aronson, & Brown, 1969a, 1969b). Those that relate to stress patterning, intonation, and rate–rhythm are included in Table 11.5. Prosodic

Table 11.5

Speech Dimensions from the Mayo Study that Relate to Various Aspects of Prosody

Stress Patterning	Intonation	Rate–Rhythm
Monoloudness	Pitch level	Rate
Monopitch	Monopitch	Increased rate in segments
Excessive loudness variation	Short phrases	Increased overall rate
Loudness decay		Variable rate
Alternating loudness		Prolonged intervals
Reduced stress		Inappropriate silences
Excess and equal stress		Short rushes of speech

Note. Adapted from "Differential Diagnostics Patterns of Dysarthria," by F. Darley, A. Aronson, and J. Brown, 1969b, *Journal of Speech and Hearing Research, 12,* 246–269.

disturbances occurred as a characteristic of all the dysarthrias studied by the Mayo Clinic group. For example, the speech dimensions monopitch and monoloudness were ranked among the 10 most deviant speech dimensions for all of the disorders studied and, along with reduced stress, among the five most deviant dimensions in parkinsonism and pseudobulbar palsy. The dimension of excess and equal stress was the second most deviant speech dimension in cerebellar lesions after the dimension of imprecise consonants. The dimensions of prolonged intervals, variable rates, and monopitch were among the five most deviant speech dimensions in chorea. Darley and colleagues (1969b) identified two general types of prosodic disruption: one was the excessiveness seen in cerebellar lesions and the other was the reduced prosody characterized by monopitch and monoloudness in parkinsonism.

ACOUSTIC CHARACTERISTICS

Patterns of dysprosody (distorted prosody) in 5 speakers with ataxia and 7 with apraxia and of aprosody (lack of normal prosody) in 20 speakers with parkinsonism and 3 with right-hemisphere damage have been studied using acoustic analysis techniques (R. D. Kent & Rosenbek, 1982). The dysprosody seen in speakers with ataxia and apraxia was characterized as follows:

1. A "sweeping" pattern—exaggerated sweeping in fundamental frequency accompanied by generally longer syllable durations

2. A "dissociated" pattern—a regularity of intrasyllabic features of duration, fundamental frequency contour, and intensity, with syllables being separated by large but constant intervals

3. A "segregated" pattern—some prosodic cohesion maintained across syllables

Kent and Rosenbek suggested that the similarities found in ataxic dysarthria and apraxia may reflect "compensations made in response to an impairment of speech production" (p. 287). The fused pattern seen in parkinsonism is characterized by a "syllable chain that is flattened or indistinct" (p. 282). Kent and Rosenbek listed the following features of a fused pattern:

1. Small and gradual fundamental frequency variation across syllables
2. Small and gradual intensity variations between syllables
3. Continuous voicing
4. Limited variation in syllable durations
5. Syllable reduction
6. Indistinct syllable boundaries because of faulty consonant articulation
7. Nasalization spread over several consecutive syllables (p. 283)

CONTRIBUTORS TO LACK OF NATURALNESS

Dysarthric speech can be unnatural for a number of reasons that usually involve complex and incompletely understood interactions between prosodic features. These include monotony, syntactic mismatches, and inconsistency across features.

Monotony

Monotony, a frequent contributor to the bizarreness of dysarthric speech, may be the result of an excessively even rhythmic patterning of syllables, an evenness of stress patterning, a minimizing of intonation contours, or a combination of all of these features. In parkinsonism, monotony takes the form of monopitch and monoloudness, or the minimization of prosody in which no syllable stands out as stressed. In ataxic dysarthria, monotony takes the form of excessive and equal patterning; each syllable is produced with such effort that none stands out from the others. Monotony can also be the result of "monopatterning." In one of the cases presented later in this chapter, short and regular breath groups, each with a simple falling intonational contour, lead to the perception of monotony.

Syntactic Mismatches

Dysarthric speech also can be bizarre because the prosodic features do not coincide with the syntactic structure of the utterance. For example, a speaker with dysarthria, who is physiologically limited to a small number of words per breath group, may inhale at syntactically inappropriate locations. Breathing every third or fourth word without regard to the syntactic structure of the utterance not only contributes to the monotony of speech but may also be perceived as unnatural because prosodic and syntactic features no longer overlap. Normal speakers have sufficient respiratory support to breathe only at syntactically appropriate boundaries so that prosodic features reinforce syntactic structures.

Inconsistency Across Features

Dysarthric speech also may be perceived as bizarre if prosodic features are in conflict with one another. For example, stress is signaled in normal speakers by a complex and subtle manipulation of fundamental frequency, duration, and intensity. Although normal speakers send consistent signals, speakers with dysarthria may produce utterances with peak fundamental frequency on one syllable, peak intensity on another, and maximum duration on still another. The net result is perceptually confusing and unnatural.

Assessment and Intervention

OVERALL RATING OF NATURALNESS

In assigning an overall rating of naturalness for a speaker with dysarthria, the first task is to determine how listeners perceive and judge a speaker's naturalness, the measure of functional limitation. Traditionally, naturalness has been rated on a 7-point equal-appearing interval scale ranging from *natural* to *very unnatural* (Darley et al., 1975). This approach is currently in widespread clinical use. Recently, Southwood (1996) has urged the use of magnitude estimation rather than interval scaling strategies for naturalness and bizarreness quantification. As these scaling procedures are clarified and standardized, they undoubtedly will become available for routine clinical use.

Once the speaker's level of naturalness is rated, the important question is whether or not this level of naturalness is of clinical concern. The disability experienced because of naturalness issues usually depends on the social role that an individual wishes to maintain and the extent of the unnaturalness. For example, for a speaker with dysarthria who wishes to maintain or establish a role as a public speaker, such as a lawyer, teacher, priest, or salesperson, a modest level of unnaturalness is of concern. Similarly, a teenager with dysarthria secondary to traumatic brain injury, who feels that she is being disvalued because of her speech, would be quite concerned about a modest level of unnaturalness. In contrast, an older individual living with family members, who were able to understand his messages, probably feels accepted and is not concerned about an extensive degree of unnaturalness. If the level of naturalness demonstrated by a speaker is of clinical concern, then additional questions regarding this dimension should be addressed.

ASSESSMENT OF COMMUNICATIVE FUNCTIONS

As mentioned earlier in this chapter, prosody serves several communicative functions, such as conveying linguistic distinctions (interrogative and neutral sentences), assigning stress (importance), and signaling syntactic structure. The second phase of an assessment should focus on the extent to which a speaker achieves these various functions of prosodic control in conversational speech and on specific assessment tasks. Robin and colleagues (1991) provided several tasks designed to assess prosody. Specifically, tasks are presented to assess a speaker's ability to adjust prosody to signal emotional speech, emphatic stress, and syntactic junctures. These stimuli are presented in Table 11.6. The tasks assess prosody in a single context, whereas the disability-level assessment of naturalness might include a variety of contexts including conversational speech, speech in groups, public speaking, and speech in noise. Obviously, these contexts should be chosen to correspond to the participation patterns of the speaker. Finally, the impact of a speaker's naturalness on his or her listeners can be assessed through interviews or questionnaires.

SPEAKER'S UNDERSTANDING OF THE TASK

The next phase in assessment of the prosodic aspects of dysarthric speech is to confirm the speaker's understanding of the task. Because prosodic patterning is used to signal meaning, clinicians need to confirm the cognitive and language skills of the speaker with dysarthria. This can be done either by reviewing available neuropsychological and language testing results or by confirming the speaker's understanding of the tasks used to sample speech prosody. For example, when assessing stress patterning, an emphatic stressing task is often employed. For normal individuals, the task is cognitively simple. The speaker is asked to read a written sentence aloud, and then to read it in response to questions that are designed to elicit particular stressing patterns. Table 11.7 contains some examples of stimulus and response utterances designed to sample emphatic stress patterning. These particular sentences were selected for ease of acoustic analysis; that is, consecutive phonemes are readily segmentable from the raw acoustic waveforms. After each sentence is recorded, the speaker is asked, "What word did you wish to make the most important in that sentence?" If the speaker does not correctly identify the word that should be targeted for primary stress, the clinician stops there, at least for the moment, and either trains the recognition task or explores the use of other cognitively simpler stress patterning tasks.

HABITUAL AND MAXIMUM BREATH GROUP LENGTH

As described earlier, the breath group theory of intonation suggests that words are grouped into units based on breath groups. The breath group is marked for

Table 11.6
Stimuli Used for Assessment of Prosody

I. Emotion (Happy Sad, Angry, Question, Neutral)
1. The bird flew away.
2. Tomorrow I'm leaving for Chicago.
3. My horse jumped over the fence.
4. We sold our cottage last month.

II. Emphatic Stress
1. <u>Don</u> shot the <u>puck</u> to <u>Kent</u>.
2. <u>Sheila</u> took the <u>money</u> from <u>Chip</u>.
3. <u>Stan</u> paid the <u>check</u> for <u>Peg</u>.
4. The <u>salesman</u> sold the <u>couch</u> to my <u>Father</u>.
5. <u>Mary</u> typed the <u>paper</u> for <u>Kate</u>.
6. <u>Chuck</u> ate <u>supper</u> with <u>George</u>.

III. Syntactic Juncture Sentence Pairs
1a. If Harry went to the bank, Ann will be very angry.
1b. Uncle Harry went to the bank Ann went to yesterday.
2a. If Jerry kicked his mother, we'll be upset.
2b. If Jerry kicked, his mother will be upset.
3a. Roger went to the concert with Chuck, and Laura went with Rob.
3b. Roger went to the concert with Chuck and Laura and Rob.
4a. Ellen called Philip, Bob called Jim, and Sally called Kate.
4b. Ellen called Philip, Bob, and Jim, and Sally called Kate.
5a. If the teacher forgot, Jim will remind him.
5b. If the teacher forgot Jim, we'd remind him.
6a. I went skiing with Jack, and Mike met us there.
6b. I went skiing with Jack and Mike last year.
7a. When John left Cindy, we were upset.
7b. When John left, Cindy was upset.
8a. If Jimmy used the truck, Sharon will be angry.
8b. Cousin Jimmy used the truck Sharon used yesterday.

Note. From "Neurogenic Disorders of Prosody," by D. A. Robin, G. V. Klouda, and L. N. Hug, 1991, in *Treating Disordered Speech Motor Control: For Clinicians by Clinicians* (p. 249), by M. P. Cannito and D. Vogel (Eds.), Austin, TX: PRO-ED. Copyright 1991 by PRO-ED, Inc.

intonation and stress. Because analysis of intonation and stress patterning involves comparison within and not across breath group units, breath groups must be identified. The importance of breath groups can be illustrated by comparing an emphatically stressed sentence produced by a normal speaker with one produced by a speaker with dysarthria. Figure 11.2 contains a fundamental frequency and intensity × time plot of the sentence "Show SAM some snow" as produced by a normal speaker. Note that the fundamental frequency contour is represented

Table 11.7
Examples of Questions and Expected Responses for Sampling Emphatic Stress Patterning

Stimulus	Response
To whom should I show the snow?	Show SAM some snow.
Should I show Sam all the snow?	Show Sam SOME snow.
What should I show Sam?	Show Sam some SNOW.
What should I do with the applesauce?	SAVE some applesauce.
Should I save all of the applesauce?	Save SOME applesauce.
Should I save the applebread?	Save some appleSAUCE.

by the dashed line. A line of declination has been drawn from the peak fundamental frequency of the first syllable of this declarative sentence to the peak fundamental frequency of the final syllable. Note the generally falling fundamental frequency pattern, except for the word that receives the primary stress. Cooper and Sorenson (1981) suggested that there is a generally falling fundamental frequency pattern within a breath group unit in declarative sentences. Fundamental frequency is reset, after a breath group, to the higher level. In nor-

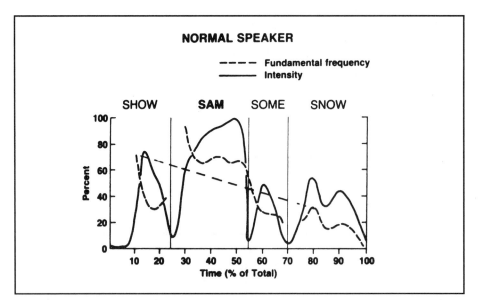

Figure 11.2. A fundamental frequency and intensity × time tracing for a normal speaker producing the emphatically stressed sentence "Show SAM some snow." A line of declination is drawn from the fundamental frequency peak of the first syllable to the peak of the final syllable.

mal speakers, stressed syllables consistently fall above this line of declination for emphatically stressed utterances such as those in Figure 11.2. Thus, the fundamental frequency of the stressed syllable may not be the highest in the sentence, but it tends to be higher than the line of declination. The fundamental frequency contour characterized by this "high-to-low-then-reset" pattern is based on the breath group unit.

Many speakers with severe dysarthria produce breath groups that are extremely restricted in length. In fact, some speakers with the most severe dysarthria produce only one or two words per breath. Other speakers, although they appear to have the physiologic potential of producing longer breath groups, treat each word as if it were a breath group. This is the case for the speaker with ataxic dysarthria whose sentence production is illustrated in Figure 11.3. Note that there is a generally falling fundamental frequency pattern for each syllable, and the fundamental frequency is reset at the beginning of each syllable. This case appears to be an example of the "dissociated" prosodic pattern (R. D. Kent & Rosenbek, 1982). Because this speaker had the underlying motor control to produce much longer breath groups, a treatment program was developed to encourage him to extend his breath group, and thus to make the entire sentence an intonational unit.

Other speakers exhibit such poor physiologic support that they can produce only a syllable or two per breath group. With these speakers, a different approach to assessment is appropriate. Stimulus material should be shortened so that the utterances are within the speaker's breath group capacity. At the same time, the clinician may wish to work on the underlying respiratory–phonatory control in order for the speaker to produce longer breath group units. To summarize briefly, the breath group may be considered the unit of prosody. Therefore, the breath groups that speakers are producing, or are able to produce, must be identified in order to adequately understand prosodic patterning.

PERCEPTUAL ASSESSMENT OF ACCURACY AND NATURALNESS

Once the speaker's cognitive understanding of the task has been established and materials appropriate for the speaker's breath group have been selected, then the "successfulness" of prosodic patterning can be assessed. When assessing stress patterning, the term *targeted stress* refers to the syllable on which the speaker intends to place primary stress, and the term *perceived stress* refers to the syllable that the listener judges to be the most prominent. The distinction is an important one clinically. If the speaker is not successful in achieving stress on the targeted syllable, then the first treatment task must be to increase the ability to signal stress.

Failure to signal locus of stress accurately may be the result of two types of errors. The first error is to send the listener no signals. In this case, speakers are

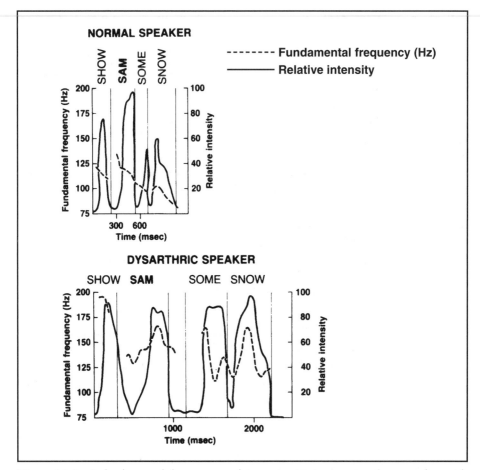

Figure 11.3. A fundamental frequency and intensity × time tracing for a speaker with ataxic dysarthria producing the emphatically stressed sentence "Show SAM some snow." Also included for comparison is an acoustic analysis of the production of a normal speaker.

not signaling prominence with any of the suprasegmental features—intensity, duration, or fundamental frequency. Such is the case in the sample of the speaker with dysarthria presented in Figure 11.3. Note that none of the acoustic features gives a clear indication of prominence.

The second error that frequently results in a failure to signal locus of stress is the sending of misleading acoustic signals. Such is typically the case in speakers with ataxia. Figure 11.4 contains the acoustic information from such a "confusing" sample. Note that duration is longest on the word "Sam," relative intensity is greatest on the word "snow," and fundamental frequency is highest on the word "show." In effect, the listener is forced to choose among a number of con-

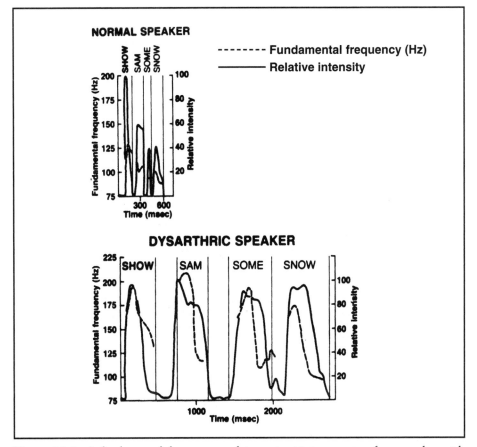

Figure 11.4. A fundamental frequency and intensity × time tracing for a speaker with ataxic dysarthria producing the emphatically stressed sentence "SHOW Sam some snow." Perceptual judgments indicate that listeners usually perceive stress on the final syllable of the utterance rather than on the target syllable.

flicting signals. Although most judges indicate that primary stress is on the syllable "snow," agreement is not unanimous.

If the speaker is able to accurately signal stress on the targeted word or syllable, the clinician next considers questions related to the naturalness of the production. A speaker may successfully signal stress at the appropriate locus yet his or her speech may be perceived to be highly unnatural. Figure 11.5 contains acoustic information from a production in which the speaker with ataxic dysarthria understood the task and was able to produce the entire utterance in one breath group, and where judges unanimously agreed about the locus of stress. However, all judges rated these productions to be highly unnatural. The goal in

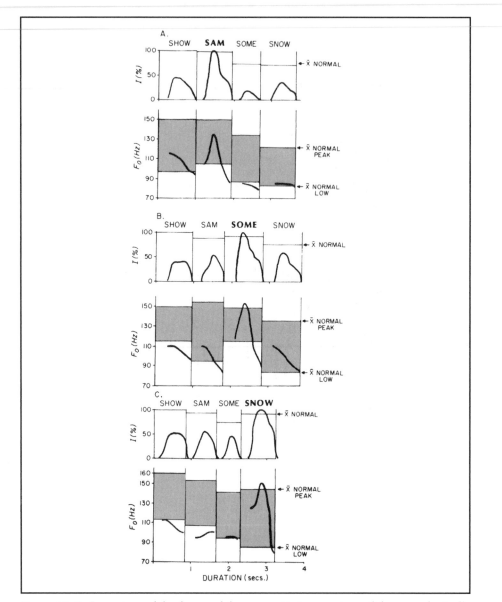

Figure 11.5. Intensity and fundamental frequency × time tracings of three emphatically stressed sentences produced by a speaker with ataxic dysarthria. Stress patterning on these sentences was judged to be accurate but highly unnatural. From "Assessment of Stress Patterning," by K. M. Yorkston, D. R. Beukelman, F. Minifie, and S. Sapir, 1984, in *The Dysarthrias: Physiology, Acoustics, Perception, Management* (pp. 131–162), by M. McNeil, J. Rosenbek, and A. Aronson (Eds.), San Diego: Singular. Copyright 1984 by Singular Publishing Group. Reprinted with permission.

training is to maximize both the naturalness and the accuracy of the prosodic pattern.

ACOUSTIC ANALYSIS OF HABITUAL PROSODIC PATTERNING

Although naturalness is a perceptually derived phenomenon, perceptual measures of naturalness may be supplemented with acoustic information. Instrumentation is becoming available in more and more clinical settings. This instrumentation allows the clinician to display fundamental frequency and intensity × time contours on an oscilloscopic screen or on a computer monitor. If perceptual judgments indicate how successful the speaker has been in signaling stress, then acoustic analysis gives some insights into how speakers are achieving the perceptual results. Fundamental frequency and intensity contours indicate what suprasegmental features or strategies are being used to signal stress. Information about suprasegmental features often helps to explain the perceived lack of naturalness.

ANALYSIS OF MODIFIED PROSODIC PATTERNING

The next step in intervention is to ask the speaker with dysarthria to modify his or her production. For example, if the speaker were using exaggerated shifts in fundamental frequency and intensity to signal stress, the instructions might be to use only durational adjustments (prolongations of the stressed syllable or pauses) to signal stress. Perceptual assessment techniques are used to indicate whether or not the speaker was achieving stress on the targeted syllable and whether or not the new strategies produced a more natural-sounding result. Acoustic analysis is used to document the features that have been changed. Thus, the sequence of training usually involves the following steps: First, the speaker is asked to modify his or her production in an effort to signal targeted stress. Initially, specific instructions are not provided regarding which parameter to change. By experience, we have realized that such instructions can yield attempts that are quite unnatural. Then, the features associated with the most natural productions are identified and the speaker is trained to consistently use those features.

In this sequence of training, a "normal" model is rarely used because suprasegmental features used by normal speakers are complex and subtle, and require a high level of motor control. Normal performance simply may not be possible for the speaker with dysarthria. Rather than normalcy, the goal is "the best possible speech," given the individual's motor control deficits. Again, as in many other treatment approaches in dysarthria, the speaker is asked to compensate for deficits rather than to produce normal speech. The following are some examples of modifications or compensatory adjustments we have asked speakers with dysarthria to make in an effort to maximize the naturalness of their speech.

For individuals with insufficient prosodic patterns, general instructions such as "make the target word stronger," "emphasize the target word," and "use extra force on the target word" may have the desired consequence of bringing into play one or more of the suprasegmental features that signal stress to the listener. For those individuals with prosodic excess, treatment may involve reducing the number of suprasegmental features that signal stress. Speakers with ataxic dysarthria are encouraged to use durational adjustments as their primary means of signaling stress. Speakers learn to prolong stressed syllables and insert pausing at appropriate locations. Instructions to signal stress using only durational adjustments have a number of benefits. First, the control and coordination to simultaneously modify three suprasegmental features is often well beyond the capabilities of speakers with more severe ataxia. Reducing the task to a single stressing feature has the effect of simplifying the speaking task. Syllable prolongation is an adjustment that is usually within the capability of the speakers. Second, exaggerated durational adjustments tend to be perceived as less bizarre than exaggerations of either intensity or fundamental frequency. We have found that fundamental frequency and intensity adjustments do not disappear when individuals with ataxia are given the instructions not to use them as stress signalers. Rather, both contours may become more natural as they are deemphasized.

COMPARISONS ACROSS BREATH GROUPS

Thus far, prosody has been perceptually and acoustically assessed within the breath group unit. The final phase of assessment involves identifying abnormalities of prosodic patterning across breath groups. Monotony is a feature that often reduces the speech naturalness of those individuals with dysarthria whose speech is intelligible but not normal. Monopitch and monoloudness both rank among the 10 most deviant dimensions in all of the seven diagnostic groups in the Mayo Clinic study (Darley et al., 1975). Both of these features rank within the five most deviant speech dimensions in parkinsonism and pseudobulbar palsy.

Recent studies have suggested that the perception of monotony may be more complex than simply reduced ranges of fundamental frequency and relative intensity. J. R. Solomon, Ludolph, and Thomson (1984) acoustically analyzed the fundamental frequency of speech samples of individuals who were judged to exhibit monopitch using the perceptual methods of Darley and colleagues (1975). Solomon and colleagues found that the range of fundamental frequency excursion was not reduced as compared to normal. This suggests that other factors contributed to the perception of monopitch.

In addition to being a phenomenon that occurs within a breath group, the perception of monotony may be the result of excessive uniformity across breath group units. For normal speakers, the breath group unit is regulated to a large extent by the syntactic demands of the utterance being produced. In Chapter 7, data were presented that illustrated the variability of breath group length as normal individuals read a passage. Although the average number of words per breath group was just less than 10 words, these speakers frequently produced breath groups of only 4 words. At other times they spoke nearly 20 words before taking a breath. These data suggest that normal individuals vary their breath group durations depending on the material they are reading. Further, their breath group duration is not restricted by the limits of their physiologic support. Speakers with dysarthria are quite different.

Bellaire, Yorkston, and Beukelman (1986) presented the case of a 20-year-old male who had suffered a closed head injury in a motor vehicle accident. His speech was intelligible at a speaking rate of 90 words per minute (wpm), but was judged to be quite monotonous. He was able to signal stress within breath groups accurately and without exaggerating any of the suprasegmental features of fundamental frequency, relative intensity, or duration. However, when prosodic patterning across breath groups was analyzed, an explanation of the monotony was found. The speaker produced breath groups that were both shorter and more regular than normal, inhaled during nearly every pause in the paragraph production, and demonstrated a restricted fundamental frequency range. Because the speaker appeared to have the physiologic support to produce more extended breath groups, a training program was undertaken in which he was asked to increase the number of words per breath and to increase the frequency of pauses without inhalation. Data obtained at the end of treatment suggested he had learned to do what was asked of him. Mean words per breath group increased from 5.1 to 9.8, and his speech was judged to be more natural. Figure 11.6 contains fundamental frequency × time tracings for a portion of a paragraph read pre- and posttreatment. Note that in the posttreatment sample, breath group lengths were extended and fundamental frequency excursions were greater than in the pretreatment tracings. This case illustrates the point that the perception of monotony may arise from a number of sources. It may be the result of monoloudness and monopitch within a breath group, or it may be the result of monopatterning across breath groups. Breath groups of equal length add to the perception of monopitch because of the repetitive fundamental frequency pattern that they create.

GENERALIZATION TO SPONTANEOUS SPEECH

The final phase of intervention for individuals with prosodic disruption involves generalization of the strategies learned during highly structured tasks to spontaneous speech. This may be accomplished using a series of steps in which feedback provided to the speaker is gradually faded and practice materials are made more complex. An intermediate step between reading of sentence and paragraph

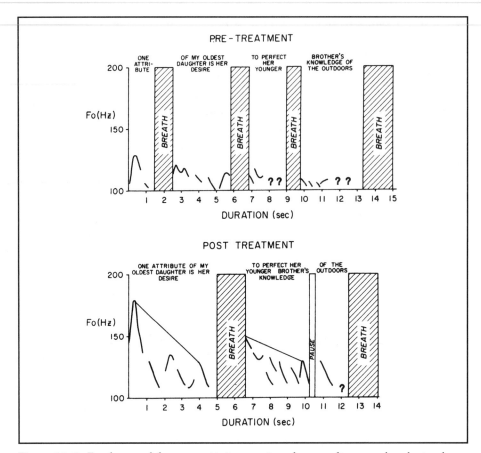

Figure 11.6. Fundamental frequency × time tracings from reading samples obtained pre- and posttreatment from "Modification of Breath Patterning to Increase Naturalness of a Mildly Dysarthric Speaker," by K. Bellaire, K. M. Yorkston, and D. R. Beukelman, 1986, *Journal of Communication Disorders, 19,* p. 277. Copyright 1986 by Elsevier Science Publishing Co. Reprinted with permission.

material and spontaneous speech is the creation of short dialogues or scripts of conversations between the individual with dysarthria and the clinician. During the generalization phase, speakers are also taught to critique their own productions. Initially, they may learn to judge the adequacy of their performance as they review an audio- or videotape. Later, they are encouraged to monitor speech in an ongoing fashion (Bellaire et al., 1986).

INDIRECT TREATMENT OF NATURALNESS

Because naturalness is an overall measure of speech performance, a clinician should expect that a variety of direct and indirect intervention procedures might impact it positively or negatively. For example, in Chapter 10 the impact of specific rate reduction intervention on naturalness was highlighted. Depending on the speaker, this impact is variable. For some speakers, the use of rigid rate control techniques, such as pacing boards and supplemented speech, causes speech to be less natural. However, for those with somewhat unnatural speech prior to a rate control intervention, speaking rate reduction minimally impacts speech naturalness (Yorkston et al., 1990). Undoubtedly, the Lee Silverman Voice Treatment program (Ramig, Pawlas, & Countryman, 1995) described in Chapter 10, in which persons with Parkinson's disease are instructed to speak with increased effort and therefore with increased loudness, has an impact on speech naturalness. Indirectly, one would expect that such an intervention would be associated with improved naturalness as well.

Because a variety of interventions can indirectly impact speech naturalness, it is necessary to monitor the multidimensional influences of intervention strategies employed with speakers with dysarthria. At times, decreases in speech naturalness must be tolerated in order to achieve other intervention goals, such as increased speech intelligibility and reduction in speaker fatigue. However, when possible, care should be taken to minimize the negative impact on speech naturalness when focusing on other treatment goals.

REFERENCES

Adams, S. G. (1994). Accelerating speech in a case of hypokinetic dysarthria: Descriptions and treatment. In J. A. Till, K. M. Yorkston, & D. R. Beukelman (Eds.), *Motor speech disorders: Advances in assessment and treatment* (pp. 213–228). Baltimore: Brookes.

Barlow, A., & Abbs, J. (1983). Force transducers for the evaluation of labial, lingual, and mandibular motor impairments. *Journal of Speech and Hearing Disorders, 26,* 616–621.

Barnes, G. (1983). Suprasegmental and prosodic considerations in motor speech disorders. In W. R. Berry (Ed.), *Clinical dysarthria* (pp. 57–68). Austin, TX: PRO-ED.

Bellaire, K., Yorkston, K. M., & Beukelman, D. R. (1986). Modification of breath patterning to increase naturalness of a mildly dysarthric speaker. *Journal of Communication Disorders, 19,* 271–280.

Beukelman, D. R., Yorkston, K. M., & Tice, R. (1997). *Pacer/tally rate measurement software.* Lincoln, NE: Tice Technology Services.

Booker, H. E., Rubow, R. T., & Coleman, P. J. (1969). Simplified feedback in neuromuscular retraining: An automated approach using electromyographic signals. *Archives of Physical Medicine and Rehabilitation, 50,* 621–625.

Caligiuri, M. P., & Murry, T. (1983). The use of visual feedback to enhance prosodic control in dysarthria. In W. Berry (Ed.), *Clinical dysarthria* (pp. 267–282). Austin, TX: PRO-ED.

Cooper, W. E., & Sorenson, L. (1981). *Fundamental frequency in sentence production.* New York: Springer-Verlag.

Daniel, R., & Guitar, B. (1978). EMG feedback and recovery of facial and speech gestures following neural anastomosis. *Journal of Speech and Hearing Disorders, 43,* 9–20.

Darley, F., Aronson, A., & Brown, J. (1969a). Clusters of deviant speech dimensions in the dysarthrias. *Journal of Speech and Hearing Research, 12,* 462–496.

Darley, F., Aronson, A., & Brown, J. (1969b). Differential diagnostics patterns of dysarthria. *Journal of Speech and Hearing Research, 12,* 246–269.

Darley, F. L., Aronson, A. E., & Brown, J. R. (1975). *Motor speech disorders.* Philadelphia: Saunders.

DeFeo, A. B., & Schaefer, C. M. (1983). Bilateral facial paralysis in a preschool child: Oral-facial and articulatory characteristics—A case study. In W. Berry (Ed.), *Clinical dysarthria* (pp. 165–190). Austin, TX: PRO-ED.

Downie, A. W., Low, J. M., & Lindsay, D. D. (1981). Speech disorders in parkinsonism: Usefulness of delayed auditory feedback in selected cases. *British Journal of Disorders of Communication, 16,* 135–139.

Duffy, J. R. (1995). *Motor speech disorders: Substrates, differential diagnosis, and management.* St. Louis: Mosby.

Finley, W. W., Niman, C., Standley, J., & Ender, P. (1976). Frontal EMG biofeedback training of athetoid cerebral palsy patients: Report of six cases. *Biofeedback Self Regulation, 1,* 169–182.

Fisher, H. B., & Logemann, J. A. (1971). *The Fisher–Logemann Test of Articulation Competence.* Boston: Houghton Mifflin.

Fry, D. (1955). Duration and intensity as physical correlates of linguistic stress. *Journal of the Acoustical Society of America, 27,* 765–768.

Hanson, W., & Metter, E. (1983). DAF speech rate modification in Parkinson's disease: A report of two cases. In W. Berry (Ed.), *Clinical dysarthria* (pp. 231–254). Austin, TX: PRO-ED.

Hardy, J. (1967). Suggestions for physiologic research in dysarthria. *Cortex, 3,* 128.

Ince, L. P., & Rosenberg, D. N. (1973). Modification of articulation in dysarthria. *Archives of Physical Medicine and Rehabilitation, 54,* 233–236.

Johns, D. F., & Darley, F. L. (1970). Phonemic variability in apraxia of speech. *Journal of Speech and Hearing Research, 13,* 556–583.

Jones, R. (1997). *Speech recognition as a practice tool for speakers with severe dysarthria due to traumatic brain injury.* Lincoln: University of Nebraska, Lincoln.

Kennedy, M. R. T., Strand, E. A., & Yorkston, K. M. (1994). Selected acoustic changes in the verbal repairs of dysarthric speakers. *Journal of Medical Speech–Language Pathology, 2,* 263–280.

Kent, J. F., Kent, R. D., Rosenbek, J. C., Weismer, G., Martin, R., Sufit, R., & Brooks, B. R. (1992). Quantitative description of the dysarthria in women with amyotrophic lateral sclerosis. *Journal of Speech and Hearing Research, 35,* 723–733.

Kent, R. D., Kent, J. F., Weismer, G., & Martin, R. E. (1989). Relationship between speech intelligibility and the slope of second-formant transitions in dysarthric subjects. *Clinical Linguistics and Phonetics, 3,* 347–358.

Kent, R. D., Kent, J. F., Weismer, G., Sufit, R. L., Rosenbek, J. C., Martin, R. E., & Brooks, B. R. (1990). Impairment of speech intelligibility in men with amyotrophic lateral sclerosis. *Journal of Speech and Hearing Disorders, 55,* 721–728.

Kent, R. D., & Rosenbek, J. C. (1982). Prosodic disturbance and neurologic lesion. *Brain and Language, 15,* 259–291.

Kent, R. D., Sufit, R. L., Rosenbek, J. C., Kent, J. F., Weismer, G., Martin, R. E., & Brooks, B. R. (1991). Speech deterioration in amyotrophic lateral sclerosis: A case study. *Journal of Speech and Hearing Research, 34,* 1269–1275.

Kent, R. D., Weismer, G., Kent, J. F., & Rosenbek, J. C. (1989). Toward phonetic intelligibility testing in dysarthria. *Journal of Speech and Hearing Disorders, 54,* 482–499.

Lehiste, I. P. (1970). *Suprasegmentals*. Cambridge, MA: MIT Press.

Lieberman, P. (1960). Some acoustic correlates of word stress in American English. *Journal of the Acoustical Society of America, 32*, 451–454.

Lieberman, P. (1967). *Intonation, perception and language*. Cambridge, MA: MIT Press.

Linebaugh, C. (1983). Treatment of flaccid dysarthria. In W. H. Perkins (Ed.), *Dysarthria and apraxia* (pp. 59–67). New York: Thieme-Stratton.

Linebaugh, C. W., & Wolfe, V. E. (1984). Relationships between articulation rate, intelligibility, and naturalness in spastic and ataxic speakers. In M. McNeil, J. Rosenbek, & A. Aronson (Eds.), *The dysarthrias: Physiology, acoustics, perception, management* (pp. 197–206). San Diego: Singular.

McNeil, M. R., Robin, D. A., & Schmidt, R. A. (1997). Apraxia of speech: Definition, differentiation, and treatment. In M. R. McNeil (Ed.), *Clinical management of sensorimotor speech disorders* (pp. 311–344). New York: Thieme.

Morton, J., & Jassem, W. (1965). Acoustic correlates of stress. *Language and Speech, 8*, 159–181.

Murry, T. (1983). The production of stress in three types of dysarthric speech. In W. Berry (Ed.), *Clinical dysarthria* (pp. 69–84). Austin, TX: PRO-ED.

Netsell, R. (1973). Speech physiology. In F. Minifie, T. Hixon, & F. Williams (Eds.), *Normal aspects of speech, hearing and language* (pp. 211–234). Englewood Cliffs, NJ: Prentice-Hall.

Netsell, R. (1985). Construction and use of a bite-block for use in evaluation and treatment of speech disorders. *Journal of Speech and Hearing Disorders, 50*, 103–106.

Netsell, R., & Cleeland, C. (1973). Modification of lip hypotonia in dysarthria using EMG feedback. *Journal of Speech and Hearing Disorders, 38*, 131–140.

Odell, K., McNeil, M. R., Rosenbek, J. C., & Hunter, L. (1991). Perceptual characteristics of vowel and prosody productions in apraxic, aphasic, and dysarthric speakers. *Journal of Speech and Hearing Research, 34*, 60–66.

O'Shaughnessy, D. (1979). Linguistic features in fundamental frequency patterns. *Journal of Phonetics, 7*, 119–145.

Platt, L., Andrews, G., Young, M., & Quinn, P. T. (1980). Dysarthria of adult cerebral palsy: I. Intelligibility and articulatory impairment. *Journal of Speech and Hearing Disorders, 23*, 28–40.

Ramig, L. O., Pawlas, A. A., & Countryman, S. (1995). *The Lee Silverman Voice Treatment*. Iowa City, IA: National Center for Voice and Speech.

Robin, D. A., Goel, A., Somodi, L., & Luschei, E. S. (1992). Tongue strength and endurance: Relation to highly skilled movements. *Journal of Speech and Hearing Research, 35*, 1239–1245.

Robin, D. A., Klouda, G. V., & Hug, L. N. (1991). Neurogenic disorders of prosody. In M. P. Cannito & D. Vogel (Eds.), *Treating disordered speech motor control: For clinicians by clinicians* (pp. 241–271). Austin, TX: PRO-ED.

Robin, D. A., Somodi, L. B., & Luschei, E. S. (1991). Measurement of tongue strength and endurance in normal and articulation disordered subjects. In C. A. Moore, K. M. Yorkston, & D. R. Beukelman (Eds.), *Dysarthria and apraxia of speech: Perspectives on management* (pp. 173–184). Baltimore: Brookes.

Robinovitch, S. N., Hershler, C., & Romilly, D. P. (1991). A tongue force measurement system for the assessment of oral-phase swallowing disorders. *Archives of Physical Medicine and Rehabilitation, 72*, 38–42.

Rosenbek, J. (1984). Treating the dysarthric talker. *Seminars in Speech and Language, 5*, 359–384.

Rosenbek, J. C., & LaPointe, L. L. (1985). The dysarthrias: Description, diagnosis, and treatment. In D. Johns (Ed.), *Clinical management of neurogenic communication disorders* (pp. 97–152). Boston: Little, Brown.

Rosenfield, D., Viswanath, N., Herbrick, K., & Nudelman, H. (1991). Evaluation of the speech motor control system in amyotrophic lateral sclerosis. *Journal of Voice, 5,* 224–230.

Rubow, R. (1984). Role of feedback, reinforcement, and compliance on training and transfer in biofeedback-based rehabilitation of motor speech disorders. In M. McNeil, J. Rosenbek, & A. Aronson (Eds.), *The dysarthrias: Physiology, acoustics, perception, management* (pp. 207–230). San Diego: Singular.

Rubow, R. T., Rosenbek, J. C., Collins, M. J., & Celesia, G. G. (1984). Reduction of hemifacial spasm and dysarthria following EMG biofeedback. *Journal of Speech and Hearing Disorders, 49,* 26–33.

Schulz, G. M., & Ludlow, C. L. (1991). Botulinum treatment for orolingual-mandibular dystonia: Speech effects. In C. A. Moore, K. M. Yorkston, & D. R. Beukelman (Eds.), *Dysarthria and apraxia of speech: Perspectives on management* (pp. 227–242). Baltimore: Brookes.

Simmons, N. (1983). Acoustic analysis of ataxic dysarthria: An approach to monitoring treatment. In W. Berry (Ed.), *Clinical dysarthria* (pp. 283–294). Austin, TX: PRO-ED.

Solomon, J. R., Ludolph, L. B., & Thomson, F. E. (1984, February). *How "mono" is monopitch: An acoustic analysis of motor speech disorders tapes.* Paper presented at the Biennial Clinical Dysarthria Conference, Tucson, AZ.

Solomon, N. P., Lorell, D. M., Robin, D. A., Rodnitzky, R. L., & Luschei, E. S. (1996). Tongue strength and endurance in mild to moderate Parkinson's disease. In D. A. Robin, K. M. Yorkston, & D. R. Beukelman (Eds.), *Disorders of motor speech: Assessment, treatment and clinical characterization* (pp. 259–274). Baltimore: Brookes.

Southwood, M. H. (1996). Direct magnitude estimation and interval scaling of naturalness and bizarreness of the dysarthria associated with amyotrophic lateral sclerosis. *Journal of Medical Speech–Language Pathology, 4*(1), 13–27.

Southwood, M. H., & Weismer, G. (1993). Listener judgments of the biazarreness, acceptability, naturalness, and normalcy of the dysarthria associated with amyotrophic lateral sclerosis. *Journal of Medical Speech–Language Pathology, 1*(3), 151–161.

Stierwalt, J. A. G., Robin, D. A., Solomon, N. P., Weiss, A. L., & Max, J. E. (1996). Tongue strength and endurance: Relation to the speaking ability of children and adolescents following traumatic brain injury. In D. A. Robin, K. M. Yorkston, & D. R. Beukelman (Eds.), *Disorders of motor speech: Assessment, treatment and clinical characterization* (pp. 241–258). Baltimore: Brookes.

Till, J. A., & Toye, A. R. (1988). Acoustic phonetic effects of two types of verbal feedback in dysarthric subjects. *Journal of Speech and Hearing Disorders, 53,* 449–458.

Yorkston, K. M. (1989). Facial anastamosis in a dysarthric speaker. In N. Helm-Estabrooks & J. L. Aten (Eds.), *Difficult diagnoses in adult communication disorders* (pp. 163–172). Boston: College-Hill.

Yorkston, K. M., Beukelman, D. R., Minifie, F., & Sapir, S. (1984). Assessment of stress patterning. In M. McNeil, J. Rosenbek, & A. Aronson (Eds.), *The dysarthrias: Physiology, acoustics, perception, management* (pp. 131–162). San Diego: Singular.

Yorkston, K. M., Beukelman, D. R., & Tice, R. (1998). *Phoneme identification task: A computer program.* Lincoln, NE: Tice Technology Services.

Yorkston, K. M., Hammen, V. L., Beukelman, D. R., & Traynor, C. D. (1990). The effect of rate control on the intelligibility and naturalness of dysarthric speech. *Journal of Speech and Hearing Disorders, 55,* 550–561.

Ziegler, W., Hoole, P., Hartmann, E., & Von Cramon, D. (1988). Accelerated speech in dysarthria after acquired brain injury: Acoustic correlates. *British Journal of Communications Disorders, 23,* 215–228.

OPTIMIZING COMMUNICATIVE EFFECTIVENESS: BRINGING IT TOGETHER

with Katherine C. Hustad

Webster's New World Dictionary has a number of definitions of the word *effective*: (1) producing a result; (2) efficient, (3) in effect; operative; active; (4) actual, not merely potential or theoretical; and (5) making a striking impression (Guralnik, 1982). In some respects, all of these definitions are appropriate when describing an "effective" communicator. That individual produces a result and is active and efficient in getting the message across. This activity is not simply possible in the clinical setting, but actually occurs in real-world social contexts. Finally, the effective communicator is impressive because he or she controls, influences, and directs the environment. The goal of optimizing communicative effectiveness is not a small one. This chapter presents some broad strategies for helping speakers with dysarthria to become effective communicators. These strategies often cross several levels of chronic disease. Out of convenience, many of the previous chapters in this text have focused on particular speech subsystems or aspects of speech performance. In this chapter, we attempt to bring together the various threads of the intervention process and to add a more complete discussion of techniques for optimizing effectiveness in natural communication settings at the levels of disability and social limitation.

A MODEL FOR OPTIMIZING COMMUNICATIVE EFFECTIVENESS

In Chapter 1, we provided a perspective that views dysarthria as a chronic disorder. In this chapter, we return to this model. Table 12.1 reiterates the definition of dysarthria at various levels from the impairment through societal limitation. The table also summarizes the general goals of intervention and provides specific examples of treatment tasks at each level. At the impairment level, the general goal of intervention is to reduce the neuromotor problem. Impairments may occur in any or all of the speech subsystems. Chapters 7, 8, and 9 contain detailed discussions of intervention for respiratory, laryngeal, and velopharyngeal speech subsystems. For example, strengthening exercises for the respiratory musculature of speakers with flaccid dysarthria associated with brain stem stroke focus on the level of the impairment. In another example, proper positioning of a child with cerebral palsy may have the effect of decreasing abnormal muscle tone and, thus, reduce the impairment.

At the level of the functional limitation, intervention focuses on the development of compensatory strategies and/or use of prostheses to optimize speech performance. Examples of the use of compensatory strategies can be found throughout this text. In Chapter 10, the use of rate control techniques is discussed. At times, these techniques involve teaching the speaker techniques to slow speech and, at other times, they involve prosthetic devices such as pacing boards and delayed auditory feedback units. Compensatory techniques may also involve specific speech subsystems. In Chapter 7, techniques were discussed for modifying the speech breathing patterns of individuals with dysarthria. The primary purpose of these techniques is not to reduce the impairment, but rather to change the speech style in an effort to compensate for the impairment. For example, a speaker with poor respiratory support may be taught to initiate speech at slightly higher than "normal" lung volume levels in order to achieve an adequate level of subglottal pressure for speech. In another example of respiratory compensation, speakers with poor respiratory support may need to accommodate by shortening the number of words per breath.

At the level of disability, the goal of intervention is to optimize communication in natural settings. In this chapter, a variety of approaches designed to reduce the disability will be presented. These techniques do not focus on the speech signal but rather on "signal-independent information," such as linguistic and environmental cues and other strategies to enhance communicative interaction. Finally, at the level of the societal limitation, treatment focuses on providing opportunities for communication and eliminating barriers to the performance of selected communicative roles. This approach to treatment also is reviewed in this chapter.

Table 12.1

Optimizing Communicative Effectiveness in Speakers with Dysarthria

	Description	General Goals of Intervention	Examples of Specific Techniques
Impairment	Slow, weak, imprecise, and/or uncoordinated movements of the speech musculature	Reduction in the neuro-motor problem in the respiratory, laryngeal, velopharyngeal, and oral articulatory musculature	• Strengthening weak respiratory muscles in flaccid dysarthria • Decreased overall muscle tone with proper positioning for a child with cerebral palsy
Functional limitation	Speech characterized by reduced intelligibility and rate and by abnormal prosodic patterns	Development of compensatory strategies and use of prostheses to optimize speech performance	• Speaking rate reduction • Modifying respiratory patterns to achieve adequate subglottal pressure for speech
Disability	Speech performance in natural communication settings	Optimizing the communication environment and development of effective interaction strategies	• Reducing environmental adversities, such as noise and poor lighting • Conversational management techniques, such as topic introduction • Listener training
Societal limitation	Performance of roles by speakers with dysarthria in social systems	Providing opportunities for communication and eliminating barriers to performing communicative roles	• Changing school district's policy • Changing nursing home procedures related to social interaction

In order for a speaker to be an effective communicator, interventions for dysarthria typically involve strategies at several levels of the chronic disease model. These strategies include (a) optimizing speech performance via reduction of the impairment and development of compensatory strategies and techniques, (b) optimizing speech comprehensibility by combining residual natural speech with contextual information independent of the speech signal, and (c) creating the opportunity to communicate by identifying and reducing potential barriers.

OPTIMIZING SPEECH PERFORMANCE

Traditionally, speech intelligibility has been defined as the accuracy with which an acoustic signal is conveyed by the speaker and recovered by the listener (Kent, Weismer, Kent, & Rosenbek, 1989; Yorkston & Beukelman, 1980; Yorkston, Strand, & Kennedy, 1996). As has been evident throughout this book, improving speech intelligibility in the face of a chronic neuromotor impairment is a primary goal of dysarthria intervention. No single approach is effective for all speakers with dysarthria. Rather, specific approaches or combinations of approaches are selected based on the results of the clinical examination (see Chapters 5 and 6), as well as examination of the various speech subsystems (see Chapters 7, 8, and 9) and other aspects of speech performance (see Chapters 10 and 11).

Multiple Approaches to Intervention

The quality of the speech or acoustic signal, and therefore speech intelligibility, is influenced by the two general speaker-related variables—speech impairment and compensatory strategies—illustrated in Figure 12.1. Obviously, impairment of the speech mechanism impacts the quality and, therefore, the understandability of speech. However, most speakers with dysarthria use compensatory strategies to accommodate for their neuromotor impairment. As was apparent from Chapters 7 through 10, some speakers with dysarthria are able to improve the quality of their speech signal through intervention focused on the reduction of impairment of individual speech subsystems and the improved coordination of multiple systems. Some achieve additional improvement of the speech signal by learning to adjust their speaking style to accommodate their impairments, for example, adopting a speaking rate appropriate for their level of motor control. Still others compensate for the impairment via the use of prosthetic devices, such as palatal lifts.

Planning treatment with the goal of improved speech intelligibility involves the selection of tasks and approaches. These are illustrated schematically in Figure 12.2. The impairment is on the right side of the scale. If the impairment is sufficiently heavy (severe), the scale will be tipped so that speech intelligibility is poor. The scale can be tipped in the favor of the speaker, that is, in the direction of improved intelligibility, if one of two things happens—either the weight (severity of the impairment) is reduced or the impact of the compensatory strategies is increased. For many speakers with dysarthria, reduction of the impairment is not a realistic possibility. Therefore, much of dysarthria intervention focuses on the left side of the scale and seeks to find ways to increase the impact of the compensatory strategies. In rare cases, a single intervention

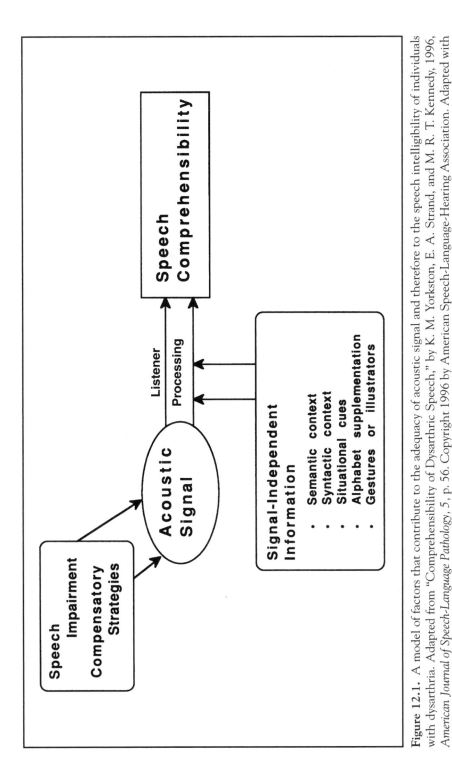

Figure 12.1. A model of factors that contribute to the adequacy of acoustic signal and therefore to the speech intelligibility of individuals with dysarthria. Adapted from "Comprehensibility of Dysarthric Speech," by K. M. Yorkston, E. A. Strand, and M. R. T. Kennedy, 1996, *American Journal of Speech-Language Pathology, 5*, p. 56. Copyright 1996 by American Speech-Language-Hearing Association. Adapted with permission.

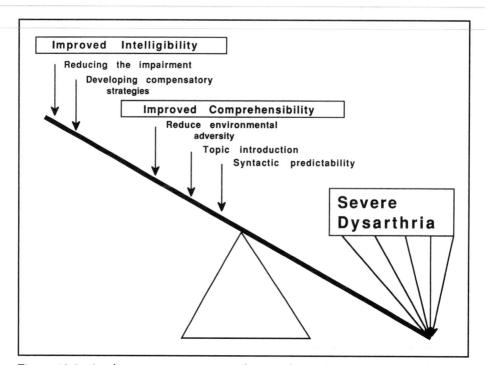

Figure 12.2. A schematic representation of approaches to intervention for individuals with severe dysarthria. From "Comprehensibility of Dysarthric Speech," by K. M. Yorkston, E. A. Strand, and M. R. T. Kennedy, 1996, *American Journal of Speech-Language Pathology, 5,* p. 62. Copyright 1996 by American Speech-Language-Hearing Association. Reprinted with permission.

strategy is so powerful that its use affects intelligibility dramatically. The reader is referred to Figure 10.1 in which the speech intelligibility of a speaker with ataxic dysarthria was improved from 36% when he spoke at 125 words per minute to over 94% at 75 words per minute. For him, a compensatory strategy—specifically, rate control—optimized his speech intelligibility and enhanced his communicative effectiveness with a rather simple, brief intervention. Many speakers with moderate and severe dysarthria are unable to achieve adequate intelligibility with a single strategy. For them, treatment planning requires understanding the impairment of the various speech subsystems, along with the ways in which the subsystems may interact. Individualized treatment programs may involve a combination of approaches that together have the power to tip the balance in favor of intelligible speech.

Changes brought about by any single intervention strategy need not be dramatic. Rather, modest changes in several subsystems may lead to important overall changes in speech performance. In an excellent example of multisystem intervention, a case study of an individual with traumatic brain injury was described (McHenry & Wilson, 1994). Marked improvement in overall speech performance was brought about by making slight adjustments in each of the subsystems.

Integrating Approaches to Treatment

Treatment programs focusing on optimizing speech performance often reflect a blending of approaches and must be responsive to changes over time in the neuromotor status of the speaker. Early in the intervention of some individuals recovering from severe dysarthria, we may focus primarily on specific speech subsystems. Occasionally, the clinician may use nonspeech tasks such as the blow-bottle technique for developing respiratory control that was described in Chapter 7. However, as quickly as possible, the focus of interventions should be shifted onto speech or at least speechlike tasks (sustaining phonation). One of the tasks of the clinician is to stage interventions in such a way that the performance of individual subsystems can receive appropriate attention, yet be appropriately integrated into the overall pattern of speech.

In the following case study, we review the experiences of a man with brain stem stroke. From time to time, we focused briefly on individual subsystems. However, this case study is a nice illustration of both changing neuromotor status and the integration of the subsystems in speech motor control. As speech became more functional, we dealt less and less with individual subsystems and more and more with an overall integrated approach to speech.

 CASE STUDY

Herman was in his 60s when he was admitted to the rehabilitation center. He had survived a stroke that left him with extensive brain stem damage. He was very weak, unable to sit without support, unable to produce voluntary phonation, and unable to swallow. Initially, he communicated using a light-tech word/alphabet board. In addition, he typed messages to be spoken using an augmentative communication system with synthesized speech. Once the augmentative communication system was in place to meet then-current communication needs, we began to focus on his natural speech. Using the blow-bottle technique to develop his ability to produce and control air pressure, he was able to improve some level of respiratory control (see Chapter 7). At times he was able to produce short voluntary phonation in the supine position, and we began to assist him in differentiating vowels (see Chapter 8). About this time, his personalized wheelchair arrived and he was able to sit at about a 120-degree angle with considerable support. He was delighted with the opportunity to view the world from a somewhat vertical position; however, during his next speech intervention session, we realized that all of his vowel sounds were severely nasalized. In fact, we were unable to differentiate the vowels that he was practicing. While Herman was in the supine position, gravity apparently positioned his very weak soft palate away from his tongue so that he was able to radiate sound through the oral cavity and differentiate vowels. However, in the more upright position, gravity positioned his soft palate on the posterior part of his tongue and he radiated all of his sound through his nasal cavity. We really had not expected to refer Herman for a palatal lift this early in his treatment, although we knew that his soft palate was so flaccid that he would probably need it at some point (see Chapter 9). Under the circumstances, we referred him for a palatal lift with a goal of simply lifting his soft palate off of his posterior tongue so that we could continue with his speech intervention program. Following his palatal lift fitting, Herman practiced differentiating vowels and producing words that contained vowels, nasals, glides, semivowels, and so on (see Chapter 11). In time, his palatal lift was modified in an effort to position his soft palate closer to the pharyngeal wall in order to create greater velopharyngeal resistance that would allow him to produce the pressure consonants. By this time, he was speaking more extensively, was stronger, and could tolerate the modification of the palatal lift prosthesis so that it effectively provided resistance to airflow through the velopharyngeal port.

As his speech became intelligible enough to carry much of his communicative load, we focused increasingly on the naturalness of his speech. Because of his early respiratory inadequacy, he had developed a speech pattern that involved very short breath group lengths, with inhalations frequently occurring at inappropriate points, syntactically. He also spoke with an excess and equal stress pattern, also a residual of his earlier difficulties. Initially, he had spoken with a one-word-at-a-time strategy in order to produce adequate respiratory support for speech. Now, he reestablished more appropriate breath group lengths and began to emphasize the words to be stressed in an utterance. As his breath group lengths were normalized, natural intonation patterns returned with little direct instruction or practice (see Chapter 11). Throughout the intervention, focus was placed at various times on respiration, phonation, velopharyngeal function, oral articulation, and speech naturalness. Despite this apparent focus on multiple aspects of speech, an attempt was always made to integrate the work with subsystems into speaking activities and to focus on one feature of speech at a time.

Intervention as a Motor Learning Task

As has been indicated throughout this text, speech is produced in a complex, integrated pattern of movement. Clinicians must be aware that most of the interventions in dysarthria involve motor learning and, therefore, need to adhere to motor learning principles. In brief, motor learning usually involves several phases, including prepractice, intensive practice, and maintenance. During prepractice, the individual is instructed regarding the task and informed about the success criteria (e.g., one or two important aspects of the movement to be practiced with at least 80% accuracy). Usually, models are provided by the clinician or the practice partner. An important component of prepractice for the individual with dysarthria is the selection of one or two important aspects of the movement to be practiced. Given the fact that all speech subsystems are impaired in many speakers with dysarthria, it is easy to make motor learning overly complex by having the individual focus on too many aspects of the motor movement. It is essential to select one or two aspects of the movement that influence the overall pattern to be influenced. An example is presented in Chapter 7, in which a young woman habitually spoke well into expiratory reserve. When she did so, her vocal quality became rough and harsh, and she became excessively fatigued. Her intervention focused on consistent inhalation to an appropriate lung volume level prior to initiating speech. This behavior nearly eliminated her tendency to speak deep into expiratory reserve, thus reducing phonatory roughness and harshness, and markedly decreasing her problems with fatigue. Thus, multiple benefits were achieved by focusing on a single aspect of speech.

During the practice phase, tasks should be distributed in such a way that a variety of different tasks are practiced in individual sessions, thereby avoiding repeated practice on a single word, single sound, or movement. During this phase, the client is provided with the knowledge of results (e.g., about vocal quality or intelligibility) rather than detailed information about performance (i.e., specific movement patterns). For example, the young woman discussed earlier was provided with information about her lung volume level at which she initiated speech; however, she was not provided information about how she managed her thorax or her abdomen or her breath group length. Depending on the judgment of the clinician, knowledge of results may be provided frequently or infrequently. This should be influenced by the individual's age, cognitive capability, and motivation. Generally, persons with dysarthria should be given substantial and systematic practice opportunities. Typically, occasional or inconsistent practice is not adequate to develop or refine motor programs. If an individual is scheduled to receive intervention only once or twice a week, it is necessary for him or her also to have a practice routine that can be implemented by caregivers in the residential, school, or employment setting.

Question: Why is it important to search for "simple" interventions?

An ideal treatment is one that is both simple and effective in modifying many aspects of speech production. Obviously, it is not always possible to develop ideal treatment strategies. The following case may help to illustrate why simplicity is important. The complexity of the motor task influences

(continues)

the speaker's ability to perform successfully. Some speakers with dysarthria achieve speech intelligibility or naturalness goals under optimal conditions, such as (a) in stress-free environments, (b) when talking with their clinicians, or (c) when producing rote or repetitive practice tasks. However, the cognitive load of overly complicated intervention strategies makes it very difficult for the individual to transfer speaking style into less optimal contexts. We are reminded of an individual with dysarthria (also discussed in Chapter 3) who had been through considerable dysarthria treatment. Prior to his conversation with us, he laid on the table in front of him a 5 × 8 card on which 12 strategies were listed, including talk slowly, talk loudly, inhale deeply, conserve your breath supply, look at your listener, don't use run on sentences, and so on. It was apparent that his intervention strategy was too complicated for him to remember without a cue card. We also noticed that, as he focused on individual strategies, he could implement them. So, at times he would look at his card and speak loudly while ignoring many of the other strategies, or he would obviously take near-maximal inhalations as he focused on that type of intervention. Clearly, the cognitive load of his intervention was excessive for him.

Finally, for motor learning to be maintained, individuals often need to engage in maintenance activities. We have found that this is particularly true if the individual is engaged in motor control strategies that are quite demanding for him or her and are at the limits of the speaker's ability. In Chapter 9, we highlight the experience of a physician with Parkinson's disease. He found it useful to engage in maintenance activities when he arrived at work in the morning, following lunch, and before social events. In his case, we audio recorded familiar passages; he would listen to the audiotape and then "speak along with the tape" as he practiced speaking loudly with appropriate effort. Additional information on the principles of motor learning can be found elsewhere (McNeil, Robin, & Schmidt, 1997).

REDUCING THE DISABILITY

Comprehensibility as a Goal of Intervention

Recently, Yorkston and colleagues (1996) used the term "speech comprehensibility" to refer to the dynamic process by which individuals share meaning using any and all information available. The notion of comprehensibility is particularly important when attempting to understand the adequacy of communication in natural settings when many sources of information are available. The concept is consistent with that of Lindblom (1990), who suggested that speakers and their communication partners achieve mutuality using two types of information: (1) information exclusively from the speech signal and (2) information about context that is independent of the speech signal. Figure 12.3 illustrates the relationships between these sources of information. When the speech signal information is rich and speech intelligibility is high, messages are comprehensible even in the face of limited contextual information. However, when the speech signal is degraded because of reduced intelligibility due to severe dysarthria, contextual information that is independent of the speech signal becomes critical for the maintenance of message comprehensibility.

In Figure 12.4, we have illustrated a framework of factors that contribute to comprehensibility. Because speech intelligibility is an implicit component of comprehensibility, all of those factors shown in Figure 12.1 are also included in the comprehensibility framework. In addition, signal-independent information

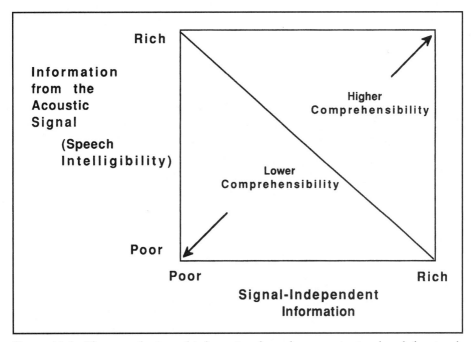

Figure 12.3. The contribution of information from the acoustic signal and the signal-independent information to the comprehensibility of speakers with dysarthria. Adapted from "Comprehensibility of Dysarthric Speech," by K. M. Yorkston, E. A. Strand, and M. R. T. Kennedy, 1996, *American Journal of Speech-Language Pathology, 5*, p. 60. Copyright 1996 by American Speech-Language-Hearing Association. Adapted with permission.

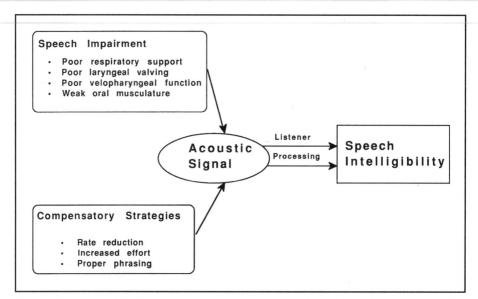

Figure 12.4. A model of factors that contribute to comprehensibility of speakers with dys-arthria. Adapted from "Comprehensibility of Dysarthric Speech," by K. M. Yorkston, E. A. Strand, and M. R. T. Kennedy, 1996, *American Journal of Speech-Language Pathology, 5,* p. 56. Copyright 1996 by American Speech-Language-Hearing Association. Adapted with permission.

of a variety of types is included in this framework. To enhance communica-tion effectiveness, this information can be provided to the listener at the time a communication is occurring, such as by providing the topic (semantic infor-mation) or the situation. Or, specialized information about the specific speaker, such as daily routines or preferences, may be available to listeners. This informa-tion may supplement information from the speech signal in order to enhance comprehensibility.

Staging Intervention for Comprehensibility

In Chapters 3 and 4, dysarthria intervention staging information was provided for speakers with a wide variety of etiologies. In this section, we describe in more detail the intervention strategies for optimizing comprehensibility that are typically included in each stage. The reader is reminded that the ordering of the stages varies depending on the course of the disease or condition. The following section is organized according to the chronology of speakers with a degenerative course. For speakers who are recovering, the order would typically be reversed.

No Detectable Speech Disorder

Many speakers who do not demonstrate a detectable speech disorder report that they notice changes in their speech production. Although speakers describe these changes in different ways, many suggest that extra attention or effort is needed to produce speech. Although their listeners may be unaware, these speakers are understandably very concerned about these changes. One of our clients was a woman who lived a very active, outdoor lifestyle. During the early stages of ALS, she complained that she could no longer talk using her habitual style. Because of insidious changes in respiratory support, she complained that she was able to speak in breath groups that averaged only 10 or 12 words in length. Given her energetic style, this was a marked reduction in her communication efficiency from her perspective.

Some individuals without detectable speech disorders also experience loss of communicative effectiveness, because other aspects of their disorder change the interaction environment. For example, those who experience mobility impairments, such that they must use a wheelchair, often complain about the changes in communication patterns that result from being positioned at a level much lower than listeners who are standing. Some need to be instructed to have their listeners sit beside them in a chair so that they can communicate face to face or to have their listeners move to the edge of a crowd, so that the person in the wheelchair is not surrounded by excessive ambient noise while sitting at a lower level than those standing nearby.

Obvious Speech Disorder with Intelligible Speech

Individuals with mild impairments often maintain intelligible speech even though dysarthria is apparent to all listeners. These individuals are often involved in a wide variety of social contexts and environments. Therefore, their communication effectiveness is challenged in ways that are not often experienced by persons with more severe speech disorders who may have fewer communication opportunities. Individuals with obvious speech disorders but with preserved speech intelligibility may well find themselves involved in employment, community activities, volunteerism, social groups, and so on. At this stage, intervention is focused on assisting these speakers to maintain or enhance their communicative effectiveness by analyzing patterns of communicative success and failure and to help them to adjust their communicative style in order to minimize communication breakdowns.

Assessment of these individuals is based on the notion that these speakers are the "experts" and perhaps the only authoritative source of information on the topic of their own communication effectiveness. Therefore, careful interviews are critical. Using a communication effectiveness assessment tool, such as the one in Appendix 12.A, also provides insights into the speakers' and important listeners' perceptions of communicative effectiveness. In addition to gathering information on common communication activities, special care should be taken to include contexts that are unique to the individual, such as speaking in groups, speaking in new environments (employment and recreation), speaking before groups of children, and speaking for long periods of time. For example, one of our clients was particularly frustrated by her inability to use the outside speaker system for ordering at a takeout restaurant. For years, she had stopped by this restaurant and ordered meals for her family. Even though her speech was intelligible in most contexts, her speech disorder was such that she had great difficulty being understood over the speaker phone. Given her mobility limitations, it was difficult for her to leave her car and enter the restaurant to order her food. Once she identified the problem, an acceptable solution was quickly developed. She began to use a portable telephone to call the restaurant from her car and to park where she could be seen from the restaurant so that employees could deliver the food to her car.

Communication diaries are often a good vehicle for understanding barriers to communication in natural environments. Many speakers with dysarthria are quite effective at analyzing communication interactions both in situations where they are successful and in those where they fail. By having individuals with mild dysarthria document these situations through writing, they can be encouraged by their successes and learn to be astute observers of factors that influence communication. Such an analysis often encourages speakers to understand those elements that are involved in communicative failures and successes. We have found that, by describing these scenarios, our clients are encouraged to experiment with strategies in difficult situations that have appeared to them to be useful in successful situations.

Even though speakers with mild dysarthria are intelligible in many interaction settings, they also experience some communicative breakdowns. Because many of them lead quite active lives, they tend not to recall during clinic visits the detail of these breakdowns. Therefore, we have found it useful for them to maintain a diary of communication breakdowns that includes information about the environment, the context, the speaking task, and the listener(s). With their clinician, they can analyze these situations to determine underlying causes of breakdowns and potential intervention options.

Question: What sort of problems or communication breakdowns can a speaker with good intelligibility experience? Aren't they easily able to "get their message across"?

At first glance, it may seem that speakers with good intelligibility will have no difficulty in real-world communication. However, speech has

(continues)

many purposes other than simply an exchange of information. For example, even mild dysarthria may impact an individual's expression of humor. Persons who enjoyed humor and engaged in verbal humor prior to the onset of their speech disorder are often frustrated at their decreasing ability to successfully tell jokes and humorous stories. This probably occurs because humor has several unique communication characteristics. First, verbal humor requires the listener to understand the details of the message. Second, successful humor typically involves unpredictable or unexpected information and language patterns. The unpredictability of this form of communication interferes with speech intelligibility because humorous messages are typically not as redundant as regular conversation. Third, some humor is based on "word play" in which words are very similar, or is based on words that are the same but are used in different ways. This puts heavy demands on speech intelligibility. Finally, some humor is dependent on, or at least supported by, the suprasegmental information (stress and intonation) with which messages are spoken. Persons with speech disorders often find the signaling of suprasegmental information difficult, which often interferes with humor. At one level, awareness of these difficulties in communicating humor may assist the speaker to understand his or her personal frustration and ineffectiveness in this area of communication. By understanding the pattern of difficulty experienced by a speaker, he or she can be encouraged to use types of humor that he or she can still manage. For example, one of our clients who loved humor began a collection of cartoons and humorous quotes that he would carry with him. He would share these with friends, laugh together, and then extend the conversation using more predictable language patterns.

REDUCTION IN SPEECH INTELLIGIBILITY

The theory of mutuality, discussed earlier in this chapter, suggests that, as the speech signal becomes more distorted (or less intelligible), signal-independent information becomes more and more important. Individuals with reduced speech intelligibility can improve their communication effectiveness in natural settings by providing their partners with this extra information. A number of the techniques to accomplish this have been investigated in research paradigms. Some of this research is reviewed in the literature (Yorkston et al., 1996) and is summarized in Table 12.2.

Clinically, it may be useful to divide techniques for enhancing comprehensibility into three general categories: those techniques that are managed by the speaker with dysarthria, those that are the primary responsibility of the

Table 12.2
Studies of Comprehensibility in Speakers with Dysarthria

Reference	Variable	Speakers	Task	Results
Hammen, Yorkston, and Dowden (1991)	Semantic context	21 adults with moderate to profound dysarthria	Single words with and without semantic context	Intelligibility scores improved with context; most improvement in the severe group (40%)
Dongilli (1994)	Semantic context	8 adults with mild to profound flaccid dysarthria	Single word and target words embedded in sentences	Speakers with severe dysarthria benefited most; largest effects in single words rather than words embedded in sentences
Dowden (1997)	Semantic cues	4 children or adolescents with severe dysarthria	Single words or two-word phrases with and without semantic cues	Partner familiarity and semantic cues influenced communication
Carter, Yorkston, Strand, and Hammen (1996)	Semantic and syntactic context	6 adults with moderate or severe dysarthria	Sentences judged with either semantic or syntactic cues	Both semantic and syntactic cues improved intelligibility of subjects with severe dysarthria
Garcia and Cannito (1996a)	Gestures and predictiveness	An adult with severe flaccid dysarthria	Sentences of varying levels of predictiveness	Intelligibility differences of as much as 70% were noted when listener's information was enhanced with gestures and predictable messages

(continues)

Table 12.2 (continued)

Reference	Variable	Speakers	Task	Results
Garcia and Cannito (1996b)	Gestures, predictiveness, contextual relatedness, and familiarity with speaker	An adult with severe flaccid dysarthria	Sentences of varying levels of predictiveness	Gestures, predictiveness, and context enhanced intelligibility when more information was provided
Beukelman and Yorkston (1977)	First-letter cues	2 adults with severe dysarthria	Sentences produced habitually or with first-letter cues	First-letter cueing improved intelligibility for both speakers even when listeners could not see the alphabet board
Crow and Enderby (1989)	First-letter cues	6 adults with mild to severe dysarthria	Single words and sentences	Both articulatory accuracy and intelligibility improved with cueing
Beliveau, Hodge, and Hagler (1995)	First-letter and word-class cues	3 adults with moderate to profound dysarthria	Single words with first-letter or word-class cues	Word-class (part of speech) cues increased the intelligibility of speakers with severe dysarthria at a magnitude similar to first-letter cueing

communication partner, and those that require interaction of both the speaker and the partner. This organization is reflected in the checklists for speakers with dysarthria and for communication partners that can be found in Appendixes 12.B and 12.C of this chapter.

Readers' Note: Readers will note a subtle change in the use of terminology. In previous sections, where intelligibility was discussed as a measure of the adequacy of speech performance, the term *listener* was used to denote

(continues)

the receiver of the information. In the following section, the term *communication partner* is used to indicate a more active role in maintaining the communication exchange. The communication partner must not only receive and interpret the acoustic signal, but also provide feedback and respond to the message. Both the speaker and the communication partner are active and share responsibility for the effectiveness of the communication interaction.

Speaker Strategies

Preparing Your Partner. Perhaps the most obvious strategy that speakers with dysarthria should adopt is to make sure that the communication partner is listening. It is impossible for anyone to understand highly distorted speech if he or she is not paying attention. Before beginning each interaction, speakers with dysarthria should alert their partners, perhaps by saying the partner's name. It also is critical to select a time when the partner is able to attend. A husband's attempt to communicate when his wife is reading the newspaper may lead to frustration on both sides of the exchange.

Setting the Topic. Individuals with dysarthria can enhance their comprehensibility by identifying the topic for their listeners prior to beginning conversation. This can be accomplished verbally, with gestures when appropriate, or in writing. In research paradigms, topic knowledge is often referred to as semantic context. Semantic context has received considerable research attention (see Table 12.2). It has been investigated using both single-word and sentence stimuli with a broad range of speakers with dysarthria who exhibit deficits in speech intelligibility. The semantic cue usually takes the form of categorical information. For example, the cue "bedding" provides semantic context for the stimulus word "sheets" (Dongilli, 1994), or the contextual cue "things children play with in the bathtub" might set the context for discussion about items such as cup, duck, bubbles, animals, soap, and so on (Dowden, 1997). Generally, the studies of semantic context suggest that providing semantic information in addition to the acoustic signal improves the intelligibility scores on both single-word and sentence tasks for speakers with a broad range of severity levels (Carter, Yorkston, Strand, & Hammen, 1996; Dongilli, 1994; Dowden, 1997; Hammen, Yorkston, & Dowden, 1991).

It is even more critical to introduce the topic whenever the speaker with dysarthria is changing from one topic to another within a conversation. It has been our clinical experience that the most common cause of communication breakdown between partners who are highly familiar with one another is changing topics without letting the partner know. This is to be expected if you believe that the best partners learn to rely heavily on contextual cues to interpret highly distorted messages. If suddenly this signal-independent information is no longer correct because the topic has changed, confusion will occur. Some speakers need to actually provide their partners with the new topic either verbally or in writing. For others, it is sufficient to indicate that there is about to be a topic change. Most speakers prefer to do this with a prearranged gesture, such as raising a finger.

Question: How can the techniques used to estimate the impact of semantic context on intelligibility be modified for children who do not read?

With individuals who possess good literacy skills, estimates are based on the speaker's reading of words or sentences, which is then played to judges who transcribe the messages either with or without semantic information. These techniques have been modified for children by Dowden (1997), who carefully constructed a listing of picturable words in over 30 semantic contexts. For example, the category "types of people children pretend to be" includes nurse, mom, dad, baby, policeman, teacher, mailman, doctor, clown, and fireman, and the category "things children like to pick up outside" includes stick, rock, sand, flower, snow, plant, grass, nuts, ant, and bug. Words are elicited from pictures using the least amount of cueing possible in the following hierarchy: (1) picture only, (2) picture plus context (e.g., "It's clothing you might wear. What is it?"), and (3) picture plus embedded model ("It's a shirt. Now you say it.").

Using Grammar To Enhance the Message. Grammatic structure is another source of information for the communication partner. For all but speakers with the most severe dysarthria, partners understand messages better if they are presented as complete sentences. Research has confirmed this idea. Judges were better able to transcribe sentences if they were provided with a grammatic frame (Carter et al., 1996). For example, "The _____ _____ the _____ was not my _____" was more accurately understood as the sentence, "The police said the collision was not my fault," than it was when no signal-independent information was provided. The syntactic structure evidently provides listeners with information about word class and word boundaries.

Speakers with dysarthria may use syntactic information to enhance comprehensibility in a number of ways. For example, they can avoid telegraphic utterances and use complete sentences instead. Further, sentence structure that is simple and predictable rather than unusual or complex is more likely to be understood. Finally, for those with more severe dysarthria, indication of the word class or part of speech might be helpful (Beliveau, Hodge, & Hagler, 1995). This could be accomplished by having the parts of speech (noun, adjective, pronoun, etc.) listed along with the alphabet on a board. Speakers can indicate the part of speech of words that partners have difficulty understanding. Some individuals with severe dysarthria use this technique as part of their breakdown resolution strategy. When a partner signals that he or she has not understood a word, the speaker repeats the word and also points to the appropriate part of speech.

Use of Gestures. Gestures that support the communicative intent of the message can also be used concurrently to supplement speech. Naturally occurring illustrators have been shown to enhance the intelligibility of speakers with severe dysarthria (Garcia & Cannito, 1996a, 1996b). Illustrators are movements that are directly tied to speech by serving to visually illustrate what is spoken verbally. For example, for the sentence "Stop and turn around where you are," the illustrators might be palm extended in a halting motion and then circular motion of the index finger. Use of gestures may also include any environmental information that is readily available and relevant to the message being expressed. Examples include pointing to nearby items, use of environmental props, and gestures to indicate that a communication breakdown occurred. In addition, forthcoming repair attempts can be indicated using gestures.

Use of Turn Maintenance Signals. Some speakers with reduced speech intelligibility complain that they have difficulty obtaining and maintaining communication turns with their family members and other communication partners whom they have known for years. We typically teach our clients signals to indicate that they wish to initiate a turn, such as leaning forward, or raising a hand or a finger. In addition, we try to have them select and use a consistent signal to maintain their conversational turn, such as positioning the palm of the hand toward the listener (to mean, "Wait, I'm not finished"), moving their finger in a circular motion ("I'm going to continue"), and so on. If these signals are to be effective, they should be used consistently. Direct instruction should be provided to listeners regarding these turn maintenance signal strategies.

Timing of Important Communication Exchanges. Speakers with reduced intelligibility may find it useful to analyze their patterns of energy expenditure and select times for important communication exchange when their energy levels are high. Some indicate that they are so fatigued late in the day that their speech is more disordered in the afternoons than in the mornings. By adjusting their schedules, events that require more precise speech are scheduled in the morning or after rest periods. Also, activities that require a great deal of energy expenditure may need to be scheduled at times when they do not interfere with subsequent communication efforts. Some speakers with reduced intelligibility learn to conserve their energy. For example, many of these speakers learn to limit their casual interaction during group activities by being "a good listener" and conserving their speech energy for "important" interactions that follow.

Selecting a Conducive Environment. Some communication environments are more difficult than others. We all have had experiences with difficulties communicating in adverse surroundings where there is too much noise and distraction and too little lighting. These environmental conditions are particularly troublesome for individuals with dysarthria. Speakers with reduced intelligibility should avoid carrying out important conversations in noisy places or in places where the communication partner cannot watch them. Trying to speak with someone who is across the room or in another room is also difficult.

Question: Are there strategies that are useful for speakers with dysarthria who need to communicate in groups?

As the question implies, communication in groups is particularly difficult for individuals with dysarthria and reduced speech intelligibility. Further, speaking in groups where discussion and interaction occur tends to be more difficult than speaking in a lecture format to a group of people. I will answer your question by recounting the experience and strategies developed by a man with ALS who continued to work as a project manager after his dysarthria became obvious. He needed to run meetings in which a small group of 4 to 6 people discussed the progress of various projects. He used a variety of techniques, many of which are modifications of the speaker strategies just discussed. First, he made sure that all of his team members knew about the nature of his speech problem and informed them to give prompt and honest feedback when they were not understanding him. In addition to establishing the "rules of the game" for interaction, prior to each meeting he provided the team members background information in writing or through electronic mail. Thus, he was setting the topics and reducing the amount of information that he needed to deliver verbally. Even though the group size was small, he also used an overhead projector to display the meeting agenda and to jot down topic words for the group. Because of his slow speech, he occasionally needed to use hand gestures to signal turn maintenance. He was amused to see that others in the group who did not exhibit dysarthria also began to

(continues)

adopt these turn maintenance gestures to hold the floor for themselves. Also, in an effort to compensate for his slow speaking rate, which he knew taxed the patience of listeners, he attempted to be brief and to-the-point in his discussions. He selected an appropriate time and place for the meetings. He scheduled them for a quiet room at a time early in the morning when he was not tired. Finally, his administrative assistant attended the meeting to take notes and occasionally served as a translator when a portion of his message was not understood. She assumed this role only when he requested a "recap." In summary, this man used a combination of strategies for enhancing his communicative effectiveness in groups.

Partner Strategies

When both partners in a communication exchange are easily understood, most of their thought goes into what they are saying and little attention is paid to consciously working to "decode the message." Communication with individuals who have significant speech impairments often requires communication partners to take on different roles in the interaction. When communicating with speakers with dysarthria, frequently communication partners must carry more than their typical share of the communication responsibility. Partners are responsible not only for communicating their own messages, but also for ensuring that they, as listeners, understand what the speaker with dysarthria is saying. This often involves employing strategies to enhance or check personal comprehension.

The following comments illustrate the perspective of an individual who interacts frequently with a speaker with dysarthria.

When Jerry calls me on the telephone, I am always ambivalent. I enjoy Jerry and appreciate what he is attempting to do despite his cerebral palsy. While I can understand his speech, his speech disorder is such that I have to work very hard to understand him over the telephone. Because he tends to call me about important things and because he speaks rather slowly, our phone conversations tend to be quite lengthy—a half hour or more. By the end of the conversations, I am fatigued.

Communication partners can employ a number of strategies to enhance comprehensibility and ensure their own understanding during interaction with a speaker with dysarthria. These strategies do not necessarily require the person with dysarthria to engage in strategic changes in his or her communication behavior. Rather, they require the communication partner to change his or her communication behavior to compensate for the speech impairment. The focus of these strategies is on bringing the process of understanding distorted speech to a level of awareness where both speaker and listener realize the potential for communication breakdown if understanding is not established and maintained.

Maintain Topic Identity. Identification of the topic was discussed previously as a speaker strategy. However, it is also an important listener strategy. Optimally, both the listener and the speaker will use topic identification strategies "to stay on the same page" during conversation. Ideally, both partners should use this strategy, with each being equally responsible for maintaining topic knowledge. The partner may employ this strategy to monitor his or her own comprehension by periodically asking or telling the speaker, "We're still talking about _____ (?)." This strategy is also effective for repairing communication breakdown. Controlled guessing based on previous topics and shared knowledge is one way that the communication partner can facilitate repair of a communication breakdown. This may take the form of a 20-questions format with topics moving from broad to narrow.

Pay Attention to the Speaker. This seemingly obvious suggestion is a simple and effective way to increase comprehensibility. Giving the communication interaction visual and auditory attention while reducing distractions as much as possible can ease the challenge of communication. This might involve communicating in a quiet environment when possible. Reducing environmental noise and distractions is likely to optimize the partner's ability to process and understand information contained in the distorted speech signal. In addition, sitting directly in front of the speaker so that his or her face is clearly visible can enhance the paralinguistic cues available through facial expressions and gestures as well as the use of environmental referents.

Piece Together Clues. Often speech produced by an individual with dysarthria is fragmented in several different ways. Thought or linguistic units may be disrupted by the underlying speech subsystem impairments. What the partner is able to comprehend from the distorted speech signal may also be fragmented, consisting of bits and pieces of information, but not a continuous whole. One important job of the listener is to take these cues and piece them together, trying to understand the meaning being conveyed. This can be likened to putting together a puzzle one piece at a time. Maintaining awareness of all the pieces is important, not only those from the speech signal, but also those that are signal-independent sources of information. As new bits of information emerge, the relations among the pieces may change. Vigilance in putting the pieces together to understand what the person with dysarthria is trying to express is important. Additionally, perseverance on behalf of the speaker is necessary.

Not infrequently, familiar communication partners, such as family members and friends, are called on to act as facilitators or interpreters for the person with dysarthria. This may involve helping other listeners piece together information to understand messages being communicated. It is important that the role of familiar partners acting as facilitators be carefully negotiated with the person with the speech impairment. Roles should be clearly delineated to maintain a comfortable level of independence for the individual with dysarthria.

Enhancing Communication Interaction

Manage Communication Breakdowns. When intelligibility is compromised to any extent, communication breakdown will occur. It is important that speakers with dysarthria and their communication partners manage these situations strategically. Breakdown resolution strategies will vary with different communication partners and contexts. Familiar partners will benefit from different repair strategies than will unfamiliar partners. In addition, the contribution of different communication partners to the repair of communication breakdown will vary with context, familiarity, topic knowledge, and shared knowledge. Several basic suggestions that the speaker with dysarthria can employ to enhance repair of communication breakdown are presented here.

The most obvious strategy and probably the most automatic one is repetition of the message if it is not understood. This is accomplished more easily in some situations than in others. For example, in conversations where frequent turn-taking occurs, communication is dependent on turn-by-turn comprehension. If this is not maintained, determining the point at which communication went awry usually is fairly clear-cut. However, in situations where the speaker is engaging in narrative discourse, such as storytelling, the listening task is different. Listeners are allowed a little more flexibility in their comprehension. They may rely more heavily on the use of keywords, and semantic and syntactic bootstrapping strategies to infer meaning. This suggests that listeners do not have to understand every word; they merely need to understand the gist. However, listeners do need to know when they do not understand enough and therefore need to request repetition or clarification. Occasionally, listeners do not have adequate insight into their own comprehension, or are uncomfortable indicating that they don't understand. This is more likely to be the case with unfamiliar listeners than with familiar ones. To assure adequate comprehension, speakers with dysarthria can probe comprehension by allowing the listener opportunity to request repetition or clarification. One suggestion for doing this is for the speaker to offer occasional pauses or actually ask the listener if he or she understands. This strategy departs from conventional wisdom whereby the speaker assumes that the listener understands unless he or she indicates otherwise. However, communication with an individual with dysarthria departs from traditional interpersonal communication in many ways.

When specific communication breakdowns are isolated, there are two important strategies that speakers with dysarthria can use to resolve them using natural speech alone. As mentioned above, repetition of the message is one mechanism. Typically, if a listener does not understand with two or three repetitions, this strategy should be abandoned. It is important to read the cues of the communication partner, however. With less familiar partners, if they do not understand the message after two or three repetitions, they probably will not. With partners who are familiar, multiple repetitions may help them put the pieces together.

When repetition fails, another useful strategy is to rephrase the message, essentially expressing the same meaning using different words. If particular words cause difficulty, the use of synonyms is often useful. In addition, circumlocution strategies can be employed to describe lexical items or ideas that present comprehensibility challenges for the listener.

When communication breakdown occurs and attempts at resolution using repetition and rephrasing have been unsuccessful, a mutually agreed upon partner scaffolding for resolving the breakdown is useful. It is important that listeners communicate to the speaker with dysarthria exactly what was understood from the message so that the speaker does not have to reiterate the entire message. Misunderstood words or phrases should be repeated one time in a final attempt at piecing together the message. One strategy that has been successful with speakers with severe dysarthria is called shadowing. This strategy involves having the listener repeat each word, phrase, or thought unit after it is produced by the speaker. This allows both the speaker and the listener to gain confirmation of their interpretation of the speech signal. If misinterpretation occurs, determining the exact point where it happened is less difficult. Shadowing should be employed only with the permission of the speaker, as it can be viewed as offensive by some. Another strategy to maintain comprehension is for the listener to periodically summarize his or her interpretation of the ideas being conveyed. Again, this serves as a useful comprehension check for both speaker and partner.

Establish Interaction Rules. Speakers with dysarthria and their partners should be encouraged to establish mutually agreeable rules or communication signals for use during interaction. These rules can be used as guidelines for the roles that speaker and listener play during communication. Rules may vary with communication partners. For example, communication signals may be used to indicate that a communication breakdown has occurred, or to indicate to the listener that the person with dysarthria wants to take a communication turn. One suggestion for managing communication breakdown is to establish natural signals that do not interrupt the person who is speaking at the moment, but that inform him or her that the message was not understood. These unobtrusive types of signals may take the form of gestures or facial expressions, allowing the speaker to reiterate or rephrase his or her message in a second attempt at comprehensibility. Listeners should be encouraged to watch closely for these interaction signals. These signals are likely to be most easily accomplished through nonverbal means, because it may require less energy than using speech of reduced intelligibility to compete for the floor.

Question: My client attempts to use conversation control signals, but a couple of listeners do not seem to get it. They ignore the signals. Do you have any suggestions?

At times we have found it useful to write out the conversational control signals and rules on a 5 × 8 card, or to post them on a wall poster. When the rules have been made explicit, some listeners are more likely to understand and comply with them. Occasionally, we have had to provide some direct instruction and "encouragement" to listeners who remained insensitive to the modified patterns of interaction preferred by a speaker with dysarthria.

RESIDUAL NATURAL SPEECH AND AUGMENTATIVE STRATEGIES

Individuals with severe functional limitation for whom natural speech alone is insufficient to meet their communication needs benefit from augmentative communication strategies to supplement or support their natural speech.

Alphabet Supplementation Strategies

Alphabet supplementation is a strategy involving simultaneous use of a light-tech alphabet board and natural speech (Beukelman & Yorkston, 1977; Crow & Enderby, 1989). The alphabet board is used for phonemic cues during speech production. Alphabet supplementation can be used for several different purposes. It has traditionally been used with the speaker simultaneously saying each word while pointing to the first letter of that word on an alphabet board (Figure 12.5). This provides the listener with additional signal-independent

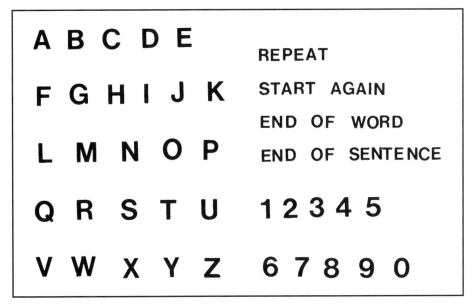

Figure 12.5. Alphabet board.

information in the form of phonemic cues identifying each word. In addition, use of alphabet supplementation results in marked decreases in rate of speech for two reasons. First, the speaker must slow his or her rate to allow adequate time for simultaneous pointing to the first letter of each word as it is spoken. Second, communication partners often engage in shadowing as discussed above, saying each word following the speaker's production to confirm correct interpretation. Alphabet supplementation has been employed to reduce rate or to provide a pacing tool for some speakers with habitual rates that are too high given their level of motor control.

Children with limited spelling skills are often able to successfully use alphabet supplementation. The literacy knowledge level required is awareness of the first letter of each word, not the complete spelling of words. Some children find the task of speaking and pointing to the first letter of each word (on an alphabet board) confusing, whereas others master the task quite easily. For all children, instruction and practice are needed. Figure 12.6 shows an alphabet board developed for a young child.

The Impact of Alphabet Board Use. The impact of alphabet board supplementation of sentence intelligibility has been illustrated with two cases (Beukelman & Yorkston, 1977). Speaker N was a 61-year-old man with severe primarily flaccid dysarthria as the result of a brain stem cardiovascular accident.

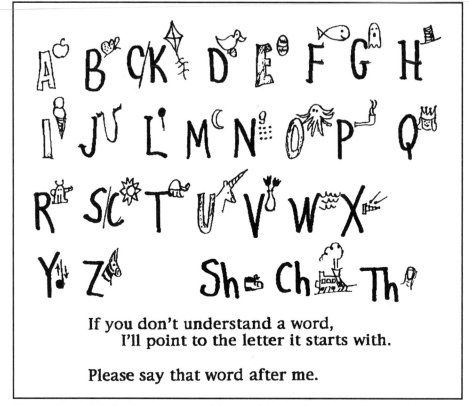

Figure 12.6. Alphabet board developed for a child (Pat Mitsuda and Marsha Adams, personal communication, September 22, 1997).

Speaker H was a 17-year-old high school student who had suffered a brain stem injury in a motor vehicle accident. Both of these individuals had sufficient language and spelling skills to support a letter-by-letter spelling approach. Figure 12.7 contains measures of sentence intelligibility in three listening conditions. In the unaided speech condition, the subjects spoke without the aid of the spelling board. In the alphabet supplementation (aided) condition, the subjects identified the initial letter of each word as they spoke. In the spelling board concealed condition, the speech samples recorded for the alphabet supplementation condition were presented to the listeners; however, the portion of the video monitor showing the alphabet board was concealed. Thus, in this condition, the listeners were unable to benefit from knowledge of the initial letter of the word despite the fact that the speech sample itself was the same as in the alphabet supplementation condition.

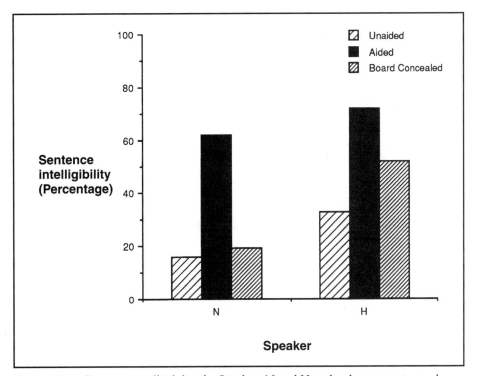

Figure 12.7. Sentence intelligibility for Speakers N and H under three experimental conditions: Unaided (habitually produced), Aided (pointing to the first letter of each word on an alphabet board), and Board Concealed (same as Aided except that the judge could not see the alphabet board). Adapted from "A Communication System for the Severely Dysarthric Speaker with an Intact Language System," by D. R. Beukelman and K. M. Yorkston, 1977, *Journal of Speech and Hearing Disorders, 42*, pp. 265–270.

Results differed somewhat for the two speakers. The alphabet board supplementation approach had the effect of increasing speech intelligibility for both speakers, as compared to the habitual condition. However, when the alphabet board was concealed, intelligibility scores for Speaker N returned to the habitual level. Apparently, the improvement in intelligibility occurred because of the signal-independent information about the first letter of each word received by the listeners. When the alphabet board was concealed from Speaker H, his intelligibility scores were higher than habitual but slightly lower than when the board was not concealed. Apparently, Speaker H changed the way in which he spoke when pointing to the first letter of each word as he spoke. The authors reported that he reduced his speaking rate considerably during the alphabet supplementation, as compared to the habitual condition.

Question: When a speaker with dysarthria uses alphabet supplementation, do you include written instructions to listeners?

Yes, on the back of the alphabet board, we provide written instructions that the speaker can present to listeners if he or she chooses to do so. The instructions read something like the following: "To help you understand me, I will point to the first letter of each word as I speak. Please say each word after me. I'll let you know if you are wrong. If you don't understand a word, let me know and I will repeat it or spell it for you. Please don't finish the sentences for me unless I ask you to do so. Thank you for your patience."

Candidacy for Alphabet Supplementation. Generally, candidates for the alphabet supplementation approach are individuals with severe dysarthria who are using an alphabet-based augmentative communication approach. These individuals have some speech, but reduced intelligibility limits the usefulness of that speech in natural communication situations. The requirements for successful use of the alphabet supplementation approach can be divided into five areas: speech, approach to letter identification, spelling, language, and interaction skills.

Minimal speech production requirements are needed for successful use of the alphabet board supplementation approach. Individuals using this approach must be able to achieve consistent, voluntary phonation. Because the first letter of each word is identified for the listener, treatment often focuses initially on vowel differentiation and later on the inclusion of final consonants for individuals who are being trained to use the alphabet board supplementation approach.

Most frequently, the individuals with dysarthria using this approach point to letters on an alphabet board. In cases where the individual with dysarthria is unable to indicate letters by direct selection, other options are available. Some speakers with minimal hand function indicate letter selection via a head-mounted light pointer (see Figure 12.8). Other individuals who use alphabet-based augmentative communication systems can turn off the devices and use them as an alphabet board while speaking.

Individuals with dysarthria who use spelling-based devices or alphabet boards must make a number of changes in their communication style as they make the transition to the alphabet board supplementation approach. It is typical for individuals who are completely dependent on letter-by-letter spelling approaches to be highly telegraphic in their utterances. Because communication rates are slow but messages are highly understandable, proficient users of such systems will increase efficiency by providing only content words and letters and allowing their partners to fill in the rest of the message. Individuals

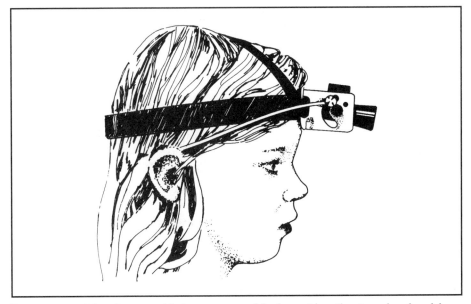

Figure 12.8. A head-mounted light pointer used for letter identification when hand function is poor.

making the transition to the alphabet board supplementation approach need to learn to do just the opposite. They are more likely to be understood if they produce grammatically complete utterances in order to increase the redundancy of their message. Often, some instruction and practice is needed for speakers with dysarthria to develop the ability to change from one style to the other when appropriate.

Many individuals with dysarthria prefer to use the alphabet board supplementation approach because it is much more rapid than a letter-by-letter spelling approach. However, the price that is paid for this increase in communication rate is often a reduction in message intelligibility. For communication partners who are good readers, a spelling-based approach to communication may approach 100% intelligibility. Severely dysarthric speech, even when it is supplemented, is typically less than 80% intelligible. Therefore, users of this approach must be skilled at "managing" their communication partners and resolving communication breakdowns. Many individuals with severe dysarthria place control phrases on the alphabet–number board. These include "end of sentence," "end of word," "start again," and "repeat." These phrases are used to facilitate the resolution of communication breakdowns. Instructions to new listeners, outlining the speaker's and listeners' roles in interaction, are mounted on the back of the board. It has been our experience that some individuals with dysarthria prefer to have their communication partners repeat each word after them. These speakers indicate that it is less fatiguing for them to resolve the breakdowns as they occur, rather than waiting for the end of the utterance only to find that the listener has misunderstood the first or second word. Word-by-word repetition is unnatural for many listeners, and some speakers with less severe dysarthria find it easier to complete the entire sentence before the listener repeats it. Some individuals with dysarthria and cognitive impairment have difficulty switching from the communication styles used with the alphabet board to supplement speech to the communication style used with the alphabet board to spell out words in their entirety when resolving breakdowns. For such individuals, we recommend the use of two different alphabet boards—one with black letters on a white background and the other with white letters on a black background. By training the speaker to use a different board for different communication tasks, confusion resulting from task shifting can be minimized.

Augmentative Communication Approaches for Topic and Situation Introduction

Using augmentative communication approaches to introduce a new topic or change the subject is another way for speakers to enhance comprehensibility. As discussed previously, topic knowledge has an important effect on a listener's ability to understand speech of an individual with dysarthria. For speakers with more severe impairments, use of augmentative communication strategies rather than use of natural speech should be employed for topic introduction. This will likely make the process of topic identification faster and easier with less opportunity for communication breakdown. Strategies for topic introduction include the use of a communication board or book containing prestored topic lists that are frequently used by the speaker. Figure 12.9 illustrates an augmentative communication-based speech supplementation board containing the alphabet, as well as control phases and a list of topics. With this board, a speaker can establish the topic before beginning to speak. The alphabet can be used for alphabet board supplementation or communication breakdown resolution as necessary. The alphabet board is used to spell out topics that have not been prestored on the board. Alternatively, speakers can use a pen and paper to write down the next topic to establish context for forthcoming messages. The most effective strategy will depend on the individual's capabilities, the communication partner, and the context. For speakers with other motor impairments, use of prestored topics is recommended to maximize speed and efficiency in accessing this information. It is important to consider energy expenditure, particularly for those with degenerative conditions. Topic setting should be as easy as possible, saving effort for the communication process itself.

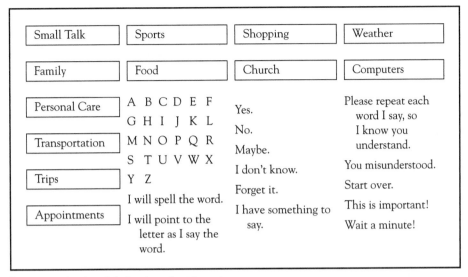

| Small Talk | Sports | Shopping | Weather |
| Family | Food | Church | Computers |

Personal Care	A B C D E F	Yes.	Please repeat each
	G H I J K L	No.	word I say, so
Transportation	M N O P Q R	Maybe.	I know you
	S T U V W X		understand.
Trips	Y Z	I don't know.	You misunderstood.
	I will spell the word.	Forget it.	Start over.
Appointments	I will point to the	I have something to	This is important!
	letter as I say the	say.	Wait a minute!
	word.		

Figure 12.9. An alphabet board with topics.

Spoken Words and Phrases Dictionary

The communication board shown in Figure 12.10 is a further expansion of the one previously shown in Figure 12.9. However, a spoken words/phrases dictionary has been added to the board. We use this strategy to assist individuals with very limited speech capability to use their residual or newly emerging speech. Initially, the speaker can point to a specific word or phrase before attempting to say it. This strategy allows the use (or practice) of marginally intelligible natural speech without risking communication breakdowns. It also provides the speaker with a way to "train" new partners to recognize his or her unique speech patterns. In time, most speakers begin to change their strategy, as they point to the word dictionary or phrase dictionary location (rather than a specific word or phrase) before attempting to speak. In this way they inform their listeners that they are attempting to say a word or phrase that is in the dictionary. By reviewing the items contained in the dictionaries, the listeners often are able to understand the word from the closed set of words or phrases.

For speakers who are attempting to add additional words to their spoken vocabulary, the dictionaries can serve a somewhat different purpose. The dictionary is filled with words that the speaker is attempting to say well enough to be understood. When listeners experience communication breakdowns involving one of these words, the speaker has several choices. He or she can point generally to the dictionary and say the word again. By indicating that the word

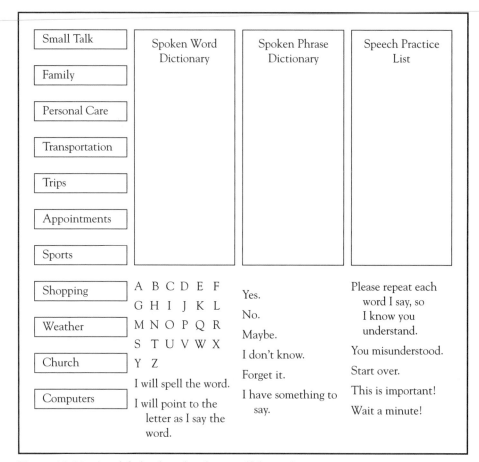

Figure 12.10. An alphabet board with a word/phrase dictionary.

is in the dictionary, the listener can attempt to understand it from the restricted word set as the word is repeated. Or, the speaker can simply point to the word in question to quickly resolve the communication breakdown.

In Figure 12.10, we also have included space for a speech practice list. By targeting the sounds, words, or phrases for practice, we find that a speaker who is attempting to develop or reestablish natural speech is reminded to practice during the course of a day and is encouraged to practice by those around him or her. Hopefully, in time, items included in the practice list can be moved into the dictionaries. As speech improves, words and phrases once included in the dictionaries become so intelligible that they can be understood with alphabet supplementation. Perhaps eventually, these messages become so intelligible that supplementation is not needed.

> *Question:* *These supplemented speech strategies seem like a lot of work. Why not just have the person with severe dysarthria use an augmentative communication system for conversational interaction until he or she is able to use natural speech to meet daily communication needs?*
>
> As we indicated earlier in this chapter, motor learning takes considerable practice. We have found that by having speakers use supplemented speech techniques, they speak much more frequently than if they talk only during treatment and practice sessions. Also, it is very encouraging for speakers and families alike to observe progressive improvements in speech performance. Finally, we strongly believe in a multimodal approach for persons with severe communication disorders. Speech, supplemented speech, and augmentative communication can all be used to achieve communication goals. Much too often, those who stress natural speech development ignore augmentative communication options and limit the communication opportunity and development of individuals who are developing speech for the first time or who are recovering natural speech. Similarly, those who stress augmentative communication often ignore the development or restoration of natural speech, thereby depriving persons with the most severe motor speech disorders the opportunity to speak.

Shifting Communication Modes

The most effective and efficient strategies for managing communication breakdown resolution involve shifting the mode of communication if speech is not readily comprehensible for the listener. Shifting modes may involve use of writing, gestures, alphabet supplementation, or letter-by-letter spelling. Essentially, shifting modes refers to using anything but speech as the primary communication tool. In addition, if the individual uses a voice output augmentative communication system to supplement his or her speech, it may be an effective tool for breakdown resolution.

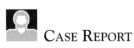 **CASE REPORT**

Betty is a woman with severe dysarthria secondary to cerebral palsy. Her intelligibility, as measured by traditional decontextualized listening tasks, is less than 25% for unfamiliar listeners. It is markedly higher for familiar listeners and when signal-independent information such as context and visual cues are available. In fact, she communicates effectively with family members and other familiar partners using primarily speech. Betty prefers to use natural speech for communication; however, she often experiences difficulty "getting her message across," particularly with unfamiliar listeners. To compensate, she uses a variety of strategies when her speech is not understood. First, if her natural speech alone is not understood in one to three repetitions, she uses alphabet supplementation strategies. This involves saying each word of her message while pointing to the first letter of that word on her alphabet board. She often requests that partners shadow her productions, saying each word after her, so that she can confirm the listener's correct interpretation. If partners do not understand particular words, she spells them out letter by letter. If partners still fail to understand main points of her messages, Betty shifts modes yet again. Betty also uses a voice output communication system. Its use is reserved primarily for unfamiliar listeners and for communication breakdown resolution. This may involve topic identification, reiteration of the entire messages she was attempting to communicate, or generating the parts of her message that her listener did not understand. Clearly, mode shifting and strategy use at this level of sophistication require the speaker with dysarthria to have good insight into his or her partner's comprehension as well as what he or she should do to compensate.

Shifting modes according to situational context is another useful strategy to ensure comprehensibility. Speakers with dysarthria should become tuned to the effects of noise and reverberation on their speech so that they can shift modes accordingly. For example, when in the acoustically taxing food court of a mall, speakers should expect that listeners will very likely have challenges understanding their speech, and should make necessary accommodations such as employing augmentative communication strategies to preempt communication breakdown.

In addition, speakers with dysarthria should be prepared to shift communication modes according to the linguistic context of their message. When speaking of past events, or other abstract topics removed in time and space from the present, linguistic predictability is likely to vary. In addition, the amount of knowledge and lived experience shared by speaker and listener will effect ease of understanding for the listener. Communication about events where the referent is not immediately present may be enhanced by use of supplementation strategies.

Providing Context for Communication

Speakers with severe dysarthria can improve their speech comprehensibility by supplementing their natural speech with information about context through the use of remnant books or photo albums (Beukelman & Mirenda, 1998). By collecting remnants associated with ongoing experiences (e.g., ticket stubs from movies, receipts from purchases, menus from restaurants, or programs from plays or concerts), a speaker can maintain a list of current topics to be used in conversations. For many, the collection of remnants is something speakers can do for themselves, so they are not dependent on family members and speech–language pathologists.

Carefully selected photographs are particularly useful to support the communication of complex narratives or procedures. Narratives, such as family vacations, trips to the zoo, family reunions, or life stories, can be illustrated with photographs that allow a speaker with severe dysarthria to engage in extended interaction. By setting the context and providing details with the photographs, natural speech can be used to carry the remainder of the discussion. Sequences of photographs are also useful to support the communication of detailed procedures, such as setting up the dock at the summer cottage, lighting the gas lamp in the front yard, testing the outdoor grill, or setting the table for guests. One of our clients was responsible for taking care of family property. Following his stroke, he became very frustrated when his extended family members took this role away from him by reassigning these tasks without asking his opinion. By providing him with photographs to illustrate the procedures involved in preparing the family cottage for the summer, he was able to maintain this role while communicating effectively with his grown children and their spouses about the work that needed to be done.

Modifying the Strategies for Children

Children with severe physical limitations often use assistive technology to manage daily needs for mobility, play, and communication. Although many of these children use augmentative communication devices, natural speech is also an important component of their communication system (Beukelman & Mirenda, 1998; Dowden, 1997). Various strategies to enhance comprehensibility have been recommended (see Table 12.3). A review of these strategies suggests that, like intervention with adults, the goal is to structure the environment to enhance signal-independent information and to teach the child strategies for supplementing speech that is difficult to understand. Remnant books are very effective with children.

Alphabet supplementation can also be modified to meet the needs of children with severe speech limitations. Children using the alphabet supplementation approach must have spelling skills that are sufficient to correctly identify initial letters of words. Although no data are available that suggest minimal grade levels, our experience has shown that this is not a demanding spelling task. C. R. Musselwhite (personal communication, 1986) has modified the approach

Text continues on page 522

Table 12.3
Speech Supplementation Strategies for Children

Enhancing Natural Communication Strategies

- Teach the child to add natural or universal gestures to repertoire (e.g., point, mime, "I don't know" shrug, and so on).

Managing Dynamics of Communication Breakdowns

- Teach the child to recognize when his partner does not understand.

- Teach the child to use a hierarchy of breakdown resolution strategies, beginning with the approach that is best for him or her and proceeding to more and more elaborate resolution strategies. Many children, for example, should begin with speech, then add gestures and signs and repeat the speech. If still not understood, the child should add contextual cues (from context boards or devices) and repeat the speech again. Last, the child should resort to specific vocabulary on communication boards or devices.

- Teach the partners to cue the child to try different strategies (if cueing is absolutely necessary) and then to withdraw the cues gradually.

- Model the use of any of these strategies for the child.

Setting the Context for Common Topics

- Teach the child better use of natural gestures and mime to set the context of a verbal message that was not understood.

- Develop a context board or program a voice output communication aid (VOCA), which says "I am talking about . . ." and then give symbols and words for the contexts of everyday life, including home, school, playground, meal/food, stores, friends, family, playing with toys, bedtime, and so on.

- Develop daily, weekly, and monthly calendars of regular activities, including school activities, family activities, routine bus rides, and so on.

- Model the use of daily and weekly calendars to set the context for common activities.

Setting the Context for Unusual Topics

We often need to teach the child and team to use novel strategies such as the following to set the context for speech:

- Collecting souvenirs from special events (e.g., a leaf from a trip to the park taken home to show Mom about the field trip).

- Developing a personal activity calendar for home and for school so the child can use it to set the context for past and future events that are unusual (e.g., when talking about a camping trip that is coming up).

(continues)

Table 12.3 (continued)

- Keeping a journal between home and school with line drawings for the child to recognize. The line drawings can set the context for speech about unusual past events (e.g., a visit by a fireman at school).

- Modeling the use of all of these strategies for the child in all environments.

Alternative Strategies for Predictable Vocabulary—Ambulatory Children

Even with speech supplementation, some vocabulary will need to be specifically represented on communication displays. For ambulatory children, this special challenge can be addressed with the following:

- Developing multiple, specific communication boards that would be posted in the location of use. For example, there could a board in a child's kitchen with school-related activities and people to supplement speech about school and a similar board regarding home and family to help at school.

- Using multiple, small VOCAs, each kept in a specific location for some specific topics where speech is particularly problematic and speech output is essential. For example, young children cannot participate in group singing or group reading activities without voice output. A device can be preprogrammed with the chorus or all parts of a song or the repetitive line of books.

- For the young child especially, these strategies should be kept in the location of use and not be carried around. In some cases for older children, they may carry a communication book and/or device, but it requires careful planning by the team to minimize the weight and maximize the organization of the vocabulary for easy access. Of course, this will become more and more feasible as technology changes.

Alternative Strategies for Unpredictable Vocabulary

When specific vocabulary needs cannot be foreseen, then the words/symbols will not be in the communication books, boards, or devices. Yet the child will still need to use that vocabulary at times (e.g., when the class takes time to talk about flooding or bad weather that has occurred overnight). The following are some strategies we have recommended:

- Drawing instant symbols and words using any supplies available (from pencil and paper to chalk boards or dry-erase boards) for communication on the spot.

- Clipping picture from today's newspaper or magazines.

- Programming "hot" buttons on VOCA for day.

With New Partners, To Aid in Familiarization Process

For some children with extremely limited repertoires and few unfamiliar partners, we can make a difference by familiarizing new partners (e.g., new babysitters, new attendants, new teacher) as quickly as possible. We have done this through:

(continues)

Table 12.3 *(continued)*

With New Partners, To Aid in Familiarization Process *(continued)*

- A communication dictionary listing the child's communication strategies and what each entry means. For example, for a child with idiosyncratic signals or nonstandard signs, the dictionary might list each signal or sign and give its meaning.

- A videotape of a child signing, with explanation of what each sign means to the child.

This approach must be used with care since it is easy to believe that we are improving the child's communication when we are actually just making particular listeners more familiar.

Investing in the Future

- Include in the school program regular opportunities for the child to communicate with unfamiliar partners, using the context-setting strategies described above to resolve breakdowns and noting the child's level of success and where intervention is necessary.

- Include regular opportunities for the child to communicate about new topics and events that are in the past or future, noting the child's success and any intervention that would facilitate more of this communication.

- Literacy must be emphasized for these children so that they can progress as far as they are able. Even if they develop only basic literacy skills, these children will be able to supplement their speech far more easily using words or first letters to resolve breakdowns than through total reliance on symbols. If the child excels in literacy, this will have a huge impact on his or her communication.

Note. From "Augmentative and Alternative Communication Decision Making for Children with Severely Unintelligible Speech," by P. A. Dowden, 1997, *Augmentative and Alternative Communication, 13,* pp. 56–57. Copyright 1997 by *Augmentative and Alternative Communication.* Reprinted with permission.

for children as young as 5 years of age. She teaches children to indicate initial sounds of words as they speak. Orthographic symbols representing initial sounds are accompanied by other symbols more meaningful for the child; for example, the sound /s/ is accompanied by a line drawing of a snake. Other letter combinations such as "th" and "ch" with appropriate symbols accompanying them can also be added to the board. Some find that arranging the alphabet so that the vowels line up on the left side of the board, as in Figure 12.11, also facilitates use by young children.

REDUCING SOCIETAL LIMITATIONS

Earlier in this chapter, social limitations were described as part of the model of chronic disease and defined as limitations in the performance of roles within a social system. The general goal of intervention at this level is to provide oppor-

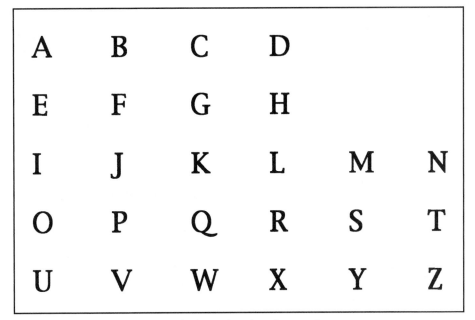

Figure 12.11. An alphabet board arranged so that the vowels are easy to access.

tunities for communication and to eliminate barriers to performance of communicative roles. Social limitation can also be thought of as the disadvantage that a speaker with dysarthria faces within the context of society. This disadvantage results from the interaction of the individual within the cultural, social, and physical environment (Peters, 1996).

The model of chronic disease as it was presented in Chapter 1 and reiterated in Table 12.1 perhaps gives a false impression that there is a linear relationship among the various levels of the model. In other words, pathophysiology leads to impairment, which in turn results in a functional limitation, disability, and societal limitation. This linear relationship would imply that the severity of the impairment would predict the severity of the functional limitation, and the functional limitation would in turn predict the disability, and so on. This notion of linearity is an oversimplification (Peters, 1996). Instead of a linear relationship, there is an interaction among the levels. Social disadvantage is the result of the interaction of an individual's impairment and disabilities with external environmental factors (Badley, 1987). For example, two individuals with mild dysarthria may face very different degrees of disadvantage. A 70-year-old man living at home with his family may participate in all the communication roles he wishes, whereas a 50-year-old college professor may be placed at great disadvantage by even mild dysarthria. Further, the interactions among the levels may be bidirectional (Peters, 1995). Consider the example of a woman with ALS and severe dysarthria who was unable to continue her work as a counselor and teacher. This inability to perform a social role in turn led to depression (i.e., a further impairment) and diminished capacity in activities of daily living (i.e., a further disability).

Effect of the Environment on Opportunities for Communication

Opportunities to participate in communicative roles are often dictated by the environment. Consider the elderly person in a nursing home whose social roles are dictated by the regimented environment. The primary social role of the individual with dysarthria in this environment is that of the patient, one who receives care (Lubinski, 1991). A child in a wheelchair who cannot participate in reading circle because of mobility limitations and physical barriers is another example of an individual whose opportunities for communication are limited by the environment.

In a discussion of the assessment of these obstacles to opportunity, four types of barriers have been identified (Beukelman & Mirenda, 1998). The first of these is *policy barriers*, which are the result of legislative or regulatory decisions that govern the situation. For example, some school districts in North America still have policies that segregate students with disabilities into classrooms or facilities that are not shared by their peers without disabilities. This type of segregation limits opportunities for communication. The second type of obstacle to opportunity is the *practice barrier*. These are procedures or conventions that have become routines in the environment (i.e., the school, workplace, or extended care facility). For example, it may be a practice for residents of a nursing home to stay in their rooms for most of the day, thus restricting the opportunities for social interaction and communication. The third type of barrier are *attitude barriers*. These occur when an individual rather than an agency presents a barrier to participation. For example, a supervisor in the workplace who does not believe that an individual with dysarthria is capable of performing the job even when the job may not have excessive demands in terms of communication. The final barrier is a *knowledge barrier*. Because these involve lack of information, these types of barrier may be quite easy to deal with once they are identified.

Lubinski (1991) clearly described how particular environments such as nursing homes reduce the opportunity for participation. Because individuals who enter nursing homes must adhere to a regimented lifestyle, they frequently have few opportunities for self-determination and choice. The routines in nursing homes are frequently established to meet the needs of the care providers rather than the residents. Lubinski suggested that nursing homes can be "communication-impaired or -deprived environments" where residents have few reasons to talk, few people of choice with whom to talk, few things to talk about that arise from stimulating activities, few private places to communicate, and a variety of rules that restrict communication opportunity.

Question: How should institutions such as nursing homes be changed to optimize communication?

Although drastic conceptual changes may be needed to achieve more opportunities for communication, Lubinski (1991) listed the following characteristics of a positive communication environment:

- Elderly and chronically ill patients want to talk, and feel that communication is important to their well-being.

- Members of the staff are the primary communication partners of the patients and thus play a crucial role in the patients' communication life.

- It is possible to change the physical environment to make it more conducive to communication.

- People need to be able to engage in activities that foster communication and to be allowed access to their choice of communication partners in order for optimal communication to occur.

Perceived Reactions of Others

Communication partners and their attitudes about the individual with dysarthria have an important impact on social limitations. These attitudes are formed in ways that are complex and poorly understood. For example, social interactions may be limited because communication partners may feel failure for not interpreting the dysarthric speech accurately (Lubinski, 1991). This feeling of failure may cause them to avoid the communication contact, which they believe will be unsuccessful and frustrating.

Peer perspectives in reaction to dysarthria in children have been investigated (Lass, Ruscello, Harkins, & Blankenship, 1993; Lass, Ruscello, & Lakawicz, 1988; Ruscello, Lass, Hansen, & Blankenship, 1992). In these studies videotaped samples of children with dysarthria are played to judges of comparable ages, who are asked to rate a number of nonspeech characteristics on a semantic differential scale containing bipolar adjectives. Even when potential communication failure is not an issue, peers rate individuals with dysarthria less favorably than individuals without dysarthria. In a case report of an 11-year-old girl with mild ataxic dysarthria, other students perceived her as frightened, nervous, tense, and unlovable (Gies-Zaborowski & Silverman, 1986). Results of this rating were used by her clinician to justify keeping her longer in the caseload.

When a group of adults with dysarthria were asked a series of questions about their perceptions of others' reactions, most endorsed items that suggested that their communication partners were helpful (Yorkston, Bombardier, & Hammen, 1994). A listing of items related to the reactions of others can be found in Table 12.4. Responses varied depending on the severity of the dysarthria. Indi-

Table 12.4
Questionnaire Items that Relate to the Perceived Reactions of Others to Speakers with Dysarthria

- People remind me to slow down or look at them when I speak.
- People work hard to make communication easy for me.
- Because of my speech problem, people treat me as if I am not very bright.
- Others get irritated with my speech.
- Others ignore me if they do not understand what I am saying.
- Others treat me like a child when it comes to communication.
- Others have taken over making telephone calls for me.
- People tend to get impatient because I speak slowly.
- Others praise me when I try to speak for myself.
- Others interrupt me when they are having difficulty understanding me.
- People treat me as if I can't do the job when I know that I am able.
- People fill in words for me before I have a chance to complete my thought.
- Others order for me in a restaurant, although I would prefer to do it myself.
- Others criticize me for the way I talk.
- People include me in conversation despite my speech problem.
- Members of my family let me know when they do not understand me.
- My family is patient when trying to communicate with me.
- People leave me out of conversations.
- People treat me as if I am hard of hearing.
- People speak louder when talking to me because they think I have a hearing problem.
- Family or friends tell me to not work so hard trying to speak.
- Others have taken over my responsibilities because of my speech problem.
- Others laugh or joke about my speech problem.
- People encourage me to speak for myself.
- When I am talking, people pretend to understand.
- Others say they will speak for me whenever I want them to do so.

Note. From "Dysarthria from the Viewpoint of Individuals with Dysarthria," by K. M. Yorkston, C. Bombardier, and V. L. Hammen, 1994, in *Motor Speech Disorders: Advances in Assessment and Treatment* (pp. 33–35, by J. A. Till, K. M. Yorkston, and D. R. Beukelman (Eds.), Baltimore: Brookes. Copyright 1994 by Paul H. Brookes Publishing. Reprinted with permission.

viduals with severe dysarthria felt that partners were more influential in communication exchanges than did individuals with mild or moderate dysarthria. Individuals with severe dysarthria also endorsed a large portion of questionnaire items that suggest that partners were solicitous (e.g., "Others order for me in a restaurant, although I would prefer to do it myself") and punishing (e.g., "Because of my speech problem, people treat me as if I am not very bright").

Integration into Assessment and Treatment

Social limitations may best be viewed from the perspective of the individual with dysarthria. This perspective has been called the *insider's perspective* and reflects the "subjective experience of living with and in spite of illness" (Conrad, 1990; Peters, 1996). It is in contrast with the *outsider's perspective*, which views disability from outside the experience itself. Lubinski (1991) listed a series of questions that may serve as a good starting point for speech–language pathologists to understand the psychological, social, and emotional impacts of dysarthria (see Table 12.5). Note that these questions elicit information about how the individual with dysarthria defines the problem and the impact of the problem on many aspects of his or her life. Questions about motivation to improve are also posed.

To assess communicative effectiveness, Sullivan, Beukelman, and Gaebler (1997) developed a questionnaire (Appendix 12.A). A review of the questionnaire reveals that communicative effectiveness is assessed by social context. The first eight contexts are typical for most individuals. However, contexts 9 through 15 may or may not be appropriate for specific individuals depending on their lifestyles and their levels of independence. To obtain a complete picture of communicative effectiveness, items that are appropriate for individual speakers should be selected, as well as contexts unique to the individual (e.g., calling Bingo games, coaching youth sports, arguing cases in court, or selling products in noisy environments). Communicative effectiveness in each context is rated on a 7-point equal-appearing interval scale.

In our practice, we try to have speakers with dysarthria, as well as important representatives from different social contexts, complete a communication effectiveness questionnaire. This is done to determine whether the perceptions of speakers are consistent with their most common listeners. At times, speakers are aware of changes in their speech motor control processes, such as increased effort or decreased respiratory support, that do not yet result in a detectable speech disorder to their listeners. These speakers may rate their communicative effectiveness as reduced because of their sensitivity to these changes. However, their listeners are often unaware of any reduction in communicative effectiveness. Because some speakers with progressive dysarthria are very sensitive to early changes in their speech performance, it is not uncommon that they overestimate

Table 12.5
Probe Questions for the Client

Definition of the Problem

- What concerns you about your speech?
- What kinds of sounds or words give you the most difficulty?
- In what situations do you feel you have the most difficulty talking?

Impact of the Problem

- How do you feel when you have difficulty being understood?
- How do others react when you have difficulty being understood?
- Do you ever avoid a situation or a person because of your speech problem? If yes,
  —What is this situation (person)?
  —Why do you think this happens?
- How has your speech problem affected your interaction with your family?
- How has your speech problem affected your social life (employment, and so on)?
- Do you think you have less opportunity to talk now than previously? If yes,
  —Why?
  —How can you change this?

Motivation to Improve

- Why would you like to improve your speech?
- What would you like to improve?
- What have you done on your own to improve your speech?
- What techniques did you find helped you talk better?
- Have you attended speech therapy sessions before this? If so,
  —Where were they held?
  —What were your goals?
  —What were the results?
- How will your family work to help you improve your speech?
- How will we know when speech therapy has been successful?
- What do you think is my role in the speech therapy situation?

Note. From "Dysarthria: A Breakdown in Interpersonal Communication," by R. Lubinski, 1991, in *Treating Disordered Speech Motor Control* (p. 159), by D. Vogel and M. P. Cannito (Eds.), Austin, TX: PRO-ED. Copyright 1991 by PRO-ED, Inc. Reprinted with permission.

the impact of these changes on their communicative effectiveness. In these situations, listener perceptions probably provide a more accurate assessment of a speaker's communicative effectiveness.

Conversely, some speakers with dysarthria appear to be largely unaware of reductions of communicative effectiveness. This is particularly true if the speaker has experienced cognitive impairments. For these individuals, accurate ratings of communicative effectiveness may be difficult because they are aware of the message and, therefore, have trouble determining how difficult it is for their listeners to understand their speech. In these situations, the speaker may indicate high levels of communicative effectiveness, whereas the frequent listeners may record a low level of communicative effectiveness. When there is a considerable difference among speakers and their communication partners regarding communicative effectiveness, interventions can be complicated. For example, when individuals with dysarthria perceive themselves as having higher communicative effectiveness than is perceived by their listener, the listener may interpret them as being difficult, lazy, or obstructionistic.

Case Note: In Chapter 10, we discuss a case history of a man who used an alphabet board to control his speaking rate and supplement his comprehensibility. Because he overestimated his communicative effectiveness, and because he found the alphabet supplementation technique rather burdensome, he had difficulty understanding the need for this strategy. Frequent listeners (his wife, children, and grandchildren) initially misunderstood his unwillingness to use alphabet supplementation, believing him to be stubborn or in denial of his disability. In time, his family realized that he simply was not aware of the extent of his speech disorder and accepted responsibility to remind him to use the supplemented speech technique.

On the other hand, when speakers with dysarthria feel themselves to be much less communicatively effective than is perceived by their listeners, it is easy for the listeners to believe that the individual is overreacting or being hypersensitive.

Perspectives of the family as "insiders" are central to this assessment of social limitations. This assessment must be viewed within the broad context of social systems. The family is perhaps the most common example of a social system (Satir, 1981). Communication is critical in families. Lubinski (1991) described the family as an interdependent, interacting system of roles in a state of dynamic equilibrium. Roles are developed over time through both verbal and nonverbal communication. For individuals with dysarthria, communication and therefore family roles may be altered. When communication skills change suddenly or gradually over time, family members may need to disturb the family's equilibrium and assume different roles within the system. These additional roles may include familial tasks such as maintaining family communication and exchange of information, interacting with medical and social services professionals, and acting as advocate for the individual with dysarthria.

Because family dynamics are often so fundamental to the success of intervention, the perspectives of the family members are critical. Lubinski (1991) outlined an approach to soliciting this information from family members. She questions families in three areas (see Table 12.6). The first relates to the issues of the demands placed on the family as the result of the dysarthria, the second to resources that are at the family's disposal, and the third to the family's definition of the problem.

Table 12.6
Probe Questions for Family Members

Demands

- What significant events were occurring in your family prior to the onset of your (dad's, mom's, husband's, wife's, etc.) chronic illness or communication difficulties?

- How have these events changed since the onset of the physical and communication problems?

- Who has primary care or responsibility for your (dad's, etc.) physical needs?

- How does this care affect (you, her, him, them)?

- How has the chronic illness or communication difficulty affected your (dad's, etc.) social life?

- How has the chronic illness or communication difficulty affected the primary caregiver's social life?

- What physical stress or strains does the primary caregiver have because of the physical problem?

- What financial problems is your family incurring related to the physical or communication problem?

- How has the primary caregiver's daily life changed since the onset of the problem?

- What physical or psychological changes have you noted in the primary caregiver since the inception of the problem?

- How did the family change immediately at the onset of the problem? How has it changed over time?

Resources

- How would you describe your family's strengths?

- What other problems did your family have in the past and how did they solve them?

- How successful do you think your family is in solving difficult problems?

(continues)

Table 12.6 (continued)

- How willing is your (dad, etc.) to seek help from friends? counselors? religious institutions? social service? others?

- During difficult times, will your family call a family conference and discuss problems? Who is likely to be the leader or take-charge person in these situations?

- Who will be the primary communication partner of your (dad, etc.)? Will this individual be available to come to therapy sessions on occasion?

Definition of the Problem

- What do you perceive as the major problem facing your family at the present time?

- Why is this problem so paramount?

- What do you think can be done about this problem?

- Should the communication problem not be mentioned, then ask the following: How does your (dad's, etc.) communication problem compare to this problem you have just defined?

- Do other members of your family define the impact of your (dad's, etc.) problem in the same way as you have just done? How is their definition different from yours?

Note. From "Dysarthria: A Breakdown in Interpersonal Communication," by R. Lubinski, 1991, in *Treating Disordered Speech Motor Control* (p. 166), by D. Vogel and M. P. Cannito (Eds.), Austin, TX: PRO-ED. Copyright 1991 by PRO-ED, Inc. Reprinted with permission.

The assessment of communicative effectiveness is an important aspect of dysarthria or motor speech intervention, because it focuses on the overall goal of most interventions, which is to assist the person to be an effective communicator. Such intervention focuses the speaker with dysarthria, important communication partners, and the clinician on the overall goals of intervention. At times, communicative effectiveness is enhanced by maintaining or improving the intelligibility and efficiency of natural speech. However, at times the provision of information in addition to natural speech improves their speech comprehensibility and allows them to be more communicatively effective. Finally, in some contexts augmentative communication options are the most effective (or only) way to enhance the communicative effectiveness for persons with the most severe communication disorders.

APPENDIX 12.A
COMMUNICATIVE EFFECTIVENESS SURVEY

Name _____ Date _____

Person completing the survey ☐ Speaker ☐ Family/Friend _____

Section 1

This is an evaluation of how effectively the speaker communicates in various social situations. Please read the statement describing each of the following situations and indicate how successfully you feel the speaker is able to communicate. If you feel that communication is very effective, circle the 7. If communication cannot occur at all in a situation, circle the 1. Feel free to use any number on the scale.

1. Having a conversation with a few friends (at home or bedside).

   Not at all able   1   2   3   4   5   6   7   Very effective

2. Participating in a conversation with strangers in a quiet place.

   Not at all able   1   2   3   4   5   6   7   Very effective

3. Conversing with a familiar person over the telephone.

   Not at all able   1   2   3   4   5   6   7   Very effective

4. Conversing with a stranger over the telephone.

   Not at all able   1   2   3   4   5   6   7   Very effective

5. Being part of a conversation in a noisy environment (social gathering).

   Not at all able   1   2   3   4   5   6   7   Very effective

6. Speaking to a friend when you are emotionally upset or when you are angry.

   Not at all able   1   2   3   4   5   6   7   Very effective

7. Having a conversation while traveling in a car.

   Not at all able   1   2   3   4   5   6   7   Very effective

8. Having a conversation with someone at a distance (across the room).

   Not at all able   1   2   3   4   5   6   7   Very effective

Section 2

Please read the statements describing the following situations. If you feel that the statement describes a frequently occurring or important communication situation for the speaker, mark the box to the left of the item number. Next, for each statement that you have chosen, circle the number that indicates how successful you feel communication is in each situation. Add contexts that are unique to your situation in Items 16 through 18.

☐ 9. Speaking in front of a small group without a microphone.

Not at all able   1   2   3   4   5   6   7   Very effective

☐ 10. Conversing with someone who is somewhat hard of hearing.

Not at all able   1   2   3   4   5   6   7   Very effective

☐ 11. Conversing through the outdoor speaker system with an employee at a fast-food restaurant or at a gas station.

Not at all able   1   2   3   4   5   6   7   Very effective

☐ 12. Having a *long* conversation (over an hour in length).

Not at all able   1   2   3   4   5   6   7   Very effective

☐ 13. Speaking outdoors.

Not at all able   1   2   3   4   5   6   7   Very effective

☐ 14. Communicating at work (specify type of work: _____).

Not at all able   1   2   3   4   5   6   7   Very effective

☐ 15. Speaking to young children.

Not at all able   1   2   3   4   5   6   7   Very effective

☐ 16. Other: _____

Not at all able   1   2   3   4   5   6   7   Very effective

☐ 17. Other: _____

Not at all able   1   2   3   4   5   6   7   Very effective

☐ 18. Other: _____

Not at all able   1   2   3   4   5   6   7   Very effective

APPENDIX 12.B
TECHNIQUES FOR IMPROVING COMPREHENSIBILITY: FOR THE SPEAKER WITH DYSARTHRIA

The following techniques may be useful for individuals whose natural speech may at times be difficult to understand. The items that are checked may be the most appropriate for you. These techniques enhance the understandability of your speech by providing your communication partner some extra cues. (Adapted from Vogel & Miller, 1991; Yorkston, Strand, & Kennedy, 1996; Yorkston, Strand, & Miller, 1995.)

☐ **Provide your communication partner context for what you are saying.** Knowing the topic of conversation makes a big difference in understanding speech that is distorted. If your speech is difficult to understand, provide the context by writing or spelling the topic of your message.

☐ **Don't shift topics abruptly.** If your speech is difficult to understand, your partners may get lost if you change from one topic to another without a transition. Let people know that you are changing topics and what the new topic is.

☐ **Use turn-taking signals.** Conversations tend to go very quickly. If your speech is slow, you may need to use clear signals that you want a turn. These signals may take the form of an eye gaze, breathing pattern, body movement, gesture, or verbal interjection. Choose one or two that work for you and make sure listeners are aware of them.

☐ **Get your listener's attention.** It is impossible for any listener to understand unless he or she is paying attention. If your speech is difficult to understand, it is even more important that listeners are paying attention. Before you begin a message, alert your communication partner by saying his or her name.

☐ **Use complete sentences.** Grammatically complete sentences are usually easier for listeners to understand. Avoid telegraphic sentences or those in which the "little" grammatical words are deleted.

☐ **Use predictable types of sentences.** Simple, grammatically predictable sentences are generally easier to understand than longer, grammatically complicated sentences.

☐ **Use predictable wording.** There are many ways to communicate a single idea. If your speech is difficult to understand, avoid unusual idioms or slang expressions. Be direct. For example, "Close the window, please," may be easier to understand than, "I wouldn't mind if you would close the window."

☐ **Watch the tone of your voice.** We communicate much information by changing the tone of voice. For example, the phrase "You really look terrific" may mean two completely different things depending on how you say it. If you have difficulty expressing subtle changes in meaning with your intonation, you'll need to express sarcasm or humor in other ways.

☐ **Rephrase your message.** If listeners have not understood you even after you've repeated the message, try communicating the thought using different words. But use a signal to let them know.

☐ **Accompany speech with simple gestures when appropriate.** At times, speech may be supplemented by simple gestures. For example, extending the palm in a halting motion, then rotating the index finger in a circular motion, may accompany the message, "Stop and turn around where you are."

☐ **Take advantage of situational cues.** Your surroundings may help you give a listener extra cues. For example, you might point to objects in the room in order to introduce a topic.

☐ **Make the environment as "friendly" as possible.** Some communication environments are more difficult than others. Avoid carrying out important conversations in noisy places or in places where your communication partner cannot watch you as you speak, for example, in dimly lit rooms or in situations where your listener is a long distance from you.

☐ **Avoid communication over long distances.** Trying to speak with someone who is across the room or in another room is difficult. If you need to call attention to yourself, a buzzer, beeper, or baby monitor may be useful.

☐ **Use alphabet board supplementation.** If your speech is very difficult to understand, you may want to point to the first letter of each word as you say it. This reduces your speaking rate, allowing weakened muscles more time to formulate the precise movements of the speech sounds. It also provides the listener with information about the word being spoken. If a word is not understood even when the first letter of the word has been identified, you can resolve the misunderstanding by spelling out the word in its entirety.

☐ **Communicate emotional messages.** Take care to communicate "emotionally loaded" messages when you are not tired and when there is plenty of time.

☐ **Have a handy backup system.** Have a highly understandable communication system handy in case of difficulty. This may be as simple as a pad of paper and pencil to write cue words. Generally, we advise speakers with dysarthria not to let their listener get absolutely lost. Understanding little or nothing of a message can be very frustrating to a listener. If you see that someone is not understanding you, stop and make sure that he or she understands before you continue.

APPENDIX 12.C
TECHNIQUES FOR IMPROVING COMPREHENSIBILITY: FOR THE COMMUNICATION PARTNERS OF THE SPEAKER WITH DYSARTHRIA

Communication is a partnership. The following techniques may make the communication process easier. The items that are checked may be the most appropriate for you. (Adapted from Vogel & Miller, 1991; Yorkston, Miller, & Strand, 1995; Yorkston, Strand, & Kennedy, 1996).

☐ **Make sure you know the general topic of the conversation.** Knowing the topic of conversation makes a big difference in understanding speech that is distorted. Encourage speakers with dysarthria to introduce topics.

☐ **Watch for turn-taking signals.** Some speakers with dysarthria for whom speech is slow have difficulty getting a turn in a conversation. Watch carefully for your partner's signals or decide in advance on some turn-taking signals.

☐ **Give your undivided attention.** Speech is usually so easy to understand that listeners can do other things and still understand what is being said. Speech that is slow and distorted is more difficult to understand and therefore requires undivided attention.

☐ **Choose the time and place for communication.** Most of us can talk all day without getting tired. Most of us can do many things while we talk. We can walk and talk, chew gum and talk, or eat and talk. Talking may be a very difficult task for a speaker with dysarthria. Avoid important conversations when the speaker is tired. Mealtimes may no longer be the best time for conversation.

☐ **Watch the speaker.** All of us get a considerable amount of information by watching a speaker. When speech is slow or distorted, it is even more important to look at the speaker's face.

☐ **Piecing together the cues.** Some people describe the task of understanding slow and distorted speech as a process of piecing together a series of cues. Some of the cues, of course, come from speech. Other cues may come from the gestures that the speaker uses or from the physical surroundings. Take advantage of whatever cues are available to you.

☐ **Make the environment work for you.** Maximize your ability to understand the speaker with dysarthria by making sure that you have enough light, that the light is on the speaker's face, and that all extraneous noise is eliminated or reduced.

☐ **Avoid communication over long distances.** Make sure to always be in the same room when you initiate conversation. It is difficult for many speakers with dysarthria to speak loudly enough to be heard in another room.

☐ **Make sure your hearing is as good as possible.** It is important that you hear well. If you suspect you have mild hearing loss, have your hearing tested. Properly fitted hearing aids may make the speech of individuals with dysarthria more understandable.

☐ **Decide on and incorporate strategies for resolving communication break-downs.** There may be times when you will not be able to understand some or all of a message. It is important to develop a plan of action to take if this happens. Some people find the following steps helpful in preventing frustration:

  ☐ Signal as soon as you don't understand. (Most people find that a nonverbal signal is best because it does not disrupt the flow of conversation.)

  ☐ Let the speaker know the parts of the message that you did understand. (In this way, the speaker will not have to repeat the entire message.)

  ☐ Let the speaker repeat the misunderstood words one time.

  ☐ If you still don't understand, ask the speaker with dysarthria to go to a predetermined "backup" plan that involves perhaps rephrasing, verbal spelling, or writing.

☐ **Establish some rules of the game.** Speakers with dysarthria may have some very definite preferences about what they would like you to do and what they wish you would not do. Knowing these preferences may reduce frustration. For example, does the speaker with dysarthria want you to guess or not? want you to finish sentences or not?

☐ **Facilitating communication with others.** Communicating with unfamiliar people is difficult for many speakers with dysarthria. You may be of assistance as a translator in some situations. Again, it is useful to have some predetermined guidelines. Does the speaker with dysarthria want you to translate misunderstood parts of the message? to provide long or elaborate responses to questions when you know what the answers are? to order food in a restaurant?

REFERENCES

Badley, E. M. (1987). The ICIDH: Format, application in different settings, and distinction between disability and handicap: A critique of paper on the application of the International Classification Impairment, Disabilities, and Handicaps. *International Disability Studies, 9*, 122–125.

Beliveau, C., Hodge, M., & Hagler, P. (1995). Effect of supplemental linguistic cues on the intelligibility of severely dysarthric speakers. *Augmentative and Alternative Communication, 11*, 176–186.

Beukelman, D. R., & Mirenda, P. (1998). *Augmentative and alternative communication: Management of severe communication disorders in children and adults* (2nd ed.). Baltimore: Brookes.

Beukelman, D. R., & Yorkston, K. M. (1977). A communication system for the severely dysarthric speaker with an intact language system. *Journal of Speech and Hearing Disorders, 42*, 265–270.

Carter, C. R., Yorkston, K. M., Strand, E. A., & Hammen, V. (1996). The effects of semantic and syntactic content on the actual and estimated sentence intelligibility of dysarthric speakers. In D. Robin, K. M. Yorkston, & D. R. Beukelman (Eds.), *Disorders of motor speech* (pp. 67–88). Baltimore: Brookes.

Conrad, P. (1990). Qualitative research on chronic illness: A commentary on method and conceptual development. *Social Science and Medicine, 30*, 1257–1263.

Crow, E., & Enderby, P. (1989). The effects of an alphabet chart on the speaking rate and intelligibility of speakers with dysarthria. In K. M. Yorkston & D. R. Beukelman (Eds.), *Recent advances in clinical dysarthria* (pp. 99–108). Austin, TX: PRO-ED.

Dongilli, P. (1994). Semantic context and speech intelligibility. In J. Till, K. Yorkston, & D. Beukelman (Eds.), *Motor speech disorders: Advances in assessment and treatment* (pp. 175–192). Baltimore: Brookes.

Dowden, P. A. (1997). Augmentative and alternative communication decision making for children with severely unintelligible speech. *Augmentative and Alternative Communication, 13*, 48–58.

Garcia, J. M., & Cannito, M. P. (1996a). Influence of verbal and nonverbal context on sentence intelligibility of a speaker with dysarthria. *Journal of Speech and Hearing Research, 39*, 750–760.

Garcia, J. M., & Cannito, M. P. (1996b). Top down influences on the intelligibility of a dysarthric speaker: Addition of natural gestures and situational context. In D. Robin, K. Yorkston, & D. Beukelman (Eds.), *Disorders of motor speech* (pp. 89–104). Baltimore: Brookes.

Gies-Zaborowski, J., & Silverman, F. (1986). Documenting the impact of a mild dysarthria on peer perception. *Speech and Hearing Services in Schools, 17*(2), 143.

Guralnik, D. B. (Ed.). (1982). *Webster's New World Dictionary* (p. 445). New York: Simon and Schuster.

Hammen, V. L., Yorkston, K. M., & Dowden, P. A. (1991). Index of contextual intelligibility: I. Impact of semantic context in dysarthria. In C. Moore, K. M. Yorkston, & D. R. Beukelman (Eds.), *Dysarthria and apraxia of speech: Perspectives on intervention* (pp. 43–54). Baltimore: Brookes.

Kent, R. D., Weismer, G., Kent, J. F., & Rosenbek, J. C. (1989). Toward phonetic intelligibility testing in dysarthria. *Journal of Speech and Hearing Disorders, 54*, 482–499.

Lass, N. J., Ruscello, D. M., Harkins, K. E., & Blankenship, B. L. (1993). A comparative study of adolescents' perceptions of normal-speaking and dysarthric children. *Journal of Communication Disorders, 26*, 3–12.

Lass, N. J., Ruscello, D. M., & Lakawicz, J. A. (1988). Listeners' perceptions of nonspeech characteristics of normal and dysarthric children. *Journal of Communication Disorders, 21*, 385–391.

Lindblom, B. (1990). On the communication process: Speaker–listener interaction and the development of speech. *Augmentative and Alternative Communication, 6*(4), 220–230.

Lubinski, R. (1991). Dysarthria: A breakdown in interpersonal communication. In D. Vogel & M. P. Cannito (Eds.), *Treating disordered speech motor control* (pp. 153–181). Austin, TX: PRO-ED.

McHenry, M., & Wilson, R. (1994). The challenge of unintelligible speech following traumatic brain injury. *Brain Injury, 8,* 363–375.

McNeil, M. R., Robin, D. A., & Schmidt, R. A. (1997). Apraxia of speech: Definition, differentiation, and treatment. In M. R. McNeil (Ed.), *Clinical management of sensorimotor speech disorders* (pp. 311–344). New York: Thieme.

Peters, D. J. (1995). Human experience in disablement: The imperative of the ICIDH. *Disability and Rehabilitation, 17,* 135–144.

Peters, D. J. (1996). Disablement observed, addressed, and experienced: Integrating subjective experience into disablement models. *Disability and Rehabilitation, 18,* 593–603.

Ruscello, D. M., Lass, N. J., Hansen, G. G., & Blankenship, B. L. (1992). Peer perceptions of normal and dysarthric children. *Journal of Childhood Communication Disorders, 14,* 177–186.

Satir, V. (1981). Family symptoms and approaches to family therapy. In G. Erickson & T. Hogen (Eds.), *Family therapy.* Monterey, CA: Brooks Cole.

Vogel, D., & Miller, L. (1991). A top-down approach to treatment of dysarthric speech. In D. Vogel & M. Cannito (Eds.), *Treating disordered speech motor control* (pp. 87–109). Austin, TX: PRO-ED.

Yorkston, K. M., & Beukelman, D. R. (1980). A clinician-judged technique for quantifying dysarthric speech based on single word intelligibility. *Journal of Communication Disorders, 13,* 15.

Yorkston, K. M., Bombardier, C., & Hammen, V. L. (1994). Dysarthria from the viewpoint of individuals with dysarthria. In J. A. Till, K. M. Yorkston, & D. R. Beukelman (Eds.), *Motor speech disorders: Advances in assessment and treatment* (pp. 19–36). Baltimore: Brookes.

Yorkston, K., Miller, R., & Strand, E. (1995). *Management of speech and swallowing disorders in degenerative diseases.* San Antonio, TX: Psychological Corporation.

Yorkston, K. M., Strand, E. A., & Kennedy, M. R. T. (1996). Comprehensibility of dysarthric speech: Implications for assessment and treatment planning. *American Journal of Speech–Language Pathology, 5,* 55–66.

TREATMENT OF DEVELOPMENTAL AND ACQUIRED APRAXIA OF SPEECH

Note to Students: In many workshops and even in college courses in communicative disorders, a common complaint is "There wasn't enough time spent on discussing treatment." This complaint is so common, in fact, that many of us who teach college wonder why this is so. Probably, it is due to the fact that it is hard to talk or write about an interaction as dynamic and complicated as that between clinician and client in a therapy setting. Those of us who have worked with individuals with communicative disorders know that the real learning happens only with the doing. It is hard for students who have yet to spend much time with individuals with apraxia of speech to integrate facts about approaches to treatment because there is little experience with which to associate that information. Yet, it is important that students be introduced to basic principles early. Developing clinical skills is a process that continues over time, throughout the course of one's career. In other words, it is appropriate to feel a bit uncomfortable at first. The concepts and procedures you will read about in this chapter will give you a knowledge base from which to start. Experience will take you the rest of the way.

> Tell me, and I'll forget. Show me, and I may not remember. Involve me, and I'll understand. (Native American saying)

This chapter focuses on treatment of apraxia of speech, even though one rarely treats apraxia in isolation without taking into account concomitant language problems. Many treatment issues presented in this chapter are applicable to both children with developmental apraxia of speech and adults with acquired apraxia. Before discussing specific issues related to these populations, we review some general principles.

GOALS OF INTERVENTION

In Chapter 12, we presented an overview of treatment for individuals with dysarthria where the goal of intervention was to optimize communication effectiveness. In that chapter, we suggested that speech intelligibility could be optimized by reducing the level of the impairment (improving physiologic support for speech) or by helping the speaker to develop techniques to compensate for the impairment. How does one design a treatment to focus on reducing the impairment in apraxia of speech? In dysarthria, it seems clear that clinicians are working to improve physiologic support for speech, such as improving vital capacity, or increasing vocal fold adduction, or perhaps improving strength of articulatory contacts. In aphasia treatment, clinicians may work to improve the person's ability to retrieve words by providing strategies such as phonemic or semantic cueing. Or, clinicians may model and provide structure that allows the individual with aphasia to use appropriate syntactic forms. In apraxia of speech, the goal or the focus of treatment is to improve the individual's ability to assemble, retrieve, and execute motor plans for speech. In order to do that, the person must be offered the opportunity to practice these motor planning processes. At first maximum cues are provided, and then they are faded, giving the speaker increasing responsibility to formulate and execute the plan on his or her own.

Question: *Does the clinician have to teach every motor plan that the speaker with apraxia will use?*

No, that would be inefficient and impractical. Rather, think of treatment as improving the person's ability to practice the "processes" of motor planning and programming. Through rehabilitation and spontaneous physiologic recovery, it is likely that speakers will be able to plan and program "on line" with more efficiency, store learned motor "schemas" that can be played out when needed, and therefore increase the number and type of utterances that they can use.

(continues)

> The amount of overall improvement in this processing will depend on severity. In fact, individuals with very severe impairment may be able to achieve only a few functional phrases. In those cases, clinicians may be teaching specific plans for each utterance that will not be carried over for use in other contexts. Many individuals with acquired apraxia, however, will be able to achieve the ability to produce utterances that were not specifically trained during therapy.

A variety of factors are important in treating both developmental and acquired apraxia of speech. These concepts are incorporated into most treatment methods that have been shown to be effective in treating both children and adults who have difficulty with motor planning and programming. When treating a motor speech disorder, one often needs to consider the complication of linguistic factors such as aphasia or acquisition of phonology and syntax. General principles of treatment include focus on movement performance drill, movement patterns, and sequences of movement. This is in contrast to linguistic approaches that focus on individual sound production or sound classes. Intensive, frequent, and systematic practice toward habituation of the movement pattern is a salient part of all treatment programs designed to improve motor skills. These approaches also include careful construction of hierarchies of stimuli, the use of decreased rate with proprioceptive monitoring, and pairing movement sequences with suprasegmental facilitators such as stress, intonation, and rhythm.

It is important to keep the word *movement* in mind as you begin to read this chapter. Students and clinicians are accustomed to thinking in terms of "sound errors" and treating "sound" production. Because speech consists of meaningful sound combinations, sound production has to be the ultimate goal in apraxia of speech treatment. However, those sounds are produced because of specific sequences of movement. This movement has to be produced in a particular way, with a specific amount of muscle contraction, with a specific speed and direction, and so on. In apraxia of speech, the difficulty is not with the sounds, but with the movement required to produce articulatory configurations and constrictions to make those sounds. Therefore, it is helpful to think in terms of treating movement sequences rather than phonemes. This is not a trivial distinction. What you believe about the nature of a disorder leads you to particular choices in devising treatment approaches. If the nature of the impairment in apraxia of speech is difficulty with movement, then one must focus treatment toward improving movement rather than teaching the child the "rules" of phonology.

The appropriate question is, How does one focus treatment on movement? If the nature of the movement impairment is one of weakness due to spasticity or flaccidity, such as might occur in dysarthria, movement is treated by improving physiologic support. The movement disorder in apraxia, however, is not due to weakness. It is characterized by difficulty achieving articulatory configurations and transitioning into and out of these configurations. Therefore, practice should focus on making those movement transitions, in the context of speech, and to perform that movement over and over again. At first, the clinician will provide maximum support by providing visual and auditory models, fading those cues over time. Throughout planning and providing this intervention, the clinician will be facilitated by paying attention to the principles of motor learning.

PRINCIPLES OF MOTOR LEARNING

It seems logical to assume that, in treating individuals who have motor speech disorders, clinicians ought to know something about how people learn motor skill. Speech–language pathologists are frequently challenged to provide intervention for improved motor performance when working with clients who have motor speech disorders. Yet, speech–language pathology training programs typically do not require courses in cognitive motor learning or kinesiology. Speech–language pathologists are beginning to turn to the cognitive motor literature as a source of information to facilitate treating communicative disorders that result from motor impairments. The principles of motor learning discussed by researchers in cognitive motor learning are especially important in treating speakers with apraxia. This section briefly covers some of the major principles of motor learning, how they can be incorporated into treatment planning, and how they can be implemented during treatment sessions. We present only a brief summary of some of these principles. Readers are encouraged to go to other sources (Schmidt, 1988, 1991; Schmidt & Bjork, 1996) for more detailed explanations of these principles in general, and for more complete descriptions of their application to apraxia of speech (McNeil, Robin, & Schmidt, 1997).

Motor learning has been defined as the "processes of acquiring the capability for producing skilled actions" (Schmidt, 1988, p. 345). It occurs as a result of experience and practice, and is influenced by a variety of factors. In treating acquired apraxia of speech, the clinician is facilitating the individual in recovering the capability for producing skilled action, whereas in treating developmental apraxia, the clinician is facilitating the child's ability to develop motor skill for speech. In either case, the goal is to provide modeling, practice, and therefore experience of the movement skills, so that learning, and eventually retention of, the motor skill occurs. The most important aspect of motor learning is that it requires experience. That means practice. Other principles important to achieving improvement in motor skills for speech include motivation, pretraining, conditions of practice, knowledge of results, and influence of rate.

Precursors to Treating Motor Speech Disorders

Before actual practice of motor skill, it is important that the clinician address factors that facilitate motor learning. These precursors to treatment enable the adult or child to be in a state that is conducive to motor learning. First, the adult or child needs to trust the clinician. Many children with developmental apraxia of speech have experienced only failure with attempts to speak. Many are frustrated, and have not had any experience that leads them to believe therapy can help. Adults, especially immediately following stroke, may be frightened and frustrated at futile attempts to speak. The clinician can help to establish trust by assuring clients that he or she understands what is wrong and can help, and by giving some success in the first meeting. This also leads clients to increased motivation. Although the desire to talk may seem a huge motivational force, the years of failure a child may have experienced, or the devastation of a stroke, can sometimes overshadow that desire. What motivates a child or adult may vary from person to person, but early success is highly motivating in encouraging further work. Other factors also facilitate motivation. The clinician should explain what he or she will be doing in treatment and why it helps. The child or adult can participate in choosing initial goals in treatment, as well as stimuli that are meaningful and useful to them.

In addition, active participation in treatment requires focused attention. Processing capacity is limited for everybody. That is, a person cannot attend to and focus effort on too many things at once. For example, the clerk checking out groceries may easily carry on a conversation while sliding the items over the automatic price reader. As soon as he or she has to punch in the code for the bananas, however, the clerk may slow down speech, make speech errors, or stop speaking altogether. This is an example of how capacity for attention is limited. Models of allocation of capacity for processing illustrate that different mental and physical activities impose different demands on a person's limited capacity for processing (Kahneman, 1973). Some activities require very little conscious processing, such as the reflexive movement that occurs when a person touches something hot. Others need more conscious effort and attention, such as threading a needle. If attention and effort do not match the processing demands required for whatever one is trying to do, performance will be degraded.

Speech involves complex rapid sequences of movement. As individuals develop and use speech, some of these movements become well practiced or habituated (e.g., counting to 10, or singing "Happy Birthday"). These familiar utterances require much less conscious processing than an utterance that is unfamiliar or phonetically difficult (e.g., saying "diadochokinesis" or "homonymous hemianopsia"). The influence of controlled versus automatic processing is an important issue in treating motor speech disorders, especially apraxia of speech.

Maintaining attention can be difficult, both with adults who have recently experienced neurologic insult, and with children who are young and distractible and who find the task difficult. Processing capacity, limited for everyone, is even more constrained for these individuals. When planning treatment, the clinician should take into account the attentional mechanisms of the adult or child, and plan ways to improve attention. These techniques will vary depending on the severity of attentional deficits, the severity of the apraxia, and the age of the individual. Specific ways to address attentional mechanisms are discussed later in the sections on treating acquired apraxia and developmental apraxia. In addition to achieving and maintaining increased attention, the clinician needs to consider processing capacity and demands when choosing stimuli for treatment. Learning of motor skills will be greatly facilitated by varying the length and linguistic complexity of stimulus materials so that enough processing capacity remains for the motor skill required.

Conditions of Practice

Issues pertinent to conditions of practice include prepractice, instructions, and modeling. Two issues especially relevant to planning and implementing treatment for apraxia of speech are the use of repetitive practice, and the concepts of massed versus distributed practice.

PREPRACTICE

Prepractice is a term used in the motor learning literature to indicate those principles important to address so that motor learning can occur. Attention, effort, motivation, and goal setting, which were discussed previously, are often considered part of prepractice. As the clinician begins sessions, it is important to make sure that the adult or child understands the task and why it is being done. This is typically done through both instruction and modeling. Modeling works better than instruction with children and with adults who have both aphasia and apraxia. In fact, complicated or long verbal instructions should be avoided because they can impede the client's ability to understand and follow through with the motor task. Techniques for instruction and modeling are presented later in the sections specific to acquired and developmental apraxia.

MASSED VERSUS DISTRIBUTED PRACTICE

The next condition of practice to consider when planning and implementing treatment is to decide whether practice should be massed or distributed. It is important in helping the client to enhance and retain motor learning. The issue of mass versus distributed practice is especially important when choosing the set size as well as the nature of the stimuli in treatment for apraxia of speech. This issue relates directly to decisions about how many stimuli to work on at one time, how many to work on in the entire course of treatment, how many to work on in a row before switching to a new stimulus, and so on. There are no hard and fast rules that help in making this decision. Students often ask, "Should I work on 10 utterances or 50?" "Should I work on only one at a time until the client can do it?" If one adheres strictly to massed practice, the clinician would take one utterance (e.g., "How are you?") and practice it the entire session. Although the client may demonstrate very good learning of that one motor pattern, the learning does not easily generalize to other contexts. It may also be difficult for the client to combine parts of that movement sequence with other movement sequences (e.g., "Are you coming?"). Thus, even though massed practice contributes to fast learning, it does not generalize well. Distributed practice results in slower learning, but that learning is better generalized and retained. In practice, the clinician probably never wants to introduce only one utterance because the client might overhabituate that utterance; however, practicing too many may not yield enough early success to give the client confidence in the treatment. In our clinical work with individuals with severe apraxia, we use a smaller set size at first, perhaps 5 to 7 utterances, and gradually increase it as the individual progresses in treatment. For those with mild apraxia, the set size may start out larger.

RANDOM VERSUS BLOCKED TRIALS

After making decisions about the set size and the content of the stimuli, the clinician has to pay attention to how and when to present stimuli. In this case, students often ask the following questions: "Should I work on 20 utterances, one time each, and then start over?" "Should I practice each one 10 times and then go to the next one?" This issue relates to the principle of random versus blocked trials. Blocked practice means that one stimulus would be practiced repeatedly. Then, practice would begin on the next stimulus, so that each one is practiced separately. In random practice, the stimuli are mixed up throughout the session. For example, consider a stimulus set of 10 words. In blocked trials, the first word would be practiced over and over for a period of time, then the second word, then the third, and so forth, so that each is practiced separately throughout the session. In random practice, the first word would be practiced a few times, then another, then another, randomly interspersed throughout the session. The cognitive motor literature has shown that random practice is better at facilitating the development of motor learning (Schmidt, 1988). It is important, then, that clinicians take this advantage into account when implementing treatment programs.

Varying the Context

Another factor relating to practice of movement is variability. By having the client practice movement sequences in different contexts and conditions, motor learning is facilitated. There are a few ways to do this. First, in choosing stimuli, one may want to have a particular movement sequence (e.g., the movement from lip closure to a vowel) represented in several stimuli, but with different coarticulatory contexts and different manners of production. For example, the set may include "me, my, baby, ball, my ball," along with other stimuli. Also, after the movement sequence is produced accurately in one prosodic context, the clinician will want to model the utterance with varied prosody and loudness.

Providing an Adequate Amount of Practice

As we stated, the most important aspect to motor learning is that it requires experience. The individual with apraxia must practice producing the movements for utterances over and over again. This repetitive motor drill can seem difficult to implement for adults who are recovering from strokes, or for young children who are distractible and have difficulty paying attention during lengthy drills. Probably the most common error made by speech–language pathologists who treat motor speech disorders, is failure to provide adequate practice in the form of hundreds of trials or responses per session. The individual needs the opportunity to practice producing correct utterances. Therefore, a sufficient number of trials per session are needed to allow acquisition and habituation of motor learning. Thus, activities should provide repeated opportunities for production of target utterances, and reinforcements should not require excessive time to deliver. Specific ways to implement motor practice will be discussed in the sections on treating acquired and developmental apraxia.

Question: What do you mean by not getting enough responses per session? What is enough?

The number of responses per session will vary from person to person, but generally in a half-hour session, one should get hundreds of responses from the client. It takes less than a second to say a word or a short phrase. It is quite easy to get hundreds of responses in a session, yet clinicians often spend too much time talking to the adult client, and using reinforcers that take time with children (e.g., taking 1 second to say an utterance, then 2 minutes to fit a puzzle piece). This reluctance to provide sufficient practice is not surprising. Although clients have difficulty talking, clinicians can talk easily. Because clinicians strive to make the situation comfort-

(continues)

able, they often take up the time talking. There are many techniques, however, as discussed later in the section on treating developmental apraxia, that can facilitate getting adequate responses per session.

Knowledge of Results

Speech–language pathologists are trained early in their careers that feedback to their clients is important. The cognitive motor researchers have shown that there are different kinds of feedback (Schmidt, 1988). When treating speakers with apraxia, two are extremely important: knowledge of results and knowledge of performance. Knowledge of results refers to giving the child or adult feedback about whether the movement sequence was correct. The clinician gives feedback about the overall "goodness" of the utterance. How one provides knowledge of results has received considerable attention in the cognitive motor literature. For example, the feedback should be given immediately. Too long a delay between the response and the feedback interferes with motor learning. After the feedback is given, the individual must be given some time, perhaps 3 seconds, to process the feedback. The next trial should then be given so that the child stays on task and the adult maintains attention. If the delay is too long, the speaker will not be able to use the feedback during the next trial.

Those who study cognitive motor learning have also shown that giving knowledge of results on every trial may not be as facilitative to motor learning as providing feedback after a number of responses. This has not yet been studied in tasks designed to improve motor skill in persons with apraxia of speech. In our experience, most individuals with apraxia know when the utterance is right or wrong, and do not need knowledge of results on every trial, but do benefit from acknowledgment that the trial was close or correct.

Individuals with apraxia often benefit from feedback on specifics of the error in the movement. This feedback is called knowledge of performance. It involves giving the speaker information such as "Close your jaw a little" or "Put your tongue back." Although too much information can be detrimental, occasional verbal and tactile feedback about specific parameters of the movement is often needed. Reports in the cognitive motor literature also suggest that adults may benefit from increased specificity of feedback, but too much specificity can actually decrease performance in children.

Although much has been learned about the role of feedback in motor learning, most of this work has focused on limb movement in subjects without neurologic impairment. No one has yet studied these parameters in treating individuals with apraxia of speech. Despite the paucity of research, the issues are important in treating motor speech disorders.

Influence of Rate

The speed–accuracy trade-off has been well documented in the law of simple movement called Fitt's law, which suggests that as one moves more rapidly, the person becomes more inaccurate in terms of the goal he or she is trying to achieve (Schmidt, 1988). Conversely, if the rate is slowed, accuracy will increase. In treating individuals with apraxia of speech, by slowing the movement while modeling it, the clinician will facilitate imitation for a number of reasons. First, speakers with apraxia may have decreased proprioceptive monitoring. Although this is not easily confirmed through any diagnostic test, slowing the rate gives the individual more time to process sensory information. The speaker has more time to "feel" the movement, and thus appreciate proprioceptive feedback. Slowing the rate also gives the individual time to think about the movement while doing it. This cognitive processing facilitates attention and effort and improves motor learning. As practice continues, modeling and practice productions can then be modified, moving toward more natural rate and prosody. Varying the rate can be an effective tool during repetitive practice of targeted utterances. This will facilitate habituation of articulatory movement accuracy while allowing variation in practice, and improved prosody.

TREATMENT APPROACHES
FOR APRAXIA OF SPEECH

Students often ask for clarification about the difference between treatment methods, treatment approaches, and treatment techniques. They ask whether those terms all mean the same thing or apply to different concepts. It is a good question, because it helps the clinician think about what he or she is really doing in treatment. In practice, the terms are often used interchangeably. In this chapter, we use the term *approach* to indicate whether the focus is on motor, cognitive, or linguistic impairment. The term *method* refers to a specific procedure for treatment, such as integral stimulation. The term *technique* refers to specific tasks that can be implemented within the treatment method.

The Approach

When making decisions about how to treat a person with a speech disorder, the clinician needs to determine which level or levels of deficit are contributing most to the disorder. Because the level of impairment in apraxia of speech is primarily motor planning, the clinician uses a motor approach when treating clients. That means that the clinician will rely heavily on the principles of motor learning, and use methods and techniques that facilitate motor skill acquisition. On the other hand, if the major impairment were aphasia, the clinician would choose a linguistic approach, focusing on phonologic, semantic, syntactic, or discourse skills. In some cases, the clinician may need to combine approaches or decide which level of deficit contributes most to the communication problem and treat that level first.

Methods of Intervention

A method is a well-described set of procedures designed to facilitate the learning or rehabilitation of specific skills. Sometimes, these are called treatment programs or even treatments. In this chapter, we focus only on methods that use a motor approach to treatment. The techniques we describe are specific tasks or procedures that may be used as part of the treatment method or program. Treatment methods that are frequently suggested for apraxia of speech fall into three categories: those that are based on articulatory movement patterns and sound production, those that focus primarily on prosodic aspects of speech production, and those that target gestural or augmentative communication. See Table 13.1 for a list of these methods and techniques. Note that methods of treatment for children and adults with apraxia overlap a great deal. Some methods devised for acquired apraxia, such as the Eight Step Continuum (Rosenbek, Lemme, Ahern, Harris, & Wertz, 1973), have been applied to children. Similarly, techniques reported first for children with developmental apraxia have been successfully applied to adults (e.g., Prompts for Restructuring Oral Muscular Phonetic Targets). Application of these methods differs somewhat for speakers with acquired and those with developmental apraxia of speech. In general, all methods use a motoric approach and are based on a hierarchy of stimuli, with carefully chosen length and phonetic complexity. All are most effective when implemented so that the client gets repetitive motor practice through systematic drill.

ARTICULATORY METHODS

The methods and techniques that focus on articulatory movement usually follow a "bottom–up" sequence of treatment. In other words, they start with phonetically simple, shorter utterances and progress to longer, more phonetically complex utterances.

Integral Stimulation

For speakers with moderate or severe apraxia, the most commonly used method to improve speech production is imitation. The clinician provides an auditory

Table 13.1
Treatment Methods and Techniques Frequently Suggested for Apraxia of Speech

Methods

Articulatory	Integral stimulation
	Eight Step continuum
	Prompts for Restructuring Oral Muscular Phonetic Targets
	Multiple Input Phoneme Therapy
	Touch-cue method
Prosodic	Melodic Intonation Therapy
	Contrastive stress
Gestural/Augmentative	Sign language
	Naturalistic gesture
	American Indian Sign

Techniques

Phonetic placement
Phonetic derivation
Tactile cueing
Rate variation
Stress variation
Intonation variation

and visual model, after asking the client to "watch me and listen to me." This is called *integral stimulation* because it emphasizes multiple input modes, especially auditory and visual. Integral stimulation works well as a motor approach to treatment, because the focus is on the movement patterns and the goal is an adequate speech signal. The clinician's models of stimuli are both auditory and visual because the clinician is producing speech while the client watches. All responses are movements, and these movements result in a target acoustic signal. This allows for the repetitive motor practice that is so important in motor learning. While the focus is on auditory and visual stimulation and repetition, gesture can often be an important facilitator. Gestural cues (e.g., moving one's hand to show the continuance of an airstream) can provide additional information for the client. Gestures can also be used by the speaker to facilitate overall movement.

The best example of a treatment method based on integral stimulation is the Eight-Step Continuum (Rosenbek et al., 1973). In this method, clinicians carefully choose a set of meaningful utterances, starting with length and phonetic complexity that will give the client early success. The utterances may be words, phrases, or sentences, depending on the severity of the individual's apraxia. The most important aspect of this method is that it begins by giving the client maximum cueing, then slowly fades those cues as the individual is able to take increasing responsibility for the assembly, retrieval, and execution of the motor plan. Table 13.2 lists the hierarchy of steps used in this approach. Note that not all steps will be used for every speaker. For example, the steps involving written stimuli would not be used for adults who do not read or for children who have not yet learned to read. In most cases, clinicians begin with direct imitation, going back to simultaneous production if a child is unable to imitate the utterance. If the child is still unsuccessful, additional steps might be added if necessary, such as providing tactile cues. Other intermediate steps

Table 13.2
Typical List of Cueing Used in the Integral Stimulation Method of Treatment

Cueing Type	Stimulus
Tactile cues	Clinician uses tactile cues to show the client how the movements should be made and provides tactile stimulation for location.
Simultaneous production	Clinician says the target utterance while the client watches and listens. Then the clinician and client say the utterance together, simultaneously, while the client continues to watch the clinician.
Mimed production	The clinician says the utterance while the client watches and listens. The client then imitates the utterance immediately after the clinician. In this step, the auditory cue is faded, but the clinician continues to mime the movement, while the client produces it.
Immediate repetition	Direct imitation without auditory or visual cues during the client's production.
Successive repetition	Direct imitation of the utterance, with several successive productions made by the client.
Delayed repetition	Client imitates the clinician's production, but must wait 1 to 5 seconds between hearing the utterance and producing it.
Reading	Presentation of written stimuli, followed by the client's oral reading with no auditory or visual cues from the clinician.
Reading with delay	Presentation of written stimuli, followed by delayed spoken production by the client.
Answering questions	The target utterance is elicited by a question.
Role playing	The target utterance is elicited during a role-play situation.

Note. Adapted from "A Treatment for Apraxia of Speech in Adults," by J. C. Rosenbek, M. L. Lemme, M. B. Ahern, E. H. Harris, and R. T. Wertz, 1973, Journal of Speech and Hearing Disorders, 38, pp. 462–472.

would include miming the utterance during the child's imitative utterance. Modifications of the method and demonstrated use with four cases have also been reported (Deal & Florance, 1978).

One important aspect of this method is the adding and fading of cues. This is done as each utterance is produced. By varying the amount of time between the clinician's stimulus and the client's imitative response (which we call "varying the temporal relationship"), the client establishes increasing autonomy in producing the movements for the utterance. We use this cueing, then fade the cues, response by response. For example, if the target utterance is "How are you?" we first model and ask for direct imitation. If the client is successful, we stay at that step until he or she easily produces the utterance with accuracy, natural rate, and varied prosody. If the speaker is not successful, we back up to a simultaneous production, having the client watch the clinician and produce the utterance simultaneously. We stay at simultaneous production until the movement is produced accurately with ease. Then we fade the simultaneous auditory model but continue the mime until accuracy occurs with little effort. Next, we move to direct imitation, adding back in the mime if the movement starts to be in error or seems effortful. If the client loses the ability to produce the utterance, we go back to simultaneous production. This back and forth, adding and fading of cues, continues until the client can spontaneously produce the utterance with normal rate and prosody. This may not occur in one or even several sessions. Thus, for any one word or phrase, many steps along the continuum of cueing may be used.

Many clinicians who first use this technique comment that they are exhausted at the end of the session. This probably reflects the fact that the technique is fast moving and elicits a large number of responses from the client. Each of these responses requires a decision on the part of the clinician. Figure 13.1 provides a schematic representation of these decisions. First, the clinician considers whether the response is correct. If the answer is no, then the clinician decides what additional cues are needed and provides these cues in the next trial. If the response was accurate, the clinician must decide whether the client has had sufficient practice to habituate the response. If this answer is no, then the clinician repeats the cueing. If the answer is yes, then the clinician must decide which cues can be faded without compromising the accuracy of the next response. These decisions are made literally hundreds of times in a treatment session.

It is not surprising that considerable clinical skill is needed to carry out the treatment called integral stimulation. The following questions are common when beginning clinicians use this type of intervention.

1. *Why is cue addition and fading so important in this method?* The answer to this question relates to the principles of motor learning reviewed earlier in this

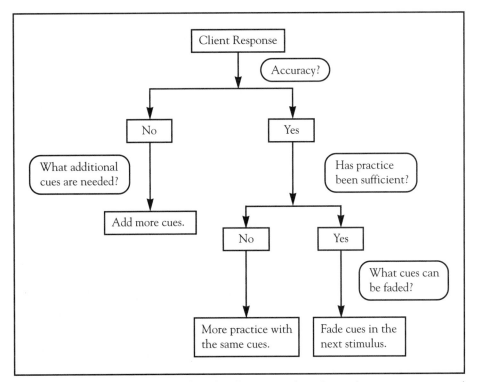

Figure 13.1. Matrix of decisions that the clinician makes after each response in integral stimulation therapy for apraxia of speech.

chapter. Consider what would happen if the clinician were at the wrong step in the cueing hierarchy. First, if the clinician is not providing enough cues and the speaker's responses are repeatedly in error, this would be violating the principles of motor learning in that the clinician is encouraging the speaker to practice the *wrong* motor skill rather than the right one. Next, if the clinician is providing too much cueing and the speaker's productions are always correct, this would also violate the principles of motor learning. Evidence suggests that adding some difficulty to the acquisition phase enhances long-term retention because it forces the learner to be an active processor (Schmidt & Bjork, 1996).

2. *Why is varying the temporal relationship between stimulus and response such an important part of the cueing hierarchy?* Many times a client with apraxia of speech will be able to repeat a word or phrase immediately after the clinician but will be unsuccessful when even a short delay of 1 or 2 seconds is imposed. The delay seems to force the speaker to hold the motor plan in a memory store. This may be a critical step in habituating the motor plan and, thus, in facilitating spontaneous production. It should be acknowledged that delays of 3 to

5 seconds seem very long in the midst of rapid stimulus–response exchanges. With children, the clinician can use an exaggerated hand signal for "stop" and make the waiting period into a game.

3. *How do you help the client develop natural sounding productions?* It is important to note that, in addition to articulatory accuracy, the clinician helps the adult or child gain the ability to produce the movement sequence with natural rate and prosody. Models may start with slow rate to achieve accuracy, and gradually move toward normal rate. As movement accuracy improves, models should vary the prosody somewhat, so that some variable practice with the movement can occur.

4. *My client is very severely involved. Can you give me an example of what additional cues you would provide to ensure an accurate response?* Two techniques that are frequently used along with integral stimulation are phonetic derivation and phonetic placement. *Phonetic derivation* involves the use of an intact nonspeech or speech gesture to elicit production of a target sound or sound combination. This concept may be familiar to speech–language pathologists by the term *progressive approximation*. *Phonetic placement* involves deriving speech sounds and sequences of sounds from intact nonspeech or speech gestures. In phonetic placement, techniques are used to help the client assume the correct position for producing a speech sound. This may be actual manipulation of the articulators, description of position where the client should feel the contacts, illustrations of where airflow is to be directed, and so on. For example, consider an adult who is working on the target "I want lunch." The clinician may be using integral stimulation, but be unable to get correct production, even in simultaneous conditions, because the "l" in lunch may be difficult. Here the clinician might go back to phonetic derivation, slowing down the stimulus presentation and using tactile stimulation or phonetic placement techniques to illustrate how and where the tongue should go. The clinician directs the client to let the tongue stay in place for 2 to 4 seconds to increase proprioceptive awareness, and then proceeds into simultaneous production of the phrase. The clinician may need to stay at the slow rate and simultaneous production for many repetitions before moving to the repeated elicitation. If maximal cueing and slow rates are required all of the time, however, the clinician may need to consider using stimuli with less phonetic complexity in order to achieve accuracy.

Multiple Input Phoneme Therapy

Another method similar to integral stimulation is Multiple Input Phoneme Therapy (MIPT). Stevens (1989) described this method, which is appropriate for those individuals with severe apraxia who have only a few verbal stereotypies. See Chapter 3 for a description of this type of individual. This method, then, is appropriate for adults with acquired apraxia, because children with developmental apraxia do not usually exhibit the same type of stereotypic utterances. In this method, the clinician identifies frequent stereotypic utterances, which are then used as initial stimuli. As in integral stimulation, the clinician models the utterance for the client. He or she begins with slowed production, and emphasizes the initial movement. A simultaneous gestural–prosodic cue (tapping of the ipsilateral arm) is performed by both the client and the clinician. After about 10 productions, the clinician fades the voice but mimes the movement and taps while the client continues to produce the target. In this way, the speaker with apraxia is able to volitionally control the movements associated with the automatic utterance. After this occurs, the clinician introduces new words, using the initial phoneme of the stereotypic utterance. If the stereotypy was the word "because," one might move to "bye," "bed," or "bye-bye." Progressively, the clinician would increase the number of targets, as well as the length and phonetic complexity of targets. This approach is also similar to integral stimulation in that, as target utterances become accurate in simultaneous production and repetition, utterances are then elicited by questions, pictures, or reading.

Prompts for Restructuring Oral Muscular Phonetic Targets

Prompts for Restructuring Oral Muscular Phonetic Targets (PROMPT) is a method originally described for use with children with developmental apraxia (Chumpelik, 1984; Hayden, 1994). It uses a motor approach to treatment, emphasizing movements into articulatory positions. This method focuses on the use of tactile cues to the face and neck to facilitate movement for speech production. The cues involve very specific placement of the fingers to cue articulatory positions as well as manner of articulation. Feedback is primarily tactile and kinesthetic. In its original form, each PROMPT (hand shapes and movements for the tactile cue) was associated with each of the phonemes of English (Chumpelik, 1984). They specify jaw height, lip contraction, tongue height and position, muscular tension, and airstream management. It is recommended that clinicians receive specific training in the use of these PROMPTS. These tactile cues are then provided serially, in order to guide sequential events for syllables and words.

The PROMPT system emphasizes the use of meaningful linguistic units, rather than nonsense syllables. Like other motor approaches, stimuli usually begin with phonetically and grammatically easy utterances and progress to more difficult stimuli. This method also emphasizes prespeech posturing for achieving the maximal physiologic support for speech movement.

Other Methods for Developmental Apraxia of Speech

The next three methods also focus on articulatory skill, and were developed for use with children with apraxia. The touch-cue method is described as being a systematic approach to improving motor skill for production of phonemes (Bashir, Grahamjones, & Bostwick, 1984). Tactile cues to the face and neck along with simultaneous auditory and visual cues are used through three stages of treatment. Stage 1 involves a series of nonsense syllable drills to teach the cues, improve movement sequencing, and facilitate self-monitoring. Stage 2 moves those learned movement sequences into monosyllabic and polysyllabic words. These include both real and nonsense words and emphasize distinctive feature contrasts. In Stage 3, the child is asked to produce multiword utterances, and then move to spontaneous speech.

Both PROMPT and touch-cue methods rely heavily on tactile cues and feedback. Other approaches, such as the Adapted Cueing Technique (ACT; Klick, 1985) use gestural cues. The clinician uses hand motions to reflect patterns of articulatory movement and manner of production. The clinician says the target utterance while moving the hand to cue tongue trajectory. Hand motions also signal air release. During vowel production both cues show the degree of jaw closure as well as the tongue movement. Signed Target Phoneme Therapy also uses visual cues to facilitate motor learning (Shelton & Garves, 1985). The hand shapes from the American Manual Alphabet are used simultaneously with an auditory model. The child then repeats the utterances without imitating the visual cue.

PROSODIC APPROACHES

Melodic Intonation Therapy

Melodic Intonation Therapy (MIT), a method that focuses on prosody, has frequently been used in treating individuals with apraxia of speech (Sparks & Deck, 1994; Sparks, Helm, & Albert, 1974). It was originally developed for speakers with acquired aphasia, usually those who fall under the category of Broca's aphasia. These speakers have fairly good auditory comprehension, but poor speech production. This method has also been proposed for use with children with developmental apraxia of speech (Helfrich-Miller, 1994). In this adaptation for children, stimuli progress from simple two- to three-word phrases to more grammatically and phonetically complex utterances.

In this method, the intonation or melodic pattern of a phrase is emphasized. For adults, the clinician models by intoning the phrase while tapping out the rhythm. The method uses a structured sequence of tasks, beginning with imitation of rhythmic tapping patterns and working toward imitation of utterances that are practiced in response to an intoned stimulus. Although the intoning or melody is based on patterns of natural speech, pitch and durational aspects of the utterances are exaggerated. Gradually, the clinician's tapping and intoning of cues are faded, while the client continues to produce the utterance. When the method is used for children, Helfrich-Miller (1994) suggests the use of symbols of signed English as the method of keeping time (in contrast to tapping out the rhythm, as is used for adults). The prosodic aspects of this method seem to facilitate motor planning and programming to improve speech production.

Contrastive Stress

Contrastive stress also uses prosodic cues and stress patterns as a major facilitator to improve both speech production and prosody. This method has been used for speakers with dysarthria (Rosenbek & LaPointe, 1985) and with apraxia (Wertz, LaPointe, & Rosenbek, 1984). In this chapter we focus on its use with speakers with apraxia. We have found this method to be most effective for those individuals with mild to moderate apraxia who need to improve speech naturalness through the use of stress patterning and intonational contour in sentence production or conversational speech. The method involves having the client produce an utterance with primary or emphatic stress on a particular word. Often the stressed word contains phonetic elements that are targeted for the individual. For example, if the clinician wanted to provide opportunities for an adult with acquired apraxia to produce the word "tomorrow" in a sentence context, he or she would elicit the utterance with a question such as "Are you going out today?" The client would then respond, "I am going out *tomorrow*." A number of elicitations using different phrases may be used, focusing on the targeted phonetic string in the same and in different word contexts. See Table 13.3 for an example. Keep in mind that this method is appropriate only after articulatory skill has been demonstrated for the targeted phonetic string. This task helps habituate and stabilize the articulatory production, with appropriate stress patterning and prosody.

The method is also effective for those speakers with apraxia needing improvement in the prosodic aspects of connected speech. The clinician would choose a number of sentences, all of which change meaning when word stress is varied. For example, as shown in the lower part of Table 13.3, the clinician would present a picture showing a boy hitting a ball. The clinician would ask the child with apraxia, "Is the girl hitting the ball?" The child would then

Table 13.3
Example of Stimuli for an Individual with Apraxia Who Is Working on Vowel + *r* or *r* + Vowel Phonetic Strings, Using Contrastive Stress Treatment

Target	Question	Sentence Context with Stressed Target
Articulatory Focus		
Tomorrow	"Are you going out today?"	"I am going out *tomorrow*."
	"Are you going out Wednesday?"	"I am going out *tomorrow*."
	"Are you going out now?"	"I am going out *tomorrow*."
	"Are you going out later?"	"I am going out *tomorrow*."
Market	"Are you going to the movies?"	"I am going to the *market*."
	"Are you going to church?"	"I am going to the *market*."
	"Are you going to school?"	"I am going to the *market*."
	"Are you going to the drug store?"	"I am going to the *market*."

(Other words that could be used to provide continued practice include *car, carpet, bar, bargain, more, here, wear,* etc.)

Target	Question	Sentence Context with Stressed Target
Focus on Intonational Contour		
Picture of a boy hitting a ball	"Is the girl hitting the ball?"	"No, the *boy* is hitting the ball."
	"Is the boy kicking a ball?"	"No, the boy is *hitting* the ball."
	"Is the boy throwing a frisbee?"	"No, the boy is hitting the *ball*."
Picture of a mom washing the dishes	"Is the mom washing the clothes?"	"No, the mom is washing the *dishes*."
	"Is the mom drying the dishes?"	"No, the mom is *washing* the dishes."
	"Is the dad washing the dishes?"	"No, the *mom* is washing the dishes."

respond, "No, the *boy* is hitting the ball." The next question might be, "Is the boy throwing a ball?" The child's response would be, "No, the boy is *hitting* the ball." Again, it is important that the speaker is able to produce each phonetic element of the sentences, and that the length of the elicited sentences be appropriate for the speaker's linguistic and motor capabilities.

Question: Do you ever use nonspeech drills for individuals with apraxia of speech and, if so, how long do you use them before beginning to work on speech?

Researchers disagree as to the appropriateness of using nonspeech movement tasks to study speech motor control (Luschei, 1991; Weismer & Liss, 1991). There is also controversy about using nonspeech exercises as part of treatment to improve speech (Love, 1992). Some nonspeech

(continues)

activities are occasionally appropriate for children with dysarthria, especially for those who will benefit from improving strength or range of motion (Strand, 1995). There are no data to indicate whether nonspeech movement activity is helpful for children who have developmental apraxia or adults who have acquired apraxia. In our experience, the only nonspeech activities that are helpful are the phonetic placement techniques and phonetic derivation that are used to help speakers make the movements toward and/or through a particular configuration. Although nonspeech activities can be used during the first few minutes of a session to increase attention to the face, increase awareness of movement, and so on, spending much of the session on nonspeech movement is probably not the best use of treatment time.

GESTURAL METHODS

The term *intersystemic reorganization* has been used to describe the use of a nonspeech system, such as hand or limb gestures, to facilitate movement for speech production (Wertz et al., 1984). The use of gesture in this context, as a facilitator, has already been discussed in conjunction with other methods, such as integral stimulation, Adapted Cueing Technique, and Signed Target Phoneme Therapy. In this section, we focus on different methods of treatment that use gesture as the primary focus of intervention. This would be appropriate for those individuals who have limited speech production capabilities, and want to use gesture to augment verbal communication.

Sign language is one form of gestural communication sometimes suggested for individuals with apraxia, especially those with developmental apraxia of speech. For adults with acquired apraxia, aphasia or hemiparesis can hamper attempts to use sign, either as an augmentative form of communication or as a facilitator. Children with developmental apraxia often learn and use signs with little difficulty. One problem with this approach is that sometimes it is introduced in lieu of treatment for speech production, even when the prognosis for developing motor planning skills for speech is good. Using sign language is also not indicated if there are few people in the child's environment who will use sign with the child. If the treatment goals are to establish some form of communication so that language development will be facilitated and so that the child will be less frustrated in attempts to convey communicative intent, the child's environment needs to be rich in opportunities for communication. If few people in the family or at school use sign, the child will be limited in communicative attempts.

Some children who are working to improve speech production need a gestural system to augment their speech. We have had good experiences teaching naturalistic gesture to children and their families. This involves identifying a set of meaningful gestures for use in particular situations. For example, laying one's head on folded hands can be the symbol for "I'm tired." Movement gestures mimicking tooth brushing, bathing, eating, and so on, work well for a variety of verbs. Children and their families usually have little difficulty determining a large set of these gestural symbols. Because they are also naturalistic, others will often understand them.

For individuals with severe acquired apraxia who are unlikely to regain functional speech production, AMERIND, a system based on American Indian sign language, has been suggested (Wertz et al., 1984). Signs used in this method are appropriate for individuals with hemiplegia because they have been modified for performance with one hand. Their meanings are often quite transparent so that they may likely be understood by untrained persons.

FROM ASSESSMENT TO TREATMENT

In this chapter, we have described many of the treatment approaches that have been suggested for apraxia of speech. It might seem as if one could go to the literature and choose a method, and read step by step exactly what to do in treatment. To some degree, this can be done, but this takes clinicians only part of the way. The literature can provide information about the nature of the disorder, and it can describe the basic steps involved in a particular method. However, because every speaker with apraxia is different, the literature cannot tell clinicians how many utterances to practice in a session, what utterances should be used, or how many times the client may have to practice one utterance before going to the next one. Those are all decisions the clinician has to make based on assessment of the child or adult, the clinician's knowledge of principles of motor learning, and the ongoing performance of the individual during treatment.

In the following section, we turn to those important, and sometimes difficult, clinical decisions that lead to successful implementation of treatment methods. These decisions involve summarizing assessment data, determining the relative contribution of motor versus linguistic deficits, determining severity and prognosis for recovery, choosing whether to use a motor or a linguistic approach to treatment, and choosing a method or methods that are congruent with that approach. At this point, we also make decisions regarding frequency of treatment, length of sessions, and choice of stimuli. Summarizing assessment data involves more than simply calculating scores on standardized tests. It involves considering all the data, including test scores, the speaker's approach to assessment tasks, the amount of delay or trial-and-error behavior that occurred, attentional factors, and performance on nonstandard protocols. In fact, when planning treatment for apraxia of speech, it is the client's performance on nonstandard testing procedures (e.g., physical examination of structure–function and motor speech examinations) that may be most helpful in planning treatment. See Chapter 5 for a discussion of this topic.

Decisions About the Approach

The first major decision is whether to choose a linguistic approach or a motor approach to treatment. The goal at this point is to determine the relative contribution of linguistic versus motor deficits. This is often difficult, both with acquired apraxia and developmental apraxia of speech. In acquired apraxia, concomitant aphasia is the rule rather than the exception. The clinician needs to determine the type and severity of the aphasia. One needs to carefully determine whether deficits in language testing may be due in part to the deficit in motor speech performance or are solely attributable to language problems. For example, naming difficulties may be the result of word retrieval problems, difficulty mapping or retrieving the phonology, or deficits in planning and programming the movement to produce the word. If the impairment is linguistic in nature, the treatment approach focuses on strategies for word and/or phonologic retrieval. If the impairment is in motor planning and programming, the treatment focus is on improving movement for sequential sound production. Determining the relative contribution of linguistic versus motor deficits is also difficult in developmental apraxia of speech. Children are still in the process of acquiring linguistic skills, and motor planning deficits will influence their acquisition of phonology. It is not surprising, then, that children with developmental apraxia of speech will exhibit phonologic errors.

If motor planning and programming deficits contribute significantly to the communicative disorder, in most cases the clinician will decide on a motor approach to treatment. For those individuals who also have significant language problems, it is appropriate to use a combination of linguistic and motor approaches. For example, an adult with acquired apraxia may have a significant syntactic deficit in addition to the apraxia of speech. The clinician might decide that the client's motor planning problem warrants a motor approach, and therefore choose a method such as integral stimulation. The clinician might then plan to include remediation of the syntactic problem by carefully framing utterances chosen for integral stimulation so that particular types of syntactic frames are systematically practiced. Tables 13.4 and 13.5 depict a short series of stimulus items that illustrate how one might include language goals when incorporating integral stimulation or another motor approach to treatment. The patient for whom the stimuli were chosen was a 62-year-old man who was 3 weeks post–left cerebrovascular accident. He exhibited moderate

Table 13.4

Example of Stimulus Set Focusing Specifically on Personal Pronouns and *Is* + Verb, Used for 2 Weeks Early in Treatment

She is washing the car.
She is doing the dishes.
She is my sister.
She is in Seattle.
She is coming on Thursday.
She is going to call back later.
He is my friend.
He is my neighbor.
He is mowing the lawn.
He is helping me today.
He is going with me.
He is coming over today.

apraxia of speech and moderate Broca's aphasia characterized by mild word finding and syntactic deficits. For example, when asked what he did that morning, the speaker may have said, "store, bread, milk." The approach used in treatment was integral stimulation, but the choice of stimuli emphasized carefully chosen syntactic targets. Table 13.4 shows the set of stimuli used early in treatment focusing on personal pronouns and *is* + verb constructions. Table 13.5 is a list of stimulus items contrasting early and later target utterances. Note that although the linguistic goals of personal pronouns, verbs, and prepositional phrases are represented, utterances are shorter and less phonetically complex in early treatment. Complexity of movements increases as treatment progresses.

For a child with severe phonologic impairment, the clinician may decide that motor planning plays a part, but that the phonologic deficit is such that a linguistic approach to treatment is desirable. In this case, the clinician would use a phonologic perspective in choosing treatment targets (e.g., particular sounds or sound classes) but also bring in the principles of motor learning. For example, the clinician would use smaller set sizes, constrain the phonologic targets to phonetically simple contexts, use meaningful utterances (rather than isolated phonemes) for practice, use phonetic derivation and phonetic placement as needed, pay more attention to rate, and pay particular attention to giving feedback regarding performance and outcome.

Severity and Treatment Planning

The rest of the decisions involved in planning treatment depend a great deal on the client's severity and prognosis and the availability of treatment. Severity is

Table 13.5

Examples of Stimulus Sets Used To Incorporate the Goal of Improving
Use of Personal Pronouns and Prepositional Phrases

Examples of Items from Early Stimulus Sets

My name is Jim.
I live in Modesto.
I have two sons.
My son's name is Tony.
I will be there at two.
How much does it cost?
What time will you be here?
He can go with us.
He took me with him.
He went home.
She is going to call back.
She is going home.
She is taking me.

Examples of Items from Later Stimulus Sets

I went to the store, and bought bread, milk, and eggs.
My grandchildren are Kristen, Joe, and Michael.
We are going to the doctor tomorrow morning.
I put the keys on the table for you.
I would like to have another piece of pie.
He should be careful with that lawn mower.
He called yesterday morning and said to call back.
He is on the Little League baseball team.
He is going to take me to the doctor on Monday.
He has to go home on Wednesday morning.
She has to go with him on Tuesday.
She is going to come for a visit next month.
She is taking her grandchildren with her.

determined both by the number of utterances or phonetic sequences that can
be produced by the client, as well as the degree of difficulty exhibited during
attempts at production. For example, if during the motor speech examination it
was necessary to go to simultaneous production with frequent tactile cueing
while sampling movement sequences for utterance production, it will take longer
to achieve initial success in producing speech. The severity of the apraxia of
speech will lead the clinician to choose a particular method. For example, integral stimulation is more appropriate for severe and moderate apraxia of speech.
Prosodic methods such as contrastive stress would more often be appropriate
for individuals with milder apraxia. Another factor related to severity is the

presence of oral apraxia. Presence of severe oral apraxia may indicate that early steps of integral stimulation will be more difficult.

In many cases, size and site of lesion, time postonset, and current severity of the disorder are major factors in the determination of prognosis. For example, if an individual has suffered a severe left hemisphere stroke involving both frontal and temporal lobes, resulting in severe aphasia and severe apraxia of speech, the prognosis for functional verbal communication may be poor. For a patient who has suffered a more focal stroke, resulting in no problems with auditory comprehension and mild or moderate apraxia of speech, it is likely that the individual will regain the ability to use speech to convey communicative intent.

Other factors may also be important for determining prognosis. For example, consider what concomitant deficits may exist that might interfere with treatment. An individual with acquired apraxia may also have linguistic, sensory, or visual deficits that would hamper some treatment methods. Children with developmental apraxia may also have other developmental (cognitive, linguistic, and/or motor) delays that would make motor approaches to treatment more difficult. In these cases, the prognosis for improvement in motor planning and programming for speech production would be worse than if those conditions did not exist. In both children and adults with neurologic disorders, severe attentional deficits can impede intervention and should be considered when determining prognosis.

Other factors relating to prognosis in acquired apraxia are time postonset and availability of treatment. If a person is more than a year poststroke, prognosis for improvement is poorer than if the stroke were recent. The following example illustrates how the availability of treatment may influence prognosis for improvement with intervention. Consider the case of a 62-year-old man seen in the acute hospital for treatment of moderate apraxia of speech and mild Broca's aphasia. He was able to attend 3 weeks of outpatient treatment and made good progress. At that time, he returned to his rural home where he saw a home health therapist only twice a month. At that point, prognosis for continued improvement was considered poorer than if he could have continued treatment twice a week. Another case illustrates someone with even poorer prognosis. A 40-year-old woman, 6 years post–left hemisphere stroke requested treatment to improve her speech. She was severely apraxic, with no functional verbal communication. Although gestural skills were good, she could not imitate even a CV combination, and used no speech other than "hi" and "oh, oh." She stated her desire to learn to produce 7 to 10 functional phrases so that she could answer the phone and do some social speaking. After the assessment was completed, we explained to her that, given the time since onset and the severity of her disorder, prognosis was very poor. To learn to produce 7 functional phrases would take months of treatment and a great amount of effort. We also explained that, due to the poor prognosis, we could not bill a third-party payer because we likely would not be able to demonstrate progress. In this particular case, the patient was willing to put in the effort to attend three 1-hour sessions per week, do the home practice, and pay privately. In 9 months, she learned to produce 5 functional phrases well within treatment sessions, and was inconsistently able to produce them at home when needed. The phrases were as follows: "Hi, I'm Sue." "Want to go to lunch?" "Chuck's not home now." "How much is it?" "See you later."

Now, consider developing a plan of treatment for a 5-year-old with severe developmental apraxia of speech. He exhibited oral apraxia, a few CV combinations, and many vowel distortions. Thus, virtually no functional verbal communication was present. Unfortunately, this child lived in a rural area with no speech–language pathologist. A consulting clinician who visited the community once a month wanted suggestions for treating his apraxia. In this case, the prognosis for functional verbal communication is very poor given the amount of intervention possible.

The severity of apraxia is also an important factor in making decisions regarding stimuli, and relates to what is known about the principles of motor learning. Several decisions need to be made regarding stimuli, including the number of utterances, the phonetic complexity of the items, and the length of stimuli. Generally, if the apraxia of speech is more severe, the clinician would use fewer stimulus items and shorter, less phonetically complex utterances than if the apraxia is less severe. The number of utterances chosen for an initial training set is based, in part, on the principle of massed versus distributed practice. For clients with severe apraxia, early success is necessary to decrease frustration and build trust. That might lead the clinician to suggest massed practice, perhaps even targeting only one word or a short phrase. Although this may help to achieve the goal of early success, the clinician also risks some unwanted effects, such as overhabituation of one movement pattern and decreased generalization. However, through distributed practice, perhaps by practicing 50 different utterances per session, motor learning will not occur as quickly. A balance needs to be reached between massed and distributed practice, thus allowing efficient motor learning. Table 13.6 shows sample stimulus lists for two children with different severity levels of developmental apraxia of speech.

No studies to date have examined the relationship of set size to improvement in speech production for either acquired or developmental apraxia. We have found that, when apraxia is severe, starting with a set size of five or so utterances works quite well. Usually within those five utterances, two might be targeted for the most practice within a session, while the other three are interspersed for distributed practice. For example, using as an example the child with severe apraxia in Table 13.6, one might practice the utterances in the following sequence:

   1. Hi, Mom.   30–40 repetitions or until an adequate utterance is produced
   2. Hi, Dad.   30–40 repetitions
   3. No!   20–30 repetitions
   4. Hi, Mom.   30–40 repetitions
   5. Hi, Dad.   30–40 repetitions
   6. Me too.   20–30 repetitions
   7. Hi, Mom.   30–40 repetitions
   8. I'm Tom.   20–30 repetitions
   9. Hi, Dad.   30–40 repetitions
  10. No!   20–30 repetitions
  11. Hi, Mom.   30–40 repetitions
  12. Hi, Dad.   30–40 repetitions

In this way, "Hi, Mom" and "Hi, Dad" are targeted for more massed practice, and the other utterances are interspersed for distributed practice. For moderate apraxia, the set size might be increased to 8 or 10 utterances and, as motor skill improves, perhaps up to 20.

Table 13.6

Initial Stimulus Lists for Two Children, One with Severe and the Other with Mild to Moderate Developmental Apraxia of Speech

Sample Items for Child with Severe Apraxia

Hi, Mom.
Hi, Dad.
Me too.
I'm Tom.
No!

Sample Items for Child with Mild to Moderate Apraxia

Can I go with you, Dad?
I want a turn!
Please help with this.
My brother's name is Jeremy.
I am in the first grade.
I go to St. Steve's School.
Can I go outside and play?

Choices regarding length and phonetic complexity also depend on the severity of the developmental or acquired apraxia. For individuals with severe apraxia of speech, highly visible and phonetically simple sounds may be the best place to start. For example, one may choose to emphasize bilabials in different coarticulatory contexts embedded in highly functional words for an initial stimulus set (e.g., *bye, my, me, mom*). Results of the motor speech examination will indicate which movement patterns for sound production are already produced by the speaker and which can be produced with maximum cueing. Those that can be produced accurately with cueing should form the initial practice set. For those clients who have moderate apraxia of speech, a greater variety of phonetic contexts and progressively longer utterances may be included. It is not necessary to always start with isolated words because the speaker may just as easily be able to imitate "I'm Bob" as "water," and the short phrase may be more functional or important. With mild apraxia of speech, sentence-level utterances, progressing quickly to short descriptive or narrative contexts will be appropriate. In these cases, phonetic complexity may be less important than the linguistic context in which the targets are elicited. As one increases the linguistic complexity from formulating a sentence, to a short description of a picture, to generating a narrative, one also increases the load put on the motor planning, programming, and execution systems.

Intensity of Treatment

After selecting a motor approach, a method suitable for motor learning, and a set of stimuli appropriate to the severity of the apraxia of speech, the clinician determines the number of sessions per week and the length of sessions. A review of the cognitive motor literature suggests that motor learning requires practice. Thus, treatment of speakers with apraxia requires frequent sessions. It is generally recommended that both adults and children should be seen at least three times per week. The rule of thumb is the more frequent, the better. For example, if the clinician has authorization for payment for 2 hours per week for an adult with apraxia, it would be better to schedule four half-hour sessions per week than two 1-hour sessions. Keep in mind that these are guidelines, and that real-world constraints often make it impossible to do what is optimum.

> *Question: In my school district, I am not allocated the amount of time that you recommend for treatment of children with developmental apraxia. Can I compensate for these time limitations by having aides or parents provide the treatment?*
>
> *(continues)*

It is difficult to answer this question for all children. The techniques involved in motor approaches require skilled clinical decisions throughout the session, which can be very difficult for parents or aides without considerable training. As a result, we typically do not have parents or aides involved in treatment of target utterances, but use their help extensively when working on generalization of utterances. The other reason it is hard to use parents to provide treatment is that this is difficult work, accompanied by some failure before success. This is often frustrating for both parents and children. On the other hand, some children will receive little or no intervention if parents or aides do not provide it. In these cases, it is important to provide as much training as possible for the trainer. It is also important for the child and the parent to work out mutually agreed-upon methods of expressing frustration.

Recording Data During Treatment

The final aspect of treatment planning is for the clinician to decide to make decisions regarding changes in the treatment program, including when to change or add stimuli, when to discontinue, and so on. In graduate training programs, students are taught to "keep data" and "measure progress" because it is important to determine when treatment needs to change and when to stop treatment. The data recorded during treatment depends on the question being asked. For example, to determine whether treatment (and not other factors such as maturation or environmental influences) caused the change in motor speech performance, single-subject design methods are available. Examples of these include the multiple-baseline design, a changing criterion design, and others (McReynolds & Kearns, 1983). These designs manipulate specific variables so that the clinician can determine if the intervention was indeed responsible for the changes noted. Although it is beyond the scope of this chapter to discuss how to do treatment efficacy research, note that important elements are to record stable baseline measurement before treatment and, in most designs, to continue to probe performance on both trained and untrained items during treatment.

Another important question is what kind of outcome was seen after the treatment. In this case, the clinician is more interested in how the speaker changed in terms of functional communication ability, rather than whether the change was due explicitly to the treatment. Functional outcome measures are more directly related to changes in communication that are achieved by the client and used in real-life situations. A complete discussion of functional outcome measures in a variety of clinical populations is available (Fratelli, 1997).

Clinicians are also interested in keeping track of progress during treatment in order to make decisions about when to move on within a particular program. Clinicians need to know with some objectivity when to add stimulus items, when to change the number of items, and when to perhaps give up on something. Many speech–language pathologists use a particular criterion that the speaker must reach in order to move on. A typical criterion would be 80% correct over three probe sessions. However, clinical research has suggested the use of a cumulative criterion when treating adults with acquired apraxia of speech (Deal & Florance, 1978). We have also used this with children with developmental apraxia and found that it facilitates generalization of motor learning that occurs during treatment sessions.

"Cumulative criterion" simply means that one keeps track of the cumulative number of correct responses over the total number of trials during probe testing. In the example presented in Table 13.7, it took 10 sessions to reach 90% accuracy using the traditional percent criterion. Using the cumulative criterion, the same 10 sessions yielded only 49% cumulative accuracy. If a 10-session criterion were used, treatment on that utterance would be discontinued. If a cumulative criterion were used, considerably more practice would have been provided. A cumulative criterion takes into account the early difficulty an individual may have producing a particular movement pattern, and allows for extra practice with that movement. We have found that generalization is enhanced when the clinician adheres to the cumulative criterion, although common sense is also needed. That is, if the client seems to have really achieved the movement pattern with accuracy, good prosody, and ease (or if the speaker is really tired of a stimulus item), the clinician does not need to push the client to achieve 80%.

Most clinicians prefer to collect data on probe samples rather than the entire session. Although it might seem desirable to record accuracy of responses throughout the session, this is unwieldy, is likely to take attention away from the task, and reduces the amount of practice the speaker might receive. Doing therapy for apraxia of speech is hard work and takes concentrated effort by both the clinician and the speaker with apraxia. Many clinicians choose to probe

Table 13.7
Example of Traditional and Cumulative Criterion for Same Data

Probe Test	1	2	3	4	5	6	7	8	9	10
Traditional percent criterion	0/10	0/10	1/10	3/10	5/10	6/10	7/10	9/10	9/10	9/10
Cumulative criterion		0/20	1/30	4/40	9/50	15/60	22/70	31/80	40/90	49/100

test on some regular interval. For example, if the client is seen four times per week, the clinician might probe every other session. Probe testing may be conducted in the last 5 to 10 minutes every other treatment session. Typically, probe testing is carried out in direct imitation only, and usually samples 10 trials of each utterance being trained. For individuals with less severe apraxia who may have larger sets for treatment, a subset is usually probed. Probe items are scored as either right or wrong and a percentage is reported for each item. We keep separate data for each utterance. As one or more utterances reach cumulative criterion, they go out of the "working" list into the "maintenance" list. Then, a new utterance is brought into the training set.

Thus far in this chapter, we have focused on topics that pertain to both children and adults with apraxia. We now move to separate discussions of treatment for acquired apraxia and for developmental apraxia, so that issues specific to each can be emphasized.

TREATING ACQUIRED APRAXIA OF SPEECH IN ADULTS

Family and Patient Education

The first important step in treating adults with apraxia is to make sure the people involved in their daily life (spouse, parent, caregiver, sibling, friend, etc.) understand the nature of the motor speech disorder, and what the speakers will likely be able to do and not be able to do. Apraxia of speech can be very difficult to understand. Families who do not understand the nature of the problem can become anxious and frustrated and may think that their spouse or parent is not even trying. For example, we met with the spouse of a man who had experienced a left CVA the week before. He was mildly aphasic, but severely apraxic. The spouse was very angry, saying, "He understands everything I say, but he won't talk to me. Why is he being so stubborn?" We explained the nature of the motor planning problem in apraxia, and that individuals can often understand speech, know exactly what they want to say, but not be able to move in the correct way to make the right sounds. After she understood the nature of the problem, she found it much easier to be patient, to offer encouragement, and to appreciate his use of gesture, pointing, and communication boards. She also observed treatment sessions so that she would understand what utterances he was able to make and which would be impossible for him at this point in treatment. She soon began to model and facilitate production of words he might attempt to speak when the clinician was not in the room.

When educating families of individuals with acquired apraxia, it is helpful to explain that different parts of the brain have specific roles in speech and language functioning. When a person has a stroke, certain areas may be deprived of oxygen and no longer function. If those areas are involved in motor planning, the individual will have apraxia of speech. We often go back to the model of speech production presented in Chapter 1 of this text, and describe where the impairment occurs using vocabulary appropriate for that family. We make sure the speaker with apraxia also understands what has happened and participates as fully as possible in treatment planning (e.g., selecting phrases that he or she wishes to practice). This often helps to decrease fear and build trust. The next step is to help the family understand, realistically, what the patient can and cannot do. This discussion often requires a compromise between realism and hopefulness.

Students reading this chapter might want to prepare answers to the following questions that are commonly asked by families of speakers with apraxia:

- Why can my husband say a word one time, and ten minutes later he can't?

- Why does he grope?

- Why can he count to ten, but he can't say "three" if it's by itself?

- When will he talk again?

Many of these questions will be answered by a careful explanation of the model, and the nature of apraxia of speech. After a complete evaluation, the clinician will be able to give an honest opinion about prognosis. It is also important to explain concomitant problems that might exist. Some will be evident and need little explanation, such as hemiplegia and fatigue. Others, such as apraxia for phonation, emotional lability, hemianopsias and other visual field deficits, and perseveration, may take more explanation.

The clinician will want to take time to make sure the client with apraxia of speech also understands the nature of the disorder. The client needs to know that the clinician understands and can help. For example, we saw a 61-year-old woman immediately after a left hemisphere stroke. She had mild right hemiparesis, mild aphasia, and a very severe apraxia of speech. The women was confused and very frightened. She knew what she wanted to say, but she could not sequentially move her lip, tongue, or jaw to make even a consonant–vowel combination. When anyone walked into her room, she pulled the sheets over her head and would not interact. She was so frustrated that she was not even willing to approach the problem. In the acute stages of treatment for this woman, it helped to just sit by her bed and validate her frustrations. We began to talk with her about apraxia. We let her know that we had experience with this problem, and that we could help her. Dealing with the client's early frustration can be frustrating for the therapist as well. Providing early support, encouraging any method of total communication, and achieving very early success facilitate building trust.

Dealing with Concomitant Problems in Apraxia Treatment

An important part of treating acquired apraxia of speech is dealing with concomitant problems frequently associated with neurologic insult. Initially, the client may be quite frustrated. In addition to the counseling described earlier in this chapter, beginning treatment at the correct level of complexity, spending a good deal of time making simultaneous movement patterns to ensure early success, and giving a lot of positive reinforcement can help reduce this frustration and build trust.

Depression, which can also occur after a stroke, may severely affect the person's ability to be motivated, focus effort, and maintain attention (Robinson, Lipsey, & Price, 1985; Stern & Bachman, 1991). Working with the family and providing early success can sometimes help. It might also be necessary to communicate with the individual's physician regarding the use of antidepressants. When medication is appropriate, we have found it to be helpful in improving the client's ability to participate in treatment.

Emotional lability is frequent soon after stroke, and is therefore common in individuals with apraxia of speech. These individuals will laugh or cry frequently, often with little or no provocation. They may be embarrassed or confused about why this happens. We explain that this inability to control emotion is frequent after injury to the brain, and has been caused by their stroke. We talk to them about techniques that have been helpful to others. Some individuals with lability find distraction techniques helpful. Some hold a small rubber ball, and squeeze it when periods of lability occur. Others simply use their fist, tightening and relaxing it over and over. Any motor act that can take attention away from the laughter or crying is sometimes helpful. Others find it helpful to perform mental activities, such as counting backward by 3s. The clinician can also change topics or divert the individual's attention from the crying or laughter. For example, during one episode, a colleague asked the patient to hold his notebook while he looked for something. After only a moment, he took back the notebook and they continued. It is important to recognize that emotional lability is occurring rather than pretend it is not happening. After it is acknowledged, one can then work through it and more quickly return to the task at hand.

Attention and effort can be significantly affected as a result of damage to the brain. Both the ability to pay attention to a task for a certain amount of time (attention span) and ability to focus attention on a particular task (selective attention) are likely to be impaired. Earlier in this chapter, the importance of attention and effort for motor learning was discussed. Decisions regarding stimuli, treatment tasks, length of session, and so on, should be made with attentional mechanisms in mind. The individual may need constant support, encouragement, and frequent reminders of the task at hand. In addition, techniques such as changing pitch or loudness, changing position, or standing up can facilitate keeping the individual's attention focused on the clinician's face and auditory models.

TREATING DEVELOPMENTAL APRAXIA OF SPEECH

Explaining the Disorder to Parents

Family education is just as important for parents of children with developmental apraxia of speech as for families of individuals with acquired apraxia. For example, parents phoned us, asking for advice about treatment for their child. Their 4-year-old son, who had only a few monosyllabic utterances, had just been diagnosed with developmental apraxia of speech. They were very concerned about the diagnosis, were anxious to know if that meant brain damage, wanted to know if he would need a special school, and were very concerned about other aspects of development. The concern they communicated bordered on panic. After much discussion about the nature of the problem, as well as how treatment would proceed, the parents were able to focus on addressing the problem. They found a therapist who had experience with motor speech disorders, and began therapy several times per week.

This case illustrates the importance of helping families understand the nature of the problem. By using a simple model (see Figure 1.1 from Chapter 1) and explaining what the child is doing well and where the deficit seems to be occurring, the clinician can help the parents to focus their attention on a plan of action instead of worrying over what the term apraxia means. We often begin our explanation by pointing out that the process of speech production, although very complicated, can be modeled such that specific levels of processing impairment can be associated with different types of speech and language disorders. We also explain that, although the vertical nature of the model gives the illusion that cognitive, linguistic, and motor processes are sequential, it is really more correct to think of them as interactive. In fact, they often occur simultaneously or overlap in time. We have found it helpful to stress that language and motor processes interact and are so inextricably linked that they cannot be separated.

Then we often go through the model, explaining the different processes involved. We might use an example, such as, "Your child runs in the house after seeing his dad's car coming down the street. He is excited and wants to tell you daddy is home." We explain that at this point, cognitive processing is occurring. He has the idea and the intent to communicate. In order to convey this intent, he needs to symbolize the thought. For talk, the symbols used are spoken words. When he begins to retrieve those words, map their phonology, and frame the syntax of the utterance, linguistic processing is occurring. We explain to parents that both cognitive and linguistic types of processing are mental. For speech to be produced, the physical act of movement must occur. Movement has to occur because the sounds of spoken language are merely the result of the shape of the vocal tract and the constriction of an airstream by the vocal folds, velum, pharynx, tongue, jaw, and lips. For the constriction of the airstream to result in the particular sounds meaningful to a language, these structures have to move in a particular direction, with a particular speed and force, and achieve a specific articulatory target. Further, the movement of each structure has to begin and continue with precise timing relative to the movements of all the other structures. The processes that make this happen are called motor planning and programming.

We explain that some children have difficulty with the development of language. They do not learn the rule-governed system of sounds (phonology), or they have difficulty developing vocabulary. Other children, such as those with cerebral palsy, have difficulty with the execution of movement because there are problems with the neuromuscular control of movement in general (dysarthria). We then point out that children who have been diagnosed with developmental apraxia of speech have difficulty at the level of motor planning and programming. It is also important to explain that, if there is a problem at the level of motor planning, programming, or execution, it is likely that motor problems will affect the acquisition of phonology. That is one reason why children who have motor planning deficits also often have phonologic deviancies.

Question: When is the ability to plan and program movements for speech developed?

We do not yet have good models of acquisition of speech motor control. That is, we do not know how and when "motor programs" are developed.

(continues)

We know that, over time, speech becomes not only more accurate, but also more automatic. It is plausible, then, that some motor plans, or "sub-routines" for planning sequences of movement, are stored and can be retrieved for use as needed. How or when this occurs during development is still a matter of speculation.

Treatment for Developmental Apraxia

Earlier in this chapter, we discussed the treatment planning and decision making for apraxia of speech, whether developmental or acquired. These decisions involved summarizing assessment data; determining the relative contribution of motor versus linguistic deficits; determining severity and prognosis; choosing whether to use a motor, linguistic, or a combined approach to treatment; and choosing a method or methods that are congruent with that approach. Decisions are also made regarding frequency of treatment, length of sessions, and choice of stimuli. In this section, we briefly discuss these decisions specific to children with developmental apraxia of speech.

DECISIONS IN TREATMENT PLANNING

If the clinician determines that the child's speech delay is significantly influenced by motor planning deficits, the clinician will probably choose a motor approach to treatment, such as integral stimulation or an approach emphasizing tactile cueing, such as PROMPT. Because motor learning occurs only with practice, it is important to schedule treatment sessions as frequently as possible. Although this is often difficult in some settings, frequent practice is mandatory for successful treatment of apraxia of speech. Principles of motor learning also influence the choice of stimuli. For nonverbal children, or children with severe motor planning deficits, the clinician strives for early success and to develop a core functional vocabulary as soon as possible. Thus, the clinician may use massed practice, keeping in mind that some distributed practice may be needed for better retention of particular motor patterns. For the child who is nonverbal or severely involved, then, the clinician might start with a set size of five or six utterances. The phonetic makeup of the early utterances involves visible movements and movement trajectories that are easily cued tactilely. For example, starting with "I'm home" or "Hi, Mom" is easier for the client than starting with "Can I go?"

For the child who has less severe apraxia, or for whom the phonologic deficit is primary but a mild motor component is contributing, more distributed practice might be appropriate. For example, the set size might be 10 to 15 utterances initially, with stimuli added to the training set as needed. For all levels of severity, it is helpful to involve the children in the choice of stimuli. For the nonverbal child or child with severe apraxia, it is important that the utterances be as functional as possible, and important to the child. For example, words such as "no" or "not now" may give the child power and be quite motivating. We worked with a child who requested that we add the utterance "Leave me alone" to her list, because she thought this would be very handy to use with her twin brother. Although the phonetic context was not what we would have chosen at that point in treatment for her severe apraxia, we included it. She mastered the utterance in simultaneous production in the first session and was able to use it by herself within a few weeks. She had no difficulty generalizing correct productions in real settings.

TREATMENT TECHNIQUES

Intervention with motor speech disorders in children poses challenges because of the practice required. We have emphasized in this chapter that motor learning happens through experience and that experience takes practice. This implies therapy "drills," a concept dreaded by both children and clinicians. It is true that, to improve motor skill in these children, the clinician must elicit hundreds of utterances per session; however, this need not be drudgery. Sessions can be fast moving, interesting, and even fun for the child. More important, when children start having success with the movement patterns, they easily become even more engaged in the drill work.

It is *not* necessary that the child be seated in a chair with hands folded on the table. It *is* necessary that the child attend to the clinician's face and remain attentive to the task. Depending on the child's age and attentional skills, the clinician may be on the floor with the child, doing whatever is necessary to make sure the child is watching the clinician's face during modeling. Sometimes the clinician must move around to keep his or her face in front of the client. Often, we have a child do 10 responses sitting, then 10 standing, 10 very quiet, 10 loud, 10 with their hands on their head, and so on. One child liked to stand, watch and listen to the model, produce the utterance, take a step, then do the next. Usually we introduce reinforcers every 10 or 20 utterances to keep up a child's motivation. It is important to remember that reinforcement should not take more time than it took to produce the utterances. Because the clinician must try to get in as much practice as possible, reinforcers should provide enjoyment to the child but take little time. Stamps, stickers, rolling a bowling ball at pins (once), and tokens that can be thrown in a can are all examples of "quick" reinforcers that can be accumulated. These types of reinforcers are more conducive to maximizing the number of responses per session than ones that take time, such as fitting in pieces of a puzzle or drawing a picture.

In addition to maximizing the number of responses per session, the clinician also must pay attention to the principles of massed versus distributed practice. For children, especially those who have little functional verbal communication, the goal is to help them acquire functional utterances as soon as possible, and massed practice facilitates faster motor learning. Even though several utterances are included in the initial set, the clinician probably wants to target one or two of these for more massed practice, so that the child will be able to use them in real situations quickly. The clinician can include three or four other phrases for distributed practice.

CONCLUSION

Treatment for apraxia of speech requires that the clinician be well aware of the motor processing involved in speech production, and the way in which those motor processes interact with language. Further, the clinician should be knowledgeable about the principles of motor learning and how application of those principles is integral to treatment planning. Although there is much overlap in the methodology of treatment for children and adults, it is important that the clinician be aware of the impact of motor deficits on speech development in children. Because of the nature of the motor deficit in apraxia of speech (planning and programming), we have emphasized the following aspects of treatment: structured hierarchy of stimuli based on length and phonetic complexity, selection of target utterances that are meaningful and useful to the child or adult, adding and fading of cues so that movement errors are kept at a minimum, systematically adding a delay between stimulus and response to provide increased opportunity for the speaker to assemble and retrieve motor plans, and providing frequent sessions and maximizing responses per session so that enough practice is provided to enhance motor learning.

REFERENCES

Bashir, A. S., Grahamjones, F., & Bostwick, R. Y. (1984). A touch-cue method of therapy for developmental verbal apraxia. In W. H. Perkins & J. H. Northern (Eds.), Seminars in speech and language (pp. 127–137). New York: Thieme-Stratton.

Chumpelik, D. (1984). The prompt system of therapy: Theoretical framework and applications for developmental apraxia of speech. Seminars in Speech and Language, 5, 139–156.

Deal, J. L., & Florance, C. L. (1978). Modification of the eight-step continuum for treatment of apraxia of speech in adults. Journal of Speech and Hearing Disorders, 43, 89–95.

Fratelli, C. (1997). Outcome measures in speech language pathology. New York: Thieme Medical.

Hayden, D. A. (1994). Differential diagnosis of motor speech dysfunction in children. *Clinics in Communication Disorders, 4*, 119–141.

Helfrich-Miller, K. R. (1994). Melodic intonation therapy for developmental apraxia. *Clinics in Communication Disorders, 4*, 175–182.

Kahneman, D. (1973). *Attention and effort.* Englewood Cliffs, NJ: Prentice-Hall.

Klick, S. L. (1985). Adapted cuing technique for use in treatment of dyspraxia. *Language, Speech, and Hearing Services in Schools, 16*, 256–259.

Love, R. J. (1992). *Childhood motor speech disability.* New York: Macmillan.

Luschei, E. (1991). Development of objective standards of nonspeech oral strength and performance: An advocate's views. In C. M. Moore, K. M. Yorkston, & D. R. Beukelman (Eds.), *Dysarthria and apraxia of speech: Perspectives on management* (pp. 3–14). Baltimore: Brookes.

McNeil, M. R., Robin, D. A., & Schmidt, R. A. (1997). Apraxia of speech: Definition, differentiation, and treatment. In M. R. McNeil (Ed.), *Clinical management of sensorimotor speech disorders* (pp. 311–344). New York: Thieme.

McReynolds, L. V., & Kearns, K. (1983). *Single subject experimental design in speech pathology.* Baltimore: University Park Press.

Robinson, R. G., Lipsey, J. R., & Price, T. R. (1985). Diagnosis and clinical management of post-stroke depression. *Psychosomatics, 26*, 775–778.

Rosenbek, J. C., & LaPointe, L. L. (1985). The dysarthrias: Description, diagnosis, and treatment. In D. Johns (Ed.), *Clinical management of neurogenic communication disorders* (pp. 97–152). Boston: Little, Brown.

Rosenbek, J. C., Lemme, M. L., Ahern, M. B., Harris, E. H., & Wertz, R. T. (1973). A treatment for apraxia of speech in adults. *Journal of Speech and Hearing Disorders, 38*, 462–472.

Schmidt, R. A. (1988). *Motor control and learning: A behavioral emphasis* (2nd ed.). Champaign, IL: Human Kinetics.

Schmidt, R. A. (1991). *Motor learning and performance: From principles to practice.* Champaign, IL: Human Kinetics.

Schmidt, R. A., & Bjork, R. A. (1996). New conceptualizations of practice: Common principles in three paradigms suggest new concepts for training. In D. A. Robin, K. M. Yorkston, & D. R. Beukelman (Eds.), *Disorders of motor speech: Assessment, treatment and clinical characterization* (pp. 3–26). Baltimore: Brookes.

Shelton, I. S., & Garves, M. M. (1985). Use of visual techniques in therapy for developmental apraxia of speech. *Language, Speech, and Hearing Services in Schools, 16*, 129–131.

Sparks, R. W., & Deck, J. W. (1994). Melodic intonation therapy. In R. Chapey (Ed.), *Language intervention strategeis in adult aphasia* (3rd ed., pp. 368–379). Baltimore: Williams & Wilkins.

Sparks, R. W., Helm, N., & Albert, M. (1974). Aphasia rehabilitation result from melodic intonation therapy. *Cortex, 10*, 303–316.

Stern, R. A., & Bachman, D. L. (1991). Depressive symptoms following stroke. *American Journal of Psychiatry, 148*, 351–356.

Stevens, E. R. (1989). Multiple input phoneme therapy. In P. A. Square-Storer (Ed.), *Acquired apraxia of speech in aphasic adults* (pp. 220–238). Philadelphia: Taylor and Francis.

Strand, E. A. (1995). Treatment of motor speech disorders in children. *Seminars in Speech and Language, 16*, 126–139.

Weismer, G., & Liss, J. L. (1991). Acoustic/perceptual taxonomies of speech production deficits in motor speech disorders. In C. A. Moore, K. M. Yorkston, & D. R. Beukelman (Eds.), *Dysarthria and apraxia of speech: Perspectives on management* (pp. 15–28). Baltimore: Brookes.

Wertz, R. T., LaPointe, L., & Rosenbek, J. (1984). *Apraxia of speech in adults: The disorder and its management*. Orlando, FL: Grune and Stratton.

AUTHOR INDEX

Subject Index